Comprehensive ENT

Series Editor
Cemal Cingi, Department of Otorhinolaryngology, Medical Faculty, Eskişehir Osmangazi University, Eskisehir, Türkiye

As technology progresses, there are continuous advances in every medical subspeciality, and otorhinolaryngology/ENT is a particularly outstanding example of this. ENT lends itself well to the development of innovative and sophisticated solutions, including those affecting the vital area of airway management. Rhinoplasty and related cosmetic procedures are now a well-established part of ENT practice, and make major contributions to patient well-being, quality of life and social function. The series also covers the key principles involved in the use of social media for advertising and sharing cosmetic outcomes, from minor procedures to full-scale surgical operations. The series gathers ENT and related sub-specialty experts from across the globe and translates their knowledge into easily accessible, well-structured summaries of the current state of knowledge, with accompanying illustrations, diagrams and summary tables. Each volume is under the leadership of editors who are thoroughly familiar with the area covered and understands exactly which information is of most relevance and interest to those entering the field for the first time or seeking to update their existing knowledge. The series both outlines precisely the current state of the art in each area of ENT practice and shows where the future of the feld may lie. The fundamental scientifc basis of various disorders is covered, including molecular and cellular aspects, as well as diagnostic practice and the appropriate use of investigations. Historical aspects will be covered where they cast light on the general direction of the specialty. The latest developments in clinical management, disease prevention and public health aspects are described. The series shows how these multiple scientifc and clinical aspects can be best understood in supporting an individual, personalized approach to patient care that fts the patient-centered ethos of twenty-frst century ENT healthcare.

Cemal Cingi • Nuray Bayar Muluk
J. Regan Thomas
Editors

Minor Interventions, Major Outcomes on the Face

Updates in Facial Plastic Surgery

Springer

Editors
Cemal Cingi
Eskisehir Osmangazi University, Medical Faculty, Department of Otorhinolaryngology
Eskisehir, Türkiye

Nuray Bayar Muluk
Department of Otorhinolaryngology
Kırıkkale University
Kırıkkale, Türkiye

J. Regan Thomas
University of New Mexico School of Medicine
Albuquerque, NM, USA

ISSN 2731-6742 ISSN 2731-6750 (electronic)
Comprehensive ENT
ISBN 978-3-032-01304-0 ISBN 978-3-032-01305-7 (eBook)
https://doi.org/10.1007/978-3-032-01305-7

This Springer imprint is published by the registered company Springer Nature Switzerland AG
The registered company address is: Gewerbestrasse 11, 6330 Cham, Switzerland

Contents

Part I

Structure of the Face: General Overview

The Beauty of the Face: Features of the Female Face

1

Oğuzhan Oğuz, Cemal Cingi, and J. Regan Thomas

1.1 The Aesthetic Ideal

Comprehending what makes faces seem beautiful is a long-standing human preoccupation. For centuries after its creation, the sculpture of Aphrodite by Praxiteles was held up as an aesthetic ideal. However, what is taken to constitute an ideally beautiful face has evolved over the centuries. Humans have built-in preferences for certain features, whilst other ideas of beauty stem from artistic representations and philosophical discussions. The contemporary media landscape is one in which our icons both inform and are informed by the prevailing aesthetic ideals [1].

In talking about facial aesthetics, it is essential to understand what makes a facial feature disharmonious or disproportionate. Disproportion occurs when the dimensions of a feature are not within two standard deviations of the mean dimension. Even where a feature exhibits disproportion, provided the overall facial features are attractive, harmony may still be preserved. Farkas et al. examined nasal measurements in 29 different women. Amongst those considered attractive, 70% had nasal proportions that fell within one standard deviation of the mean [2]. Farkas proposes that the nose pays a particularly large role in providing harmony to the facial features, where these are not of normal proportions.

It is surprising to learn that there is considerable intercultural agreement on what constitutes a beautiful face, which is the result of selective pressure whereby

O. Oğuz
Dr. Oğuzhan Oğuz Wellnose Clinic, Istanbul, Turkey

C. Cingi (✉)
Eskisehir Osmangazi University, Medical Faculty, Department of Otorhinolaryngology, Eskisehir, Türkiye
e-mail: cemal@ogu.edu.tr

J. R. Thomas
University of New Mexico School of Medicine, Albuquerque, NM, USA

C. Cingi et al. (eds.), *Minor Interventions, Major Outcomes on the Face*, Comprehensive ENT, https://doi.org/10.1007/978-3-032-01305-7_1

physical attractiveness correlates with greater biological fitness and social adjustment. A number of studies have confirmed that attractiveness in women's body features is the result of being in good health and able to reproduce and arise from the actions of oestrogen [3, 4]. Perret et al. modified digital portraits of women's faces to investigate how strongly particular features were considered preferable [5]. The adjustments to the portraits were made to make the face appear younger and fertile; the features adjusted were those on which sex hormones have an action. There was a consistent preference across cultures for the portraits where feminine traits had been exaggerated from the usual appearance. The subjects not only preferred feminised faces of women within their own culture, but also rated more highly feminised faces from different cultures [6].

Mommaerts et al. compared faces considered ideal in antiquity with those seen amongst contemporary celebrities noted for their beauty [7]. They discovered that beautiful women at present have faces with a lower value for the classical facial index than in antique representations or in men. This comes about either because the facial height is less, or because the face is wider. The sex difference is also apparent in contemporary faces when the Bruges index was applied. In contemporary men's faces, the lower face makes up 48% of the total length of the face, whereas in contemporary women, the lower face accounts for 45%. However, this result failed to reach the level of statistical significance ($p = 0.08$). In contrast, there has been minimal alteration in the facial thirds index applied to the lower face since the time of Praxiteles. The contemporary ideal for both male and female faces involves a stomion-gnathion distance, which is 70% of the subnasale-stomion distance. The mean facial length of attractive contemporary women was below men's, although the interpupillary distance differs only slightly. In ideal contemporary faces, the lower facial third is divided such that 30% of the distance is from the upper line to the bottom of the upper lip, and 70% from the top of the lower lip to the chin.

In women, the eyebrows are arched, rising, then falling as they pass laterally. The portion of the eyebrow that is most superior in ideal faces falls on a vertical line passing through the lateral limbus, or no further laterally than a vertical line passing through the lateral canthus [8].

1.2 Aesthetic Facial Analysis

The appropriate position of the patient when the surgeon performs an aesthetic facial analysis is in the Frankfort horizontal position with the ears equally visible bilaterally. The assessment begins by mentally dividing the face into three equal horizontal and five equal vertical "slices" (Fig. 1.1). The five vertical slices should each measure roughly the same distance as that between the canthi [1].

The horizontal facial slices are also valuable in evaluating how symmetrical the facial features are. The line dividing the upper and mid-third passes through the

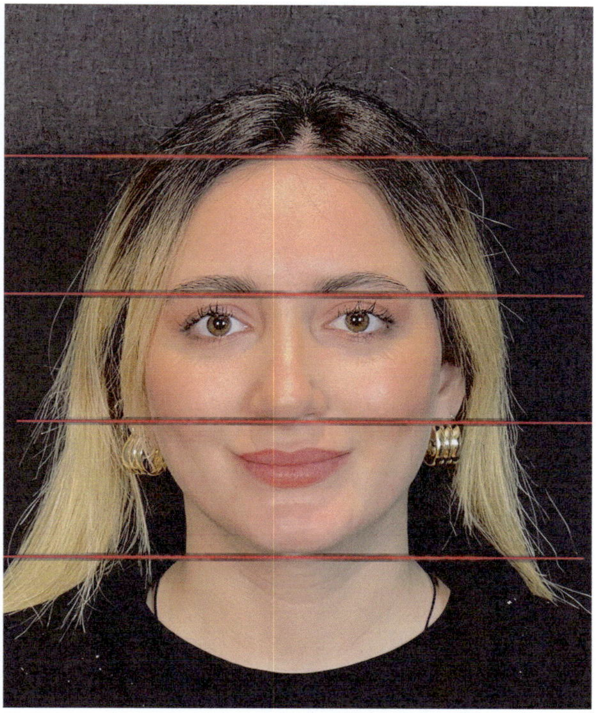

Fig. 1.1 Horizontal thirds of the face

most anteriorly located portion of the glabella. The line dividing the mid- and lower third passes through the subnasale, which is the point where the columella abuts the superior lip. Thus, the nasal structures should fall within the mid-third (Figs. 1.1 and 1.2) [1].

The nose may also be divided into thirds, proceeding from superior to inferior. The most superior portion of the nose consists of the osseous portion of the nose, the mid-third consists of the superior lateral cartilages and the dorsal septum, and the lower third consists of the nasal tip [1] (Fig. 1.3).

In an idealised nose, the base has the form of an equilateral triangle (Fig. 1.4). A further division of the base into three is again possible. The nostrils occupy the lower two of three slices, whilst the infratip lobule occupies the top third. Ideal nostrils are ovoid and exhibit symmetry. The medial crura widen to a varying degree at their footplates, and this typically means there is an indentation in the ovoid outline of the nostril. If the nostrils are asymmetrical, the reason for such an abnormality should be sought. This may arise from scarring of the ala, previous operations on the nose, a septum that is dislocated from the spine of the maxilla in its caudal aspect, or a congenital defect [9].

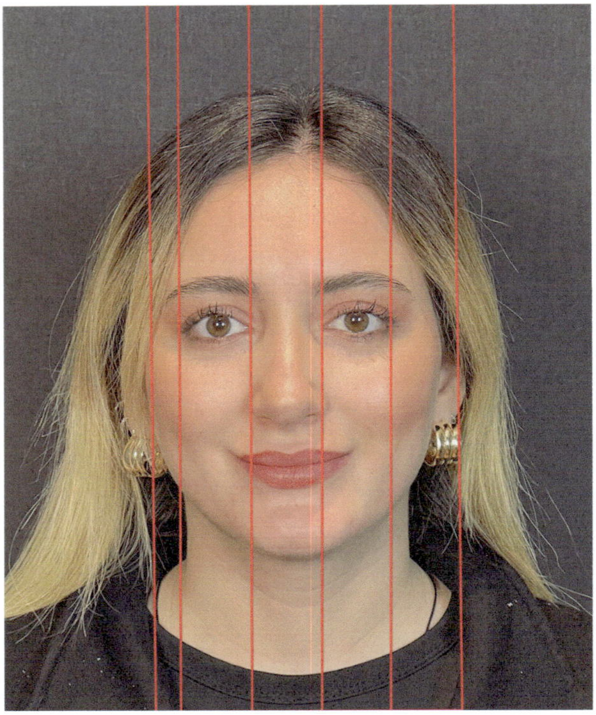

Fig. 1.2 Vertical fifths

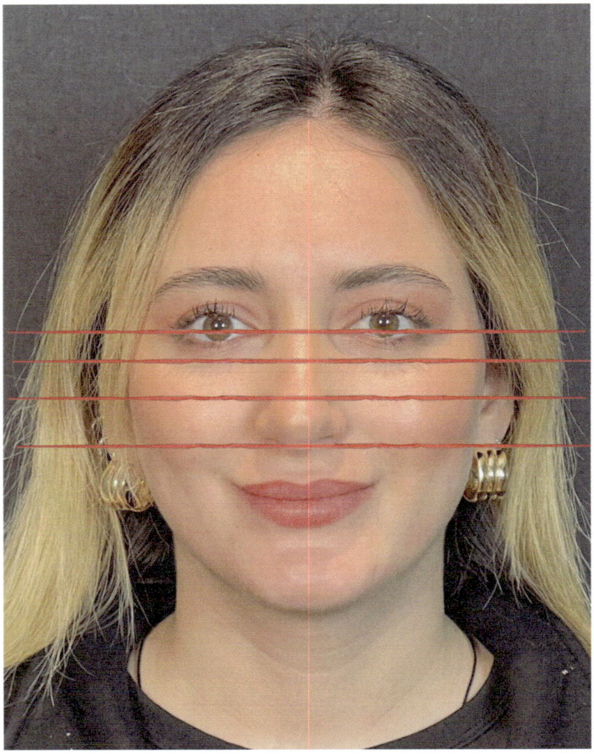

Fig. 1.3 Horizontal thirds of the nose

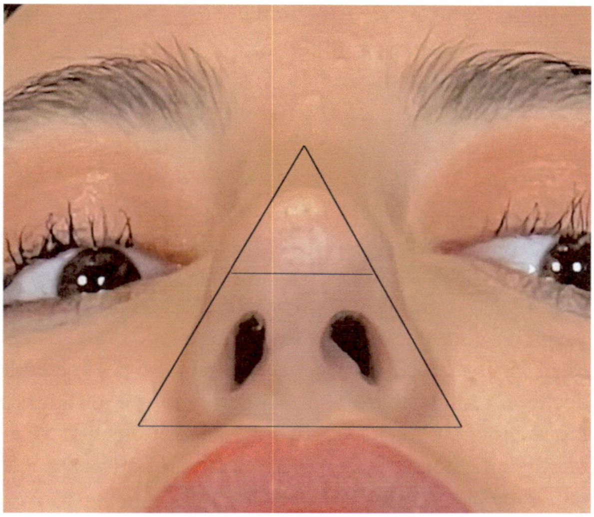

Fig. 1.4 The base of the nose, ideally forms an equilateral triangle

1.2.1 Lips

Penna and colleagues [10] employed 176 photographic portraits of Caucasian men and women. These pictures were graded by 250 volunteers on how attractive they seemed. These results were then correlated with different measurements of the lips and bottom third of the face. The faces received a grading ranging from 1 (indicating absolute attractiveness) to 7 (complete absence of attractiveness). In the portraits rated "attractive" (i.e. with a score of 1 or 2), the ratio of upper vermilion height to nose-mouth distance was 0.28, where the nose-mouth distance equates to the distance separating the subnasale from the inferior margin of the superior vermilion border. This value for the ratio is higher than in those portraits which received a score of 6 or 7 (i.e. "lacking attractiveness"). The result was at the level of statistical significance ($p < 0.05$). Furthermore, in the portraits rated more attractive, both men and women, the ratio of upper vermilion height to the distance from the subnasale to the chin (menton) was 0.09; a value above that calculated in the portraits was graded as lacking attractiveness. Figure 1.3 is a composite image illustrating the most attractive features, based on the findings of the two studies. It should be borne in mind, however, that both studies utilised portraits of Caucasian individuals only [11].

In ideal women's faces, the lower lip-to-upper lip ratio (D:C) reaches 2.00, the ratio of upper vermilion height to mouth-nose distance (C:B) is 0.28, and the ratio of upper vermilion height to subnasale-menton distance (C:A) equates to 0.09 [11].

1.2.2 The Golden Ratio

The Golden Ratio (sometimes referred to by the Greek letter ϕ) may be encountered in nature or artistic (including architectural) productions. Mathematically, its value is close to 1.618. The possibility that ϕ is reflected in aesthetically pleasing facial features has been discussed widely in the general media. Some authors have claimed to find the ratio exemplified in the ratio of nasal to oral width or tooth height to width, along with different levels of rigour evident in the attempt to prove a definite correlation [12]. According to Swift and Remington [13], ϕ can be noted in a whole set of ratios regarding the ideal face. Marquardt generated a 3d model of the perfect face, referred to as the golden decagon mask, by using ϕ for various ratios [14]. Whilst there are suggestions that ϕ and the golden decagon mask may offer some utility in analysis of faces, they may be impracticable to apply in ordinary aesthetic practice. One problem is that the non-specialist press has overhyped the utility of ϕ, such that it seemingly applies to multiple ratios in facial analysis, and this leads to suspicion that the value is found by chance rather than genuinely being present in ideal faces. A further difficulty is that whilst some authors do argue that the golden decagon representation helps to embody the different ratios that exist in attractive faces, other authors assert that the mask looks like a Caucasian woman of somewhat manly appearance and is not reflective of attractive faces from women of different ethnicities [15–19].

References

1. Winkler AA. Prerhinoplasty facial analysis. In: Meyers AD, editor. Medscape. Updated: 20 Feb 2020. https://emedicine.medscape.com/article/842545-overview#a5. Accessed online at 13 Apr 2021.
2. Farkas LG. Linear proportions in above- and below-average women's faces. In: Anthropometric facial proportions in medicine. Springfield: Thomas; 1987. p. 119–29.
3. Singh D. Ideal female body shape: role of body weight and waist-to-hip ratio. Int J Eat Disord. 1994;16(3):283–8.
4. Barber N. Secular changes in standards of bodily attractiveness in women: tests of a reproductive model. Int J Eat Disord. 1998;23(4):449–53.
5. Perrett DI, Lee KJ, Penton-Voak I, et al. Effects of sexual dimorphism on facial attractiveness. Nature. 1998;394(6696):884–7.
6. Manevska I, Pavlic A, Katic V, Trinajstic Zrinski M, Drevensek M, Spalj S. Satisfaction with facial profile aesthetics: are norms overrated? Int J Oral Maxillofac Surg. 2018;47(1):72–8.
7. Mommaerts MY, Moerenhout BA. Ideal proportions in full face front view, contemporary versus antique. J Craniomaxillofac Surg. 2011;39(2):107–10. https://doi.org/10.1016/j.jcms.2010.04.012. Epub 2010 Jun 12. Erratum in: J Craniomaxillofac Surg. 2013 Dec;41(8):705.
8. Prendergast PM. Facial proportions. In: Erian A, Shiffman MA, editors. Advanced surgical facial rejuvenation. Berlin Heidelberg: Springer-Verlag; 2012. p. 15–22. http://www.springer.com/978-3-642-17837-5. Accessed online at 13 Apr 2021.
9. Grossbart TA, Sarwer DB. Psychosocial issues and their relevance to the cosmetic surgery patient. Semin Cutan Med Surg. 2003;22(2):136–47.
10. Penna V, Fricke A, Iblher N, et al. The attractive lip: a photomorphometric analysis. J Plast Reconstr Aesthet Surg. 2015;68:920–9.
11. Hashim PW, Nia JK, Taliercio M, Goldenberg G. Ideals of facial beauty. Cutis. 2017;100(4):222–4.
12. Prokopakis EP, Vlastos IM, Picavet VA, et al. The golden ratio in facial symmetry. Rhinology. 2013;51:18–21.
13. Swift A, Remington K. BeautiPHIcation™: a global approach to facial beauty. Clin Plast Surg. 2011;38:247–77.

14. Marquardt SR, Dr. Stephen R. Marquardt on the Golden decagon and human facial beauty. interview by Dr. Gottlieb. J Clin Orthod. 2002;36:339–47.
15. Veerala G, Gandikota CS, Yadagiri PK, et al. Marquardt's facial Golden Decagon mask and its fitness with South Indian facial traits. J Clin Diagn Res. 2016;10:ZC49–52.
16. Holland E. Marquardt's phi mask: pitfalls of relying on fashion models and the golden ratio to describe a beautiful face. Aesth Plast Surg. 2008;32:200–8.
17. Alam MK, Mohd Noor NF, Basri R, et al. Multiracial facial golden ratio and evaluation of facial appearance. PLoS One. 2015;10:e0142914.
18. Kim YH. Easy facial analysis using the facial golden mask. J Craniofac Surg. 2007;18:643–9.
19. Bashour M. An objective system for measuring facial attractiveness. Plast Reconstr Surg. 2006;118:757–74. discussion 775–776.

Beauty of the Face: Features of the Male Face

2

Zeynel Öztürk, Nuray Bayar Muluk,
and Emmanuel Prokopakis

2.1 Introduction

The face in human beings is the entire region in front of the pinnae, stretching from the hairline above to the chin below. The upper face consists of the frontal region, which extends from the hairline to the supercilium. The shape of the forehead is created by the frontal bone, which is overlying, with adipose tissue pads between the skin and muscle layers and underneath the muscle. The glabella consists of a slight inter-superciliary prominence. When the procerus or corrugator muscles contract here, hyperdynamic wrinkles may appear. In men, the eyebrows are horizontal and over the supraorbital ridges [1].

Several soft tissue landmarks are on the midline, used as reference points in cephalometry, extending from the glabella above to the neck below. The reference points are employed when analysing the proportions of facial features and when calculating angles. The external nose has the form of a pyramid, the base of which covers the pyriform aperture within the skull. The nasal radix is below the glabellar prominence in the midsagittal plane, overlying the frontonasal suture. The nation is the posteriormost point on the external nose. The rest of the nose then projects in an

Z. Öztürk
Istanbul Nişantaşı University, Health Services Vocational School, Department of Audiology, Istanbul, Turkey

N. Bayar Muluk (✉)
Faculty of Medicine, Department of Otorhinolaryngology, Kırıkkale University, Kırıkkale, Türkiye

E. Prokopakis
Department of Otorhinolaryngology, Medical School, University of Crete, Heraklion, Crete, Greece
e-mail: Emmanuel@prokopakis.gr

C. Cingi et al. (eds.), *Minor Interventions, Major Outcomes on the Face*, Comprehensive ENT, https://doi.org/10.1007/978-3-032-01305-7_2

anteroinferior direction towards the nasal apex (i.e. nasal tip). The nasal dorsum is the region that lies between the nasion and tip. It has an osseous skeleton in the superior portion, which resists movement, and a more flexible cartilaginous skeleton in the inferior portion. The nose is widest at the nostrils (alae), which form the entrance to the vestibular portion of the interior nose. Between the nostrils lies the columella, which extends from the nasal tip to the philtrum. The philtrum is within the cutaneous portion of the superior lip. The vermillion border is where the red-coloured portion of the lips abuts the normal skin, and running right next to this border, in parallel with the lip, lies the tubular white roll. There is an anterior projection of the superior lip in the midline, referred to as the tuberculum labii superioris. The labiomental sulcus divides the lip and chin. The nasolabial folds bilaterally, which extend from the alar prominence to the ipsilateral corner of the mouth, show the boundary between the cheek and the superior lip [1].

In the superolateral aspect of the cheek, the soft tissues overlie the cheekbones (i.e. the zygomatic arch). In most cultures, cheekbones are considered an important aspect of a beautiful face. The convex outline of the cheek and smooth transition of the eyelid to the cheek depend upon infraorbital fat pads and inframuscular fat pads lying within the cheeks. In a more inferolateral direction, a buccal pad of fat causes children, in particular, to have rounded or chubby cheeks [1].

2.2 Features of the Face

In Caucasians, there is a tendency for the midfacial height to be less than the height of the top and bottom facial thirds [2]. This tendency has also been noted in black men [3, 4].

The lower face is divisible into three equal-sized horizontal slices. The top third extends from the subnasale to the stomion (defined as the middle of the oral fissure with closed lips). The distance from the station to the mention then represents the mid- and bottom third of the lower face [3] (Fig. 2.1).

2.2.1 Vertical Fifths

From a neoclassical perspective, the facial width can be divided into five equally sized slices [5] (Fig. 2.2). The outermost slice bilaterally extends from the most lateral point on the ear rim to the lateralmost corner of the eye (i.e. the exocanthus). The next slice, moving inwards, extends from the outer to the inner corner of each eye. The innermost fifth extends from the inner corner of the right to the left eye (i.e. the intercanthal distance). The intercanthal distance matches the interalar width, reflecting how wide the nose is. The distance between the right and left corners of the mouth should be 50% greater than the interalar width. These neoclassical proportions apply equally to men and women [5].

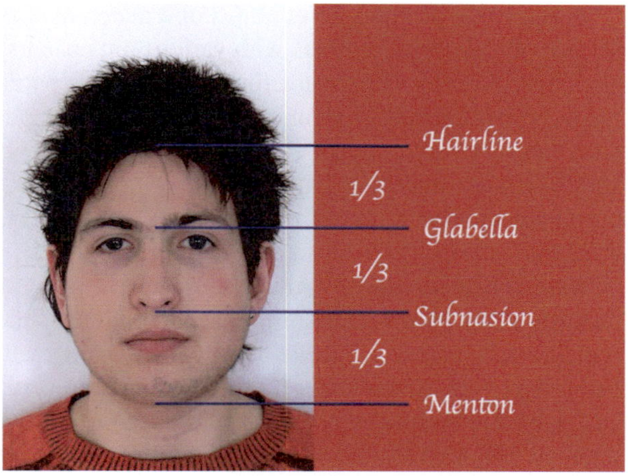

Fig. 2.1 Male face divided into equally spaced horizontal thirds

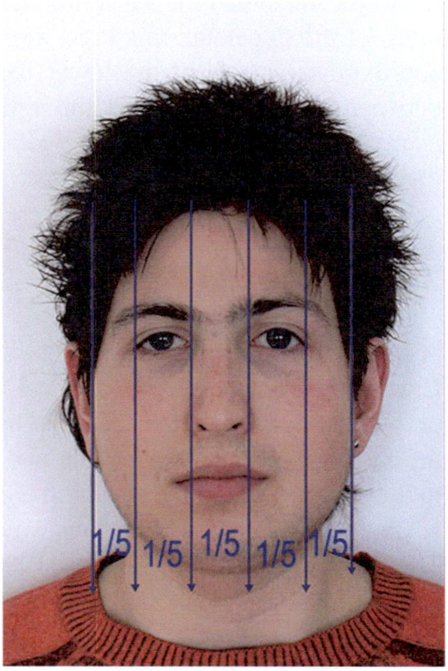

Fig. 2.2 Male face divided into equally spaced vertical fifths

2.3 Lips

The lips play a major role in determining how attractive the lower third of the face is deemed. There has been extensive discussion, in both mass and social media, about lip augmentation, whereby the lips may appear attractively plump and full [6]. What a culture considers to constitute ideal lips changes over time. Still, several recently published studies have attempted to supply a quantitative basis for how the attractiveness of lips is perceived.

In the study of Popenko et al. [7], the materials used were digitally composited images of Caucasian females with various dimensions for the lips and lower facial elements. Focus groups were formed from 400 participants, who were asked to grade how attractive they found the faces. The images that exhibited the greatest attractiveness had an upper lip height of half the lower lip height, while the faces adjudged least attractive had the inverse proportions. In the faces with the most appealing lips, the lips covered around 10% of the surface area of the bottom facial third [7].

Research undertaken by Anic-Milosevic et al. [8] examined the ratio of the facial features of the bottom third of the face in both men and women. In both males and females, the largest facial element was the chin, with the smallest measurement being the height of the lower lips. Comparing the vermilion heights of the superior and inferior lips showed no systematic difference in proportion between males and females, although the absolute vermilion heights of both lips were greater in men. For men and women, the vermilion height of the upper lip was exceeded by that of the lower lip. When the vermilion height was calculated relative to the surface distance of the upper lip, this ratio was higher in women. The lips generally occupy approximately 40% of the lower facial width, which is the same length as that between the medial limbus of the right eye and left eye. The usual height of the face is around 33% greater than the width, and the closer to an oval, the more ideal the face is deemed.

2.4 Nose and Nasal Tip

A description of how the nose, including its tip, should project has been provided by Crumley and Lanser [9]. In an ideal nose, a right-angled triangle with sides in the proportion 3:4:5 is found, with the hypotenuse represented by the line connecting the nasion and apex and the other two sides formed by the lines connecting the apex to the alar crease and the nasion to the alar crease. The degree to which the tip projects may be evaluated in various ways. One such way is to utilise the Baum ratio. Three lines are needed. The nasal length (defined as the distance from nasion to apex) is measured. Then, an imaginary line is drawn vertically from the nasion passing through the subnasale. Finally, a line at right angles to the vertical line and passing through the apex is drawn (forming the short side of a right-angled triangle). The Baum ratio is the hypotenuse of this triangle divided by the shortest side. An alternative to the Baum ratio is the Simons ratio, which is the distance between the subnasale and apex over the distance between the subnasale and the upper lip. Powell and Humphreys state that in idealised Caucasian faces, the Baum ratio is 2.8:1 and the Simons ratio is 1. Nasal rotation is indicated by the nasolabial angle, formed by the intersection of a line passing from the columella to the subnasale with a line joining the subnasale and the mucocutaneous margin of the superior lip. Leach [10] criticises using the nasolabial angle as a measure of nasal rotation in cases where the maxilla exhibits excessive protrusion or the incisors deviate from a vertical orientation. Leach therefore proposes using an imaginary line drawn at right angles to the Frankfort horizontal plane rather than the line connecting the subnasale to the superior lip. Viewed from its base, the nose is divisible into thirds. The columella-lobule ratio in an ideal nose is 2:1.

2.5 The Golden Ratio

It is easy to tell what types of faces are beautiful, but reducing this perceived beauty to exact values is easy. Nonetheless, the subjective sense of attractiveness may partly be quantified in numbers and using geometrical idealisations [11]. It is remarkable to find that in a wide variety of investigations of aesthetics stretching back more than two thousand years, a particular ratio recurs. This Golden Ratio (often referred to as φ (the Greek letter phi)) is so often encountered in investigations of harmonious proportion and beauty that it has achieved near legendary status. The actual numerical value of φ (an irrational number) is around 1.618033988. It is the solution to the equation $a + b/a = a/b$. There is evidence that the Ancient Indian mathematicians were interested in the Golden Ratio. Still, its first appearance in writing dates to the Greek geometer Euclid's *Elements*, first published around 300 BCE [12]. An alternative term for φ is the 'divine proportion'. It is popularly thought to unlock the mysterious nature of aesthetic attraction, including that exemplified in the human form [13]. Studying this ratio has fascinated and enchanted scholars and scientists in many different disciplines, such as mathematics, science, architecture, art, and aesthetic medicine, from the flourishing of Hellenic culture through the Renaissance and up to the present. Ricketts has applied to explain the relationship between many features of facial beauty [14–17]. Examples include the ratio of the nasal and oral widths, the ratio of the distance between the lateral canthi and the oral width, and the ratio of the mentopupillary distance to the distance between the hairline and pupils. Marquardt [18] has developed a mathematical model wherein the Golden Ratio is used to generate aesthetically satisfying idealised faces [18].

References

1. Prendergast PM. Facial proportions. In: Erian A, Shiffman MA, editors. Advanced surgical facial rejuvenation. Berlin Heidelberg: Springer-Verlag; 2012. p. 15–22. http://www.springer.com/978-3-642-17837-5. Accessed online on 13 Apr 2021.
2. Farkas LG, Hreczko TA, Kolar JC, et al. Vertical and horizontal proportions of the face in young-adult North-American Caucasians: revision of neoclassical canons. Plast Reconstr Surg. 1985;75:328–38.
3. Hashim PW, Nia JK, Taliercio M, Goldenberg G. Ideals of facial beauty. Cutis. 2017;100(4):222–4.
4. Porter JP. The average African American male face: an anthropometric analysis. Arch Facial Plast Surg. 2004;6:78–81.
5. Vegter F, Hage JJ. Clinical anthropometry and canons of the face in historical perspective. Plast Reconstr Surg. 2000;106:1090–6.
6. Powell N, Humphreys B. Proportions of the aesthetic face. New York: Thieme-Stratton; 1984.

7. Popenko NA, Tripathi PB, Devcic Z, et al. A quantitative approach to determining the ideal female lip aesthetic and its effect on facial attractiveness. JAMA Facial Plast Surg. 2017;19:261–7.
8. Anic-Milosevic A, Mestrovic S, Prlic A, Slaj M. Proportions in the upper lip–lower lip–chin area of the lower face as determined by photogrammetric method. J Craniomaxillofac Surg. 2010;38(2):90–5.
9. Crumley RJ, Lanser M. Quantitative analysis of nasal tip projection. Laryngoscope. 1988;98(2):202–8.
10. Leach J. Aesthetics and the Hispanic rhinoplasty. Laryngoscope. 2002;112(11):1903–16.
11. Atiyeh BS, Hayek SN. Numeric expression of aesthetics and beauty. Aesthet Plast Surg. 2008;32(2):209–16.
12. Vegter F, Hage J. Clinical anthropometry and canons of the face in historical perspective. Plast Reconstr Surg. 2000;106(5):1090–6.
13. Bashour M. History and current concepts in the analysis of facial attractiveness. Plast Reconstr Surg. 2006;118(3):741–56.
14. Ricketts RM. Esthetics, environment, and the law of lip relation. Am J Orthod. 1968;54(4):272–89.
15. Ricketts RM. The biologic significance of the divine proportion and Fibonacci series. Am J Orthod. 1982;81(5):351–70.
16. Ricketts RM. The golden divider. J Clin Orthod. 1981;15(11):752–9.
17. Ricketts RM. Divine proportion in facial aesthetics. Clin Plast Surg. 1982;9(4):401–22.
18. Marquardt SR. Dr Stephen Marquardt and the golden decagon of human facial beauty. Interview with Dr Gottlieb. J Clin Orthod. 2002;36(6):317–8.

Facial Anatomy: Muscles

3

Orhan Tunç, Cemal Cingi, and Jeffrey C. Bedrosian

3.1 Facial Muscles

The muscles of the face serve a dual purpose. In addition to regulating the opening and narrowing of the various spaces in the front, they also communicate information about a person's psychological and emotional state. Thus, they are essential in conveying messages via body language [1].

The facial musculature consists of a score of flat, striated muscles underlying the skin of the head and face. Most of these muscles have an origin connected to bones or fibrous structures of the skull with a tendinous attachment to the overlying skin. Unlike other groups of striated muscles, except the buccinator, there is no investing fascial sheath. The forces of the face either surround the oral, ocular, nasal, and otic openings or connect different parts of the skull and neck. Their positioning permits these muscles to perform a range of facial gestures. The forces act together to create the full range of expressions, including smiling, grimacing, etc [1].

O. Tunç
Gaziantep University, Medical Faculty, Department of Otorhinolaryngology, Gaziantep, Turkey

C. Cingi (✉)
Eskisehir Osmangazi University, Medical Faculty, Department of Otorhinolaryngology, Eskisehir, Türkiye
e-mail: cemal@ogu.edu.tr

J. C. Bedrosian
Rhinology and Skull Base Surgery, Specialty Physician Associates, St. Luke's Medical Center, Bethlehem, PA, USA

C. Cingi et al. (eds.), *Minor Interventions, Major Outcomes on the Face*, Comprehensive ENT, https://doi.org/10.1007/978-3-032-01305-7_3

3.1.1 Facial Musculature

The following muscles are all considered facial muscles: occipitofrontalis, orbicularis oculi, corrugator supercilii, procerus, nasalis, orbicularis oris, levator labii superioris, zygomaticus minor, buccinator, zygomaticus major, levator anguli oris, risorius, depressor anguli oris, depressor labii inferioris, mentalis, and platysma.

Blood supply

The vascular supply to all these muscles is via the facial artery.

Nerve supply

The seventh cranial nerve supplies all these muscles.

Function

These muscles are unlike other voluntary muscles in that they do not act on articulations but instead move the overlying skin. The muscles surrounding the mouth's principal actions are raising and lowering the corners of the mouth, forcing the superior and inferior lips, and opening and closing the external entrance to the oral cavity [1].

In addition, the levator labii superioris alaeque nasi muscles raise the nasal openings, widening the entrance to the nasal cavity [1].

The muscles that play a crucial role in laughter are the risorius, zygomaticus major, and zygomaticus minor. The nasal muscles can pucker the nose and partially close external openings [1].

3.2 Oral Musculature

The mouth's musculature moves the lips and the mouth itself. It consists of the following individual or pairs of muscles: orbicularis oris, buccinator (paired), triangularis, caninus, risorius, zygomaticus major and minor, quadratus labii superioris, levator labii superioris alaeque nasi, quadratus labi inferioris, mentalis, and platysma [2, 3].

- The orbicularis oris forms a circle around the external oral opening.
- The buccinators lie between the maxilla superiorly and the mandible inferiorly and extend toward the corners of the mouth. These muscles form the muscular component of the cheeks.
- The quadratus labii superioris connects the upper lip to the area of the infraorbital foramen.
- The quadratus labii inferioris connects the mandible below the level of the mental foramen to the inferior lip.

- The levator labii superioris alaeque nasi connects the superior lip and the alae to the medial margin of the orbit.
- The mentalis produces the crease lying under the lip and above the chin.
- The risorius connects the cheek to the corner of the mouth. Its Latin name, musculus risorius, translates as "laughing muscle."
- The canines connect the mouth's corner to an area lying below the orbit.
- The triangularis is also inserted in the corner of the mouth, connecting this to the inferior mandibular margin.
- The zygomaticus major and zygomaticus minor extend between the zygomatic arch and the corner of the mouth [1].

3.2.1 Orbicularis Oris

The orbicularis oris encircles the oral fissure. Its circular pattern resembles a sphincter.

Origin

- This muscle originates on the medial portion of the maxilla, mandible, and modiolus [4].

Insertion

- The muscle inserts into the skin, which encircles the lips.

Action

- As the orbicularis contracts, it furrows the lips and seals off the oral fissure.

Nerve supply

- The nerve supplying this muscle is the buccal branch of the seventh cranial nerve [4].

Vascular supply

- This is via the facial artery's labial branches, both superior and inferior [4].

3.2.2 Buccinator

This muscle lies between the maxilla superiorly and the mandible inferiorly. The cheek gets its outline from the power both anteriorly and laterally. The forces provide the wall of the oral cavity. The buccinator is pierced at several points by the salivary duct of the parotid gland, the salivary glands located opposite the molar teeth, and the buccal branch of the mandibular nerve [2].

Origin

- The muscle originates on the mandibular and maxillary alveolar ridges and the pterygomandibular ligament [2].

Insertion

- The buccinator inserts into the muscular fibers of the orbicularis oris and the modiolus [2].

Action

- When the buccinator contracts, it presses the inner wall of the cheek against the teeth, which assists in chewing. It is also essential to be able to whistle [2].

Nerve supply

- Innervation is via the buccal branch of the seventh cranial nerve [4].

Vascular supply

- The muscle is supplied via the maxillary artery's buccal branch [4].

3.2.3 Triangularis

Origin

- This muscle originates on the mandibular mental tubercle [3].

Insertion

- It inserts into the modiolus and the corner of the mouth.

Action

- When the triangularis contracts, it depresses the mouth's corner, as occurs when a person frowns.
- Contraction of the triangular counteracts the effect of the canines [2].

Nerve supply

- The muscle is innervated by the buccal branch and mandibular branch of the seventh cranial nerve [2].

Vascular supply

- The blood supply to this muscle is via the facial and maxillary arteries (mental branches).

3.2.4 Caninus

Origin

- This muscle originates in the maxillary canine fossa [4].

Insertion

- It inserts into the modiolus and corner of the mouth [2].

Action

- When the canines contract, they lift the lateral portion of the oral fissure, which is part of smiling [3].

Nerve supply

- It is innervated by branches of the seventh cranial nerve, i.e., zygomatic and buccal [2].

Vascular supply

- Arterial supply occurs via the facial artery (superior labial branch) and the maxillary artery (infraorbital branch) [3].

3.2.5 Risorius

Origin

- This muscle originates in the parotid fascia [2].

Insertion

- It inserts into the modiolus [2].

Action

- Contraction of the risorius pulls the corner of the mouth in a posterior direction [3].

  Nerve supply

- Innervation is via the buccal branch of the seventh cranial nerve [3].

  Vascular supply

- The artery supplying the muscle is the facial artery's superior labial branch.

3.2.6 Zygomaticus Major

Origin

- The zygomaticus major originates in the zygoma [2].

  Insertion

- It inserts into the modiolus.

  Action

- Its action is essential when an individual smiles, as it pulls the corners of the mouth upwards and outwards [2].

  Nerve supply

- It is innervated by branches of the seventh cranial nerve (zygomatic and buccal).

  Vascular supply

- Its arterial supply is via a branch of the facial artery, the superior labial [4].

3.2.7 Zygomaticus Minor

Origin

- This muscle originates in the zygoma [4].

  Insertion

- It has its point of insertion in the skin surrounding the lateral portion of the superior lip [2].

Action

- Contracting helps raise the superior lip [2].

Nerve supply

- It is innervated by branches of the seventh cranial nerve (zygomatic and buccal).

Vascular supply

- Its arterial supply is via a branch of the facial artery, the superior labial [4].

3.2.8 Quadratus (Levator) Labii Superioris

Origin

- This muscle originates on the maxilla and the portion of the zygoma lying above the infraorbital foramen [2].

Insertion

- Its insertion points are the skin and muscles comprising the superior lip [4].

Action

- When it contracts, it raises the superior lip [2].

Nerve supply

- It is innervated by branches of the seventh cranial nerve (zygomatic and buccal) [4].

Vascular supply

- Its arterial supply is via the facial artery, a branch of the maxillary artery, and the infraorbital [2].

3.2.9 Levator Labii Superioris Alaeque Nasi

Origin

- This muscle originates in the maxillary frontal process.

  Insertion

- It inserts into the skin overlying the nasal alar cartilage and the skin of the superior lip [4].

  Action

- When this muscle contracts, the individual appears snarling since it widens the external nasal apertures and lifts the alae and superior lip [2].

  Nerve supply

- It is innervated by branches of the seventh cranial nerve (zygomatic and buccal) [2].

  Vascular supply

- Its arterial supply is via the facial artery, a branch of the maxillary artery, and the infraorbital [3].

3.2.10 Depressor Labii Inferioris

Origin

- This muscle originates from between the mandibular symphysis and the mental foramen.

  Insertion

- It inserts into the skin, covering the inferior lip—the fibers of depressor labii inferioris insert among the muscular fibers making up the orbicularis oris.

  Action

- When it contracts, it lowers the inferior lip.

  Nerve supply

- It is innervated by a branch of the seventh cranial nerve (mandibular) [2].

  Vascular supply

- Its arterial supply is via a branch of the facial artery (inferior labial) and of the maxillary artery (mental) [2].

3.2.11 Mentalis

Origin

- This muscle originates from the anterior portion of the mandibular bone [3].

Insertion

- It inserts into the skin overlying the chin.

Action

- When the muscle contracts, the inferior lip protrudes. The skin overlying the chin also puckers as it is raised [2].

Nerve supply

- It is innervated by a branch of the seventh cranial nerve (mandibular) [2].

Vascular supply

- Its arterial supply is via a branch of the facial artery (inferior labial) and of the maxillary artery (mental) [2].

3.2.12 Platysma

Origin

- This muscle originates in the skin and fascial layers above and below the clavicle.

Insertion

- It inserts into the lower part of the mandible, the skin overlying the cheeks and inferior lip, the corner of the mouth, and the orbicularis oris [3].

Action

- Contraction of the platysma pulls the angles of the mouth inferiorly. This causes the face to appear sad.
- If the jaw is also clenched, the cervical skin becomes taut [4].

- It pulls the mandible inferiorly [4].

Nerve supply

- It is innervated by the cervical branch of the seventh facial nerve [3].

Vascular supply

- Arterial supply is via multiple arteries branching off the submental and suprascapular roadways [3].

3.3 Muscles of the Nose

The nose's muscles allow the nose and adjacent skin to move. The nasal musculature mainly consists of three major forces: the nasalis, procerus, and depressor septi nasi [2].

The nasalis muscle connects the maxilla to the cartilage of the nose.

The procerus muscle connects the intersuperciliary skin to the bridge of the nose [1].

3.3.1 Nasalis

The nasalis is the most substantial of the nose's muscles—a bipartite muscle with an alar and transverse part [4].

Origin

- It takes its head from the maxillary incisive fossa [3].

Insertion

- It inserts into the aponeurosis overlying the nasal bridge. This aponeurosis joins the left and right nasalis. Furthermore, it inserts into the skin surrounding the alae [2].

Action

- It compresses the skin overlying the bridge of the nose.
- It lowers the nasal tip [2].
- It can close off the nostrils.

Nerve supply

- It is innervated by the buccal branch of the seventh cranial nerve [4].

Vascular supply

- The arterial supply is via a branch of the facial artery (superior labial) and the maxillary artery (infraorbital) [2].

3.3.2 Procerus

Origin

- This muscle originates in the fascia superficial to the lower portion of the nasal bone and the upper part of the lateral nasal cartilage [3].

Insertion

- It inserts into the skin in the lower frontal region and around the glabella.

Action

- As the procerus contracts, it pulls the medial end of the eyebrow downwards, an action seen when a person frowns [3].

Nerve supply

- It is innervated by branches of the seventh cranial nerve (temporal and lower zygomatic) [3].

Vascular supply

- The facial artery supplies the muscle via its angular and lateral nasal branches.

3.3.3 Depressor Septi Nasi

Origin

- The depressor septi nasi originates on the maxillary incisive fossa.

Insertion

- It inserts into the nasalis' fibers and the nose's septum [4].

Action

- As it contracts, it makes the nose's external opening larger [2].

Nerve supply

- It is innervated by a branch of the seventh cranial nerve (buccal) [4].

Vascular supply

- Its arterial supply is via the superior labial artery, which branches off the facial artery [2].

3.4 Muscles of the Eyelid

- The orbicularis oculi forms a circle around the orbit.
- The depressor supercilii connects the medial canthal region to the superciliary skin.
- The corrugator supercilii connects the area above the nasal radix to the superciliary skin [1].

When the orbicularis oculi fully contracts, it seals off the palpebral fissure by closing the blephara, while partial contraction permits the individual to squint and helps tears flow more freely. Contraction of the depressor supercilii and corrugator supercilii lowers the eyebrows and puckers the frontal skin. The occipitofrontalis has the opposite action of lifting the eyebrows and the pinnae. Contraction of the platysma draws the angles of the mouth in a lateral and inferior direction and makes the skin taut. The form of the auricular muscles varies from individual to individual, which explains the varying ability to wiggle the ears when asked [1].

3.4.1 Orbicularis Oculi

Three muscles constitute the orbicularis oculi: the orbital, palpebral, and lacrimal orbicularis [4].

Origin

- The origin is on the nasal part of the frontal bone, the maxillary frontal process, the medial canthal tendon, the lacrimal crest, and the lacrimal bone [3].

Insertion

- It inserts into the skin surrounding the eye socket, the palpebral ligament, the temporal aspect of the eye socket, and the malar skin in its lower portion.

Action

- The principal action is to seal off the palpebral fissure [3].

- The palpebral orbicularis is under voluntary control but may also contract due to an involuntary impulse, as occurs when the individual blinks.
- The orbital orbicularis is only under voluntary control.
- Contraction of the lacrimal orbicularis pumps tears toward the lachrymal sac [2].

Nerve supply

- The temporal branch innervates it, and the zygomatic branch of the seventh cranial nerve [4].

Vascular supply

- The blood supply occurs via vessels branching off the facial artery, superficial temporal artery, maxillary artery, and ophthalmic artery [4].

3.4.2 Corrugator Supercilii

Origin

- The origin is located at the medial pole of the superciliary arch [2].

Insertion

- It inserts into the frontal skin near the eyebrow [2].

Action

- When the corrugator supercilii contracts, the frontal skin becomes puckered, and the eyes are protected from dazzle by the movement of the eyebrows in an anteromedial direction [4].

Nerve supply

- It is innervated by the seventh cranial nerve branch, the temporal [3].

Vascular supply

- It receives blood from the ophthalmic artery and vessels branching off the superficial temporal artery [3].

References

1. Karunaharamoorthy A. Facial muscles. https://www.kenhub.com/en/library/anatomy/the-facial-muscles. Accessed online on 2 Aug 2020.
2. Shennan J. Muscles of facial expression. Anatomy of the head and neck. https://geekymedics.com/muscles-of-facial-expression/. Accessed online at 2 Aug 2020.
3. Gilroy AM. Anatomy – an essential textbook. 2nd ed. Thieme Medical Publishers; 2017.
4. Drake RL, Wayne Vogl A, Mitchell A. Gray's anatomy for students. 2nd ed. Elsevier Health Sciences; 2009.

Facial Anatomy: Nerves

4

Onur Erdoğan, Nuray Bayar Muluk, and Dennis Chua

4.1 Introduction

There are three principal origins in the head and neck region providing the nervous supply to the superficial structures of the face and scalp [1]:

- The seventh cranial nerve (facial nerve) supplies motor nerves to the facial musculature.
- The fifth cranial nerve (trigeminal) supplies sensory nerves for the facial region. It has three divisions, i.e. the ophthalmic (V1), maxillary (V2) and mandibular (V3).
- The nerves derived from the cervical plexus supply the scalp region.

4.1.1 The Seventh Cranial Nerve

This nerve supplies the facial musculature. There are five divisions of this nerve, i.e. the temporal, zygomatic, buccal, mandibular and cervical branches [1].

O. Erdoğan
Department of Otorhinolaryngology, Silifke Olbamed Hospital, Mersin, Turkey

N. Bayar Muluk (✉)
Faculty of Medicine, Department of Otorhinolaryngology, Kırıkkale University, Kırıkkale, Türkiye

D. Chua
Department of Otorhinolaryngology, ENT Surgeons Medical Centre, Mount Elizabeth Hospital, Mount Elizabeth, Singapore

C. Cingi et al. (eds.), *Minor Interventions, Major Outcomes on the Face*, Comprehensive ENT, https://doi.org/10.1007/978-3-032-01305-7_4

4.1.1.1 The Ophthalmic Division of the Trigeminal Nerve (V1)

This nerve supplies the superior facial third, including the superior blephara, ocular conjunctivae and frontal skin. It divides forming the supraorbital, supratrochlear, external nasal and infratrochlear nerves [1].

4.1.1.2 The Maxillary Division of the Trigeminal Nerve (V2)

This nerve supplies the mid-facial third, including the nose and the skin overlying the cheekbones. It divides into the zygomaticofacial, zygomaticotemporal and infraorbital branches [1].

4.1.1.3 The Mandibular Division of the Trigeminal Nerve (V3)

This nerve supplies the inferior facial third, including skin in the peri-auricular and mental regions. It divides into the auriculotemporal, buccal and mental branches [1].

4.1.2 Cervical Plexus

This is the origin of nerves supplying the skin of the mastoid, scalp and parotid gland. It gives rise to the great auricular and greater and lesser occipital nerves [1].

4.2 Facial Nerve

In general terms, the muscles involved in producing different facial expressions are all ultimately supplied by the seventh cranial nerve (=facial nerve). This nerve springs from the brainstem at the level of the pontomedullary junction, inferolateral to the origin of the sixth cranial nerve and superomedial to the origin of the eighth cranial nerve [1].

The facial nerve consists of three types of fibres, motor, sensory and autonomic (secretomotor, i.e. parasympathetic), which supply numerous structures of the head and neck. Three nuclei within the central nervous system give rise to the fibres of the seventh cranial nerve, namely [2]:

- The facial motor nucleus
- The superior salivary nucleus
- The facial sensory nucleus

4.2.1 Structure and Function

The seventh cranial nerve fulfils four main roles:

- It innervates the muscles of the face via general somatic efferent fibres.

- It innervates the facial salivary glands (submandibular and sublingual), as well as the lacrimal gland. Thus, it also carries visceral efferent fibres of the parasympathetic division of the autonomic nervous system.
- It innervates the anterior and mid-third of the tongue, supplying special visceral afferent input to the brain.
- It innervates the auricular skin and the external ear canal. Thus, it provides somatic afferent input to the brain [2–4].

4.2.2 Motor Pathway

The upper motor neurones are situated in the precentral gyrus, within the motor area representing the face. The axons pass within the corticobulbar tract to the inferior pontine region without decussating, after which the majority of fibres do decussate before descending on the contralateral side towards the lower motor neurones of the pathway. The lower motor neurones are located in four distinct subnuclei, namely, the dorsal, intermediate, lateral and medial nuclei. Fibres originating from the dorsal motor nucleus supply the muscles of the face within the superior quadrant on the same side as the nucleus. There is bilateral input from the corticobulbar tracts to the dorsal motor nucleus. The lateral motor nucleus, in contrast, receives input via the corticobulbar tract of the opposite side alone. Fibres from the lateral motor nucleus supply facial muscles within the inferior quadrant on the same side as the nucleus [5, 6]. This neuroanatomical configuration explains why a facial palsy involving upper motor neurones is confined to the inferior facial quadrant on the opposite side to the lesion, whereas a facial palsy affecting the lower motor neurones causes both the superior and inferior facial quadrants on the same side as the lesion to be paralysed. The main motor nucleus is the origin of conscious control of the muscles of the face. Furthermore, it sends fibres to the auricular muscles, the posterior belly of the digastric muscle, the stapedius muscle and the stylohyoid muscle. Face expressions that occur in response to various emotional states involve different mechanisms, with involvement of both the limbic lobe and the extrapyramidal tract [2, 7].

4.2.3 Parasympathetic Pathway

The superior salivatory nucleus, a portion of which is the lacrimal nucleus, contributes parasympathetic outflow to the seventh cranial nerve. This nucleus lies in the inferior pontine region behind and lateral to the facial motor nucleus. It receives projections from the hypothalamus, as well as gustatory information from the nucleus of the solitary tract. The superior salivatory nucleus sends efferent fibres to the sublingual salivary glands and submandibular salivary glands, in addition to the glands of the palate and those within the nose. The lacrimal nucleus receives two types of input. The hypothalamus mediates crying in response to strong emotion, whereas crying brought about by ocular irritation is triggered via the sensory division of the fifth cranial nerve. Parasympathetic efferent outflow from the brainstem within the seventh cranial nerve passes in the glossopalatine nerve [2, 3].

4.2.4 Sensory Pathway

The motor nucleus and pontine parasympathetic nuclei lie anteromedial to the sensory nucleus, which receives gustatory input originating in the palate, the base of the oral cavity and the anteriormost and mid-third of the tongue. The geniculate ganglion is the location of the first-order gustatory neurones, which form a synaptic connection with the second-order neurones in the nucleus of the tractus solitarius, lying within the medulla oblongata. These second-order neurones decussate prior to their ascent to the thalamus via the medial lemniscus. In the thalamus, they have a synaptic connection to axons of third-order neurones, which ultimately terminate in the gustatory cortical region within the insula and post-central gyrus, having passed through the internal capsule and the corona radiata. A few fibres terminate within the hypothalamus [8].

The pathway carrying general sensory information consists of first-order neurones with their cell bodies in the geniculate ganglion, with the second-order neurones in the spinal trigeminal nucleus. The axons of the seventh cranial nerve carrying sensory and parasympathetic information are bound together, forming the glossopalatine nerve (also termed the nervus intermedius) [2, 4].

4.2.5 The Course of the Axons of the Seventh Cranial Nerve Within the Brainstem

The seventh cranial nerve consists of motor neurones arising from the motor root and the bundled sensory and parasympathetic axons making up the glossopalatine nerve. The motor portion passes in a backwards direction, skirting around the nucleus of the sixth cranial nerve before traversing the facial colliculus located on the floor of the fourth ventricle. It then exits at a point on the anterolateral medulla just inferior to the pons, the pontomedullary junction. The glossopalatine nerve also exits the brainstem at the same location [8].

4.2.6 Segments of the Seventh Cranial Nerve

The initial segment of the seventh cranial nerve is referred to as the intracranial or cisternal portion. The nerve contains the motor root and the glossopalatine nerve, which exit the pons as described above. These two roots enter the posterior cranial fossa at the cerebellopontine angle. They are accompanied by the eighth cranial nerve at this point. The two cranial nerves pass into both the temporal bone and the internal auditory canal [2].

The second segment is termed the meatal or canalicular portion. At this stage, the seventh cranial nerve is contained in the upper quadrant of the internal auditory canal [2].

The third segment of the seventh cranial nerve is the labyrinthine portion, which commences at the point where the two roots exit the internal auditory canal and enter the facial canal. The roots both bypass the cochlea and vestibular apparatus and turn in a posterior direction after joining the geniculate ganglion. Here, the motor root and glossopalatine nerve combine. There the third segment divides into three, forming the greater superficial, lesser and external petrosal nerves. The first of these carries parasympathetic information to the tear glands and gustatory fibres which extend to the palate [2].

The fourth portion of the seventh cranial nerve is the tympanic segment. This segment extends from the point where the nerve progresses in a posterior direction after the geniculate ganglion and is contained in the medial wall of the middle ear space. It is just under the lateral semicircular canal [2].

The mastoid segment is the term applied to the fifth portion of the seventh cranial nerve. This section of the nerve starts with an inferior flexion of the nerve at the pyramidal eminence of the middle ear space. It passes within the facial canal as far as the stylomastoid foramen. The mastoid portion of the seventh nerve divides three times: once to supply the stapedius muscle, a second time to form the chorda tympani and a third time to give off sensory fibres which blend with the auricular nerve (a branch of the tenth cranial nerve). The chorda tympani supplies the parasympathetic control to the sublingual and submandibular salivary glands, whereas the sensory fibres which join the auricular nerve carry general somatic sensory information from the external ear and ear canal [2].

The extratemporal segment then forms the last section of the seventh cranial nerve. The start of the segment is the point where the seventh cranial nerve leaves the temporal bone by passing through the stylomastoid foramen. At this point, the nerve branches twice, giving rise to the posterior auricular and digastric nerves. The former innervates the posterior and superior auricular muscles, plus the occipital belly of the occipitofrontalis, whilst the latter innervates the posterior belly of the digastric and the stylohyoid muscles. The seventh cranial nerve then passes through the parotid gland, where it again divides, resulting in two principal trunks, the superior temporofacial and inferior cervicofacial. Together, the trunks represent the origin of the parotid plexus. The parotid plexus then gives rise to five branches: the temporal (frontal), zygomatic, buccal, mandibular and cervical. It is these branches which provide motor innervation to the muscles of the face [3, 4, 8, 9].

4.2.7 Extratemporal Divisions of the Seventh Cranial Nerve

The seventh cranial nerve consists of five main divisions supplying the face. These divisions are the temporal, zygomatic, buccal, mandibular and cervical [1].

The temporal division of the seventh cranial nerve may also be termed its frontal division. On its path towards the temporal facial region, it goes across the zygomatic arch, where a branch heads off to the auricularis anterior. Fibres also connect to the mandibular nerve's auriculotemporal branch and the maxillary nerve's zygomatico-temporal branch. The branches of the frontal division lying most anterior within the face innervate the corrugator supercilii, frontalis and orbicularis oris. Fibres also supply the efferent portion of the corneal (blink) reflex arc [1].

Another term for the zygomatic division is the malar division. The nerves cross over the zygoma on their way towards the lateral angle of the eye. The lateral angle is the point where fibres enter the orbicularis oculi and some fibres attach to the lacrimal nerve [1].

The buccal region of the face, which refers to the region of the cheek, perioral and infraorbital regions, is supplied by the seventh cranial nerve, too. There are fibres found just deep to the skin, as well as over the outside of the superficial facial musculature. The seventh cranial nerve innervates such muscles, one of which is the procerus. At the medial angle of the eye, it accompanies fibres originating from the frontal division of the fifth cranial nerve, specifically the infratrochlear and nasociliary branches. The small muscles in the nose are innervated by deeper running fibres of the facial nerve. The deeper fibres are deep to the quadratus labii superioris and the zygomaticus muscles, both of which they supply. These fibres contribute to an infraorbital plexus, to which the maxillary nerve's infraorbital branch also contributes. The deep fibres also innervate the buccinator and orbicularis oris muscles [1].

The marginal mandibular branch also arises from the seventh cranial nerve. It travels deep to the platysma and anguli oris muscles, innervating the chin and inferior lip. It also connects to a branch of the inferior alveolar nerve, the mental branch.

The cervical division of the seventh cranial nerve is the most inferior division. It follows a path passing deep to the platysma. The path of this branch is unusual, as it consists of arched segments as it traverses the suprahyoid region and the neck proper. It gives off branches to the platysma and the depressor anguli oris. One of its branches, the cervical cutaneous nerve, forms a junction with the cervical plexus [1].

The posterior auricular nerve also branches off the seventh facial nerve as it exits the stylomastoid foramen. This is where it is joined by a ramification of the greater auricular nerve, itself a branch of the tenth cranial nerve. The posterior auricular nerve passes upwards with the mastoid process on one side and the external ear canal on the other, before bifurcating to form the occipital branch and the auricular branch. The latter innervates the superficial muscles intrinsic to the external ear, along with the auricularis posterior. The former extends for a lengthier course, passing backwards along the superior nuchal line. This landmark is on the occipital bone and represents the continuation laterally of the external occipital protuberance. The occipital branch innervates the occipitalis [1].

4.3 Trigeminal Nerve (Fifth Cranial Nerve)

The facial sensory nerve supply is provided by the fifth cranial nerve. This is the sole cranial nerve to have a direct origin from the pons. The nerve forms three divisions, namely, the ophthalmic (V1), maxillary (V2) and mandibular (V3), each of which innervates a particular facial territory. The muscles of the face involved in chewing, i.e. the medial pterygoid, lateral pterygoid, temporalis and masseter, are also innervated by the fifth cranial nerve [1].

4.3.1 Nerves Belonging to V1 (Ophthalmic Division)

The supraorbital nerve divides from the last portion of the frontal nerve. It exits via the supraorbital foramen, giving off branches supplying the superior blephara (palpebral branches). In addition, it provides innervation to the ocular conjunctivae, transparent structures which extend over the inner blepharal surface and cover the white-coloured orbit, as well as the frontal skin up to the mid-scalp region and the frontal sinus [1].

The frontal nerve branches off V1, then itself gives rise to the supratrochlear nerve. This branch passes upwards above the pulley mechanism of the superior oblique muscle, after which a delicate branch arises which forms a junction with the infratrochlear nerve. This latter is a branch of the nasociliary nerve. At this point, the supratrochlear nerve passes in a superior fashion, curving slightly, along the frontal region. The path crosses between two of the facial muscles, the frontalis and corrugator supercilii, where it enters the body of the muscle and divides to innervate the skin of the superior blepharon, the frontal skin, the glabellar skin and the ocular conjunctivae [1].

The anterior ethmoidal nerve is another branch of V1. It gives rise at its end to the external nasal branches, which supply cutaneous sensation to skin overlying the portion of the septum composed of cartilage and the inferior 50% of the nose [1].

The nasociliary nerve also branches off V1. Its terminal branch is the infratrochlear nerve, which begins at the point where the anterior ethmoidal nerve enters its namesake foramen. The course of this branch is in an anterior direction, following the upper margin of the medial rectus. As described above, it is usual for a junction to be formed with a slender branch coming off the supratrochlear nerve, in the vicinity of the pulley formed by the superior oblique muscle. The course is then in a medial direction, providing innervation to the kin overlying the nasal bridge, the upper blepharal skin, the caruncle and the lacrimal sac [1].

4.3.2 Nerves Belonging to V2 (Maxillary Division)

The zygomaticofacial nerve arises from V2 and supplies cutaneous innervation to the skin covering the temporal and zygomatic bones. This nerve passes through the orbit. There is commonly confusion between the zygomaticofacial and the zygomatic nerve arising from the seventh cranial nerve. However, the latter supplies motor, rather than sensory, innervation [1].

The maxillary nerve has another, slender branch, the zygomaticotemporal nerve. The path it follows is along the orbital wall laterally within its own groove in the zygoma. It also forms a junction with one of the diminutive branches of the lacrimal nerve. Before passing into the temporal fossa, the nerve goes through its namesake foramen within the zygoma, after which its path is deep to the temporalis muscle and superficial to the temporal bone. At a point above the zygomatic arch, it penetrates the temporal fascia before forming several branches which provide sensation to the lateral frontal skin. After the zygomaticotemporal nerve penetrates into the fascia, its path is between the two fascial layers up to the point where it enters the eye socket at the lateral angle. There are connections between this nerve and the seventh cranial nerve, as well as the auriculotemporal nerve, which comes off V3.

At a point where V2 goes into the infraorbital canal, the infraorbital branch arises. This nerve provides sensation to the inferior blepharon, inferior lip, the maxillary infraorbital foramen and the vestibule of the nose [1].

4.3.3 Mandibular Division (V3) Branches

The auriculotemporal nerve is a branch of V3 which follows the general direction taken by the superficial temporal vessels, i.e. both the artery and vein. (The superficial temporal artery is the last branch given off by the external carotid artery). The auriculotemporal nerve provides cutaneous sensation to the side of the head.

The nerve providing cutaneous sensation to the inner cheek within the oral cavity is the buccal nerve, which also branches off V3. This nerve should not be confused with the buccal branch of the seventh cranial nerve, which is a motor nerve supplying the buccinator. The fifth cranial nerve also supplies cutaneous sensation to the rest of the facial region. The last branch given off by the inferior alveolar nerve, itself a branch of V3, is the mental nerve, which passes out of the mandible through the mental foramen and supplies sensory innervation to the chin region [1].

4.4 Nerves of the Cervical Plexus

From the cervical plexus, there arises the great auricular nerve. Its roots are C2 and C3. This nerve provides cutaneous sensation to the mastoid process, external ear and the region overlying the parotid gland [1].

The cervical plexus also gives rise to a spinal nerve, the great occipital nerve, which originates in the medial branch of the dorsal primary ramus of C2. The point of emergence is between the first and second cervical vertebrae, where the lesser occipital nerve also emerges. The suboccipital triangle is formed by the rectus capitis posterior major, the obliquus capitis inferior and the obliquus capitis superior. The nerve passes inferior to the obliquus capitis inferior, which forms the base of the suboccipital triangle and penetrates the trapezius. Its path is thereafter in a superior direction. This nerve supplies cutaneous sensation to the posterior scalp, the auricle and the region overlying the parotid gland [1].

The lesser occipital nerve is sometimes referred to by the term 'small occipital nerve'. Its root is C2 alone, and the point of emergence lies below the first cervical vertebra, as described above for the greater occipital nerve. This nerve supplies cutaneous sensation to the side of the head lying behind the ear [1].

References

1. Bengochea K. Superficial nerves of the face and scalp. Last reviewed: July 13, 2020. https://www.kenhub.com/en/library/anatomy/superficial-nerves-of-the-face-and-scalp. Accessed online at 2 Aug 2020.
2. Seneviratne SO, Patel BC. Facial nerve anatomy and clinical applications. StatPearls [Internet]. Treasure Island: StatPearls Publishing; 2020. Last Update: January 24, 2020. https://www.ncbi.nlm.nih.gov/books/NBK554569/. Accessed online at 2 Aug 2020.
3. Takezawa K, Townsend G, Ghabriel M. The facial nerve: anatomy and associated disorders for oral health professionals. Odontology. 2018;106(2):103–16.
4. Phillips CD, Bubash LA. The facial nerve: anatomy and common pathology. Semin Ultrasound CT MR. 2002;23(3):202–17.
5. Jenny AB, Saper CB. Organization of the facial nucleus and corticofacial projection in the monkey: a reconsideration of the upper motor neuron facial palsy. Neurology. 1987;37(6):930–9.
6. Kuypers HG. Corticobular connexions to the pons and lower brain-stem in man: an anatomical study. Brain. 1958;81(3):364–88.
7. Gothard KM. The amygdalo-motor pathways and the control of facial expressions. Front Neurosci. 2014;8:43.
8. Myckatyn TM, Mackinnon SE. A review of facial nerve anatomy. Semin Plast Surg. 2004;18(1):5–12.
9. Kochhar A, Larian B, Azizzadeh B. Facial nerve and parotid gland anatomy. Otolaryngol Clin N Am. 2016;49(2):273–84.

Facial Anatomy: Vessels

5

Aliye Filiz, Nihat Susaman, and Suela Sallavaci

5.1 Introduction

The anatomy of the vessels which supply the face and scalp is complex and is challenging to master in its entirety, on account of the large number of small calibre vessels supplying the skin and particular muscles. Nonetheless, this complexity should not obscure the basic pattern whereby all these small arteries arise from the major vessels lying deep within the neck. An example is the facial artery, which arises as the fourth branch off the external carotid artery in the region of the head. This vessel then divides multiple times to provide the many superficial vessels supplying the face. The most useful picture is of a network of vessels spreading outwards from a central point, the heart, with branches and interconnections at various points [1].

The common carotid artery is a branch of the aorta. It then divides, forming the internal and external carotid vessels. The internal carotid artery does not usually branch at all until it enters the skull, albeit this pattern does not apply in rare instances. It is the external carotid artery which gives rise to all the vessels supplying the face and scalp [1].

The middle portion of the face has an abundant vascular supply thanks to the musculocutaneous perforating arterial branches arising from the facial artery. Furthermore, the superficial temporal artery anastomoses at several points with the

A. Filiz (✉)
Department of Otorhinolaryngology, Gölbaşi State Hospital, Ankara, Türkiye

N. Susaman
Department of Otorhinolaryngology, Health Sciences University, Elazig Fethi Sekin City Hospital, Elazig, Türkiye

S. Sallavaci
Department of Otorhinolaryngology, University Hospital Centre "Mother Teresa,", Tirana, Albania

C. Cingi et al. (eds.), *Minor Interventions, Major Outcomes on the Face*, Comprehensive ENT, https://doi.org/10.1007/978-3-032-01305-7_5

musculocutaneous branches, as does the ophthalmic artery [2, 3]. Meanwhile, the facial mid-third is the location of a number of key arteries, notably the angular, superior and inferior labial and infraorbital arteries. The arterial supply to this region therefore benefits from a well-developed network of vessels and, frequently, a dual blood supply. The surgeon can take advantage of this situation by creating flaps in the midfacial region more aggressively than would be possible elsewhere, without the usual consequence of skin being sloughed away [4, 5].

The region below the chin is supplied by the perforating submental artery. Procedures aimed at rejuvenating the face may result in haemorrhage from the vessel [6]. The submental perforator artery begins at the midpoint between the mandibular angle and menton, according to Hwang et al [2, 6]

5.1.1 Arteries

The following vessels all branch off the external carotid artery:

Superior thyroid
Ascending pharyngeal
Lingual
Facial
Occipital
Posterior auricular
Maxillary
Superficial temporal [1].

5.1.2 Veins

The following vessels empty into the jugular veins (interior, external or anterior):

Facial
Supraorbital
Supratrochlear
Superficial temporal
Transverse facial
Angular
Posterior auricular [1].

5.2 Arteries

5.2.1 External Carotid Artery

The major portion of the facial vascular supply is via vessels arising from the external carotid artery, with the internal carotid artery providing the remaining portion. The facial artery originates from the external carotid artery at a point deep to the mandible and in proximity to the pharynx. The path of this vessel passes in front of the masseter, and it may be palpated at this location. It then passes superiorly and medially before becoming the angular artery, in the vicinity of the medial canthus. There are a number of vessels which branch off the facial artery, including the labial arteries (inferior and superior) and small arterial vessels supplying the nose [7].

5.2.2 Internal Carotid Artery

The blephara, superior and dorsal nasal regions, the inferior frontal region and the scalp receive arterial blood via branches of the internal carotid artery. The most significant branch of this vessel is the ophthalmic artery, which itself divides to form the supraorbital, supratrochlear, infratrochlear, dorsal nasal and external nasal arteries. This network of vessels may anastomose with the supply ultimately originating from the external carotid by forming connections with the angular artery [7].

5.2.3 Facial Artery

The lips and middle of the face receive their vascular supply from the facial artery. The final section of this artery forms an anastomotic connection with the ophthalmic artery. In this way, a key anastomotic linkage is provided with vessels originating from the internal carotid artery [7].

The occipital artery and the posterior auricular artery both arise from the external carotid artery before its final branches are formed. These two vessels provide blood to the posterior scalp and behind the ears. The superficial temporal artery and the internal maxillary artery are the last branches to arise from the external carotid artery [7].

The fourth vessel to branch from the external carotid is the facial artery. The point where it arises lies within the carotid triangle. The path followed by this artery is highly convoluted, a feature which allows it not to hinder the head when it moves, nor to get in the way of the expanding pharynx during deglutition. The artery can accommodate movement of the cheeks, lips and jaws, too. The origin is superior to the ascending pharyngeal artery. It then follows a diagonal path, passing superiorly deep to the stylohyoid muscle and the digastric muscle. The submandibular gland is indented where the facial artery passes behind it [1].

After passing the submandibular gland, the facial artery arches upwards around the body of the mandible, passing close to the inferior portion of the masseter. Its path is then in a superoanterior direction over the buccal region until it gets to the stomal angle, where it assumes a path heading superiorly parallel to the external nose. The vessel continues as the angular artery, ending in the vicinity of the medial canthus [1].

The facial artery arises from the external carotid artery. The superficial structures of the face receive their vascular supply from this vessel. The point where the facial artery originates is within the carotid triangle, a region delineated by three muscles:

the upper belly of the omohyoid, sternocleidomastoid and posterior belly of the digastric. The origin lies under the platysma muscle, but its path is superficial shortly after it begins. By following a convoluted path, the artery can accommodate movements, e.g. chewing, which tend to stretch the vessel. Its path takes it under the posterior belly of the digastric muscle and the stylohyoid muscle, before passing behind the submandibular gland [8, 9]. Its path then takes it in a superior, curving direction across the mandibular body and along the edge of the masseter on its anterior and inferior aspect. Where the artery traverses the mandible, it is possible to palpate it and feel it pulsating. Its path is then upwards, angled obliquely as it crosses the buccal region before passing to the angle of the mouth. The artery then passes superiorly just lateral to the external nose, and its final section, by now termed the angular artery, terminates at the medial commissure of the eye [10].

The facial artery branches repeatedly, providing blood to multiple structures. The vessel passes superior to the buccinator and levator anguli oris, giving off branches that supply these muscles. The path of the facial artery can take it either over or through the body of the levator labii superioris [11]. A number of other muscles also receive their vascular supply from the facial artery, in particular the levator veli palatini, masseter, mentalis, mylohyoid, nasalis, palatoglossus, palatopharyngeus, platysma, procerus, risorius, styloglossus plus the transverse portion of the nasalis. Other structures which are supplied by the facial artery include the tonsils within the palate, the velum, the pterygoid and digastric muscles and the submandibular gland [9].

The cervical branch of the facial artery itself branches four times prior to reaching the face, forming the ascending palatine, tonsillar, submental and glandular arteries. There are also four divisions of this vessel within the facial region, giving rise to the inferior labial, superior labial and lateral nasal arteries. This last supplies the nasalis muscle. The final section (branch) is the angular artery [12].

5.2.4 Procedures Involving the Facial Artery

Facial reconstruction often needs to make use of the facial artery and its branches, which are employed to provide vascularisation to a number of different types of flap, such as local, regional or random flaps [13]. Some flaps that are frequently formed and rely on supply from the facial artery are submental, platysma muscle, nasolabial, buccinator myomucosal or musculomucosal flaps [7]. Reconstruction of the face utilising a flap of this kind may be required if a neoplasm has been excised from the head and neck region. The rich supply the facial artery can provide is important to the survival of flaps formed on the head and neck [9].

5.2.5 Complications Associated with the Facial Artery

There are a number of complications arising from surgery to the face that are linked to the facial arterial configuration. Avoiding damage to the facial artery is a key consideration. Accordingly, surgeons should avoid retracting more than is absolutely necessary. When the submandibular gland requires excision, there is a risk of bleeding from the facial artery [14]. Repair to a fractured mandible, when approached externally, may also call for the facial artery to be ligated, and, where ligation is performed, the surgeon should document it unambiguously in the surgical notes so that clinicians who carry out subsequent procedures are aware of it. Where there is haemorrhage from this vessel, it can be controlled by the application of pressure at the mandibular angle, which then allows time to identify where the vessel was ruptured and thus to staunch the flow [9].

Furthermore, when surgical procedures are undertaken close to the facial artery, the operating surgeon needs awareness of the nerves, especially the twelfth cranial nerve, that pass close to the vessel. The path of the nerves should be identified at an early stage so as to avoid inadvertent injury complicating the procedure [9].

5.2.6 Clinical Significance

It is possible to palpate the pulsatile motion of the facial artery as it passes over the mandibular bone at the masseteric anteroinferior angle, since the artery is superficial at this point [9].

There are records in existence showing that, even where the internal carotid artery is occluded, the angular artery (which represents the last stage of the facial artery) continues to pulsate powerfully in around 70% of patients [15]. The angular artery provides anastomotic linkage to the medial branches of the infraorbital artery, which is itself ultimately supplied via the external carotid artery. Another vessel to which the angular artery is anastomotically joined is the ophthalmic artery, via its dorsal nasal branch and supratrochlear branch [15]. These anastomotic linkages are, however, of restricted assistance in diagnosis given that 10% of individuals with chronic high blood pressure have these linkages after the age of 55 years [9, 15].

The formation of atheroma leading to narrowing of the common carotid artery puts individuals at risk of forming vascular emboli and thus leading to ischaemic events. Muscular weakness affecting the superficial muscles of the face is potentially due to the facial artery being constricted. Emboli may pass from the common carotid and eventually lodge in one of the distal vessels originating from the facial artery, but this is not a common consequence of atheromatous carotid arteriosclerosis [9].

5.2.7 Angular Artery

In effect, the angular artery is the final stage of the facial artery. The latter is the fourth vessel to branch off the external carotid artery. The angular artery gives off vessels which are in close attachment to the levator (quadratus) labii superioris at its angular head. The angular vein follows the same path as the angular artery [1].

The angular artery gives off narrow calibre vessels which form an anastomotic linkage with the infraorbital artery. These vessels are in the buccal region. The last stage of the artery provides blood to the orbicularis oris and the lacrimal sac before its terminal portions form an anastomotic linkage with a branch of the ophthalmic artery, the nasal artery. The ophthalmic artery itself is the fourth vessel to come off the external carotid artery [1].

5.2.8 Inferior Labial Artery

The inferior lip receives its vascular supply via the inferior labial branch of the facial artery. The origin of this vessel is in the vicinity of the stomal angle. Its path is superoanterior deep to the depressor anguli oris muscle (i.e. the triangularis). Having passed into and out of the orbicularis oris, it then follows a winding path taking it inferior to the inferior margin of the lower lip. It lies deep to the mucosa and the orbicularis oris. There is an anastomotic link to a branch of the inferior alveolar artery, the mental artery. The inferior labial artery provides blood to the muscles acting on the inferior lip and the lip mucosa [1].

5.2.9 Superior Labial Artery

The facial artery also gives off a branching vessel which provides vascular supply to the superior lip, septum and alae of the nose, the superior labial artery. The superior labial artery both is of a larger calibre and has a more winding course than the inferior labial artery. Its path resembles that of the inferior labial artery. It is deep to the mucosal membrane and superficial to the orbicularis oris muscle, continuing superior to the superior margin of the upper lip. In this case, the vessel provides blood not only to the upper lip, but additionally gives off vessels which supply nasal structures. The septal branch of the superior labial artery has a territory extending right up to the tip of the nose, as well as the externally located nasal alae [1].

5.2.10 Branches of the Maxillary Artery

The maxillary artery is the seventh vessel to branch from the external carotid artery. It gives rise, in turn, to the infraorbital artery. Furthermore, the orbital arteries and the anterior superior alveolar artery also originate from the maxillary artery. The orbital arteries provide blood to the rectus inferior and inferior oblique muscles. The lacrimal sac is also supplied by these vessels. The superior incisors and canines, plus the mucosal lining of the maxillary sinus, are supplied via the anterior superior alveolar artery. The path of this vessel is downwards, passing through the anterior alveolar canal [1].

At the point where the external carotid artery branches to form the superficial temporal artery, another deeply located artery arises—the internal maxillary artery.

This vessel rarely affects surgical procedures on the superficial structures of the face. The internal maxillary artery gives off the infraorbital and inferior alveolar arteries. The latter has a course which passes via the mental foramen, becoming the mental artery, which supplies the chin region [7].

5.2.11 Buccal Artery

The buccinator muscle and the buccal region generally receive its vascular supply via the buccal artery. This vessel divides off from the second portion of the maxillary artery and is a vessel of small calibre. The maxillary artery's origin is described above.

5.2.12 Inferior Alveolar Artery

The maxillary artery has five principal branches, one of which is the inferior alveolar branch. This vessel provides blood to the mandibular dental alveoli. The inferior alveolar artery also branches three times: once forming the incisor artery, which supplies the dental incisors, once more to form the mental artery, with a path going through the mental foramen, and finally the mylohyoid artery immediately prior to the inferior alveolar artery's entry into the mandibular foramen. This last vessel has a path within its namesake sulcus and provides vascular supply to the mylohyoid muscle [1].

5.2.13 Submental Artery

At a point immediately before it enters the submandibular gland, the facial artery gives rise to its largest branch within the neck region, the submental artery. Its path takes it over the mylohyoid, underneath the mandible and deep to the digastric muscle. This vessel provides blood to the muscles of the submental region.

The frontal skin, scalp, frontal sinus, superior blephara, diploe and levator palpebrae superioris are all supplied by the supraorbital artery. This vessel originates from the ophthalmic artery.

The ophthalmic artery's final branch forms the supratrochlear branch, the terminal branches of which form anastomotic linkages with the supraorbital artery [1].

5.2.14 Other Branches of the External Carotid Artery

5.2.14.1 Posterior Auricular Artery

The posterior auricular artery, a vessel of small calibre, is the sixth vessel to divide off from the external carotid artery. Its origin can be located by identifying the stylohyoid muscle and the digastric muscle, which are inferior to its origin. The usual origin lies opposite the tapering point of the styloid process. Its path takes it upwards, with the parotid gland superficial to it and in the line of the styloid process. It then continues with the mastoid process and the cartilaginous pinna on either side. This vessel then provides blood to the scalp posterior to the auricle, as well as the auricle itself [1].

5.2.14.2 Occipital Artery

The fifth vessel to arise from the external carotid artery is the occipital branch. It typically originates opposite the point where the facial artery divides off. Its path then takes it deep to the posterior belly of the digastric muscle, after which it reaches the occipital region. This artery provides blood to the sternocleidomastoid muscle, the scalp at the back and several muscles lying deep within the neck or back [1].

5.2.14.3 Superficial Temporal Artery

The origin of the superficial temporal artery is within the parotid gland. The facial nerve branches lie deep to it. Its path takes it upwards to a point 2 cm below the zygoma, where it branches to form the horizontal transverse facial artery, which anastomoses with the facial artery. The superficial temporal artery moves in a superior direction, getting closer to the surface. At a point behind the temporomandibular joint and in front of the auricle, it can be palpated [7].

The terminal branches of the vessel form the parietal and frontal arteries, providing a vascular supply to the scalp region. Before these final branches, it also supplies the side of the face, temporal and frontal skin and the scalp. There are a number of small calibre vessels, the middle temporal and zygomaticotemporal branches, which provide blood to a number of structures found in the middle of the face [7].

The last time the external carotid artery branches is to form the superficial temporal artery. This is the eighth division of the vessel. This large calibre vessel (at least within the head and neck) is useful in anaesthetic practice as its pulsations may be easily palpated in the temporal region, beginning superior to the zygomatic arch and the level of the tragus. The superficial temporal artery gives rise to the transverse facial artery, which provides blood to the parotid gland and its duct, in addition to the masseteric muscle [1].

The superficial temporal artery, at a point superior to the zygomatic arch, gives rise to the middle temporal artery, which penetrates the fascia of the temples and supplies the temporalis muscle. There are also anastomotic linkages to branches arising from the internal maxillary artery, the deep temporal arteries. Sometimes, the zygomatico-orbital artery arises from the middle temporal artery; at other times, it branches off the superficial temporal artery. The zygomatico-orbital artery follows a path that passes along the zygomatic arch on its superior margin, sandwiched between the temporal fascial layers. The orbicularis oculi receives its supply from this artery, which forms anastomotic linkages to branches of the ophthalmic artery, the lacrimal and palpebral [1].

5.3 Facial Veins

The veins draining the facial region generally reflect the pattern of the arteries in their layout, with the difference that the veins are typically less winding and tend towards straightness. The path of the facial vein is alongside its namesake artery, and it empties into the internal jugular vein. It carries blood away from the mid-face. The veins within the so-called dangerous triangle (i.e. the medial facial region) carry blood away from the superior lip and around the nose. This is the region in which the facial vein in some patients is in direct communication with the cavernous sinus through the intervening ophthalmic vein or empties into the cavernous sinus having first entered the pterygoid plexus. The sides of the face and scalp have drainage provided by the superficial temporal vein and the retromandibular vein. Both these vessels drain into the external jugular vein [7].

5.3.1 Facial Vein

The facial vein is a vein of considerable size, the path of which, unlike that of the namesake artery, is relatively straight. Its path commences from a point lateral to the nose. The facial artery lies anterior to it. The external palatine vein is a tributary to the facial vein, which itself drains into the retromandibular vein, after which the common facial vein is formed. Drainage of the inferior lip and the superior lip is via the inferior labial and superior labial veins, respectively. The deep facial vein is connected to the anterior facial vein. The former is a relatively large calibre vessel which arises from the pterygoid venous plexus [1].

5.3.2 Supraorbital Vein

The origin of the supraorbital vein is in the frontal region. Blood from the frontal region, supercilium and superior blepharon drains into this vessel [1], which connects to the superficial temporal vein via its frontal branch. The path is in an inferior direction, above the frontalis muscle. The usual arrangement is that the supraorbital and frontal veins combine in the vicinity of the medial angle of the orbit, thereafter continuing as the angular vein.

5.3.3 Supratrochlear Vein

An alternative term for the supratrochlear vein is the frontal vein. This vessel arises out of a venous plexus before joining with tributaries of the superficial temporal vein. These vessels combine in their entirety to produce one trunk vein, located in the vicinity of the midline, generally in parallel with the contralateral trunk vessel. The nasal arch is a vessel which runs transversely, connecting the two trunks. It is in the vicinity of the nasal root. There are generally also a few small veins which join the nasal arch from the nose. A less common anatomical arrangement is where the left and right supratrochlear vessels form a joint trunk. In this case, the paired angular veins are connected at the root of the nose [1].

5.3.4 Superficial Temporal Vein

A venous plexus on the side of the skull is where the superficial temporal vein starts. To this plexus, the supraorbital and frontal veins are also connected. The superficial temporal vein is joined by the occipital and auricular veins, and it comes together with the contralateral namesake vessel. In the vicinity of the zygomatic arch, there are several veins which unite into a trunk vessel. This trunk vessel and the middle temporal vein join together and pass out from the temporalis muscle. The path of the venous trunk is into the parotid gland. Here, the internal maxillary vein drains into the trunk, which continues as the posterior facial vein [1].

5.3.5 Transverse Facial Vein

The origin of the transverse facial vein is a venous plexus located laterally on the skull, to which a number of vessels contribute, namely the supraorbital, posterior auricular, occipital, frontal and opposite transverse facial veins. To the plexus, there are also contributions from the parietal and frontal veins. Above the arch of the zygoma, these vessels all combine as a single trunk, into which the middle temporal vein also drains, having passed out of the temporalis muscle. It then crosses over the zygomatic arch at the posterior end and penetrates the parotid gland, where it joins with the internal maxillary vein before continuing as the posterior facial vein, a vessel of substantial calibre [1].

5.3.6 Angular Vein

The frontal vein and the supraorbital vein combine in the vicinity of the eye, giving rise to the angular vein. This vessel is relatively slender. Its path is downwards from the origin on the side of the nasal root up to the eye socket. Thereafter, it continues as the anterior facial vein. The nasal veins are tributaries to this vessel. The nasal veins pass by the nasal alae before joining with the superior ophthalmic vein and the nasofrontal vein. This venous system provides an alternative route for drainage from the cavernous sinus and the anterior facial vein [1].

5.3.7 Posterior Auricular Vein

The origin of the posterior auricular vein is found on the lateral skull. It is connected to the occipital vein and the superficial temporal vein through a venous plexus. The vein proceeds inferiorly behind the auricle, forming a communication with the posterior portion of the posterior facial vein. Thereafter, the external jugular vein commences. There is also drainage from a number of vessels leading from the external ear, as well as the stylomastoid vein.

References

1. Shahid S. Superficial arteries and veins of the face and scalp. Last reviewed: June 25, 2020 https://www.kenhub.com/en/library/anatomy/superficial-arteries-and-veins-of-the-face-and-scalp. Accessed online at 2 Aug 2020.
2. de la Torre JI. Facelift anatomy. In: Narayan D (Ed). Medscape. Updated: Oct 30, 2013. https://emedicine.medscape.com/article/1294682-overview#a7. Accessed online at Aug 2, 2020.
3. Blanco-Dávila F, Arrendondo G, De La Garza O, Montemayor R, Gregori OU, Vásconez HC. Anatomical study of the blood supply to the skin in rhytidectomy. Aesth Plast Surg. 1995;19(2):175–81.
4. Whetzel TP, Mathes SJ. Arterial anatomy of the face: an analysis of vascular territories and perforating cutaneous vessels. Plast Reconstr Surg. 1992;89(4):591–603. discussion 604-5
5. Gruber RP, Levine SM, Levine JP. Facial topography: clinical anatomy of the face. Plast Reconstr Surg. 2013;132(1):249.
6. Hwang K, Han JY, Chung RS, Chung IH. Submental perforating artery: a culprit of bleeding during facelift. J Craniofac Surg. 2005 Jan;16(1):3–5.
7. Orengo I. Facial anatomy in cutaneous surgery. In: Elston DM (Ed). Medscape. Updated: Jul 21, 2015. https://emedicine.medscape.com/article/1127307-overview#a9. Accessed online at Aug 2, 2020.
8. Meegalla N, Sood G, Nessel TA, Downs BW. Anatomy, head and neck, facial arteries. StatPearls (Internet). Treasure Island: StatPearls Publishing; 2020 Jan-. Last Update: April 13, 2020. https://www.ncbi.nlm.nih.gov/books/NBK536932/. Accessed online at 2 Aug 2020.
9. Vadgaonkar R, Rai R, Prabhu LV, Bv M, Samapriya N. Variant facial artery in the submandibular region. J Craniofac Surg. 2012;23(4):e355–7. (PubMed)
10. Niranjan NS. An anatomical study of the facial artery. Ann Plast Surg. 1988;21(1):14–22. (PubMed)
11. Lee JG, Yang HM, Choi YJ, Favero V, Kim YS, Hu KS, Kim HJ. Facial arterial depth and relationship with the facial musculature layer. Plast Reconstr Surg. 2015;135(2):437–44. PubMed.
12. Lee HJ, Won SY, Jehoon O, Hu KS, Mun SY, Yang HM, Kim HJ. The facial artery: a comprehensive anatomical review. Clin Anat. 2018 Jan;31(1):99–108.
13. Mashrah MA, Zhou SH, Abdelrehem A, Ma C, Xu L, He Y, Zhang CP. Oropharyngeal reconstruction with a pedicled submandibular gland flap. Br J Oral Maxillofac Surg. 2016 May;54(4):388–93.
14. Pedroletti F, Johnson BS, McCain JP. Endoscopic techniques in oral and maxillofacial surgery. Oral Maxillofac Surg Clin North Am. 2010 Feb;22(1):169–82.
15. Fisher CM. Facial pulses in internal carotid artery occlusion. Neurology. 1970 May;20(5):476–8.

6 Effects of Aging on the Face

Ela Akbulut Harbalioglu, Nuray Bayar Muluk, and Jeffrey C. Bedrosian

6.1 Introduction

The processes by which the face ages are dynamic and affect both the soft tissues and the underlying facial skeleton. The loss of facial soft tissue volume that accompanies aging is well understood. The epidermis tends to become thinner, with lower amounts of dermal collagen, which explains why the elastic recoil of the skin lessens. Adipose tissue is also lost from the face. Together with gravitational forces and the effects of muscular contraction, all these effects produce wrinkled skin and the appearance of dynamic lines [1].

Alterations to the facial skeleton due to aging have also been demonstrated. Numerous studies have jointly concluded that the way the orbit and middle region of the face age results from contracting structures and an alteration in morphology. The resulting loss of bony tissue and the projecting features are further elements that make the face appear old [1].

E. A. Harbalioglu
Department of Otorhinolaryngology, Iskenderun State Hospital, İskenderun, Hatay, Turkey

N. Bayar Muluk (✉)
Faculty of Medicine, Department of Otorhinolaryngology, Kırıkkale University, Kırıkkale, Türkiye

J. C. Bedrosian
Rhinology and Skull Base Surgery, Specialty Physician Associates, St. Luke's Medical Center, Bethlehem, PA, USA

C. Cingi et al. (eds.), *Minor Interventions, Major Outcomes on the Face*, Comprehensive ENT, https://doi.org/10.1007/978-3-032-01305-7_6

6.2 Age-Related Skin Alterations

In many cases, the skin alterations we associate with aging stem from harmful exposure to sunlight. These changes include altered pigment levels, a sallow appearance, and deep wrinkles. Accordingly, parts of the skin that see the most sun are those in which an aged appearance most frequently appears. Such areas are the face and neck, the top of the chest, hands, and forearms. The observation that the skin of those working indoors differed in appearance from those engaged in farming or sailing was made at least as far back as the 1800s [2]. It was observed that those whose occupations kept them outside had skin that was browner and thicker where it faced the sun and that such altered appearances correlated with a higher incidence of skin tumors [2, 3].

6.2.1 Alterations Seen at Microscopy and the Mechanisms Involved

There are thus two basic processes by which aging occurs: chronological aging and photoaging. These processes produce different histological appearances. Chronological aging leads to atrophy of the epidermis, with a less undulating junction between the epidermis and underlying dermis and fewer rete pegs [4]. The dermal layer is less thick than usual, and fibroblasts are less numerous. Collagen content is reduced [5]. Photoaging may make the epidermis thicker or lead to a very noticeable atrophic appearance. However, the critical microscopical feature is that elastin accumulates immediately underneath the junction of the epidermis and dermis. This change is referred to as solar elastosis [6]. There is a noticeable disorganization of dermal collagen, constituting 90% of all proteins in the skin [7].

Collagen is a critical structural component in the skin of humans. Its presence largely accounts for the strength of skin. Fibroblasts within the dermis synthesize procollagen, the precursor to collagen. Two key molecules function to regulate the synthesis of collagen, namely TGF-β (transforming growth factor beta) and AP-1 (activator protein-1) [3]. The former (TGF-β) is classed as a cytokine that stimulates collagen synthesis [8]. By contrast, AP-1 prevents the synthesis of collagen and increases collagen degradation. It is a transcription factor [9]. The dermal collagen is constantly remodeled through new synthesis and degradation, primarily controlled by TGF-β and AP-1. TGF-β stimulates collagen synthesis, whereas AP-1 orchestrates collagen degradation by increasing the expression of matrix metalloproteinases (MMPs), which catalyze collagenous breakdown [3].

When sunlight strikes particular molecules within the skin, ultraviolet radiation from sunlight can give rise to reactive oxygen species (ROS), which may cause oxidative injury to parts of the cell, such as lipids within intracellular compartmental membranes, the mitochondria, or the DNA. ROS also influences particular biochemical pathways. A study that examined skin from the buttock region in humans found that a specific ROS, H_20_2, was raised in under 15 min following skin exposure to ultraviolet A and B at a level twice the MED. (The MED is the minimal erythema dose, i.e., the level at which redness of the skin first appears) [10]. AP-1 levels also rise in the same interval, staying high for 24 h or more after the skin has been exposed to UVA/UVB. AP-1 catalyzes the degradation of dermal collagen. Confirming this action, the MMPs are significantly overexpressed with 1 day of sunlight exposure [11]. One episode of exposure to ultraviolet light is sufficient to reduce the dermal collagen content in less than 1 day [12].

In summary, therefore, collagen starts being degraded following exposure to ultraviolet light due to the formation of ROS, the raised expression of AP-1, and the more remarkable synthesis of MMPs. Furthermore, this exposure also inhibits the synthesis of one of the TGF-β signaling molecules, i.e., TGF-β2. As described above, these signaling molecules promote collagen synthesis. The fall in the level of TGF-β thus means synthesis is inhibited. The fact that procollagen is not being manufactured at the usual level has been shown experimentally [13]. Photoaging, therefore, in essence, consists of an imbalance in collagenous remodeling, favoring degradation. Whenever the skin is exposed to ultraviolet light, collagen is degraded, and the subsequent remodeling results in initially imperceptible "solar scarring." Over time, as the exposure accumulates in an individual's life, this scarring process becomes perceptible in skin wrinkles [14].

6.2.2 The Mechanism of Skin Aging

Overall, photoaging essentially represents an accelerated and amplified form of normal chronological aging [15]. Skin showing aging features has a higher level of AP-1 when compared with skin from younger individuals [16]. Furthermore, MMPs are more active in skin samples showing aging and have a four times greater degree of collagenous degradation than in skin from younger individuals [15]. There is also a lower level of manufacture of procollagen types I and III in aged skin [5]. The balance of collagen remodeling tips in favor of degradation rather than manufacture, and accordingly, the amount of dermal collagen in aging skin is reduced compared to young skin. The molecular alterations seen in aged skin are similar to those observed where photoaging has occurred, which reinforces the hypothesis that photoaging exaggerates the mechanisms involved in chronological aging [3].

The evidence suggests a multifactorial etiology for chronological aging. The formation of ROS is likely to be of significant significance in the process. One theory explaining aging, the free radical hypothesis, proposes that aging occurs as an oxidative injury due to ROS accrues repeatedly over an individual's lifetime. These ROS are generated by aerobic metabolism [17]. Higher levels of ROS are found in aged skin, and ROS plays a significant role in the molecular mechanisms that underlie collagenous degradation, as described above. The free radical hypothesis satisfactorily accounts for the molecular alterations that occur as part of chronological aging [3].

6.3 Structural Alteration in the Aging of the Face

How the face ages indicates effects that accumulate over time and interact dynamically, altering the skin, soft tissues, and deeper anatomical facial structures. The alterations in the skin's texture and the decreased facial volume act in synergy to produce an aged appearance. In many cases, the age-related changes seen in the face can be attributed to gravity, increasingly resorbed bony structures, less elastic recoil in the tissues, and changes in the pattern of fullness in the face [18].

It is often helpful to divide the face into horizontal thirds when evaluating how aging has altered facial morphology. In this scheme, the superior facial third consists of the forehead and eyebrows, the mid-third is the middle of the face and nasal region, and the inferior third comprises the mental area, jaws, and neck. The middle of the face is especially crucial in how beautiful faces are judged since such judgments center on the central facial triangle, formed by the eyes, nose, lips, and cheekbones. In aesthetic surgery, the mid-face needs to be evaluated three-dimensionally, not simply from one viewpoint. In procedures aiming to rejuvenate the face, the main aim is to recreate the topographic configuration of a younger person in this area, as viewed in three dimensions [18].

6.3.1 Skeletal Structure

As the craniofacial bones age, they undergo osseous atrophy, and the balance between osteogenesis and resorption alters [19]. The height of the face reduces to a noticeable extent, primarily due to maxillary and mandibular alterations. Somewhat less apparent is a tendency for the face to become broader and more profound. While the dimensions of the orbit increase, the maxillary sizes decrease. These changes result in the malar fat pad moving downwards, resulting in a more prominent nasolabial crease [20]. As the maxilla reduces in mass, the tissues of the superior lip become less well-supported; thus, the skin around the mouth may appear wrinkled. Mandibular resorption around the alveolar ridge is especially noticeable in edentulous individuals. The chin profile and the degree to which it projects are also altered through the effects of aging. The bumps on the lower jaw become coarser where the muscles used for chewing are inserted, such as at the mandible's angle and the zygomatic process's lower margin. In contrast, the rest of the bone becomes smoother overall [18].

6.3.2 Subcutaneous Fat Distribution

Typically, the face of a younger person has fat spread widely around the facial area, both in more profound and more superficial areas, and this results in the facial structures possessing a smoothly rounded appearance in three dimensions. The topography is dominated by curving designs in two or three dimensions [21, 22]. When seen from the front, the jaw forms a smoothly turning line, the temporal regions are convex, and several arcs make up the labial outline. When viewed from the side, the features that most mark a face as young-looking are as follows: The line connecting the inferior eyelid to the cheek forms an uninterrupted reverse (ogee) curve; the line of the jaw curves toward the mentum from the lateral mandibular region; and the frontal area also arches smoothly [23].

As the face ages, particular regions become less full, such as around the eyes, frontally, around the cheeks, temples, lower jaw, chin, mid-forehead, and around the mouth, while in other regions, fat continues to be present, or even increases, such as under the chin, in the lateral nasolabial creases and the labiodental fold, the jowls, the area under the eyes, and the malar fat pad [24, 25]. A study based on MRI (magnetic resonance imaging) has claimed that fat gain in the upper facial third compared to the middle third was significantly higher in older patients when contrasted with younger individuals [25]. The drawback to this conclusion is that patients undergoing MRI must lie prone, and thus, the force of gravity acts in a different direction from the regular position patients adopt, i.e., upright. It can be anticipated that the fullest area within the cheek will be lower in a standing position than that shown on MRI. It would be helpful if future studies using MRI undertake sequential scans of the same individuals at different points in their lives, allowing a deeper appreciation of exactly how the aging of the face results in the redistribution of facial fat [18].

6.3.3 Morphological Changes

6.3.3.1 Upper Third (Forehead and Brows)

With advancing age, there is a loss of subcutaneous tissue in various parts of the face, which makes these areas appear hollow and the underlying hard tissue anatomy more prominent. Such sites include the frontal region, brow, temporal region, and superior blephara. The craniofacial skeletal structures are accentuated, as are the corrugator and procerus muscles attached to the brow. The path passed through the temples by blood vessels becomes ever more convoluted [24]. The brow appears to droop, an impression produced by a combination of laxity in the temples, which no longer hold up the lateral aspects, and loss of volume in the superior blephara [24]. Thus, the eyebrows appear to rest on the upper rim of the eye socket or even below it [26]. The orbital septum becomes less able to retain the intraorbital fat as the individual ages, which may result in herniation of the fat, making the eye socket outline more prominent [18].

6.3.3.2 Middle Facial Third

The middle facial third undergoes a reduction in subcutaneous soft tissue due to aging, resulting in the malar prominence appearing less full and the cheeks appearing steadily more hollow. Thus, the face has a less healthy appearance. The loss of subcutaneous fat and soft tissue within the eye socket means that the tension in the orbicularis oculi muscle is transferred to the covering skin, which appears as "crow's feet" wrinkles. With advancing age, there is increasing prominence of the lower margin of the same muscle, and this is one component behind the formation of a malar crescent overlying the zygoma in a lateral direction, along with the formation of a nasojugal fold in a medial direction. The fat pads lying inferior to the orbit in younger individuals are not visible due to the fullness below the orbit. However, as this diminishes with age, bags appear under the eyes, and the tear-trough deformity becomes apparent. This last one runs from the side of the nose near the medial canthus in an infero-oblique direction toward the mid-cheek. The end is inferior to the blepharal midpoint. In addition, in younger individuals, there is a very slight transverse depression just under the eyelashes. This depression becomes deeper as the individual ages and runs toward the lower margin of the orbit [18].

As subcutaneous tissue is lost in the face, the fat within the orbit tends to be displaced inferiorly due to the laxity of the orbital septum. The eye socket looks deeper and broader, and the inferior blepharon develops a double convex deformity [27]. The orbicularis oris muscle lies closer to the surface due to loss of infraorbital fullness, and the skin takes on a darker hue underneath the eyes, making the aged individual appear tired. Another reason for this discoloration to occur is when melanin is deposited in the dermis [28]. The malar adipose droops downwards, accentuating the nasolabial fold and adding to the already hollow appearance of the cheeks caused by loss of fullness in the malar region [18].

6.3.3.3 Lower Facial Third (Chin, Jawline, and Neck)

As the skin ages, it loses its tension, and, together with the loss of adipose in the cheeks and around the mouth, the effect is for the skin to be loose, overlying the lower facial third. This makes the outline of the jawless distinct. The masseteric ligament becomes less able to support the facial adipose, which now drops toward the border of the mandible. Jowls now appear [29]. The inferior margin of the mandible moves superiorly due to bony resorption, and this reveals the structures lying under the chin, such as the submandibular gland. The mandible projects less markedly in a lateral direction, and, in aging individuals, there is a loss of the mandibular angle, so that the buccal region and neck appear connected. The chin loses volume laterally and inferiorly, so that the middle of the chin appears to jut out more. Loss of bone from the sides of the chin means the overlying soft tissues droop, and this may give the impression that the chin is actually getting wider, as seen from the front [18].

References

1. Kahn DM, Shaw RB. Overview of current thoughts on facial volume and aging. Facial Plast Surg. 2010;26(5):350–5. https://doi.org/10.1055/s-0030-1265024. Epub 2010 Sep 17
2. Urbach F, Forbes PD, Davies RE, Berger D. Cutaneous photobiology: past, present and future. J Invest Dermatol. 1976;67(1):209–24.
3. Helfrich YR, Sachs DL, Voorhees JJ. Overview of skin aging and Photoaging. Dermatol Nurs. 2008;20(3):177–83.
4. Kurban RS, Bhawan J. Histologic changes in skin associated with aging. J Dermatol Surg Oncol. 1990;16(10):908–14.

5. Varani J, Warner RL, Gharaee-Kermani M, Phan SH, Kang S, Chung JH, et al. Vitamin a antagonizes decreased cell growth and elevated collagen-degrading matrix metalloproteinases and stimulates collagen accumulation in naturally aged human skin. J Invest Dermatol. 2000;114(3):480–6.
6. Lavker RM. Cutaneous aging: chronologic versus photoaging. In: Gilchrest B, editor. Photodamage, vol. 1. Cambridge: Blackwell; 1995. p. 123–35.
7. Bernstein EF, Chen YQ, Kopp JB, Fisher L, Brown DB, Hahn PJ, et al. Long-term sun exposure alters the collagen of the papillary dermis. Comparison of sun-protected and photoaged skin by northern analysis, immunohistochemical staining, and confocal laser scanning microscopy. J Am Acad Dermatol. 1996;34(2 Pt 1):209–18.
8. Massague J. TGF-beta signal transduction. Annu Rev Biochem. 1998;67:753–91.
9. Kang S, Fisher GJ, Voorhees JJ. Photoaging and topical tretin oin: therapy, pathogenesis, and prevention. Arch Dermatol. 1997;133(10):1280–4.
10. Kang S, Chung JH, Lee JH, Fisher GJ, Wan YS, Duell EA, et al. Topical N-acetyl cysteine and genistein prevent ultraviolet-light-induced signaling that leads to photoaging in human skin in vivo. J Invest Dermatol. 2003;120(5):835–41.
11. Fisher GJ, Datta SC, Talwar HS, Wang ZQ, Varani J, Kang S, et al. Molecular basis of sun-induced premature skin ageing and retinoid antagonism. Nature. 1996;379(6563):335–9.
12. Fisher GJ, Wang ZQ, Datta SC, Varani J, Kang S, Voorhees JJ. Pathophysiology of premature skin aging induced by ultraviolet light. N Engl J Med. 1997;337(20):1419–28.
13. Quan T, He T, Kang S, Voorhees JJ, Fisher GJ. Ultraviolet irradiation alters transforming growth factor beta/smad pathway in human skin in vivo. J Invest Dermatol. 2002;119(2):499–506.
14. Kang S, Fisher GJ, Voorhees JJ. Photoaging: pathogenesis, prevention, and treatment. Clin Geriatr Med. 2001;17(4):643–59.
15. Fisher GJ, Kang S, Varani J, Bata-Csorgo Z, Wan Y, Datta S, et al. Mechanisms of photoaging and chronological skin aging. Arch Dermatol. 2002;138(11):1462–70.
16. Chung JH, Kang S, Varani J, Lin J, Fisher GJ, Voorhees JJ. Decreased extracellular-signal-regulated kinase and increased stress-activated MAP kinase activities in aged human skin in vivo. J Invest Dermatol. 2000;115(2):177–82.
17. Hensley K, Floyd RA. Reactive oxygen species and protein oxidation in aging: a look back, a look ahead. Arch Biochem Biophys. 2002;397(2):377–83.
18. Coleman SR, Grover R. The anatomy of the aging face: volume loss and changes in 3-dimensional topography. Aesthet Surg J. 2006;26(1_Supplement):S4–9. https://doi.org/10.1016/j.asj.2005.09.012.
19. Bartlett SP, Grossman R, Whitaker LA. Age-related changes of thecraniofacial skeleton: an anthropomorphic and histologic analysis. Plast Reconstr Surg. 1992;90:592–00.
20. Pessa JE, Zadoo VP, Yuan C, Ayedelotte JD, Cuellar FJ, Cochran CS, et al. Concertina effect and facial aging: nonlinear aspects of youth-fulness and skeletal remodeling and why perhaps infants have jowls. Plast Reconstr Surg. 1999;103:635–44.
21. Hamra ST. The role of orbital fat preservation in facial aestheticsurgery. Clin Plast Surg. 1996;23:17–28.
22. Donofrio LM. Fat distribution: a morphologic study of the aging face. Dermatologic Surg. 2000;26:1107–12.
23. Little JW. Volumetric perceptions in midfacial aging with altered pri-orities for rejuvenation. Plast Reconstr Surg. 2000;105:252–66.
24. Coleman SR. Structural fat grafting. St. Louis: Quality Medical Publishing; 2004.
25. Gosain AK, Klein MH, Sudhakar PV, Prost RW. A volumetric analysisof soft-tissue changes in the aging midface using high-resolution MRI: implications for facial rejuvenation. Plast Reconstr Surg. 2005;115:1143–52.
26. Sherris DA, Larrabee WF. Anatomic considerations in rhytidectomy. Facial Plast Surg. 1996;12:215–22.
27. Ellenbogen R, Youn A, Yamini D, Svehlak S. The volumetric face lift. Aesth Surg J. 2004;24:514–22.

28. Lowe NJ, Wieder JM, Shorr N, Boxrud C, Saucer D, Chalet M, Infraorbital pigmented skin. Preliminary observations of laser therapy. Dermatologic Surg. 1995;21:767–70.
29. Özdemir R, Kilinc H, Ünlü E, Cağri Uysal A, Sensöz O, Nazmi BC. Anatomicohistologic study of the retaining ligaments of the face anduse in face lift: retaining ligament correction and SMAS placation. Plast Reconstr Surg. 2002;110:1134–47.

Beauty of the Face: Effects on Interpersonal Communication

7

Can Cemal Cingi

7.1 Introduction

Natural selection works on particular physical characteristics of humans and how they perceive them since these features affect how many offspring an individual may leave behind. There are differences in the strategies males and females adopt to maximize their attractiveness and the reasons for finding specific characteristics attractive. Despite these differences, there is considerable agreement between different cultures and males and females regarding which individuals possess beauty. Furthermore, the pattern is repeated globally: individuals judged attractive garner a higher share of resources and produce more offspring than their less beautiful peers. At least three mental modules are involved in evaluating the beauty of faces. These modules are embodied in various parts of the central nervous system. The systems identified so far are an identification module, an interpretation module, and a valuation module. The factors that influence the outcome include age, how healthy the individual appears, how symmetrical the face is, how similar to average the facial proportions and those of the body generally are the color of the face and skin texture [1].

7.2 Biology of Beauty

According to evolutionary biological theory, if a gene or genes may enhance the possessor's ability to survive and reproduce and thus transmit a copy to future generations, natural selection will tend to prefer that gene or those genes. Therefore, the

C. C. Cingi (✉)
Faculty of Communication Sciences, Department of Communication Design and Management, Anadolu University, Eskisehir, Turkey
e-mail: ccc@anadolu.edu.tr

C. Cingi et al. (eds.), *Minor Interventions, Major Outcomes on the Face*, Comprehensive ENT, https://doi.org/10.1007/978-3-032-01305-7_7

frequency in the population will increase over time. At some point, the phenotype produced by the gene(s) will be found in virtually all individuals within the people and thus may be considered a fixed phenotypic manifestation [1].

Phenotypic expression of specific genotypes may make it easier for an individual to receive adequate nutrition, such as the ability to run for a lengthy period or to possess a greater degree of manual dexterity. It is those phenotypes with a direct influence on the ability to reproduce, for example, those that determine sexual attractiveness or that help ensure assistance in caring for subsequent offspring, which are subject to maximum selection pressure. This results from the fact that genes directly involved with reproductive success are the ones that instantly guarantee their transmission to subsequent generations [1].

7.2.1 Reproductive Strategy

The reproductive strategies of males and females differ and would have developed for thousands of years before historical records began. The female system typically involves finding a male partner with healthy genes and the ability to provide for the mother and any offspring. In contrast, the male strategy consists of finding one or more women with healthy genes to whom they may supply some resources. In the case of both men and women, they display themselves to potential reproductive partners, as well as other members of their sex, seeking to show themselves as possessing reproductive value [2]. Displaying sexually appealing characteristics constitutes sexual attraction or simply being beautiful [1].

7.2.2 Attractiveness

There is an unexpected degree of concordance when males or females, or different groups, are asked to rate attractiveness. A meta-analysis that pooled the results from 919 trials involving 15,000 observers found a generally high level of agreement, both interculturally and intraculturally, in judgments about which faces are attractive or unattractive [3]. The attractiveness rating does not differ between males and females, nor is it related to age. These findings prove that the ability to judge attractiveness is innate and genetically determined. These judgments have been present since an early stage in human evolution. However this may be, it is clear from studies where the time spent by infants aged 6 months gazing at different faces was measured that beautiful or handsome adult faces already attract more attention than plain ones, even from early childhood [4].

7.2.3 Attractive People Succeed

Assessing how attractive a potential partner is has meaningful consequences insofar as a pretty face implies the possessor is in good health and thus likely has a healthy set of genes and will be able to work to raise a child. How attractive a person is correlates the most strongly among all factors with winning the favor of the preferred partner [5]. Indeed, being physically attractive continues to determine the likelihood of reproductive success, even in the modern world [6]. Females whose partner possesses healthy genes and has resources at his disposal continue to enjoy more reproductive success than those whose partner lacks such attributes [7].

7.2.4 Gender Differences in Features of Attractiveness and How They Are Perceived

The body characteristics in shaping perceptions of attractiveness are controlled by the sex hormones, i.e., testosterone in males and estrogen in females. These hormones also affect the brain and the way an individual assesses attractiveness. At puberty, the levels of sex hormones increase, and boys and girls begin to develop into the appropriate adult phenotype. For males, the shoulder width to waist width increases, facial hair grows, and the jaws become more powerfully delineated. In females, the mammary glands develop, the hips become more comprehensive than the waist, and the face is generally softened, including the jawline. Several parts of the central nervous system carry receptors sensitive to estrogen, progesterone, or androgens. Accordingly, from puberty onwards, male and female brains begin to develop in different directions [7].

The female brain is so well able to assess male faces that women can place men in the order of increasing testosterone level (measured in saliva) by examining photographs [8]. Women's preferences for the level of testosterone in a partner depend on whether the woman wishes for a short-term or long-term relationship. For a short-term relationship, a high level of apparent testosterone is preferred, while men with somewhat less noticeable effects of testosterone are generally preferred for longer-term relationships. The parents of such a woman tend to like even less apparent effects of testosterone in a partner for their daughter, which may be because a male with a higher level of testosterone may be more likely to leave them responsible for an abandoned grandchild [9]. When photographs of males are enhanced to indicate a more significant effect of testosterone, their attractiveness lessens rather than increases [10].

7.2.5 Facial Proportions

Human behavior is partly controlled by examining other people's facial reactions, which may reveal their thoughts or emotions. It is an integral feature of human sociability. Human beings additionally view facial features as key to judging attractiveness and, therefore, desirability as a sexual partner. As mentioned above, males and females in most cultures agree in assessing how beautiful or handsome a face appears. The features of the face that confer attractiveness develop partially under the influence of sex hormones, such as how a jutting jaw appears and how large the eyes are [11].

To some extent, however, judgments of attractiveness are subconscious. One study prepared sets of photographs of university students consisting of more attractive and less attractive individuals [10]. When pairs of pictures were compared, there was an agreement between the ratings, but the raters could not express how they had decided in any particular case.

When people interact socially and decide how attractive someone is, they pay particular attention to that person's eyes. A dedicated brain region, the superior temporal sulcus, integrates information about other people's eye movements and works out in what direction they are looking [12]. This part of the brain undergoes development in early life, such that an infant only a few months old can figure out where its mother is looking [13]. Recognizing eye movements involves pathways that connect with the amygdala, a region involved in basic emotional regulation [14].

Unlike the eyes, the nose and the ears do not have the same direct role in determining attractiveness. This is probably because their length is not fixed; rather, they tend to lengthen as a person advances in age.

7.3 Beauty and Communication

Human beings are a species where social relations play a dominant role, and people often exchange social information in virtually all parts of their lives. The face is highly adapted to communicate a rich and complex array of social signals. These signals let other people rapidly and straightforwardly deduce information about who someone is, whether they are male or female (socially or biologically), how old they are, what race or ethnic group they belong to, their sexual preferences, how healthy they are, their beauty or handsomeness, how they are feeling, what their character is like, whether they are experiencing pain or pleasure, how trustworthy they may be, and even their position in a social hierarchy. As the world moves toward ever greater levels of digitization, globalization, and richer intercultural exchange, it has become more important to appreciate how the face functions to facilitate social interactions and how this system can unexpectedly go wrong. This is a key design feature for those designing digital avatars or robots that communicate with people. However, this is a complex topic since facial expressions involve multiple dimensions and relay information dynamically. This complexity cannot be readily modeled using cognitive psychology nor correlated directly with neuroimaging. Thus, facial analysis needs to be more realized in digital applications. However, as novel techniques and methodologies are spreading and interdisciplinary approaches in scientific research become more commonplace, there is new hope that the subject can be better understood. One such hybrid, interdisciplinary approach utilizes the latest digital graphics technologies, psychophysics, the science of vision, and cultural and social psychology to indicate where knowledge of this topic is becoming more profound. Drawing on cutting-edge research, this approach has illuminated the possible path for research in facial communication between human beings, including where individuals from different cultures interact [15].

When people interact socially, information is exchanged dynamically, aiming for all parties to understand the messages exchanged and either act or think in a desired way. This exchange is bounded by culture and other contextual factors. Agonistic behavior is designed to send a threatening, aggressive, or placatory message, which is intended to stop the interaction from progressing into actual violence. It is thus of potential benefit to all the parties involved in the communicative act [16]. The usually beneficial effects of communication are highlighted by observing what happens when communication fails, such as when emotion cannot be shown or expressions are not recognized. In such situations, social relationships may be damaged; individuals may find themselves ostracized [17–19] or may come to harm physically or mentally. As human beings adapted and spread worldwide, the cognitive demands placed on them grew [20], and multiple cultures evolved, resulting in increased sophistication in how social interactions occurred, including those involving language [21].

7.4 A High-Dimensional Dynamic Information Space of Facial Variations

Faces vary in three dimensions: dynamic activity, morphological features, and complexion. The face has many voluntary (striated) muscles [22], which humans may contract or relax, alone or in combination, to varying degrees and for different lengths of time. This arrangement allows the face to produce complicated facial patterns expressing different meanings. The face also varies morphologically from individual to individual, i.e., the shape and structural aspects differ. There are numerous other parameters involved, some of which are the facial breadth, height, how prominent the jaw and the brows are, how wide the jaw is, the distance between the medial canthi, how wide the mouth is, how thick the lips are, how tall the forehead is, and several other parameters [23, 24]. The final dimension of variability is in complexion. This consists of the color, degree of facial pigmentation [25], pallor or erythema, and the texture of the skin, affected by rhytides, scars, skin conditions, and how fat the individual is. Each aspect of the complexion conveys information. A further way that facial communication occurs is through deliberate modification of the facial appearance, such as using make-up or warpaint, tattoos, piercings, wearing jewelry, hairstyles, clothing, and various ways teeth may be altered by filing or dyeing them. These alterations may communicate membership of a group or be designed to enhance attractiveness by changing the apparent morphology or improving the facial texture [26]. The multiple dimensions of variability ensure that all human beings have different facial features. This indicates a profound degree of information that can be encoded facially since it is estimated that, up to now, 106 billion humans have been born, each of whom has a unique facial appearance [27].

7.5 Dynamic Face Information

The expressions formed on the face do not deliver the message all at once but rather in a dynamic fashion over time. How the face expresses particular emotions is an evolved feature in humans and seems to involve a specific facial movement with a biological purpose, being co-opted to convey a social message [28–30]. A more profound knowledge of the "grammar" of facial expressions may help understand how facial communication functions. The word fear on the face usually involves the eyes opening wide and the nostrils becoming flared. It can be seen how this also makes a fight-or-flight response easier since the eyes can search for a place to flee, and the airway can carry the maximum oxygen to the lungs. Thus, the biological and social functions are intertwined. Likewise, people show disgust by partly closing their eyes and wrinkling up their noses, which may reduce the chance of pathogenic microbes entering the body. Since adopting such expressions confers an adaptive advantage [29], the origins of facial expressions may lie in the swift deployment of facial muscle movements that support physiological needs. Modern humans may benefit from the role of facial expressions in social communication thanks to the elaboration of a basic set of responses initially serving a purely biological function but later developed for an essentially communicative purpose. When models that dynamically capture the six classic expressions shown by faces were analyzed, it was revealed that there was a hierarchy of information and that this information was transmitted over some time, revealing a hitherto unsuspected complexity in communication, divisible into a set of categories of greater and greater specificity [31].

7.6 Facial Attractiveness and Beauty

While particular morphological features are strongly linked to matters of social significance, e.g., appearing attractive, dominant, or trustworthy to others [32, 33], individuals can adopt expressions that override these usual effects, which may form the basis of manipulating others to create a particular impression. It has been demonstrated in psychophysical experiments that facial expressions are more important than morphological features in determining how a person is perceived. When social evaluations were examined, it appeared that dynamic facial changes could displace judgments that would otherwise be formed based on morphological features of the face. An example case is where a face that seemed to belong to a highly submissive individual, when adopting an expression associated with dominance, came to be seen as belonging to a dominant individual [34].

References

1. Yarosh DB. Perception and deception: human beauty and the brain. Behav Sci (Basel). 2019;9(4):34. https://doi.org/10.3390/bs9040034. PMID: 30934856; PMCID: PMC6523404

2. Bovet J. The evolution of feminine beauty. In: Kapoula Z, Volle E, Renoult J, Andreatta M, editors. Exploring Transdisciplinarity in art and sciences. Heidelberg: Springer; 2018. p. 327–57.
3. Langlois J, Rubenstein A, Larson A, Hallam M, Smoot M. Maxim or myths of beauty? A meta-analytic and theoretical review. Psychol Bull. 2000;126:390–423. https://doi.org/10.1037/0033-2909.126.3.390.
4. Ramsey J, Langlois J, Hoss R, Rubenstein A, Griffin A. Origins of a stereotype: categorization of facial attractiveness by 6-month-old infants. Dev Sci. 2004;7:201–11. https://doi.org/10.1111/j.1467-7687.2004.00339.x.
5. Halberstadt J. Proximate and ultimate origins of a bias for prototypical faces. In: Forgas J, Haselton M, von Hippel W, editors. Evolution and the social mind. Sydney: Psychology Press; 2007. p. 245–62.
6. Jokela M. Physical attractiveness and reproductive success in humans: evidence from the late 20th century United States. Evol Hum Behav. 2009;30:342–50. https://doi.org/10.1016/j.evolhumbehav.2009.03.006.
7. Thornhill R, Gangestad SW. The evolutionary biology of human female sexuality. Oxford: Oxford University Press; 2008.
8. Roney J, Hanson K, Durante K, Maestripieri D. Reading men's faces. Proc Biol Sci. 2006;273:2169–75. https://doi.org/10.1098/rspb.2006.3569.
9. Kruger D. Male facial masculinity influences attributions of personality and reproductive strategy. Pers Relatsh. 2006;13:451–63. https://doi.org/10.1111/j.1475-6811.2006.00129.x.
10. Ito A, Fujii T, Abe N, Kawasaki I, Hayashi A, Ueno A, Yoshida K, Sakai S, Mugikura S, Takahashi S, et al. Gender differences in ventromedial prefrontal cortex activity associated with valuation of faces. Neuroscience. 2016;328:194–200. https://doi.org/10.1016/j.neuroscience.2016.04.047.
11. Little A, Jones B, DeBruine L. Facial attractiveness: evolutionary based research. Philos Trans R Soc B. 2011;366:1638–59. https://doi.org/10.1098/rstb.2010.0404.
12. Santhouse A, Howard R, ffytche D. Visual hallucinatory syndromes and the anatomy of the visual brain. Brain. 2000;123:2055–64. https://doi.org/10.1093/brain/123.10.2055.
13. D'Entremont B, Hains SMJ, Muir DW. A demonstration of gaze following in 3- to 6-month-olds. Infant Behav Dev. 1997;20:560–72. https://doi.org/10.1016/S0163-6383(97)90048-5.
14. Whalen P, Kagan J, Cook R, Davis FC, Kim H, Polis S, McLaren D, Somerville L, McLean A, Maxwell J, et al. Human amygdala responsivity to masked fearful eye whites. Science. 2004;306:2061. https://doi.org/10.1126/science.1103617.
15. Jack RE, Schyns PG. The human face as a dynamic tool for social communication. Curr Biol. 2015;25(14):R621–34.
16. Dukas R. Cognitive ecology: the evolutionary ecology of information processing and decision making. 1st ed. Chicago: University of Chicago Press; 1998.
17. Hawkley LC, Cacioppo JT. Aging and loneliness: downhill quickly? Curr Dir Psychol Sci. 2007;16:187–91.
18. Baron-Cohen S, Leslie AM, Frith U. Does the autistic child have a "theory of mind"? Cognition. 1985;21:37–46.
19. LeMoult J, Joormann J, Sherdell L, Wright Y, Gotlib IH. Identification of emotional facial expressions following recovery from depression. J Abnorm Psychol. 2009;118:828–33.
20. Dunbar RI. Coevolution of neocortical size, group size and language in humans. Behav Brain Sci. 1993;16:681–93.
21. Fay N, Garrod S, Roberts L, Swoboda N. The interactive evolution of human communication systems. Cogn Sci. 2010;34:351–86.
22. Drake RL, Vogl A, Mitchell AW. Gray's anatomy for students. Philadelphia: Elsevier Health Sciences; 2014.
23. Goldstein AG. Race-related variation of facial features: anthropometric data I. Bull Psychon Soc. 1979;13:187–90.
24. Goldstein AG. Facial feature variation: anthropometric data II. Bull Psychon Soc. 1979;13:191–3.

25. Pathak MA, Jimbow K, Szabo G, Fitzpatrick TB. Sunlight and melanin pigmentation. Photochem Photobiol Rev. 1976;2:211–39.
26. Cohen MM. Perspectives on the face. Oxford University Press; 2006.
27. Haub C. How many people have ever lived on earth? WORLD. 2002;6:983–7.
28. Darwin C. The expression of the emotions in man and animals. 3rd ed. London: Fontana Press; 1999/1872.
29. Susskind JM, Lee DH, Cusi A, Feiman R, Grabski W, Anderson AK. Expressing fear enhances sensory acquisition. Nat Neurosci. 2008;11:843–50.
30. Andrew RJ. Evolution of facial expression. Science. 1963;142:1034–41.
31. Jack RE, Garrod OG, Schyns PG. Dynamic facial expressions of emotion transmit an evolving hierarchy of signals over time. Curr Biol. 2014;24:187–92.
32. Oosterhof NN, Todorov A. The functional basis of face evaluation. Proc Natl Acad Sci USA. 2008;105:11087–92.
33. Todorov A, Said CP, Engell AD, Oosterhof NN. Understanding evaluation of faces on social dimensions. Trends Cogn Sci. 2008;12:455–60.
34. Gill D, Garrod OG, Jack RE, Schyns PG. Facial movements strategically camouflage involuntary social signals of face morphology. Psychol Sci. 2014;25:1079–86.

Part II

Neurotoxins on the Face

Botulinum Toxin: History, Function, Usage on the Face

8

Taylan Çil, Felicia Manole, and Nuray Bayar Muluk

8.1 Introduction

A bacterium, *Clostridium botulinum*, synthesizes botulinum toxin. Spores from this bacterial species are detectable in almost all natural environments, both on land and at sea. The spores have been detected in soil, fruit, vegetables, sea floors, and seafood. As these organisms grow, they synthesize botulinum, a substance with high neurotoxic potential. Indeed, botulinum is sometimes considered the compound with the greatest toxicity currently known. Toxicity arises because it prevents acetylcholine from being secreted from nerve terminals; thus, neuromuscular transmission cannot occur. The muscle involved undergoes flaccid paralysis [1].

Botulinum toxin exists in seven different forms, which may be distinguished by serology. The forms are termed A, B, C1, D, E, F, and G. Allergan marketed the first form in the USA, type A, under the name Botox® [1].

The seven botulinum serotypes differ in terms of molecular mass, their activity, and the mechanism for the action. Several different forms of the botulinum toxin are marketed for clinical use, and they possess different characteristics. The molecular mechanisms underlying these differences in clinical characteristics are currently the subject of intensive research [1].

Botulinum A toxin is commercially available as onabotulinumtoxinA, abobotulinumtoxinA, incobotulinumtoxinA, and prabotulinumtoxinA, whereas type B is available as rimabotulinumtoxinB. There are a variety of proprietary names used for

T. Çil
Department of Otorhinolaryngology, Mersin Tarsus State Hospital, Mersin, Türkiye

F. Manole
Faculty of Medicine, Department of ENT, University of Oradea, Oradea, Romania

N. Bayar Muluk (✉)
Faculty of Medicine, Department of Otorhinolaryngology, Kırıkkale University, Kırıkkale, Türkiye

C. Cingi et al. (eds.), *Minor Interventions, Major Outcomes on the Face*, Comprehensive ENT, https://doi.org/10.1007/978-3-032-01305-7_8

these preparations, namely Botox®/Botox® Cosmetic (OnabotulinumtoxinA), Dysport® (abobotulinumtoxinA), Xeomin® (incobotulinumtoxinA), Jeuveau® prabotulinumtoxinA), and Myobloc® (rimabotulinumtoxinB) [1].

Botulinum toxin is only beneficial for wrinkles produced when a muscle contracts. It is not suitable for treating rhytides secondary to sun damage or other degeneration that affects the skin layers [1].

8.2 Definition

Botulinum is a naturally occurring exotoxin synthesized by the *C. botulinum* bacterium, which is among the most potent of all known poisons. It acts on nervous tissue. The toxin is synthesized in eight different forms, which may be distinguished based on the different epitopes each bear. These forms are denoted by A, B, C1, C2, D, E, F, and G. All of these toxins exert their toxicity through inhibition of secretion of acetylcholine into the neuromuscular end-plate, which prevents the muscle from contracting, that is, it causes muscular paralysis. This blockade typically persists for around 3 months when botulinum toxin A is clinically injected. The clinical applications for botulinum toxins have greatly expanded, and they are a key therapeutic modality in a range of different disorders, in particular strabismus, focal dystonias, hemifacial spasm, spasticity of various causes, cephalgia, excessive salivation or sweating, and certain persistent conditions which can only partly be treated at present [2].

Type A has the highest toxic potency of the eight botulinum serotypes (A, B, C1, C2, D, E, F, and G). Type B and type F are the next most toxic. When systemic botulism occurs in humans, the usual culprits are types A, B, or E [3]. The serotypes share the common characteristics of an unbranched chain of polypeptides, each with lengthy sequences shared by other toxins in the group. Their typical molecular mass is around 150 kDa; when first synthesized, they do not possess full potency. There are both a heavy (H, molecular mass approximately 100 kDa) chain and a light (L, molecular mass approximately 50 kDa) chain, which are bonded to each other via a disulfide linkage [4]. There are associations of the botulinum exotoxins with several other protein molecules which lack toxicity but have potential haemagglutination abilities [5].

8.3 History

The potential for botulinum toxin to be used in aesthetic medicine was discovered when it was noted that patients with blepharospasm who were treated with botulinum noted an improvement in the wrinkles of the glabellar region [1].

Botulinum toxin, which has achieved notoriety on account of its extremely toxic potency, is sometimes referred to as the "miraculous poison." [6] The *C. botulinum* bacterial species responsible for its production is classified as a Gram-positive anaerobe. It has a rod-like morphology and produces spores. It may be free-living on plants, soil, or water or may exist within the gut of animals. Botulinum toxin A was the first type to be used clinically. Scott used this agent to manage patients with strabismus [7]. The use of this toxin clinically then spreads to various other conditions where spasticity occurs [6], in addition to numerous other applications. At present, scarcely any medical specialty has yet to fund an application for botulinum toxin. The use of botulinum toxin type A (as Botox®) in aesthetic medicine dates from its US Food and Drug Administration (FDA) licensing approval in 2002 to indicate temporary reversal of wrinkles in the glabellar region [2].

8.4 Function

Botulinum toxin is used dermatologically to improve the cosmetic appearance of wrinkles produced by the contraction of underlying facial muscles. The lay terms used for such wrinkles are "crow's feet," "frown lines," or "laughter lines." [1]

Contraction of the facial musculature in various combinations contributes to facial expression. The contraction of particular muscles, which may occur consciously or unconsciously, leads to the expression of emotions on the face. Thus, a person may appear afraid, anxious, angry, and so on. Despite this beneficial role in communication, some individuals may be distressed by the appearance or social consequences of deeply etched facial lines [1].

Hyperhidrosis refers to excessive sweating resulting from overactive cholinergic transmission to sweat glands. This may produce social discomfort as well as potentially hinder specific activities that individuals regularly undertake. An example of the latter is when palmar hyperhidrosis makes it difficult to hold fine tools or safely grasp a vehicle's steering wheel. [1]

Botulinum toxin may be used to treat hyperhidrosis or rhytides through the same mechanism: inhibiting acetylcholine release at the synapse [1].

Various types of botulinum toxin act in this same way. The principal neurotransmitter involved in muscular contraction is acetylcholine. When botulinum toxin is injected into a muscle, it achieves its clinical effect of paralyzing the muscle by preventing the release of acetylcholine from the neuron into the muscle end-plate [8]. There are four potential groups of targets for botulinum to act upon, namely the muscle end-plate, ganglia of the autonomic nervous system, postganglionic parasympathetic nerve fiber terminals, and postganglionic sympathetic nerve fiber terminals [5]. These are the locations where cholinergic transmission usually occurs. The specific molecular target is the high-affinity receptor found on the terminal plasma membrane of cholinergic neurons. Binding occurs selectively to the H chain on the toxin and cannot be reversed. The receptor, now bound to the toxin, is drawn into the cell by an endocytotic mechanism. The toxin contains a disulfide linkage that joins the L and H portions of the molecule. This bond is broken within the cytoplasm. The L chain can now interfere with various cytoplasmic molecules, notably the synaptosomal-associated protein molecule, vesicle-associated membrane protein, and syntaxin. The effect of this interference is that vesicles packed with the neurotransmitter can no longer fuse with the membrane and thus undergo release into the synaptic gap [5, 9]. The maximum clinical benefit is observed between 4 and 7 days after injecting the toxin. The botulinum toxins marketed all specify the dose as units of biological activity. One unit of biological activity is calculated as the median amount needed to kill female Swiss-Webster mice when injected into the peritoneum, that is, the intraperitoneal lethal dose (LD_{50}) [10]. Although the toxin does not cause any structural alteration in the neuronal bouton, the function of the nerve cell is irreversibly disrupted. The restoration of normal transmission occurs when the cell eventually (around 2 to 3 months later) produces an alternative synaptic terminal connection with its target muscle.

The paralysis of voluntary muscle by botulinum toxin occurs via the toxic effect on the alpha motor neuron terminal in the region of the muscle end-plate. Thus, botulinum toxin is used therapeutically in patients where the muscles exhibit excessive activity, as occurs in dystonia. As botulinum toxin also prevents cholinergic transmission from the gamma neurons within muscle spindles, it is potentially beneficial when the reflexes are overactive [11]. Moreover, cholinergic transmission can be inhibited in nerve cells belonging to the parasympathetic system and post-ganglionic nerve terminals in the sympathetic system. This ability suggests a role in disorders involving smooth muscle overactivity, such as in achalasia or where exocrine glandular tissue is overstimulated, as in hyperhidrosis [6].

The onset of therapeutic action occurs about 1 to 2 days after administration of the toxin, which is the result of the disrupted process of synaptosome formation. Although highly unusual, the full clinical benefit may not present in certain patients before 5 days have elapsed. The peak effect is apparent on around the tenth day and persists for between 8 and 12 weeks [2].

8.5 Indications

The indications for which the US FDA (Food and Drug Administration) has granted a license are as follows. Note that some jurisdictions may permit wider use than laid out here [1].

The indications for Botox® (on botulinum toxin A) are as follows:

- In cases of cervical dystonia where the aim is to improve the position of the head and reduce pain arising from the condition.
- Primary axillary hyperhidrosis, if treatment with topically applied medications has proven insufficient.
- Hyperactive detrusor muscle.
- Urinary bladder overactivity.
- Persistent migrainous headache.
- Strabismus and blepharospasm in association with dystonia. This encompasses both benign idiopathic blepharospasm and facial nerve palsy in patients aged at least 12 years [1].

The licensed indication for Botox® Cosmetic (on botulinum toxin A) is to temporarily reduce the appearance of wrinkles of at least moderate severity in the region of the glabella, where these are linked to the contraction of one or both of the corrugator and procerus muscles. It is for use in adults aged up to 65 years. Further indications are to temporarily reduce the appearance of wrinkles of at least moderate severity in the region of the lateral canthi, where these are linked to contraction of the orbicularis oculi muscle, and for the same purpose with wrinkles linked to contraction of the frontalis muscle. The indication in both these latter cases is in adult patients [1].

The licensed indication for Dysport® (abobotulinumtoxinA) is to treat cervical dystonia and spasticity of the lower limbs, generally in adult patients. In aesthetic medicine, it is used to temporarily reduce the appearance of wrinkles of at least moderate severity in the region of the glabella, where these are linked to contraction of one or both of the corrugator and procerus muscles. Patients must be no older than 65 years for the latter indication [1].

The licensed indication for Jeuveau® (prabotulinumtoxinA) is to temporarily reduce the appearance of wrinkles of at least moderate severity in the region of the glabella in adults, where these are linked to contraction of one or both of the corrugator and procerus muscles [12].

There are two licensed indications for Xeomin® (incobotulinumtoxinA). The first is in cervical dystonia, where it may allow the head to be in a less severely abnormal position and reduce cervical discomfort. Here, it may be used both in patients previously exposed to the treatment and those who are taking it for the first time. The second indication is to treat blepharospasm in adult patients who have already been treated with onabotulinumtoxinA. In aesthetic medicine, it is used to temporarily reduce the appearance of wrinkles of at least moderate severity in the region of the glabella, where these are linked to contraction of one or both of the corrugator and procerus muscles [1].

There is a licensed indication for Myobloc® (rimabotulinumtoxinB) in treating cervical dystonia, where it may allow the head to be in a less severely abnormal position and reduce cervical discomfort.

Botulinum toxin A is frequently employed in treating wrinkles associated with movement of the facial muscles, such as occurs in the glabellar region [13, 14], as lines across the forehead, for crow's feet (i.e., near the lateral canthi) [15], and for face lifts of the medial brow and lateral brow.

There are experts who use botulinum toxin for reducing wrinkles in a variety of facial regions, notably the superior lip, to reduce scrunching of the nose and flaring, to prevent marionette lines, necklines, and bands overlying the platysma [16], chin creasing, and dimpling. Given that some of these uses may cause complications that compromise physiological function, it has been advised by other experts that they not be attempted. Besides these cosmetic applications, botulinum toxin may be used to treat excessive sweating affecting the armpits or palms of the hand, where previous topical or systemic therapy has failed to resolve the issue [17–19].

Botulinum toxin finds many unlicensed applications, a number of which are described in the literature, such as alleviating the symptoms of hyperhidrosis affecting the hands or feet, focal dystonias, spasticity, hemifacial spasm, tics, tremors, tension headaches, and migraine [20]. In such cases, the use of botulinum toxin is essentially a limited clinical trial [21].

References

1. Trizna Z. Dermatologic use of botulinum toxin. In: Elston DM, editor. Medscape. Updated: Feb 07, 2019. https://emedicine.medscape.com/article/1126453-overview. Accessed online at 13 Apr 2021.
2. Nigam PK, Nigam A. Botulinum toxin. Indian J Dermatol. 2010;55(1):8–14. https://doi.org/10.4103/0019-5154.60343. PMID: 20418969; PMCID: PMC2856357
3. Ellenhorn MJ, Barceloux DG, editors. Diagnosis and treatment of human poisoning. New York: Elsevier; 1988. Medical Toxicology. p. 1185–7.
4. Brin MF. Botulinum toxin: chemistry, pharmacology, toxicity, and immunology. Muscle Nerve Suppl. 1997;20:146–68.
5. Sellin LC. The pharmacological mechanism of botulism. Trends Pharmacol Sci. 1985;6:80–2.
6. Münchau A, Bhatia KP. Uses of botulinum toxin injection in medicine today. BMJ. 2000;320:161–5.
7. Scott AB. Botulinum toxin injection of eye muscles to correct strabismus. Trans Trans Am Ophthalmol Soc. 1981;79:734–70.
8. Burgen AS, Dickens F, Zatman LJ. The action of botulinum toxin on the neuro-muscular junction. J Physiol. 1949;109:10–24.
9. Stanley EF, Drachman DB. Botulinum toxin blocks quantal but not non-quantal releasee of ACh at the neuro-muscular junction. Brain Res. 1983;261:172–5.
10. Hoffman RO, Helveston EM. Botulinum in the treatment of adult motility disorders. Int Ophthalmol Clin. 1986;26:241–50.
11. Priori A, Berardelli A, Mercuri B, Manfredi M. Physiological effects produced by botulinum toxin treatment of upper limb dystonia: changes in reciprocal inhibition between forearm muscles. Brain. 1995;118:801–7.
12. Jeuveau (prabotulinumtoxinA) (package insert). Santa Barbara: Evolus, Inc. 2019.
13. Carruthers JD, Carruthers JA. Treatment of glabellar frown lines with C. botulinum-A exotoxin. J Dermatol Surg Oncol. 1992 Jan;18(1):17–21.
14. Macdonald MR, Spiegel JH, Raven RB, Kabaker SS, Maas CS. An anatomical approach to glabellar rhytids. Arch Otolaryngol Head Neck Surg. 1998 Dec;124(12):1315–20.
15. Elridy AS, Zaki RGE, Elshinawy RF. Comparison of the clinical efficacy of Abobotulinumtoxin A (ABO) and Onabotulinumtoxin A (ONA) in the treatment of crow's feet wrinkles: a split-face study. Semin Ophthalmol. 2017;33(6):739–47.
16. Matarasso A, Matarasso SL, Brandt FS, Bellman B. Botulinum A exotoxin for the management of platysma bands. Plast Reconstr Surg. 1999;103(2):645–52. discussion 653–5
17. Farrugia MK, Nicholls EA. Intradermal botulinum A toxin injection for axillary hyperhydrosis. J Pediatr Surg. 2005 Oct;40(10):1668–9.
18. Heckmann M, Ceballos-Baumann AO, Plewig G. Botulinum toxin A for axillary hyperhidrosis (excessive sweating). N Engl J Med. 2001;344(7):488–93.
19. Naver H, Swartling C, Aquilonius SM. Palmar and axillary hyperhidrosis treated with botulinum toxin: one-year clinical follow-up. Eur J Neurol. 2000;7(1):55–62.
20. Schulte-Mattler WJ, Wieser T, Zierz S. Treatment of tension-type headache with botulinum toxin: a pilot study. Eur J Med Res. 1999;4(5):183–6.
21. Kern U, Kohl M, Seifert U, Schlereth T. Botulinum toxin type B in the treatment of residual limb hyperhidrosis for lower limb amputees: a pilot study. Am J Phys Med Rehabil. 2011;90(4):321–9.

Botulinum Toxin Injections: Cosmetic Applications: Overview

9

Mustafa Ibas, Nuray Bayar Muluk, and Alwyn D'Souza

9.1 Relevant Anatomy

Several key anatomical structures should be considered, along with how their function affects cosmetic appearance [1].

Vertically oriented wrinkles due to the corrugator supercilii and procerus muscle

After the corrugator supercilii contracts, most of its mass lies medially to the eyebrow. This muscle originates from where the nasal bone joins the frontal bone, in the vicinity of the superior medial orbital rim. Most corrugator supercilii lies on a coronal plane passing through the middle of the eyebrows. To achieve maximum clinical benefit and to prevent inadvertently piercing the orbital septum, when injecting botulinum toxin, the point of injection should lie on or just superior to this plane, aiming for where the muscle is broadest, that is, on the medial aspect of the supraorbital ridge. The injection site should be no further lateral than the midpupillary line [1]. The medial part is injected deep muscular and the laterally should be more superficial as the muscle becomes superficial.

M. Ibas
Department of otorhinolaryngology, Etimesgut Şehit Sait Ertürk State Hospital, Ankara, Türkiye

N. Bayar Muluk (✉)
Faculty of Medicine, Department of Otorhinolaryngology, Kırıkkale University, Kırıkkale, Türkiye

A. D'Souza
Private practice, London Facial Surgery, London, UK
e-mail: ad@londonfacialsurgery.org

C. Cingi et al. (eds.), *Minor Interventions, Major Outcomes on the Face*, Comprehensive ENT, https://doi.org/10.1007/978-3-032-01305-7_9

Horizontally oriented wrinkles due to the procerus muscle

The procerus muscle is slender and lies in the nasal midline, typically between 1 and 4 mm deep to the skin. Female patients usually have a longer procerus than male patients. The ideal site to inject botulinum toxin is a point on the midline slightly below the nasal radix [1]. The depth of injection should be deep intramuscular.

Horizontally oriented wrinkles due to the frontalis muscle

Prior to toxin injection into the frontalis, horizontal lines should be drawn on the overlying skin. The injections are into the broadest portion of the muscle at intervals of between 1.5 and 2 cm. On the lateral aspect, begin injecting some way superior to the brow, so that the facial expression is still preserved laterally. Injections that are too close to the supraorbital ridge cause ptosis, so should not be performed [1]. Depth of injection is deep subcutaneous.

Crow's feet caused by contraction of the orbicularis oculi

The injection procedure begins by marking the correct site. The lateral canthal lines should be drawn 1 cm laterally from the canthi. By asking the patient to squint, the squint lines can be identified superior and inferior to the lateral canthal lines. Injection into the orbicularis oculi follows a symmetrical placement bilaterally. If injections are placed very close to the eyelid margin (blephara), the patient may experience difficulty in closing the eyes, so this should be avoided [1]. The depth tends to be deep dermal, as there is no subcutaneous tissue between the orbicularis and skin of the eyelid.

Perioral rhytides due to contraction of the orbicularis oris and mentalis muscles

The injections should occur midway between the inferior lip's vermilion border and the lower mental margin, at a point lying between half and 1 cm medially from the oral commissure. The injection must not be sited too near to the lips, and the dose needs to be kept low [1].

Platysmal bands—platysma muscle

The muscle bands are pinched gently using the noninjecting hand, and multiple injections are placed about 2 cm apart. Electromyography may be used to define the area where injection should occur in challenging cases. The needle position is perpendicular to the muscular long axis [1].

Axilla

To reveal the areas within the armpit where hyperhidrosis occurs, iodine can be applied to test for starch. Iodine turns a deep blue or black in the affected areas.

The toxin needs to enter the dermis, and to achieve this, the injection needle is held at 45 degrees to the skin, and bevel up to avoid leakage. The injections may be placed in an even distribution. Each point where injection occurs produces a surrounding circle of around 2 cm diameter. Usually, no more than 50 U botulinum toxin should be used for the entire axilla. It is best not to indicate the sites to inject by drawing with ink as, if the needle passes through the ink, it may leave a permanent ink tattoo behind [1].

9.2 Formulation

The sole botulinum toxin serotype marketed for clinical applications at present is serotype A, albeit there is a growing body of evidence to support the use of preparations containing the B, C and F serotypes [2]. Serotype A is commercially available in many brands though two common brands are: Dysport® and Botox®. The units defining the dose, which are based on biological action, unfortunately, may be somewhat confusing when comparing preparations [3, 4]. It appears that dose is calculated on the basis of the LD_{50}, which is the mass of toxin needed to kill half of the animals in a group consisting of female Swiss-Webster mice and each weighing between 18 and 20 g. Despite this apparent equivalency, it appears that Botox® possesses a superior potency for a given dose. Indeed, a recent report in the literature indicates that it possesses threefold greater potency than an equivalent dose of Dysport® [4]; however, this is because of confusion in comparing the potency based on number of units. The best option is to follow manufacturer's guidelines. Dysport® is a preparation containing toxin of serotype A, which is marketed in Europe and certain other countries. Its manufacture calls for column-based purification. The preparation comes in vials containing 500 U. Although both Botox® and Dysport® contain botulinum toxin of serotype A, they may not be substituted for each other. The different profiles probably arise as a result of different bacterial strains used for manufacture, differences in how the toxin is prepared, the diffusibility characteristics and how the product is assessed for biological activity [5].

Myobloc is a preparation consisting of botulinum toxin of serotype B [6].

9.3 Preparations

9.3.1 Botulinum Toxin Type A (BOTOX®)

Botox® (produced by Allergan, Irvine, California, USA) consists of serotype A. It was the initial product to receive marketing authorisation in the USA. The safety characteristics of this product are well understood. It suffers from the disadvantage that, having been reconstituted, the agent begins to lose some of its biological activity [5].

9.3.2 Dysport® (Ipsen pharmaceuticals) (Botulinum Toxin Type A)

Botulinum toxin serotype A is also available as Dysport®. This is manufactured by Speywood Biopharm Ltd., UK. The unit of biological activity used to dose Botox is around fourfold more potent than that used to dose Dysport [5].

9.3.3 Xeomin®

Xeomin is a further preparation of serotype A which has marketing authorisation within the UK. This product differs from other preparations containing serotype A in the fact that it contains toxin without the proteins which are usually complexed to it. This is achieved through purifying the toxin. Thus, unlike the other preparations on the market, Xeomin consists of the 150 kDa botulinum toxin only [5].

9.3.4 Neurobloc®

This product is produced by Solstice Neurosciences Inc., San Francisco, California, USA. It first appeared in the UK in 2001 and is a botulinum toxin of serotype B with complexed proteins that is extracted from *Clostridium botulinum*. Up to now, the evidence base for usage is limited and there is no jurisdiction where it has been granted marketing authorisation for cosmetic purposes [5].

9.3.5 Myobloc®

Following reconstitution of Myobloc, it remains safe to be used for more than a year, which is of benefit to clinicians when planning their patient schedules. Nevertheless, more of this preparation than of Botox is required to produce the same effect. As the preparation contains a large volume of potentially antigenic protein, it is possible sensitisation may develop following its use [5].

9.4 Contraindications

There are a number of situations or conditions, both local and systemic, in which the use of botulinum toxin is contraindicated [1], as follows:

- Rhytides not secondary to muscle activity.
- Neuromuscular conditions.
- The patient is known to be sensitive to botulinum toxin or another component of the preparation.
- If the patient is pregnant or nursing an infant.

- The patient's expectations are too high.
- There may be an occupational or social disability caused by less facial expression, as may happen to artistes.
- The site where injection is planned is infected [1].

9.5 Applications

When injecting botulinum toxin into target muscles or glandular tissue, a fine 30-gauge needle which is 25 mm long is utilised. The dosage depends on the indication and patient characteristics, as well as the volume of the muscle involved. A bulkier muscle requires more toxin. If a patient already has some degree of muscular weakness or is female, the dose may need to be reduced [5].

The needles used have a teflon-coated bore and are placed directly into the muscle, which it is intended to weaken/paralyse. If a small area of muscle is the intended target and where there needs to be a high level of accuracy, the injection may be performed under electromyographic control [5].

Once the muscle(s) to be targeted has/have been identified, the broadest portion of the muscle is selected for injection of between 2 and 4 units of Botox or another preparation. For other preparations, dose adjustment will be required to achieve equivalent effect.

There are two injection techniques. The needle may be inserted perpendicularly or parallel to the muscle fibres. For platysma bands, parallel injection under electromyographic control is usually preferred, and the injection is delivered as the needle is slowly withdrawn from the muscle [1].

As botulinum toxin may be dispersed by massaging the injected muscle, this should be avoided, both by the clinician and the patient. Patients should be discouraged from reapplying make-up for a period afterwards and advised to rest on the day of injection [1].

Patients who have undergone such procedures should be followed up between 7 and 14 days afterwards, though current literature suggests 21 days is preferred. A photographic record should be obtained of the patient before and after the procedure, bearing the same expressions. As the effect begins to fade, further botulinum toxin may be injected to maintain the improvement [1].

9.5.1 Aesthetic Applications

There has been an enormous increase in the use of botulinum toxin in aesthetic applications over the last few years, especially after serotype A (Botox) was licensed to treat rhytides in the region of the glabella. It is only recently that cosmetic practitioners have extended the use beyond the upper facial third. Currently, the toxin is used for a wide variety of applications, including reduction of wrinkles in any facial location, the mental or cervical regions or on the chest, to paralyse the depressor anguli oris, to flatten the nasolabial creases, to paralyse the mentalis muscle, to lift the brow, either medially or laterally, to diminish facial shadows and to make the jaws and cheeks appear smoother in outline when viewed from any angle. Furthermore, dermatologists have found it a useful treatment in cases of hyperhidrosis affecting the axilla or palms, when other treatments, whether topical or systemic, have failed [5].

9.6 Complications

It is usual for patients to tolerate botulinum toxin injections well and the incidence of adverse effects is low. On rare occasions, a generalised idiosyncratic reaction may occur, but these are typically of mild and short lived. Side effects, where they do occur, consist of mild pain at the site of injection, localised swelling, redness, brief loss of sensation, headache, feeling generally unwell or slightly nauseous. These effects are usually confined to the site of injection, albeit they may affect adjacent muscles or other anatomical structures. The side effect of greatest concern is transient paresis or paralysis of adjacent muscles due to the spread of the toxin. In such cases, resolution generally occurs within a few weeks to months, or, in certain individuals, within weeks. The degree to which resolution occurs depends on where the injection was made, what dose was involved and which muscle is affected. In between 1 and 3% of patients, there may be transient ptosis of the superior blepharon or the brow, which occurs if toxin diffuses to the levator palpebrae superioris muscle [5].

The side effects of botulinum toxin injection as a whole are localised and eventually disappear. Nonetheless, they may have a serious adverse impact on daily activities, as may occur with drooling. The pain, slight bruise formation and risk of infection are no different from that seen with other injections. As side effects generally result from toxin spreading to adjacent structures, the patient should be cautioned against massaging the injected area.

Ptosis of the brow is a side effect which can happen if the toxin is injected in too lateral a position (i.e. lateral to the midpupillary line) or too near the supraorbital ridge. Brow ptosis may be corrected by injecting under the ptostic brow into the orbicularis muscle but usually resolves quickly. If lid ptosis is experienced because of the leavator weakness, the use of phenylephrine apraclonidine (Iopidine) ocular drops, which is helpful in augmenting the action of the leavator thus minimising the effects of ptosis, until it recovers spontaneously. If, when aiming for the orbicularis oculi muscle overlying the temples, the injection is placed too near to the blephara, the eye may close too slowly, blinking may be reduced and there may be excessive lacrimation. The face may end up appearing asymmetrical if the injections are made differently on each side, or the doses differ. To avoid the development of drooling, an injection site should be chosen away from the lips [7].

Where ptosis does develop, it usually persists for between 2 and 6 weeks. Eye drops containing apraclonidine 0.5% are suitable for treatment. This agent acts on alpha-adrenoceptors on the superior tarsal muscle and causes the superior eyelid to rise upon application of the drug. The degree of elevation ranges from 1 to 3 mm.

Treatment is one or two drops three times a day for the period that ptosis persists. However, ptosis should not occur if the injection site is 1 cm superior to the eyebrow and no further laterally than the midpupillary line. Apraclonidine may not be used if the patient has a known hypersensitivity. The alternative treatment is phenylephrine 2.5% [5].

Paresis may develop in the inferior blepharon or the lateral rectus muscle when the lateral orbicularis muscle is injected with botulinum toxin. Where inferior blepharal paresis is of severe degree, there is the risk of exposure keratitis. Paresis of the lateral rectus may result in diplopia. Treatment consists of palliation [5].

In cases where botulinum toxin is being used to treat torticollis, there is a risk of difficulty swallowing if the toxin leaks into the oropharynx. This side effect is typically transient, lasting at most a few days or weeks. However, in certain cases, a soft diet will be needed. Whilst dysphagia alone does not indicate systemic toxic effects of botulinum, where this is of high severity, the patient may potentially aspirate food into the airways. In certain individuals, the cervical muscles may be weak, which may be observed as the patient tries to lift his/her head when lying down [5].

A further localised side effect can be contusion, which is especially likely if the needle passes through a small vein or the patient is taking non-steroidal anti-inflammatory drugs (NSAIDs), including aspirin or vitamin E. Where feasible, these medications should be paused for a fortnight before injection of botulinum toxin. Whilst headaches are also seen following Botox, it seems, on the basis of a study carried out by Carruthers et al. [8], that the rate is the same as with placebo. Thus, headaches probably arise because of the injection itself, rather than being caused by botulinum toxin per se, which has a very favourable safety profile overall.

Botulinum toxin has the potential to cause systemic side effects. Although there are reports of headaches, these generally last only briefly. So far, there are no reports of patients exhibiting hypersensitivity. However, there are reports indicating that antibodies do develop to the toxin in some cases where it is used at a high dose, such as in therapy for torticollis or dysphonia. Once these antibodies arise, treatment resistance develops [9]. In a single case, a patient with immunodeficiency developed necrotising fasciitis following botulinum toxin injection [10].

In procedures used to treat hyperhidrosis, local anaesthetics may be utilised, which may result in complications such as paralysis of certain muscles. Patients may be alarmed if they are briefly unable to use their hands properly [1].

In theory, an overdose of toxin could occur if there is inadvertent injection of too high a dose or the toxin is swallowed. Where this is suspected, there needs to be clinical observation lasting potentially a few weeks to identify early signs of paralysis of systemic paresis. If it is definitely established that an overdose has occurred, an antidote is available, although this agent cannot reverse paralysis that has already occurred [1].

9.7 Outcome and Prognosis

Once botulinum toxin has been injected, it is necessary to wait before any effect can be observed. Usually, the full effect is noted between 3 and 7 days postinjection, and it peaks at approximately 1 month. The improvement in rhytides persists for 4–6 months, after which they gradually start becoming visible once more [1].

There is a cumulative effect from repeated injections of the toxin, such that the effect lasts longer with each round of treatment. There is possibility that the muscles targeted will atrophy after a number of repeated injections. Where this occurs, the rhytides usually permanently disappear.

A photographic record taken prior to the first injection and then at follow-up appointments is useful to demonstrate how effective the procedure has been [1].

When cases of hyperhidrosis are treated with botulinum toxin injection, the results are generally very satisfying. This improvement may be shown definitively to have occurred by reperforming the iodine test for the presence of starch. For hyperhidrosis, the treatment interval ranges between 4 and 6 months [1].

It has been proven that treating patients suffering from social anxiety disorder and hyperhidrosis with botulinum toxin has a beneficial effect on both social function and the general level of disability of the patient [11].

There have been trials recently comparing onabotulinumtoxinA (Botox) with abobotulinumtoxinA (Dysport) using a split-face technique. One trial employed random treatment allocation and double blinding. The treatments compared were either 10 U of onabotulinumtoxinA or 30 U of abobotulinumtoxinA. The indication was wrinkles of the lateral orbit. It was demonstrated that Dysport was more beneficial than Botox for this indication, a result that achieved statistical significance [12].

References

1. Trizna Z. Dermatologic use of botulinum Toxin. In: Elston DM, editor. Medscape. Updated: Feb 07, 2019. https://emedicine.medscape.com/article/1126453-overview. Accessed online at April 13, 2021.
2. Jankovic J, Brin MF. Botulinum toxin: historical perspective and potential new indications. Muscle Nerve Suppl. 1997;20:129–45.
3. Marion MH, Sheehy M, Sangla S, Soulayrol S. Dose standardization of botulinum toxin. J Neurol Neurosurg Psychiatry. 1995;19:102–3.
4. Odergren T, Hjaltason H, Kaakkola S, Solders G, Hanko J, Fehling C, et al. A double blind, randomised, parallel group study to investigate the dose equivalence of Dysport® and Botox® in the treatment of cervical dystonia. J Neurol Neurosurg Psychiatry. 1998;64:6–12.
5. Nigam PK, Nigam A. Botulinum toxin. Indian J Dermatol. 2010;55(1):8–14. https://doi.org/10.4103/0019-5154.60343. PMID: 20418969; PMCID: PMC2856357
6. Brin MF, Lew MF, Adler CH, Comella CL, Factor SA, Jankovic J, et al. Safety and efficacy of NeuroBloc (botulinum toxin type B) in type A-resistant cervical dystonia. Neurology. 1999;53:1431–8.
7. Matarasso SL, Matarasso A. Treatment guidelines for botulinum toxin type a for the periocular region and a report on partial upper lip ptosis following injections to the lateral canthal rhytids. Plast Reconstr Surg. 2001;108(1):208–14. discussion 215–7

8. Carruthers JD, Lowe NJ, Menter MA, Gibson J, Eadie N Botox® Glabellar Lines II Study Group. Double-blind, placebo-controlled study of the safety and efficacy of botulinum toxin type a in patients with glabellar lines. Plast Reconstr Surg. 2003;15:1089–98.
9. Smith ME, Ford CN. Resistance to botulinum toxin injections for spasmodic dysphonia. Arch Otolaryngol Head Neck Surg. 2000 Apr;126(4):533–5.
10. Latimer PR, Hodgkins PR, Vakalis AN, Butler RE, Evans AR, Zaki GA. Necrotising fasciitis as a complication of botulinum toxin injection. Eye. 1998;12(Pt 1):51–3.
11. Connor KM, Cook JL, Davidson JR. Botulinum toxin treatment of social anxiety disorder with hyperhidrosis: a placebo-controlled double-blind trial. J Clin Psychiatry. 2006 Jan;67(1):30–6.
12. Nettar KD, Yu KC, Bapna S, Boscardin J, Maas CS. An internally controlled, double-blind comparison of the efficacy of OnabotulinumtoxinA and AbobotulinumtoxinA. Arch Facial Plast Surg. 2011 Nov;13(6):380–6.

Botulinum Toxin Injections: Forehead 10

Gozde Gunay, Felicia Manole, and Jarrod Keeler

10.1 Introduction

Injected botulinum toxin enjoys widespread application as a treatment for rhytides caused by excessive contraction of facial muscles. A number of studies have shown that botulinum toxin can be safely and effectively used on the upper face as a way to remove wrinkles [1–3]. So long as this agent is employed in an appropriate manner, it is rare for complications to occur, and there are no reports indicating either persistent or potentially fatal side effects stemming from its use in aesthetic procedures [4, 5].

With advancing age, rhytides may start to be visible in the frontoglabellar region. If an individual tends to frown a lot, or the muscles in this region are especially active, rhytides tend to appear, even from a young age. The degree of wrinkles correlates with how active the muscles of the upper facial third are. If the frontalis is especially active, rhytides appear in a horizontal orientation. The corrugator supercilii muscle exerts an inferomedial pull on the skin, thus hyperactivity of this muscle results in the formation of wrinkles in an oblique or vertical orientation. Meanwhile, contraction of the procerus draws the glabellofrontal skin downwards, hyperactivity then leading to rhytides overlying the nasal radix and orientated horizontally. As the condition progresses, the muscular fascial covering shrinks and thus wrinkles remain even in the absence of muscular contraction [6–8].

G. Gunay (✉)
Department of Otorhinolaryngology, Seyrantepe Hamidiye Etfal State Hospital, İstanbul, Türkiye

F. Manole
Faculty of Medicine, Department of ENT, University of Oradea, Oradea, Romania

J. Keeler
Otolaryngology & Facial Plastic and Reconstructive Surgery, Specialty Physician Associates, St. Luke's Medical Center, Bethlehem, PA, USA

C. Cingi et al. (eds.), *Minor Interventions, Major Outcomes on the Face*, Comprehensive ENT, https://doi.org/10.1007/978-3-032-01305-7_10

The injection of botulinum toxin to diminish rhytides in this region presents few difficulties and typically produces satisfactory results. If there are also glabellar rhytides present, the underlying muscles may also be injected with the toxin [9].

Yeilding and Fezza [10] conducted a trial in which Botox® (onabotulinumtoxinA) or Xeomin® (incobotulinumtoxinA) were used for the treatment of dynamic rhytides in the upper facial third (i.e. glabellar lines, crow's feet or forehead wrinkles). These agents were both demonstrated to be safe and effective, although Botox, at the doses employed in the trial, had superior efficacy at 3 days, 2 weeks, 3 months and 4 months postinjection [10].

The initial report on the use of botulinum toxin serotype A dates from 1993 and is by Blitzer et al [11] Since then, there have been several trials which indicated the efficacy of the type A toxin on rhytides on the superior facial third [12–14]. This procedure is suitable to perform on outpatients and is well tolerated by most patients. The patient does not need to convalesce following injection. The appropriate dose can be achieved through titrating the dose against response. There have been no persistent complications reported in cases treated with botulinum toxin for blepharospasm or dystonia affecting the cervical or head muscles [15, 16]. The clinical benefit persists for between 4 and 6 months, but can be prolonged by repeated administrations of the agent [6].

10.2 Anatomy

The frontalis muscle is a two-bellied muscle found in the anterior scalp region. It is quadrilateral in form. Its origin is the galea aponeurotica, located in the line of the coronal suture, or anterior to it. It inserts into the muscle fibres in the glabellar region. The frontalis fibres on the medial aspect interdigitate with those of the procerus, and the intermediate fibres interdigitate with those of the corrugator supercilii or the orbicularis oculi muscles. There is a variable amount of interlacing of the two bellies of the frontalis superior to the nasal radix.

Laterally, the margin of the frontalis muscle is, in the majority of cases, close to or slightly lateral to the temporal fusion line, or the superior temporal line, which continues in the same direction [17]. The lateral margin of the muscle is somewhat oblique, with the upper part of the muscle lateral to the lower portion. The fibres are oriented vertically, and when they contract, the effect resembles a bellow spring. This contraction moves both the origin (the scalp) and the insertion (the eyebrow) at the same time, so that the net effect is that the forehead shortens [18].

Thus, the action of the frontalis is to lift the eyebrows and the frontal skin. The vertical orientation of the frontalis muscular fibres means that frontal rhytides run in a horizontal direction. The origin of the muscle lies on the galea aponeurotica in the vicinity of the coronal suture. Its insertion is the supraorbital margin and the skin of the brow. Its fibres form interdigitations with fibres of muscles which pull down on the brow, namely, the procerus, corrugator supercilii and orbicularis oculi muscles [9].

The fibres of the medial frontalis contain a greater amount of fibrous tissue than those on the lateral aspect, and accordingly, a lower dose of botulinum toxin is used on the medial than lateral portions of the muscle. If the frontalis is allowed to become completely paralysed, the supraorbital margin may undergo ptosis and the face become expressionless, therefore partial paralysis should be aimed for. There is also a danger of lateral eyebrow ptosis if the clinician injects too near to the lateral aspect of the eyebrow [9].

The superior facial third is made up of the forehead, from the nasion to the hairline in the midline (i.e. trichion). A study conducted by Farkas et al. [19, 20] noted that for men, the mean forehead height (defined as trichion to glabella) was 57 mm (range 50–64 mm), whilst for women, it was 53 mm (range 47–59 mm). Hence, if the height of the forehead does not reach 60 mm in male patients or 55 mm in females, this distance is considered undesirably short and thus a forehead lift may be indicated. The height of the forehead considered in this way fits well with the other way of deciding if forehead lift is indicated, the Mckinney criteria, according to which the operation may be indicated where the distance between the mid-pupil and the brow is less than 25 mm [21].

10.3 Clinical Application

Botulinum toxin should be injected between 4 and 5 cm superior to the rim of the orbit, which guarantees that only the superior portion of the frontalis is paralysed. This leaves the rest of the muscle, especially laterally, free to move, which allows facial expression to be preserved. Individuals who tend to raise their eyebrows or blephara commonly by contracting the frontalis muscle may find that rhytides that were not present before the procedure now appear at the point where nonparalysed fibres abut paralysed muscle. The muscles acting on the glabella may also become much more active in the medial frontal region as they too compensate for the missing contraction of the frontalis fibres [4].

Botulinum toxin serotype A has received a licence from the US FDA for the following indications: strabismus, blepharospasm, hemifacial spasm, adductor spasmodic dysphonia, oromandibular or cervical dystonia [22]. There are reports by Keen et al., as well as Blitzer et al., indicating that the toxin is both safe and efficacious in treating rhytides caused by muscular hyperactivity [11–13]. Nonetheless, at present, the use of botulinum toxin A to remedy wrinkles on the face is not licensed.

When patients are offered botulinum toxin injection for an aesthetic indication, they should be fully informed and give written consent, before the procedure is undertaken [6].

Botulinum toxin is absolutely contraindicated in cases where the patient has a documented hypersensitivity to the toxin or any excipient in the preparation intended to be used, or if the site of injection is infected. The toxin is relatively contraindicated in patients with neuromuscular diseases, for example, myasthenia gravis or Lambert-Eaton myasthenic syndrome [13], where there is abundant scarring, or if the patient has previously been treated with fillers. However, previous surgical procedures on the forehead are not a reason to avoid use of the toxin. There is a risk of potentiation with certain other medications, especially antibiotics of the aminoglycoside type [23]. Preparations of toxin marketed commercially indicate dosage in units of biological activity (IU). Botulism may present acutely in human patients who receive doses in excess of 500 IU at one time. However, the median dose causing fatality in human subjects has been calculated as 2730 IU [12].

10.4 Technique

In the USA, botulinum toxin is marketed commercially as Botox (Allergan Inc., Irvine, California, USA). This preparation is supplied in vials containing 100 IU. It requires refrigeration at minus 20 °C prior to use. To prepare the injection, the lyophilised toxin is mixed with sterile saline solution. For this use, saline that contains preservative agents should not be used. The usual volume of saline is $4cm^2$, which then gives 25 IU/mL[1]. A photographic record should be obtained at the initial appointment, and the patient should be supplied with written information about the toxin and its use. Prior to injection, the patient should provide signed, informed consent. In some centres, patients receive premedication with a sedative agent and painkiller by mouth and an anaesthetic agent may be applied topically, such as EMLA (Astra Inc., Westborough, Massachusetts, USA). It is possible to carry out the procedure with the patient sitting up or lying down [6].

If botulinum toxin injections are performed as a series of small doses, it is possible to produce weakness that falls short of complete paralysis. The way to achieve this is to inject between 3 and 5 times either side of the midline, each dose containing on average 2 IU (between 1 and 3 IU) Botox. The distance between each injection is between 1 and 2 cm. The first site should be around 1 cm superior to the eyebrow, in line with the medial canthus. Frequently, 3 injection sites are chosen on each side, and they form a "V" shape, the tops of which are close to the hairline. If required, up to three extra injections may be performed in the midline or one or two towards the lateral aspect, as indicated by the individual case [9].

If the rhytides stretch as far as the temples, injections may be placed laterally. However, no injection should be further lateral than the lateral canthus, as doing so may paralyse or weaken the temporalis muscle. It is important to inject cautiously if an individual has wrinkles which reveal muscular activity preventing ptosis of the superior blepharon [9].

When botulinum toxin is used on the superior portion of the face or around the eyes, generally speaking, it is better for the patient to be sitting up. After the injections, the patient should also not lie down for at least 2–3 h, so that toxin does not inadvertently seep through the orbital septum [9].

10.4.1 Dosage

To paralyse the frontalis muscle, some centres use a mean dose of 40 IU botulinum toxin, divided into 16 injections, each containing 2.5 IU. To avoid ptosis of the blephara from occurring, the injections should be placed no closer than a finger width from the eyebrow. For rhytides of the glabella, between 7.5 and 10 IU are injected on each side. The toxin is also an efficacious treatment for crow's feet affecting the area around the lateral canthi. In such cases, the dose applied to each side varies from 7.5 to 12.5 IU [6].

10.5 Efficacy

It generally takes between 1 and 3 days before the clinical effect from botulinum injection can be observed. These effects persist for between 2 and 6 months. It may be necessary to perform top-up injections after 10–14 days, to ensure the effect looks more natural and is symmetrical. Once it has been observed how much clinical effect was observed from the first doses, further treatments may be more accurately titrated. It has been observed clinically that, following the administration of multiple courses of treatment, the effect tends to lengthen, so that repeat treatments may occur as far apart as 9 months. The cosmetic indication (hyperfunctional rhytides) was suggested following observation of the benefit in cases with primary facial dystonias [11].

A study carried out by Keen et al. [12], which compared injection of botulinum toxin with a placebo consisting of saline and utilised double blinding, found that 9 out of 11 subjects receiving active agent experienced a significant reduction in frontal rhytides or crow's feet, evaluated by comparing both sides of the face. A report by Guyuron and Huddleson [14] noted 9 cases where botulinum toxin was successfully utilised to eliminate wrinkles.

10.6 Complications

Till date, there are no reports of serious adverse events, for example, double vision or loss of vision, in patients receiving botulinum injections for wrinkles of the face. One side effect that is sometimes seen is ptosis of the superior blepharon, which is a result of the injection being too near to the superior blepharon. However, this can generally be avoided if injections to the frontalis are at least one finger width away from the eyebrow. Besides, this ptosis is not permanent. The injection site may bleed a small amount in 1 in 10 patients, although applying pressure readily restores haemostasis. There are reports of other side effects, notably bruising or oedema, but these were of mild degree [11–14].

It is possible that hair loss may occur over the forehead when botulinum toxin of type A is repeatedly injected into the frontalis, as noted by Di Pietro and Piraccini [24].

10.7 Glabellar Rhytides

The frontalis muscle is large and thin. It adheres firmly to the overlying skin. The medial fibres coalesce in the area of the glabella and interdigitate with the procerus fibres. The muscle fibres centrally and laterally interdigitate with the corrugator supercilii and the inner portion of the orbicularis oculi. When the frontalis contracts, it elevates the eyebrows as well as the superior blepharon, which may result in wrinkles forming horizontally across the frontal region [25]. The bottom portion of this muscle (between 2.5 and 4 cm) raises the eyebrows. When this occurs for years, wrinkles begin to appear [4].

The most frequent aesthetic indication for botulinum toxin is the reduction of rhytides in the glabellar region.

10.7.1 Anatomy

Wrinkles and skin folds in the frontal region arise by repeated contraction of the depressor muscles, in particular, the corrugator supercilii, depressor supercilii, orbicularis oculi and the procerus [9].

The following muscles are responsible for vertical glabellar rhytides: corrugator supercilii, the part of the orbicularis oculi lying medially and those fibres of the depressor supercilii which have a vertical orientation [9].

The corrugator supercilii adducts the eyebrow, which results in inferomedial movement of the eyebrow. The origin of this muscle is the nasal bone at a point slightly superior to the level of the orbital rim, to which it lies medial. It extends superolaterally and the insertion is the skin in the region of mid-eyebrow. The frontalis, procerus and orbicularis oculi muscles are all superficial to the corrugator. The medial origin of the orbicularis oculi is the medial margin of the orbit, in front of where the corrugator originates. These muscle fibres form interdigitations with the other three muscles. Another muscle, the depressor supercilii, has its origin on the frontal bone, at the nasal process. Its insertion is the skin located medial to the eyebrow [9].

Frown lines which form in the glabellar region and over the nasal radix are produced by contraction of the procerus muscle, which has its origin on the superior cartilaginous portion of the nose and the inferior nasal bone. This muscle runs in an inferior-superior direction. The insertion is the skin bordered by the eyebrows and the frontal belly of the occipitofrontalis muscle. There are interdigitations with the muscle fibres of the orbicularis, frontalis and corrugator [9].

10.7.2 Technique

There are generally five points at which botulinum toxin injections are used. Injections are placed bilaterally, to include the corrugator (one on each side), the orbicularis oculi and depressor supercilii at the same time (also one each side) and a single midline injection to paralyse the procerus [9].

The dose to use depends on the particular preparation. The following gives specific advice [9]:

- OnabotulinumtoxinA (BOTOX® Cosmetic)—20 IU altogether, consisting of 5 intramuscular injections of 4 IU each time.
- AbobotulinumtoxinA (Dysport®)—50 IU altogether, consisting of five intramuscular injections of 10 IU each time.
- IncobotulinumtoxinA (Xeomin®)—20 IU altogether, consisting of five intramuscular injections of 4 IU each time.
- PrabotulinumtoxinA (Jeuveau®)—20 IU altogether, consisting of five intramuscular injections of 4 IU each time.

The first step is to get the patient to frown and scowl, so that palpation of the appropriate muscles is possible. The first muscle to be injected is the corrugator. The injection occurs where the muscle originates slightly superior to the medial canthus and the supraorbital ridge. The needle is introduced until the tip encounters bone, after which the clinician should withdraw the needle a slight distance. The tip can be advanced in a superolateral direction, following the muscular belly until it reaches the medial superciliary third. This is 1 cm above the supraorbital margin. The injection occurs as the needle is being gradually taken out [9].

The second place to inject is a spot approximately 10 mm superior to the medial aspect of the superciliary arch. The injecting needle passes vertically, pointing towards the hairline. As the needle is being withdrawn, the botulinum toxin may be injected into the orbicularis oculi and depressor supercilii muscles. When one side of the forehead is complete, proceed to the other side [9].

Once the forehead has been injected bilaterally, the final injection targets the belly of the procerus muscle, with the aim of removing dynamic wrinkles with a horizontal orientation occurring over the nasal radix. To find the centre of the nasal radix, a line may be drawn on both sides at 45 degrees to the midline, starting from the medial pole of the eyebrows. These lines will cross at the desired location, slightly above a line connecting the two medial canthi. In male patients, there is a risk that the eyebrow may appear excessively arched, so a further injection may be required to compensate for this. In such cases, inject toxin 10 mm superior to the superciliary arch, at the midpoint of the eyebrow (Figs. 10.1, 10.2, and 10.3) [9].

Hankins et al., in their 1998 trial involving 46 female patients being treated for rhytides of the glabella, report that the dose needed when using Botox was between 2.5 and 4 IU for each injection. Thus, the total dose will range from 12.5 to 20 IU [26].

The "spread test" is a useful procedure to gain an insight into how effective botulinum toxin may be in removing glabellar rhytides. This is performed by spreading the rhytides apart with the thumb and second digit. If the patient has skin that is thick and sebaceous, or there are deep scars, and the spread test does not change the appearance much, botulinum toxin is likely to offer minimal benefit. However, if the

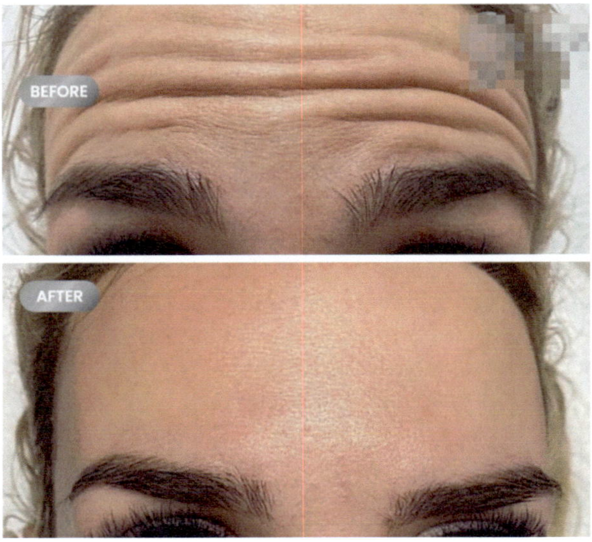

Fig. 10.1 Case 1: Botulinum toxin injection to forehead, before and after view. (Courtesy of Murat Songu MD)

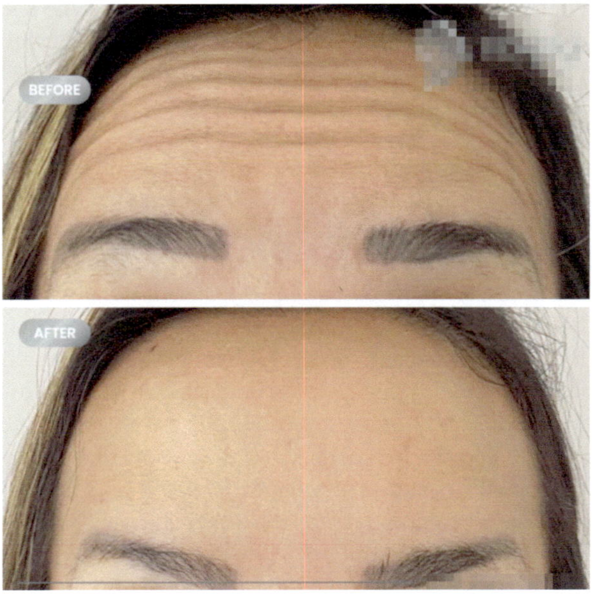

Fig. 10.2 Case 2: Botulinum toxin injection to forehead, before and after view. (Courtesy of Murat Songu MD)

first attempt at solving the issue through injections proves disappointing, electromyography potentially offers a more precise way to identify the target musculature [9].

In certain cases, there is a possibility of medial fibre recruitment from the midbrow, usually because the orbicularis oculi muscle fibres slightly inferior to the mid-eyebrow are overly active. In these individuals, botulinum toxin injection may produce an undesirable result, with the medial and lateral portion of the brow exhibiting ptosis [27].

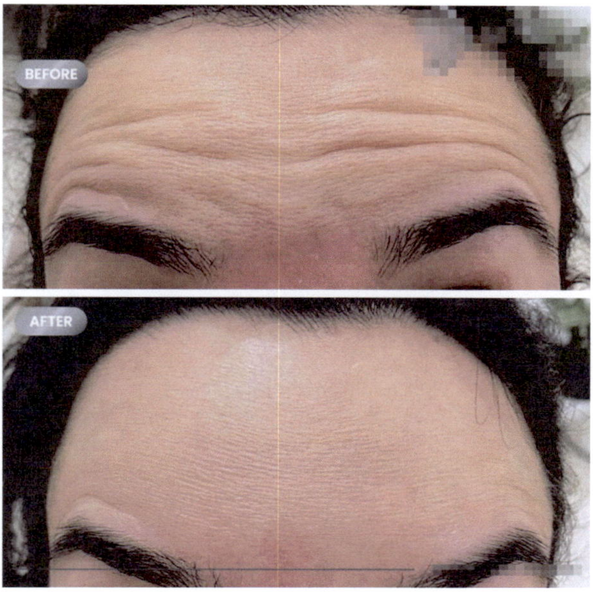

Fig. 10.3 Case 3: Botulinum toxin injection to forehead, before and after view. (Courtesy of Murat Songu MD)

Recently, trial data have shown that removal of rhytides of the glabella calls for three injections, encompassing the procerus and corrugator muscles. When five rather than three injections were performed frontally, there was no significant additional benefit [28].

It has also been shown that removing rhytides in the area of the glabella using botulinum toxin can make a person more easily appear happy and relaxed [29].

References

1. Carruthers A, Carruthers J, Cohen J. A prospective, doubleblind, randomized, parallel- group, dose-ranging study of botulinum toxin type a in female subjects with horizontal forehead rhytides. Dermatologic Surg. 2003;29:461–7.
2. Carruthers JA, Lowe NJ, Menter MA, Gibson J, Nordquist M, Mordaunt J, et al. A multicenter, double-blind, randomized, placebo-controlled study of the efficacy and safety of botulinum toxin type a in the treatment of glabellar lines. J Am Acad Dermatol. 2002;46:840–9.
3. Carruthers JA, Lowe NJ, Menter MA, Gibson J, Nordquist M, Mordaunt J, et al. One-year, randomized, multicenter, two period study of the safety and efficacy of repeated treatments with botulinum toxin type a in patients with glabellar lines. J Clin Res. 2004;7:1–20.
4. Kang SM, Feneran A, Kim JK, Park O, Kim JE, Won CH, Chang S, Lee MW, Choi JH, Moon KC, Youn CS, Cho S, Lee SH. Exaggeration of wrinkles after botulinum toxin injection for forehead horizontal lines. Ann Dermatol. 2011 May;23(2):217–21.
5. Hambleton P, Moore AP. Botulinum neurotoxins: origin, structure, molecular actions and antibodies. In: Moore P, editor. Handbook of botulinum toxin treatment. 1st ed. Oxford: Blackwell Science; 1995. p. 16–27.
6. Khosh MM, Keen MS. Botulinum toxin a injection for forehead rhytids. Oper Tech Otolaryngol Head Neck Surg. 1995;6(4):324–6.
7. Pitanguy I. Indications for the treatment of frontal and glabellar wrinkles in the analysis of 3,404 consecutive cases of rhytidectomy. Plast Reconstr Surg. 1981;67:157–68.

8. Adamson PA, Johnson CM, Anderson JR, et al. The forehead lift: a review. Arch Otolaryngol. 1985;111:325–9.
9. Hauser RA. Botulinum toxin injections in plastic surgery. de la Torre JI, editor. Medscape. Updated: Feb 08, 2019. https://emedicine.medscape.com/article/1271380-overview#a3. Accessed online at 13 Apr 2021.
10. Yeilding RH, Fezza JP. A prospective, Split-face, randomized, double-blind study comparing OnabotulinumtoxinA to IncobotulinumtoxinA for upper face wrinkles. Plast Reconstr Surg. 2015 May;135(5):1328–35.
11. Blitzer A, Brin MF, Keen MS, Aviv JE. Botulinum toxin for the treatment of hyperfunctional lines of the face. Arch Otolaryngol Head Neck Surg. 1993;119(9):1018–22. https://doi.org/10.1001/archotol.1993.01880210108015.
12. Keen MS, Bhtzer A, Aviv JE. Botulinum toxin A for hyperkanetic facial lines. Results of a double-blind, placebo controlled study. Plast Reconstr Surg. 1994;94:94–9.
13. Keen MS, Blltzer A, Binder WJ, et al. The management of hyperfunctional facial lines with botulinum toxin: a collaborative study of 210 lnjectton sites in 162. In: Patients presented at the academy of facial plastic and reconstructive surgery meeting. Minneapolis; 1993.
14. Guyuron B, Huddleston SW. Aesthetic indications for botulinum toxin injections. Plast Reconstr Surg. 1994;93:913–8.
15. Borodlc GE. Ferranter: Orblcularis muscle histology after repetitive injections of botuhnum toxin A. Atlanta: Presented at the annual meeting of the American Academy of Ophthalmology; 1990.
16. Lang DH, et al. Distal effects of locally injected botulinum toxin. Incidences and course. Adv Neurol. 1988;50:609–13.
17. Knize DM. An anatomically based study of the mechanism of eyebrow ptosis. Plast Reconstr Surg. 1996;97(7):1321–33.
18. Cohen S, Artzi O, Heller L. Forehead lift using botulinum toxin. Aesthet Surg J. 2018;38(3):312–20.
19. Farkas LG, Katic MJ, Forrest CR, et al. International anthropometric study of facial morphology in various ethnic groups/races. J Craniofac Surg. 2005;16(4):615–46.
20. Farkas LG, Kolar JC. Anthropometrics and art in the aesthetics of women's faces. Clin Plast Surg. 1987;14(4):599–616.
21. McKinney P, Mossie RD, Zukowski ML. Criteria for the forehead lift. Aesth Plast Surg. 1991;15(2):141–7.
22. National Institute of health consensus development conference clinical use of botulinum toxin, 1990; 8:1–20.
23. Wang YC, Burr DH, Korthals GJ, et al. Acute toyacity of ammoglycoside antibiotics as an aid in detecting botulism. Appl Environ Microbiol. 1984;48:951–5.
24. Di Pietro A, Piraccini BM. Frontal Alopecia after repeated Botulinum Toxin Type A injections for forehead wrinkles: an underestimated entity? Skin Appendage Disord. 2016;2(1–2):67–9. https://doi.org/10.1159/000448380. Epub 2016 Aug 5. PMID: 27843928; PMCID: PMC5096242
25. Ascher B, Talarico S, Cassuto D, Escobar S, Hexsel D, Jaén P, et al. International consensus recommendations on the aesthetic usage of botulinum toxin type A (Speywood unit)- Part I: upper facial wrinkles. J Eur Acad Dermatol Venereol. 2010;24:1278–84.
26. Hankins CL, Strimling R, Rogers GS. Botulinum A toxin for glabellar wrinkles. Dose and response. Dermatol Surg. 1998;24(11):1181–3.
27. Beer K, Cohen JL, Carruthers A. Cosmetic uses of botulinum toxin. Ward AB, Barnes MP. Clinical uses of botulinum toxin. Cambridge, MA: Cambridge University Press; 2007.
28. Rzany B, Ascher B, Fratila A, Monheit GD, Talarico S, Sterry W. Efficacy and safety of 3- and 5-injection patterns (30 and 50 U) of botulinum toxin A (Dysport) for the treatment of wrinkles in the glabella and the central forehead region. Arch Dermatol. 2006;142(3):320–6.
29. Charles Finn J, Cox SE, Earl ML. Social implications of hyperfunctional facial lines. Dermatologic Surg. 2003 May;29(5):450–5.

Botulinum Toxin Injections: Periorbital Region

11

Elvin Alaskarov, Cemal Cingi, Shriya Airen, and Jarrod Keeler

11.1 Introduction

The changes in facial appearance that reveal aging involve alterations in the pigmentation of the skin, a loss of dermal elasticity, the appearance of wrinkles and loss of facial volume [1, 2]. Due to particular characteristics of the tissues that surround the eye, the periorbital area is one where features of aging are especially likely to be present. One significant factor is that the skin overlying the blephara is extremely thin, only 0.3 to 0.5 mm thick. Only in a few other regions is such thin skin seen [3]. The blepharal skin lacks subcutaneous fat, which may disguise any eyelid irregularity and compensate for prolapsed adipose tissue, which often appears as patients grow older. The delicate nature of the skin in this region means it is somewhat transparent, so pigmentation (whether of the skin or from circulating molecules), muscle alterations and blood vessels may all appear on the eyelid. The dermis contains fewer collagen and elastin fibres than elsewhere in the body; thus, this region is more susceptible to damage, including the development of wrinkles. Furthermore, the blepharal skin and the skin around the eyes move a great deal, with the muscles of facial expression, such as the corrugator, orbicularis oculi and

E. Alaskarov
Esenler Hospital, Department of Otorhinolaryngology, Medipol University, Istanbul, Turkey

C. Cingi (✉)
Eskisehir Osmangazi University, Medical Faculty, Department of Otorhinolaryngology, Eskisehir, Türkiye
e-mail: cemal@ogu.edu.tr

S. Airen · J. Keeler
Otolaryngology & Facial Plastic and Reconstructive Surgery, Specialty Physician Associates, St. Luke's Medical Center, Bethlehem, PA, USA
e-mail: shriya.airen@sluhn.org

C. Cingi et al. (eds.), *Minor Interventions, Major Outcomes on the Face*, Comprehensive ENT, https://doi.org/10.1007/978-3-032-01305-7_11

procerus, exerting a force on it virtually continuously. This may explain why rhytides develop early in this region of the face [4].

Alongside the propensity to ageing due to the anatomical characteristics outlined above, this region is also prone to external factors which makes ageing occur at an earlier age. Exposure to sunlight is a key factor and may cause deep wrinkles to form, excessive pigmentation to be deposited and the skin to resemble leather [2]. Patients generally fail to protect their eyelids when they go out in the sun, even when they use sunscreen elsewhere on exposed areas. Ultraviolet light exposure leads to the production of oxygen-containing free radicals, and this eventually leads to collagenous degradation and reduced expression of new collagen in the skin. A further key contributor to ageing of the skin, and one that is modifiable, is smoking. Like over exposure to ultraviolet light, smoking also stimulates free radical formation, with similar downstream consequences [4–6].

11.2 Anatomy

It is vital that clinicians have a firm grasp of the anatomy of the eyebrows and eyelids to be able to utilise botulinum toxin effectively in cosmetic indications. This agent is of benefit both in reducing rhytides and for face lifts or realignment of structures. The musculature acting on the brows can separated into a group of elevator muscles and one of depressor muscles. If either the elevators or depressors are paralysed, the pull of the other group will encounter minimal resistance and a structure may move in a particular direction [7]. Soft tissue structures may become malpositioned when their supporting ligaments are weakened through the prolonged action of muscles, or potentially arise through the structure becoming exposed or being acted upon by gravitational forces. Whilst there may be considerable similarity in the exact anatomical form in two cases, there are usually at least some respects in which they differ. Thus, aesthetic procedures based on chemically mediated paralysis need to take into account the anatomical variations that may exist and the potentially different doses required [8].

The only muscle which acts to elevate the brow is the frontalis. When this muscle contracts, it may lead to horizontally oriented wrinkles overlying the forehead. The fibres of the frontalis at the lower pole form interdigitations with the muscles which depress the brow, in particular, the procerus, corrugator, depressor supercilii and the orbicularis oculi on its lateral aspect. The procerus muscle is medial and low down below the brow. When it contracts, horizontally oriented wrinkles may form over the bridge of the nose, referred to colloquially as "bunny lines." The corrugator and depressor supercilii muscles also lie medially and under the supraorbital ridge. Contraction of this pair of muscles may lead to frown lines, that is, vertically oriented rhytides in the glabellar region. The depressor originates at the frontal process of the nasal bone and is at greater depth than the corrugator. Thus, it may not be adequately paralysed if botulinum toxin is injected at too shallow a depth [9]. The orbicularis oculi muscle has three portions, that is, the pretarsal, preseptal and orbital portions. The first (pretarsal) portion is located just superior to the tarsal plate. It is responsible for subconscious blinking. This portion of the muscle has a limited effect on the formation of rhytides or malposition of soft tissues. The preseptal part wraps around the pretarsal portion of the muscle. It permits blinking and the lids to close gently. The levator palpebrae and Müller muscles have the opposite action. The final part of the muscle (outermost orbital) contracts forcefully to close the eyelids. The upper part of this portion of the muscle depresses the brow, and its contraction may produce crow's feet (wrinkles around the eyes). At the same time, this portion of the muscle raises the inferior eyelid. When the orbital portion of the orbicularis oculi contracts, it may give rise to wrinkles around the lateral canthi and the inferior blepharon. The muscle may hypertrophy over the inferior blepharon and weaken laterally and in the area of the canthi [10]. Both the levator palpebrae and Müller muscle elevate the superior blepharon. Meanwhile, another muscle of facial expression, the zygomaticus major, draws the corners of the mouth upwards and to the side, or in a posterior direction, when the patient laughs or smiles. If this muscle pulls sufficiently strongly, radial wrinkles will be more evident and soft tissue may gather around the lateral canthi.

Thus, to conclude, an appreciation of the anatomical configuration of the facial muscles is a prerequisite for a clinician to be able to utilise botulinum toxin effectively and with minimal risk to remedy cosmetic defects of the blephara and brow [34]. (Fig. 11.1).

11.3 Botulinum Neurotoxin (BoNT)

Botulinum neurotoxin (BoNT) is an exotoxin normally expressed by *Clostridium botulinum*. This organism is a bacillary bacterial anaerobe which stains positively on Gram staining and is capable of producing spores. BoNT causes botulism, which is the systemic form of botulinum toxin poisoning. At present, no more potent toxin in humans than BoNT is known [11, 12].

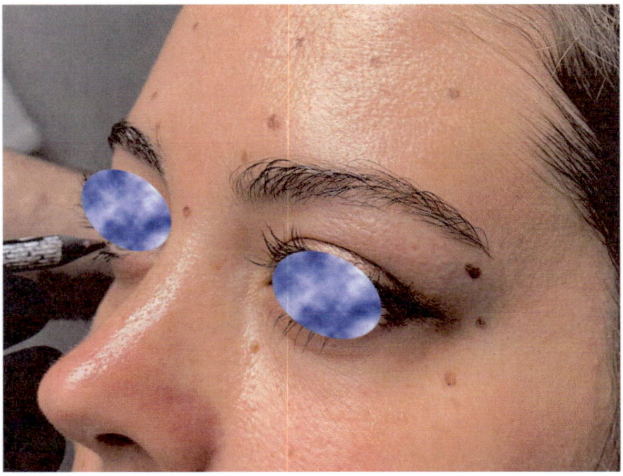

Fig. 11.1 Marking for periorbital injections. (Courtesy of Murat Songu MD)

There are seven serotypic variants of *C. botulinum*, types A through G, which differ in their antigenic profiles. The neurotoxin secreted by each subtype differs in molecular mass, the lightest having a mass of 300 kDa, whereas the heaviest is around 900 kDa. The toxin consists of a light chain, with a molecular mass of 50 kDa, bound by disulfide bridges to a heavy chain of mass 100 kDa [10]. Botulism may result from types A, B, E, F or G [13]. The toxin with the highest potency is type A, and this is the variant which is used with the highest frequency in commercial applications. The mechanism by which it exerts its toxic effect is inhibition of acetylcholine secretion into the synaptic cleft. However, acetylcholine is not the sole neurotransmitter which is blocked by BoNT—it also interferes with noradrenergic, dopaminergic, serotonergic and GABAergic transmission, as well as blocking the release of glycine and met-enkephalin [14].

11.4 Application

There are reports indicating benefit from local anaesthesia and ice packs at the time of BoNT injection. To calculate the dose required, both the area of the body involved and the specific muscle(s) to be paralysed need to be borne in mind. The mass of the muscle needs to be taken into account. Male patients tend to have a greater muscle mass than female patients; thus, the number of units needed may increase. The degree to which a muscle is able to contract helps to guide the dose chosen [15]. An injection technique that places the toxin more superficially makes bruising less likely, potentially increases efficacy of the toxin and causes less haemorrhage. It also means that the toxin may spread more evenly over the muscle it is intended to immobilise. If the muscle is bulky and more deeply located, it may be preferable to target the belly of the muscle, even though this carries an additional risk of bruising, loss of toxin by haemorrhage and a less uniform inhibition of the action of muscle fibres [16].

BoNT is now routinely offered in cosmetic indications to replace surgery for vertically oriented rhytides of the glabella, horizontally oriented deep wrinkles of the frontal region and crow's feet around the lateral canthi. An alternative to the conventional ways to treat wrinkles around the eyes, BoNT may be injected subdermally to remediate wrinkles of the inferior blepharon. The injection site is the lateral preseptal portion of the inferior blepharon and the dose needed is low—1 IU in 0.1 mL saline [17]. The bunching up of soft tissue that can occur in the region of the lateral canthus when the zygomaticus major contracts can also be treated with BoNT, as reported by Fagien and Brandt [17]. Where there are periocular rhytides and redundant soft tissue, this can be rectified by injecting 2.5 IU (i.e. low dose) in the region of the mid or lateral malar eminence. Performed in this way, the risk of paralysing the superior lip is minimised [34].

11.5 Periorbital Rhytides (Crow's Feet)

The orbicularis oculi encircles the eye in a lateral direction. As the lateral portion of the muscle contracts, rhytides may be seen radiating outward from a focus at the lateral canthus [18].

Periorbital rhytides are frequently caused by ageing and solar exposure. The rationale for using onabotulinumtoxinA to remediate periorbital wrinkles is that muscular hyperactivity may be contributing to the problem [18].

Crow's feet appear when an individual smiles. They are dynamic rhytides that arise from the contractile activity of the orbicularis oculi muscle. The injection site is placed 10 mm to the side of the orbital lateral margin, so as to prevent inadvertent paralysis of the lateral rectus muscle caused by diffusion of BoNT into adjacent structures [19]. (Fig. 11.2).

The efficacy of using either Botox 12 IU or Dysport 30–36 IU in total, as three divided doses, has been shown in trials [20, 21]. The site injected is key to success: overly superior to the lateral orbital margin and there is the risk of ptosis of the upper blepharon; whereas too inferior an injection site may cause the zygomaticus muscle to become paralysed and the lips to appear asymmetrical (in other words, labial ptosis) [22].

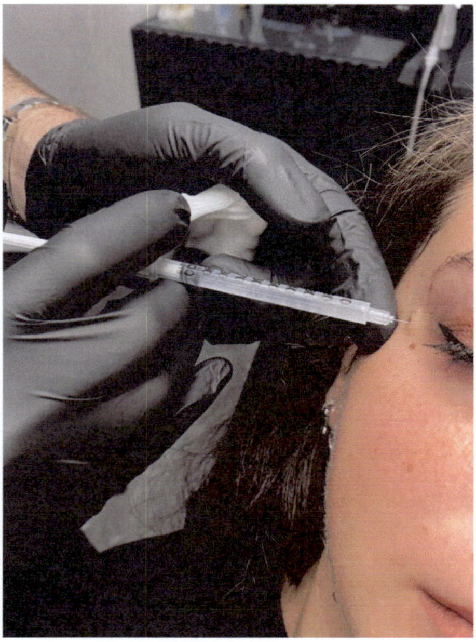

Fig. 11.2 Injection for crow's feet. (Courtesy of Murat Songu MD)

11.5.1 Technique

OnabotulinumtoxinA is injected subcutaneously at 3 or 4 sites 10 mm lateral to the lateral margin of the orbit. Each injection contains between 2 and 3 IU; thus, 6–12 IU are injected in total on each side. The distance between injection sites should be between 5 and 10 mm, and they may form a straight, vertically oriented line, or be a gentle curve. If the dose is excessive or the site is located too far medially, blepharal ptosis or double vision may develop [8, 18] (Figs. 11.2, 11.3, and 11.4).

11.6 Benign Essential Blepharospasm

Essential blepharospasm refers to a dystonic condition of the skull which is focused on the eyelids and muscles of the forehead. The characteristic feature of this disorder is frequently occurring contraction of the orbicularis oculi muscle, which the patient cannot control, and leads to the eyes being tightly closed. As the contraction of the muscle cannot be prevented by the patient, he or she may become functionally blind, with severe consequences both in terms of daily life and occupational fitness [24]. The disorder is more frequent in women than men, [25] and symptoms in females are more severe. In other respects, however, the disorder presents identically in both sexes [26].

The toxin is placed just under the skin, to diffuse into the orbicularis oculi muscle. The usual choice of injection site is medially and laterally in the preseptal portion of the orbicularis oculi muscle, within the superior and inferior blephara, which

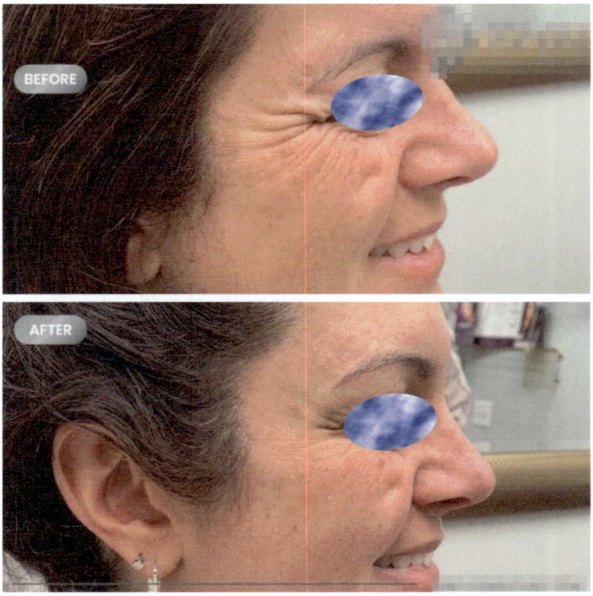

Fig. 11.3 Preinjection and postinjection (female patient). (Courtesy of Murat Songu MD)

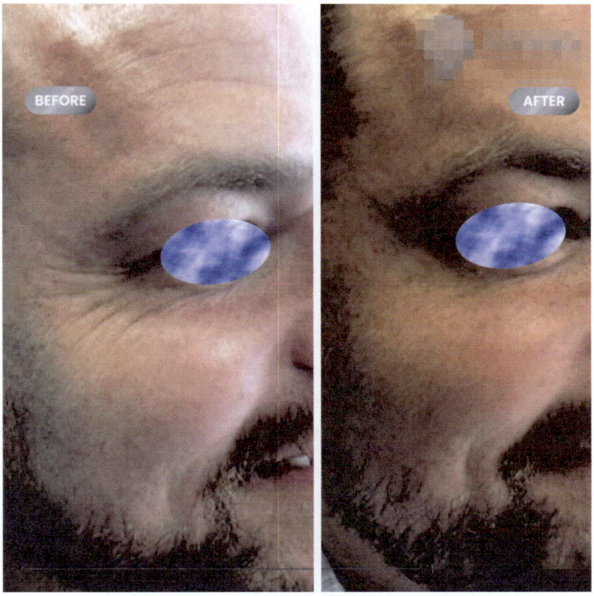

Fig. 11.4 Preinjection and postinjection (male patient). (Courtesy of Murat Songu MD)

makes ptosis unlikely to occur. Typically, the dose range for each side is Botox 12.5 to 25 IU or Dysport 50–100 IU [27].

11.7 Hemifacial Spasm

Hemifacial spasm is a condition in which half of the face undergoes repeated muscular contractions of a tonic or clonic type. The affected muscles are those controlled by the seventh cranial nerve. The condition generally begins in a patient's forties or fifties and affects one side only. A differentiating feature from blepharospasm is that hemifacial spasm is seen even when the patient is asleep. There are rare instances where hemifacial spasm is seen on both sides of the face simultaneously [27].

Treatment consists of injection with Botox 25–35 IU [28, 29] or Dysport 47–92 IU [30–32]. There have been studies which looked at the long-term outcomes of treatment with botulinum toxin serotype A.

11.8 Superior Blepharal Retraction

Superior blepharal retraction can be treated short term using BoNT. When 2.5–10 IU toxin was injected transconjunctivally at a level slightly superior to the superior margin of the tarsus into the muscular complex consisting of the levator and Müller muscle, the height of the palpebral fissure returned temporarily to a more normal level [33–35]. The safety and efficacy of treating eyelid retraction with 20 IU

Dysport was discussed by Salour et al [36] The injection was made at the midpoint of the upper margin of the tarsus and targeted the levator aponeurosis and Müller muscle. In treating this condition, a mild degree of ptosis and double vision may occur.

11.9 Lacrimal Gland Hypersecretion

Gustatory lacrimation, sometimes referred to as crocodile tears syndrome, is where taste sensation triggers excessive lacrimation. It is an autonomic synkinesis syndrome. The cause is frequently unknown or may be due to faulty reinnervation occurring after a facial palsy of traumatic type. In such cases, the facial or glossopharyngeal nerves are the nerves implicated. In a minority of cases, treatment is needed, and for this purpose, botulinum toxin A has proven efficacy [37]. This is accomplished by injecting 2.5 IU of Botox transconjunctivally directly into the palpebral lobe of the lacrimal gland. The benefit persists for 6 months [38, 39].

11.10 Contraindications

Botulinum toxin is not suitable in pregnant patients as the FDA considers it a category C agent. The level of secretion into breast milk is not known; thus, it should also be avoided in nursing mothers. The other situations in which the agent is contraindicated are as follows: a patient below the age of 12 years; known hypersensitivity to toxin or any of the excipients; patients with bleeding disorders and those with neuromuscular disorders, such as myasthenia gravis, multiple sclerosis or Lambert-Eaton syndrome [23, 33].

References

1. Coleman SR, Grover R. The anatomy of the aging face: volume loss and changes in 3-dimensional topography. Aesthet Surg J. 2006;26:S4–9.
2. Helfrich YR, Sachs DL, Voorhees JJ. Overview of skin aging and photoaging. Dermatol Nurs. 2008;20:177–83. quiz 84
3. Ha RY, Nojima K, Adams WP Jr, Brown SA. Analysis of facial skin thickness: defining the relative thickness index. Plast Reconstr Surg. 2005;115:1769–73.
4. Lee WW, Levitt AE. Periocular rejuvenation with neurotoxin and dermal filler. Plast Aesthet Res. 2018;5:43. https://doi.org/10.20517/2347-9264.2018.39.
5. Keaney TC. Aging in the male face: intrinsic and extrinsic factors. Dermatologic Surg. 2016;42:797–803.
6. Morita A. Tobacco smoke causes premature skin aging. J Dermatol Sci. 2007;48:169–75.
7. Blitzer A, Binder WJ. Cosmetic uses of botulinum neurotoxin type A: an overview. Arch Facial Plast Surg. 2002;4:214–20.
8. Balikian RV, Zimbler MS. Primary and adjunctive uses of botulinum toxin type A in the periorbital region. Otolaryngol Clin N Am. 2007 Apr;40(2):291–303.

9. Chen AH, Frankel AS. Altering brow contour with botulinum toxin. Facial Plast Surg Clin North Am. 2003;11(4):457–64.
10. Fagien S. Botulinum toxin type A for facial aesthetic enhancement: role in facial shaping. Plast Reconstr Surg. 2003;112(5):6S–18S.
11. Başar E, Arıcı C. Use of Botulinum neurotoxin in ophthalmology. Turk J Ophthalmol. 2016;46(6):282–90. https://doi.org/10.4274/tjo.57701. Epub 2016 Dec 1. PMID: 28050326; PMCID: PMC5177786
12. Dhaked RK, Singh MK, Singh P, Gupta P. Botulinum toxin: bioweapon & magic drug. Indian J Med Res. 2010;132:489–503.
13. Dowell VR. Botulism and tetanus: selected epidemiologic and microbiologic aspects. Rev Infect Dis. 1984;6(Suppl 1):202–7.
14. Maio M. Therapeutic uses of botulinum toxin: from facial palsy to autonomic disorders. Expert Opin Biol Ther. 2008;8:791–8.
15. Carruthers J, Fagien S, Matarasso SL. Consensus recommendations on the use of botulinum toxin type A in facial aesthetics. Plast Reconstr Surg. 2004;114(6 Suppl):1S–22S.
16. Choi JC, Lucarelli MJ, Shore JW. Use of botulinum toxin in patients with high risk of wound complications following eyelid reconstruction. Ophthalmic Plast Reconstr Surg. 1997;13:259.
17. Fagien S, Brandt FS. Primary and adjunctive use of botulinum toxin typeA(Botox) in facial surgery. Clin Plast Surg. 2001;28:127.
18. Hauser RA. Botulinum Toxin Injections in Plastic Surgery. de la Torre JI, editor. Medscape. Updated: Feb 08, 2019. https://emedicine.medscape.com/article/1271380-overview#a3. Accessed online at 13 Apr 2021.
19. Terzioğlu A, Tuncalı D, Barutçu AY, Başer NT, Aslan G. Botulinum toxin A: cosmetic use and literature review. Türk Plast Rekonstr ve Est Cer Derg. 2005;13:185–90.
20. Ascher B, Rzany BJ, Grover R. Efficacy and safety of botulinum toxin type A in the treatment of lateral crow's feet: double-blind, placebo-controlled, dose-ranging study. Dermatologic Surg. 2009;35:1478–86. (PubMed) (Google Scholar)
21. Prager W, Wissmuller E, Kollhorst B, Boer A, Zschocke I. Treatment of crow's feet with two different botulinum toxin type A preparations in split-face technique. Hautarzt. 2011;62:375–9.
22. Matarasso SL, Matarasso A. Treatment guidelines for botulinum toxin type A for the periocular region and a report on partial upper lip ptosis following injections to the lateral canthal rhytids. Plast Reconstr Surg. 2001;108:208–14.
23. Klein AW. Complications and adverse reactions with the use of botulinum toxin. Semin Cutan Med Surg. 2001;20:109–20.
24. Başar E, Pazarlı H, Kayıran A. Chemical denervation for the treatment of functional blindness due to essential blepharospasm. Cerrahpaşa J Med. 2003;34:24–7.
25. Grandas F, Elston J, Quinn N, Marsden CD. Blepharospasm: a review of 264 patients. J Neurol Neurosurg Psychiatry. 1988;51:767–72.
26. Lee MS, Johnson M, Harrison AR. Gender differences in benign essential blepharospasm. Ophthalmic Plast Reconstr Surg. 2012;28:169–70.
27. Dutton JJ, Fowler AM. Botulinum toxin in ophthalmology. Surv Ophthalmol. 2007;52:13–31.
28. Ababneh OH, Cetinkaya A, Kulwin DR. Long-term efficacy and safety of botulinum toxin A injections to treat blepharospasm and hemifacial spasm. Clin Experiment Ophthalmol. 2014;42:254–61.
29. Flanders M, Chin D, Boghen D. Botulinum toxin: preferred treatment for hemifacial spasm. Eur Neurol. 1993;33:316–9.
30. Jitpimolmard S, Tiamkao S, Laopaiboon M. Long term results of botulinum toxin type A (Dysport) in the treatment of hemifacial spasm: a report of 175 cases. J Neurol Neurosurg Psychiatry. 1998;64:751–7.
31. Bentivoglio AR, Fasano A, Ialongo T, Soleti F, Lo Fermo S, Albanese A. Outcome predictors, efficacy and safety of Botox and Dysport in the long-term treatment of hemifacial spasm. Eur J Neurol. 2009;16:392–8.
32. Francart J, Mourin S, Kollmann P, Laterre EC. Five-year experience in the treatment of focal movement disorders with low-dose Dysport botulinum toxin. Muscle Nerve. 1995;18:720–9.

33. Morgenstern KE, Evanchan J, Foster JA, Cahill KV, Burns JA, Holck DE, Perry JD, Wulc AE. Botulinum toxin type a for dysthyroid upper eyelid retraction. Ophthalmic Plast Reconstr Surg. 2004;20:181–5.
34. Hekimhan PK. Botulinum toxin applications in periocular pathologies. Türkiye Klinikleri J Surg Med Sci. 2007;3:56–61.
35. Kaynak P, Karabulut ÖG, Öztürker C, Yıldırım Y, Alagöz N, Akar S, Gökyiğit B, Demirok A. Upper eyelid retraction management with subconjunctival ınjection of botulinum toxin type a in patients with thyroid eye disease. MN Oftalmoloji. 2013;20:272–8.
36. Salour H, Bagheri B, Aletaha M, Babsharif B, Kleshadi M, Abrishami M, Bagheri A. Transcutaneous dysport injection for treatment of upper eyelid retraction associated with thyroid eye disease. Orbit. 2010;29:114–8.
37. Baranano DE, Miller NR. Long term efficacy and safety of botulinum toxin A injection for crocodile tears syndrome. Br J Ophthalmol. 2004;88:588–9.
38. Nava-Castaneda A, Tovilla-Canales JL, Boullosa V, Tovilla-y-Pomar JL, Monroy-Serrano MH, Tapia-Guerra V, Garfias Y. Duration of botulinum toxin effect in the treatment of crocodile tears. Ophthalmic Plast Reconstr Surg. 2006;22:453–6.
39. Wabbels B, Forl M. Botulinum toxin treatment for crocodile tears, spastic entropion and for dysthyroid upper eyelid retraction. Ophthalmologe. 2007;104:771–6.

Botulinum Toxin Injections: Middle Third of the Face

12

Yavuz Sultan Selim Yildirim, Oğuzhan Oğuz, and İbrahim Cukurova

12.1 Introduction

Human facial anatomy involves a complicated arrangement of various muscles, through the action of which both essential physiological functions are accomplished and facial expressions are produced. Armed with a detailed knowledge of the anatomical composition of the face, cosmetic practitioners can select muscles or groups of muscles to weaken or paralyse using botulinum toxin so as to improve the facial appearance of patients [1].

Botulinum toxin acts to prevent acetylcholine from being released into the synapse, i.e. denervation by chemical means. At muscle endplates, acetylcholine is secreted from the presynaptic neuron. Cholinergic transmission depends on vesicles containing acetylcholine being able to dock with the plasma membrane and discharge into the synaptic cleft [2], a process that involves a number of molecular interactions, in particular those involving *N*-ethylmaleimide-sensitive fusion protein (NSF). This molecule is found within the cellular cytoplasm and is one of several molecules that fuse together. Other cytoplasmic molecules, known as SNAPs (soluble NSF attachment proteins), bind to NSF and stabilise the complex. There are receptors for SNAPs both on the cytoplasmic vesicles and the cell outer membrane, such as VAMP (vesicle-associated membrane protein), as well as SNAP-25 and syntaxin, which circulate in plasma. VAMP is also referred to as synaptobrevin [3].

Y. S. S. Yildirim (✉)
Health Sciences University, Elazig Fethi Sekin City Hospital, Department of Otorhinolaryngology, Elazig, Turkey

O. Oğuz
Dr. Oğuzhan Oğuz Wellnose Clinic, Istanbul, Turkey

İ. Cukurova
İzmir University of Health Sciences, Tepecik Training and Research Hospital, Department of Otorhinolaryngology, İzmir, Turkey

C. Cingi et al. (eds.), *Minor Interventions, Major Outcomes on the Face*, Comprehensive ENT, https://doi.org/10.1007/978-3-032-01305-7_12

Botulinum toxin is classified as a zinc-dependent endoproteinase that consists of a light chain and a heavy chain, which are bound to each other by disulfide bridges. The light chain has a molecular mass of 50 kDa, whilst the heavy chain's mass is 100 kDa [3].

12.2 Botulinum Toxin to the Facial Mid-Third

The bottom third and mid-third of the face are very active regions, which accomplish a variety of functions, such as mastication, laughter, speech, whistling and expressing emotion. There is an expanding demand for treatments that reduce wrinkles that form in this facial region due to ageing of the skin and facial muscle hyperactivity. Currently, botulinum toxin is amongst the most popular and frequently utilised treatments available to reduce the visible signs of ageing [4].

Botulinum toxin may be utilised to improve the aesthetic appearance in several ways in the mid-third of the face. Rhytides that appear dorsally or laterally over the nose, which may be termed “bunny lines”, can be treated by injecting toxin into the superior portion of the nasalis muscle. The usual dose required for using onabotulinumtoxinA ranges from 2 to 4 IU on each side. Another possible agent is abobotulinumtoxinA. In the latter case, the dose ranges from 10 to 20 IU [5].

Clinical experience suggests that flaring of the nostrils can be reduced by using onabotulinumtoxinA on the inferior portion of the nasalis. The dose is between 5 and 10 IU. If it is desired to raise the tip of the nose, this may be achieved by injecting a low dose of onabotulinumtoxinA (around 2 or 3 IU) into the depressor septi nasi muscle [1].

Patients frequently complain about having overly noticeable nasolabial folds. These extend from the lateral portion of the alae to a point lateral to the corner of the mouth. Soft tissue fillers are often used to remedy the problem, as is resurfacing by laser. The superior portion of these folds reduces significantly in depth when a suitable preparation of botulinum toxin, such as onabotulinumtoxinA, is injected at a low dose into the muscles responsible for raising the lip. Doing so, however, does run the risk of increasing the vertical height of the superior lip, which may add to the appearance of ageing. Accordingly, botulinum used in this way is only really suitable if the patient already has a short vertical lip height. Possibly the most efficacious way to address prominent nasolabial folds involves a combination of botulinum toxin, soft tissue fills and resurfacing by laser [1].

It is important that botulinum toxin be used cautiously in treating cosmetic defects of the facial mid-third. Only some patients actually experience cosmetic improvement, and it is easy to overtreat an individual. When used in this region, chemical denervation persists for up to 6 months. Never inject toxin exactly where the nasolabial fold occurs, since doing so can cause a lopsided smile and ptosis of the lip [6].

12.2.1 Wrinkled Appearance of the Superior Lip

The best way to address wrinkling of the upper lip when there are many small wrinkles is by injecting (collagen-containing) fillers. An alternative is to resurface the area to mid-depth or even more deeply. Finely wrinkled skin does not generally improve in appearance after use of onabotulinumtoxinA, in addition to which the superior lip may suffer from weakness. If there are deep rhytides (at least 2–3), botulinum toxin may, however, be appropriate, in which case a low dose (0.5–1 IU for each injection), placed shallowly, should be utilised. Care is still needed, nonetheless, to ensure paresis of the superior lip does not occur [3].

12.2.2 Nasolabial Folds

Carruthers and Carruthers utilised onabotulinumtoxinA in small amounts (between 2 and 3 IU) to improve the appearance of nasolabial folds. Their aim was to weaken the levator labii superioris alaeque nasi [7]. Electromyographic guidance was employed. In some patients where the nasolabial folds softened, the superior lip grew in length. Typically, improving the appearance of nasolabial creases is challenging [3].

12.2.3 Masseteric Hypertrophy

The masseter may become hypertrophied for a variety of reasons, such as bruxism (grinding of the teeth), disorders affecting the temporomandibular joint, misalignment of the upper and lower jaws, or it may be an inherited trait. The result is that the jaws appear boxy, and there may be a degree of asymmetry. The traditional approach to this problem involved jaw surgery.

The evidence base supporting the effectiveness of botulinum toxin to reduce the boxiness of the jaw consists of reported cases and trials performed without control cases for comparison [8–11]. If the toxin is injected bilaterally into the masseter, this muscle becomes around 50% thinner, an effect that persists for between 3 and 6 months (and even longer in certain cases) [12–15]. Not only does this allow a more flattering jawline to be sculpted, but it also reduces the severity of bruxism [15, 16]. When the toxin is repeatedly injected into the masseter, the muscle mass shows a tendency to reduce, and thus progressively lower doses are needed [17]. There may, however, be a number of undesirable consequences to this procedure, such as a less powerful bite, disturbed speech articulation, myalgia, an asymmetrical facial appearance and prominence of the zygomata. Such effects are transient [18].

12.3 Application and Treatment

Technical competence in this area depends on a thorough familiarity with the anatomy of the face and knowing how the muscles of the face work. Incorrect technique may lead to cosmetic defects or disability related to impaired muscular activity. If the frontalis muscle, for instance, is too aggressively targeted in an attempt to remove horizontally oriented frontal rhytides, brow ptosis may occur, which is cosmetically unacceptable [19].

12.3.1 Preparation Before Treatment

Before commencing treatment, doctors need to decide if botulinum toxin injection will be suitable to achieve the desired change in appearance. The toxin is effective where an unsightly appearance comes about through overactivity of particular muscles. If there are other types of cosmetic problems, e.g. lentigo formation, telangiectasias, alterations in skin texture or excessively loose skin, other cosmetic techniques will be needed to achieve an adequately rejuvenated appearance [19].

Where the clinician identifies an aesthetic issue that is amenable to treatment with botulinum toxin, and there are no features in the case that would be contraindicative, the patient can be counselled about how long improvement may potentially last, when a further treatment will be called for, and any anticipated potential side effects/complications. If a patient sets his or her expectation at an unrealistic level, the result, however satisfactory from the clinician's viewpoint, is bound to be a disappointment to the patient. It is generally wise to obtain a photographic record indicating the appearance prior to and following the intervention, to permit some objectivity in evaluating outcomes [19].

Since botulinum toxin exerts its effect on any muscle, it is important to consider in advance how weakness of particular muscles may affect individuals undergoing treatment. Woodwind or brass instrument players may be unable to play following injections intended to reduce perioral rhytides, for example [19].

12.3.2 Reconstituting the Toxin for Injection

Sterile saline is used for reconstitution of botulinum toxin before injection. The exact degree of dilution depends on the clinician's preferences. The package inserts for onabotulinumtoxinA, incobotulinumtoxinA, prabotulinumtoxinA and abobotulinumtoxinA make recommendations as follows [19]:

- OnabotulinumtoxinA and incobotulinumtoxinA. If a 100 IU vial is used, mix with 2.5 mL sterile NaCl 0.9%, or for a 50 IU vial, mix with 1.25 mL sterile NaCl 0.9%. The resulting concentration in either case is 4 IU per 0.1 mL. For glabellar lines, 20 IU will be needed, i.e. 0.5 mL of reconstituted product.

- PrabotulinumtoxinA. A 100 IU vial is used. Mix with 2.5 mL sterile NaCl 0.9%. The resulting concentration is 4 IU per 0.1 mL.
- AbobotulinumtoxinA. A 300 IU vial is used. Mix with either 2.5 mL or 1.5 mL sterile NaCl 0.9%. In the former case, 0.08 mL will contain 10 IU toxin, whilst in the latter, 0.05 mL will contain 10 IU.

Clinical experience suggests that using a relatively small volume of saline when reconstituting botulinum toxin offers several advantages, especially in terms of improving the precision of delivery to a specific area. When toxin is less diluted, the effect lasts longer, and the tendency to diffuse into tissue adjacent to the target is reduced [20]. The authors' own preferred concentration for onabotulinumtoxinA is 100 IU/mL. If it is necessary to paralyse an extensive region, a greater volume of diluent may be called for [21].

The firms that produce onabotulinumtoxinA, abobotulinumtoxinA, incobotulinumtoxinA and prabotulinumtoxinA all recommend the use of sterile saline without preservatives for reconstitution of botulinum toxin. Despite this recommendation, it is common practice in the USA and Canada to use a mixture of saline and benzyl alcohol for this purpose, since injection is thereby rendered less painful [22]. A trial involving small numbers of patients with dynamic wrinkles in the superior facial region compared onabotulinumtoxinA reconstituted in saline with or without preservative agents. The patients in whom saline containing preservatives was used reported a lower level of discomfort but the efficacy was equal in both conditions [23]. A similar trial in which abobotulinumtoxinA was the agent used reported findings that were consistent with the other trial [24]. If clinicians do decide to use saline containing preservatives, it is important to enquire first about allergies, especially to benzyl alcohol.

There is not complete consensus on whether it is acceptable to use reconstituted botulinum toxin after a delay [22]. The package inserts included with onabotulinumtoxinA, abobotulinumtoxinA, incobotulinumtoxinA and prabotulinumtoxinA all state that the products should be stored chilled at a temperature of 2 to 8 °C. The manufacturers state that the toxin should be safely disposed of if still unused 24 h (or 4 h) after being reconstituted. Despite this recommendation, it is common practice for cosmetic practitioners to keep reconstituted toxin in the refrigerator for longer than this. One study examined 85 cases where patients underwent injections of onabotulinumtoxinA. Reconstitution was performed with non-preserved sterile saline 0.9%, after which the product continued to be used up to 6 weeks later. No alteration over time in how efficacious the agent was could be observed [25]. Furthermore, there are other studies involving randomisation that have shown no decrease in efficacy for botulinum toxin serotype A, which was left refrigerated for between 1 and 2 weeks before injection [26–28].

References

1. Carruthers J. Botulinum toxin for cosmetic indications: Treatment of specific sites. Dover JS, Ofori AO (EdS). UpToDate. Last updated: Jun 07, 2019.
2. Ferrari A, Manca M, Tugnoli V, Alberto L. Pharmacological differences and clinical implications of various botulinum toxin preparations: a critical appraisal. Funct Neurol. 2018;33(1):7–18.
3. Hauser RA. Botulinum toxin injections in plastic surgery. de la Torre JI (Ed). Medscape. Updated: Feb 08, 2019. https://emedicine.medscape.com/article/1271380-overview#a1. Accessed online at 14 April 2021.
4. Grullón LM, Ávila JR. Botulinum toxin for middle third of the face. In: Costa A, editor. Minimally invasive aesthetic procedures. Cham: Springer; 2020. https://doi.org/10.1007/978-3-319-78265-2_29.
5. Kane M, Donofrio L, Ascher B, et al. Expanding the use of neurotoxins in facial aesthetics: a consensus panel's assessment and recommendations. J Drugs Dermatol. 2010;9:s7.
6. Carruthers J, Carruthers A. Aesthetic botulinum A toxin in the mid and lower face and neck. Dermatologic Surg. 2003;29:468.
7. Carruthers A, Carruthers J. Clinical indications and injection technique for the cosmetic use of botulinum A exotoxin. Dermatologic Surg. 1998;24(11):1189–94.
8. Yu CC, Chen PK, Chen YR. Botulinum toxin a for lower facial contouring: a prospective study. Aesth Plast Surg. 2007;31:445.
9. Baş B, Ozan B, Muğlali M, Celebi N. Treatment of masseteric hypertrophy with botulinum toxin: a report of two cases. Med Oral Patol Oral Cir Bucal. 2010;15:e649.
10. Al-Muharraqi MA, Fedorowicz Z, Al Bareeq J, et al. Botulinum toxin for masseter hypertrophy. Cochrane Database Syst Rev. 2009;CD007510
11. Fedorowicz Z, van Zuuren EJ, Schoones J. Botulinum toxin for masseter hypertrophy. Cochrane Database Syst Rev. 2013;CD007510
12. To EW, Ahuja AT, Ho WS, et al. A prospective study of the effect of botulinum toxin A on masseteric muscle hypertrophy with ultrasonographic and electromyographic measurement. Br J Plast Surg. 2001;54:197.
13. von Lindern JJ, Niederhagen B, Appel T, et al. Type A botulinum toxin for the treatment of hypertrophy of the masseter and temporal muscles: an alternative treatment. Plast Reconstr Surg. 2001;107:327.
14. Park MY, Ahn KY, Jung DS. Botulinum toxin type A treatment for contouring of the lower face. Dermatologic Surg. 2003;29:477.
15. Liew S, Dart A. Nonsurgical reshaping of the lower face. Aesthet Surg J. 2008;28:251.
16. Chikhani L, Dichamp J. Bruxism, temporo-mandibular dysfunction and botulinum toxin. Ann Readapt Med Phys. 2003;46:333.
17. Kim NH, Park RH, Park JB. Botulinum toxin type A for the treatment of hypertrophy of the masseter muscle. Plast Reconstr Surg. 2010;125:1693.
18. Kim KS, Byun YS, Kim YJ, Kim ST. Muscle weakness after repeated injection of botulinum toxin type A evaluated according to bite force measurement of human masseter muscle. Dermatologic Surg. 2009;35:1902.
19. Carruthers J. Overview of botulinum toxin for cosmetic indications. Dover JS, Ofori AO (Eds). UpToDate. Last updated: Jul 22, 2019.
20. Klein AW. Complications, adverse reactions, and insights with the use of botulinum toxin. Dermatologic Surg. 2003;29:549.
21. Hsu TS, Dover JS, Arndt KA. Effect of volume and concentration on the diffusion of botulinum exotoxin A. Arch Dermatol. 2004;140:1351.
22. Liu A, Carruthers A, Cohen JL, et al. Recommendations and current practices for the reconstitution and storage of botulinum toxin type A. J Am Acad Dermatol. 2012;67:373.

23. Alam M, Dover JS, Arndt KA. Pain associated with injection of botulinum A exotoxin reconstituted using isotonic sodium chloride with and without preservative: a double-blind, randomized controlled trial. Arch Dermatol. 2002;138:510.
24. Allen SB, Goldenberg NA. Pain difference associated with injection of abobotulinumtoxinA reconstituted with preserved saline and preservative-free saline: a prospective, randomized, side-by-side, double-blind study. Dermatologic Surg. 2012;38:867.
25. Hexsel DM, De Almeida AT, Rutowitsch M, et al. Multicenter, double-blind study of the efficacy of injections with botulinum toxin type A reconstituted up to six consecutive weeks before application. Dermatologic Surg. 2003;29:523.
26. Hui JI, Lee WW. Efficacy of fresh versus refrigerated botulinum toxin in the treatment of lateral periorbital rhytids. Ophthalmic Plast Reconstr Surg. 2007;23:433.
27. Lizarralde M, Gutiérrez SH, Venegas A. Clinical efficacy of botulinum toxin type A reconstituted and refrigerated 1 week before its application in external canthus dynamic lines. Dermatologic Surg. 2007;33:1328.
28. Yang GC, Chiu RJ, Gillman GS. Questioning the need to use Botox within 4 hours of reconstitution: a study of fresh vs 2-week-old Botox. Arch Facial Plast Surg. 2008;10:273.

Botulinum Toxin Injections: Lower Third of the Face

13

Hasan Cetiner, Tarik Yagci, and J. Regan Thomas

13.1 Introduction

The use of injectable botulinum toxin on the inferior facial third is widespread [1, 2]. Nonetheless, clinicians need to act cautiously when injecting toxin around the mouth so as to prevent laxity of the cheek, the inability to close the mouth tightly or development of a lopsided smile. Furthermore, injecting botulinum toxin in this area may cause problems for people whose occupation involves singing or blowing wind instruments and who therefore make extensive use of the muscles of the lower face.

13.2 Perioral Labial Wrinkles

A frequent patient complaint is the appearance of vertically oriented wrinkles perorally. They may arise from the hyperactivity of the orbicularis oris muscle or may be due to loss of facial volume, sunlight exposure or other causes [3]. Frequently these rhytides are treated with injectable fillers or by resurfacing the skin with a laser, but these procedures have the disadvantage that the benefit is soon lost. It is probable that the intense muscular activity in this region of the face is what causes rhytides to reappear so quickly [4].

H. Cetiner
East Anatolia Hospital, Department of Otorhinolaryngology, Elazıg, Turkey

T. Yagci (✉)
Medical Faculty, Department of Otorhinolaryngology, Bilecik Seyh Edebali University, Bilecik, Turkey

J. R. Thomas
University of New Mexico School of Medicine, Albuquerque, NM, USA

C. Cingi et al. (eds.), *Minor Interventions, Major Outcomes on the Face*, Comprehensive ENT, https://doi.org/10.1007/978-3-032-01305-7_13

Low dose injected botulinum toxin may be indicated for treatment where muscles are the reason for wrinkles to appear. The site of injection is alongside the vermillion border and lateral to the philtral columns. A report on a case series consisting of 18 individuals with perioral wrinkles who were administered onabotulinumtoxinA indicated that the wrinkles were softened, and the superior lip appeared more everted following the procedure [5, 6].

The authors' usual practice is to divide the lips into four quadrants. In each quadrant, two injections are used, delivering 1 IU of onabotulinumtoxinA each time. It has also been suggested elsewhere in the literature that, when abobotulinumtoxinA is used, 8 IU in total is needed for the superior lip area, delivered as four separate injections, whilst 4 IU suffices for the inferior lip, delivered as two injections [7]. To produce an even better result, chemical denervation may be combined with injection of soft tissue filler [8, 9].

A possible hazard from treating perioral rhytides with botulinum toxin is that of severe paresis affecting the lips. In some cases, proprioceptive sensation for the lips is impaired, although this does not usually prevent eating, drinking or singing. If relatively low doses are employed and the injections are placed at shallow depths, the risk of adverse outcomes is reduced. Nonetheless, it may be best to use an alternative treatment if the patient is someone who uses their lower facial muscles an above average amount, such as singers, public speakers or wind players [6].

Two perioral locations that should be avoided when injecting are the corners of the mouth and the philtrum, since there is a possibility of creating a downturned mouth or a flat Cupid's bow [2].

13.2.1 Anatomical and Physiological Considerations

The key muscle implicated in producing hyperdynamic perioral rhytides is the orbicularis oris. There are, nonetheless, a number of other muscles found within the same region that have interdigitations with the orbicularis oris. When targeting the orbicularis oris with botulinum toxin, clinicians may inadvertently weaken or paralyse these other muscles, such as the levator labii superioris, levator anguli oris, depressor anguli oris and depressor labii inferioris. The risk of this occurring increases when higher doses are employed [2, 10].

13.2.2 Dilution

Botulinum toxin for injection periorally should be reconstituted in such a way as to create a medium level of dilution. This is required to facilitate diffusion over the area at a lowish concentration, such as 0.5 IU, rather than 2 IU, as elsewhere [11]. A vial of Botox containing 100 IU may appropriately be reconstituted with between 1 and 3 mL of sterile saline [2].

13.2.3 Locations of Injection and Dosage

There are two different ways in which botulinum toxin can be applied in the area of the lips. If there are severe or moderately severe rhytides affecting the superior lip, each quadrant of the lip, upper and lower, may be injected with between 1 and 2 IU of Botox. The ideal location is at least 3 mm and not more than 5 mm away from the vermilion border. It is highly advisable to provide multiple injections of 1 IU each time [10].

An alternative method is to inject twice or three times in each lip quadrant, slightly within the vermilion border of the upper lip, and use between 0.5 and 1 IU for each injection. This produces fullness of the superior lip, which resembles the effect of injectable fillers in the same area. The lip appears hypertrophied. The same method may also be applied to the inferior lip. However, rhytides of the lip cannot be softened in this way, since the toxin works only in the immediate vicinity of the vermilion border [10].

13.2.4 Adverse Effects and Complications

The adverse effects that patients are most prone to experience are the following [10]:

- Patients frequently complain of pain at the site of injection.
- It is unusual for bruising or discolouration of the skin to occur.
- Impaired function of the lips is an adverse effect of significance, as it may make it hard to drink, eat or speak [11]. If an overly high dose of botulinum toxin is used, it tends to diffuse into the other muscles in the same region, resulting in a lopsided smile, a degree of dysarthria and a tendency to make sucking movements [12].

13.3 Mouth Frowning and Melomental Folds

The action of the depressor anguli oris muscle is, as its name suggests, to depress the angle of the mouth. The muscles that perform the opposite action are the zygomaticus major and minor. If the angle of the mouth is generally downward turned, this makes the patient seem unfriendly and as if unhappy. It is possible, using botulinum toxin, to induce paresis of the depressor anguli oris, which then favours the action of the zygomaticus major and minor, with the result that the angle of the mouth no longer points downwards. Caution should, however, be exercised in suggesting this treatment to individuals who use the muscles around the mouth a great deal, such as wind players or singers. This situation is the same with treating perioral wrinkles of the lip [6].

The site of injection in treating mouth frown is chosen to avoid inadvertently inducing paresis in the adjacent depressor labii inferioris muscle. It lies on the posterior border of the depressor anguli oris and near the anterior masseteric border.

Typically, the dose chosen is onabotulinumtoxinA 2–3 IU bilaterally. Contraction of the mentalis muscle makes a further contribution to mouth frowning, so it is also chemically denervated using onabotulinumtoxinA 3 IU where the paired muscles insert bilaterally [6].

Melomental folds (which may sometimes be referred to as "marionette lines") are also worsened by the activity of the depressor anguli oris. The conventional approach to treating melomental folds has relied on injectable fillers. However, there is only a brief duration of noticeable benefit from doing so. When injection of fillers is combined with chemical denervation of the muscles underneath, the benefit may be increased. One study used split face photographs from 22 individuals treated for melomental folds. The images were in random order. When the images were evaluated, it appeared that combining fillers with botulinum toxin had a more long-lasting effect than when filler was the sole treatment modality, with a median duration of benefit of 39 weeks for combination treatment vs 32.5 weeks for filler only [13]. This apparent difference was not maintained when evaluation was carried out on actual patients rather than photographic images. Further research is needed to delineate the precise role for combined treatment of melomental folds [6].

13.4 Chin, Mental Crease and Peau D'orange Chin

It is common for patients to have folds or creases form in the middle of their chin whilst they are speaking or showing facial expressions. A term used to describe the wrinkled appearance is "peau d'orange". The action of the mentalis muscle contributes to this phenomenon [14]. It has recently been shown that chemical denervation of the mentalis muscle has efficacy in reducing this unsightly appearance of the chin [10].

When the mentalis contracts, a horizontally oriented fold appears beneath the inferior lip and superior to the mental prominence. The authors' clinical experience is that this fold can be reduced by injecting onabotulinumtoxinA into the mentalis. The dose required is 3–5 IU bilaterally. The site of injection is slightly in front of the bony mentum on either side of the midline. Clinicians should not inject at the level of the fold, since this may inadvertently lead to chemical denervation of the orbicularis oris muscle. If this occurs, patients may find they cannot close their mouth tightly, and the effect will persist for up to 6 months. Ageing in the chin region may lead to lower levels of collagen in the dermis and loss of adipose tissue. Coupled with the action of the mentalis, this may appear as peau d'orange, as described above. Another situation where this arises is in patients with Bell's palsy, including in the recovery phase. The use of botulinum toxin for treatment of peau d'orange on the chin has already been mentioned, including the additional benefit obtainable by combining chemical denervation with injection of fillers. The usual dose range of onabotulinumtoxinA is 5–10 IU, divided into one or more injections. It has also been reported that abobotulinumtoxinA at a dose between 5 and 20 IU may be used to weaken the mentalis. Two separate injections are used [7].

13.4.1 Anatomical and Physiological Considerations

The origin of the mentalis muscle is the lower incisive fossa, and its insertion is the mental skin [2]. The principal way the mentalis functions is elevating the skin of the chin [10].

13.4.2 Dilution

The depressor labii inferioris and the depressor anguli oris lie next to the mentalis muscle [15]. If toxin diffuses into these adjacent muscles, the smile may become lopsided [10]. The best way to avoid this occurrence is by using small volumes of Botox when injecting, e.g. 3 mL of saline or less (minimum 1 mL) when reconstituting a 100 IU vial [16].

13.4.3 Sites of Application

Injection into the mentalis muscle can be carried out in two different ways. If a single injection is to be employed, its location is at the midpoint of the mentalis, at the apex of the mentum. This is therefore the inferior margin of the ramus of the mandible. Where two injections are to be used, they are placed at the same level as the single injection but somewhat off-centre (i.e. laterally). Use of two injections may potentially allow a better diffusion of Botox over the entire mentalis muscle [10].

13.4.4 Dosages

The dosage required is influenced both by how large the chin is and how forcefully the mentalis contracts. The range is between 2 and 10 IU, which may be delivered as a single injection or as two separate injections [17].

13.4.5 Adverse Effects and Complications

The following are the adverse effects which occur with the highest frequency [10]:

- Bruise formation and swelling.
- Transient pain.
- If the toxin is inadvertently applied to the other muscles in the vicinity of the mentalis, a lopsided smile may be produced and patients may struggle to eat or speak.

13.5 Corners of the Mouth (Oral Commissures)

Individuals who possess powerful depressor anguli oris muscles have a tendency to look rather miserable since the angles of the mouth usually point downwards. In such individuals, weakening this downward pull by toxin administration has the beneficial effect of letting the corners of the mouth be horizontal, with a more pleasing resting facial expression. Furthermore, the same procedure softens the wrinkled skin overlying the chin [10].

13.5.1 Anatomical and Physiological Considerations

The origin of the depressor anguli oris lies on the mandibular oblique line. This muscle is at a slight angle to the mentalis, which lies medial and deep to it and is smaller. The insertion points are the skin and fibres of the orbicularis oris at the oral commissure. The effect of muscular contraction is to pull the oral angles downwards. Downturned corners of the mouth contribute to an impression of unhappiness [18].

13.5.2 Dilution

It is of vital importance that the injected volume of Botox be low when used in this part of the face. A 100 IU vial of toxin can be reconstituted using 1–2 mL of sterile saline. If clinicians are careful to deliver precise doses and thus small, precise volumes of Botox, there is less risk that the toxin will be inadvertently applied to nearby muscles as a result of diffusion from the injection site [2].

13.5.3 Sites of Application

Injection of Botox needs to occur directly into the muscular belly of the depressor anguli oris. This can be arranged using electromyographic guidance. Alternatively, the correct position may be ascertained by tracing an imaginary line from the nasolabial fold to the mandibular border. Where the muscle crosses the ramus of the mandible, it is safe to perform the injection [10].

13.5.4 Dosage

The necessary dose of Botox to prevent mouth frowning and improve the melancholic appearance of individuals whose depressor anguli oris is very powerful is between 4 and 8 IU [2].

13.5.5 Adverse Effects and Complications

There are a number of adverse effects and complications that occur frequently, as follows [10]:

- Pain, bruise formation and skin discolouration due to bleeding may all be experienced at the site of injection.
- If the mouth becomes asymmetrical, this is due to following an incorrect procedure for injection or because Botox has diffused into the adjacent musculature, in particular the orbicularis oris, depressor labii inferioris or both together [11].
- Where the mouth does become asymmetrical, it will be hard to close the lips fully, which creates difficulty when the patient tries to eat, drink or talk [10]. This is a temporary problem.

13.6 Gingival (Gummy) Smile

There are a number of individuals who present complaining of revealing too much of the superior gingiva when they smile. If this exposure of the gingiva exceeds 3 mm, they may be described as suffering from a "gingival smile" or "gummy smile" [19]. There are treatments available of a surgical and orthodontic kind, as well as the injection of botulinum toxin, which may avoid the need for a surgical operation [19–21].

One study followed up the outcome in 16 patients treated for gummy smile. No controls were available for comparison. These patients all received injectable abobotulinumtoxinA, targeting at least one of the two muscles, the levator labii superioris alaeque nasi or zygomaticus. In every case, gingival exposure when smiling was reduced [19]. The only adverse events recorded were of low severity. Two individuals experienced an abnormality in their smile, but this was able to be corrected using further botulinum toxin. Another study which followed up 30 individuals suffering from a gingival smile, also without control patients, followed up outcomes after onabotulinumtoxinA 2.5 IU was injected in areas where the levator labii superioris alaeque nasi and the levator labii superioris overlapped, as well as areas where both the levator labii superioris and zygomaticus minor could be targeted at the same time. Thus, four sites of injection were involved. This procedure was noted to be efficacious and usually well tolerated. Some adverse effects were noted, in particular four individuals with a painful injection site, one individual with headache and one instance of vertigo [10].

References

1. Carruthers J, Carruthers A. Aesthetic botulinum A toxin in the mid and lower face and neck. Dermatologic Surg. 2003;29:468.

2. Carruthers J, Carruthers A. BOTOX use in the mid and lower face and neck. Semin Cutan Med Surg. 2001;20:85.
3. Fagien S. Botox for the treatment of dynamic and hyperkinetic facial lines and furrows: adjunctive use in facial aesthetic surgery. Plast Reconstr Surg. 1999;103:701.
4. Fagien S. Botulinum toxin type A for facial aesthetic enhancement: role in facial shaping. Plast Reconstr Surg. 2003;112:6S.
5. Semchyshyn N, Sengelmann RD. Botulinum toxin A treatment of perioral rhytides. Dermatologic Surg. 2003;29:490.
6. Carruthers J. Botulinum toxin for cosmetic indications: Treatment of specific sites. Dover JS, Ofori AO (Eds). UpToDate. Last updated: Jun 07, 2019.
7. Kane M, Donofrio L, Ascher B, et al. Expanding the use of neurotoxins in facial aesthetics: a consensus panel's assessment and recommendations. J Drugs Dermatol. 2010;9:s7.
8. Carruthers A, Carruthers J, Monheit GD, et al. Multicenter, randomized, parallel-group study of the safety and effectiveness of onabotulinumtoxinA and hyaluronic acid dermal fillers (24-mg/ml smooth, cohesive gel) alone and in combination for lower facial rejuvenation. Dermatologic Surg. 2010;36(Suppl 4):2121.
9. Carruthers J, Carruthers A, Monheit GD, Davis PG. Multicenter, randomized, parallel-group study of onabotulinumtoxinA and hyaluronic acid dermal fillers (24-mg/ml smooth, cohesive gel) alone and in combination for lower facial rejuvenation: satisfaction and patient-reported outcomes. Dermatologic Surg. 2010;36(Suppl 4):2135.
10. Atamoros FP. Botulinum toxin in the lower one third of the face. Clin Dermatol. 2003;21(6):505–12. https://doi.org/10.1016/j.clindermatol.2003.11.014.
11. Markey AC. Botulinum A exotoxin in cosmetic dermatology. Clin Exp Dermatol. 2000;25:173–5.
12. Brandt F, Bellman B. Cosmetic use of botulinum toxin for the aging neck. Dermatologic Surg. 1998;24:1232–4.
13. Custis T, Beynet D, Carranza D, et al. Comparison of treatment of melomental fold rhytides with cross-linked hyaluronic acid combined with onabotulinumtoxina and cross-linked hyaluronic acid alone. Dermatologic Surg. 2010;36(Suppl 3):1852.
14. Binder WT, Blitzer A, Brin MF. Treatment of hyperfunctional lines of the face with botulinum toxin A. Dermatologic Surg. 1998;24:1198–205.
15. Moore KL, Dalley AF. Clinical oriented anatomy. In: Kelly PJ, editor. Muscles of the face. 4th ed. Baltimore: Lippincott Williams & Wilkins; 1999. p. 850–6. ch 7.
16. Benedetto A. The cosmetic use of botulinum toxin type A. Int J Dermatol. 1999;38:641–55.
17. Lowe NJ. Botulinum toxin type A for facial rejuvenation: United States and United Kingdom perspectives. Dermtol Surg. 1998;24:1216–8.
18. Farkas LG, Kolar JC. Anthropometrics and art in the aesthetics of women's faces. Clin Plast Surg. 1987;14:599–615.
19. Mazzuco R, Hexsel D. Gummy smile and botulinum toxin: a new approach based on the gingival exposure area. J Am Acad Dermatol. 2010;63:1042.
20. Polo M. Botulinum toxin type A (Botox) for the neuromuscular correction of excessive gingival display on smiling (gummy smile). Am J Orthod Dentofacial Orthop. 2008;133:195.
21. Polo M. Botulinum toxin type A in the treatment of excessive gingival display. Am J Orthod Dentofacial Orthop. 2005;127:214.

14 Botulinum Toxin Injections: Neck

İsmail Salcan, Nuray Bayar Muluk, Shriya Airen, and Jarrod Keeler

14.1 Introduction

Medical interest in *Clostridium botulinum* dates back to 1897, when it was discovered that this Gram-positive bacillus synthesized a toxin causing botulism [1, 2]. There are now seven forms of the botulinum toxin, produced by different bacterial strains, which can be distinguished serologically. These serotypes are as follows: A, B, C1, D, E, F, and G. These serotypes have differences in their pharmacology. Toxins A and B are generally used in clinical applications [3–5], but in cosmetic use, toxin A predominates.

The first clinical application of botulinum toxin was to remedy strabismus [6]. Since then, it has been used to treat a number of other disorders in which muscles contract excessively, such as blepharospasm [7], hemifacial spasm [8, 9], and spasmodic torticollis [10, 11].

İ. Salcan
Binali Yıldırım University, Mengücek Gazi Training and Research Hospital, ENT Department, Erzincan, Turkey

N. Bayar Muluk (✉)
Faculty of Medicine, Department of Otorhinolaryngology, Kırıkkale University, Kırıkkale, Türkiye

S. Airen · J. Keeler
Otolaryngology & Facial Plastic and Reconstructive Surgery, Specialty Physician Associates, St. Luke's Medical Center, Bethlehem, PA, USA
e-mail: shriya.airen@sluhn.org

C. Cingi et al. (eds.), *Minor Interventions, Major Outcomes on the Face*, Comprehensive ENT, https://doi.org/10.1007/978-3-032-01305-7_14

14.2 Anatomy of the Platysma

The inferior origin of the platysma muscle is the pectoralis and the fascia of the deltoid. The platysma crosses over the margin of the sternocleidomastoid in the mid-lateral cervical region at the nerve point. Three-quarters of patients have interdigitation of the platysma with the contralateral muscle at a point between 1 and 2 cm under the chin. In 15% of patients, the fibers are interlaced over the thyroid cartilage, while the area under the chin is a single band of muscle. The remaining 10% of patients have a platysma muscle on each side, which remains separated from the contralateral platysma [12].

The muscular fibers located on the lateral aspect of the platysma play a role in forming facial expressions since they exert a downward pull on the inferior labial angle. The platysmal bands are posteriorly continuous with the facial superficial musculoaponeurotic system (SMAS). Anteriorly, four deeply situated individual muscles form an "M" shape, the middle part formed by the twin mentalis muscles, and the ends formed by the twin depressor anguli inferioris muscles. At a more superficial depth, there is another "M" shape, which is more comprehensive and consists of two depressor anguli oris and lateral commissure muscles [12].

14.3 How Aging Affects the Neck

The way the neck ages depends on several factors, such as genetics, damage to actin filaments, and alterations in weight. As individuals age, the chronic effect of the platysma pulling downwards is the formation of vertically oriented bands of fibrous tissue. Meanwhile, horizontally oriented wrinkles form due to the skin overlying the platysma and becoming laxer over time. The most oversized fat pad under the chin herniates between the platysma's free margins due to the platysma and SMAS pulling downwards, coupled with degeneration of the skin and muscle that occurs with aging [12].

14.4 What Is the Mechanism by Which Botulinum Toxin Exerts an Effect?

Botulinum toxin is a valuable agent for treating several conditions thanks to its ability to inhibit muscular contraction by preventing the secretion of acetylcholine into the neuromuscular end-plate [13]. All serotypes of botulinum toxin contain both a single heavy and light chain. The heavy chain engages with receptors located on the presynaptic membrane, following which the neuron endocytoses the entire toxin. The toxin then acts on the SNARE (soluble *N*-ethylmaleimide-sensitive factor attachment protein receptor) complex, causing it to break apart. Without intact SNARE, acetylcholine cannot be released into the synaptic cleft. Different serotypes attack the SNARE complex at various points. Serotypes A, C1, and E attack the SNAP-25 protein, a molecule with a molecular mass of 25 kDa associated with the synaptosome. The other serotypes (B, D, F, and G), on the other hand, attack synaptobrevin, also known as VAMP (vesicle-associated membrane protein) [10].

Once the SNARE complex breaks apart, acetylcholine can no longer be released at the end-plate, and therefore, the muscular receptor for this molecule remains unstimulated. Thus, botulinum toxin achieves denervation by chemical means. This denervation is of transient duration, with recovery of muscular contraction frequently becoming apparent clinically around 3 months after the toxin was injected. To a degree, the resumption of neuromuscular transmission can be attributed to new nerve buds taking the place of the original terminal synapse. Nonetheless, such additional buds seem not to be permanent, and the original end-plate gradually begins to function once more [14].

There are several preparations of serotype A toxin which are marketed in the USA and Canada, such as onabotulinumtoxinA, abobotulinumtoxinA, incobotulinumtoxinA, and prabotulinumtoxinA [13]. Serotype B botulinum toxin is known as rimabotulinumtoxinB [10].

14.4.1 OnabotulinumtoxinA

The most intensively researched preparation produced with serotype A is onabotulinumtoxinA (marketed as Botox by Botox Cosmetic under the proprietary names Vistabel and Vistabex). OnabotulinumtoxinA comes as a powder containing serotype A toxin (either 50 IU or 100 IU) with human albumin and NaCl. It is prepared by cryodessication and does not contain preservative agents. The US FDA has licensed this agent for treating wrinkles of the glabella, crow's feet (lines radiating from the lateral canthi), and frontal rhytides. The same agent is also extensively utilized off-label to treat rhytides elsewhere and to improve the contours of the face [15].

14.4.2 AbobotulinumtoxinA

AbobotulinumtoxinA first received regulatory approval in Europe. It is produced by Dysport. It is prepared from serotype A toxin and is also intended for cosmetic applications. The vials contain cryodessicated toxin (either 300 IU or 500 IU) together with serum albumin and lactose. This agent began to be marketed in the USA and Canada in 2009 and now has been licensed by the US FDA for treating glabellar rhytides [10].

14.4.3 IncobotulinumtoxinA

IncobotulinumtoxinA is also prepared using serotype A toxin and has come onto the market more recently. It has regulatory approval for use in treating glabellar rhytides in the USA and a number of other jurisdictions. The preparation consists of cryodessicated serotype A neurotoxin (either 50 IU or 100 IU), together with human albumin and sucrose. One difference with this product is that the toxin is supplied without the proteins that usually form a complex with it. This is said to lessen the chances that a patient develops hypersensitivity and allergy to the agent [16, 17].

14.4.4 PrabotulinumtoxinA

This agent has been marketed in the USA as Jeuveau since 2019, when FDA regulatory approval was granted. It is for treating glabellar rhytides of at least moderate degree in adult patients. It comes as a vial containing 100 IU of cryodessicated botulinum toxin [10].

14.4.5 RimabotulinumtoxinB

This agent is marketed under the proprietary names Myobloc and Neurobloc. Myobloc is available as a liquid with a concentration of 5000 IU/mL of serotype B toxin and is marketed in the USA, Canada, and South Korea. The excipients are human serum albumin, sodium succinate, and NaCl. Myobloc is the first-line neurotoxin used in cases of spasmodic torticollis. There is a more slender evidence base for using serotype B in cosmetic applications than serotype B. Nonetheless, it has been reported that wrinkles of the face are improved by using rimabotulinumtoxinB [18–21].

14.4.6 Topical Preparations of Serotype a Neurotoxin

The topical application of serotype A neurotoxin to treat dynamic wrinkles appears promising [22–24]. A topical gel with serotype A neurotoxin was ranged against placebo in a trial involving 36 adult patients with rhytides of the lateral canthi. Treatment allocation was random. The agent was applied for 30 min, followed by a 4-week waiting period. This topical treatment was superior to placebo [22]. Further research is needed to clarify exactly how topical preparations of botulinum neurotoxin can be best used in cosmetic applications [10].

14.5 Botulinum Toxin Injections: Neck

There is a limited evidence base concerning treatment of cosmetic issues in the cervical region by means of botulinum neurotoxin. The neurotoxin does offer benefit, it seems, in cases where surgical platysmaplasty is inappropriate or patients desire another option. It appears beneficial, too, where there are still visible platysmal bands following surgical operations aiming to rejuvenate the cervical region. Botulinum neurotoxin has also been utilized in treating horizontally oriented cervical rhytides. The rationale for both these applications is that hyperactivity of the platysma muscle creates both the horizontally oriented rhytides and the vertical banding [25].

The types of cases where botulinum neurotoxin in the cervical region is likely to be most beneficial are elderly patients who present an anesthetic risk, elderly patients where operations aimed at rejuvenation of the cervical region have remained successful and the skin laxity is not unduly marked, and in young individuals where the platysmal bands are very prominent but overall they do not fit the criteria for surgical intervention. Toxin injection may also be employed adjunctively following rhytidectomy. The best results are observed in younger individuals and in elderly patients who have first undergone operative interventions. The benefit is more apparent when patients are actively animating their features than when facial movements are minimal. We may note Kane's conclusion in a study dating from 1999 [26]: "Although most of the patients were very happy with their results, even the best results in no way approached the most disappointing results obtained by means of surgical manipulation of the platysma and neck skin."

14.5.1 Anatomical and Physiological Considerations

The origin of the platysma muscle is in the superficial thoracic fascia on its superior aspect. Posteriorly, the platysma has an insertion in the depressor anguli oris and risorius muscles, whilst anteriorly the insertion is into the periosteal covering of the medial mandible [27–32]. This anatomical configuration means that the platysma causes vertically oriented cervical bands to appear, as well as horizontally oriented rhytides in the neck region [25].

14.5.1.1 Dilution

The cervical region covers a large area, and thus Botox needs to be at a relatively low concentration, which allows the neurotoxin to be diffused over the whole region. A suitable dilution is achieved by using between 1 and 5 mL of sterile saline to reconstitute a vial containing 100 IU of neurotoxin [28].

14.5.1.2 Injection Sites

To treat platysmal bands, a dose of between 2 and 5 IU is needed at each site of injection. The number of sites where an injection is to be performed is determined by the size of the cervical region in particular patients. If a patient has a long neck and the band is bulky, there may be a requirement for at least 4 or 5 injection sites [25].

The anterior approach may also be employed when using botulinum neurotoxin in the cervical region. With this technique, the clinician starts at the cervical midline, choosing injection sites at 2 cm intervals along the line of the horizontally oriented rhytides. In this way, the number of injections is typically 3 or 4. Toxin should not be injected any further posteriorly than the anterior margin of the sternocleidomastoid muscle, which lies laterally in the cervical region, since there is a danger of inadvertently inducing chemical denervation of the cervical strap muscles. If this occurs, the patient may be unable to swallow [25].

14.5.2 Dosages

To treat horizontally oriented bands in the platysma, a dose of between 2 and 5 IU is administered at each site of injection. Thus, the total dosage required is between 15 and 45 IU. To treat horizontally oriented rhytides, 3–5 IU is injected at each site, resulting in a total dosage of between 30 and 60 IU [25].

14.5.3 Adverse Effects and Complications

Adverse events arising in connection with botulinum toxin injection into the cervical region are generally those that may occur with any injection, such as skin discoloration and pain. Dysphagia may develop if the muscles involved in deglutition become inadvertently affected by toxin, generally as a result of a faulty injection technique. Somewhat unusually, patients may complain of myalgia or cervical discomfort, find they cannot easily raise their head from the pillow when lying down, or experience a headache. These adverse events are seldom seen and are temporary [25].

14.5.4 Platysmal Bands

Platysmal bands, which are vertically oriented straight bands in the neck, become increasingly prominent as an individual grows older (Fig. 14.1). They are more obvious when the muscles of the neck are actively contracting. The bands themselves are formed when the platysma contracts. The muscles separate from each other and protrude along their anterior margins [33].

The evidence base for how effective injected botulinum neurotoxin is in treating platysmal bands is confined to case series and case reports [34–38]. The authors of a case series involving 1500 individuals who were injected with onabotulinumtoxinA at various doses for an indication of latysmal bands indicated that most of these individuals had a result ranging from good to excellent [34]. It was noted that the following features seemed to correlate with better outcomes: where the platysma was flaccid, where neck wrinkles had a horizontal orientation, and where the degree of laxity of the skin was no more than moderate. Outcomes ranging from good to excellent were noted in 99% of cases where these features were present.

The adverse effect that occurs with the highest frequency in treating platysmal bands by chemical denervation is bruising [34]. It is also possible to observe swelling, redness of the skin, myalgia, and cervical discomfort. Cervical weakness and difficulty swallowing are possible but seldom occur [34].

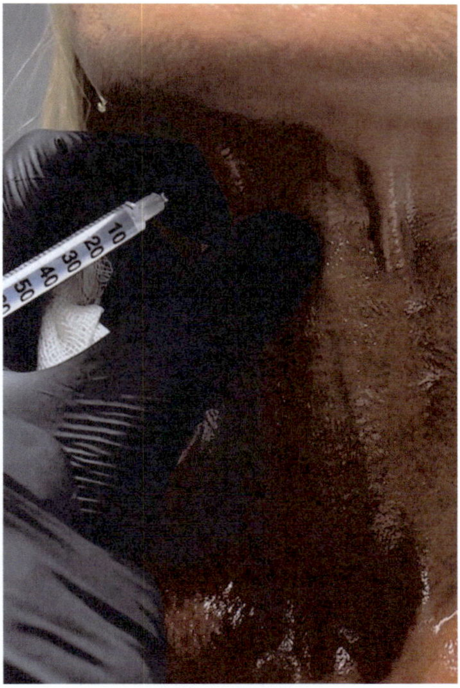

Fig. 14.1 Botulinum toxin injection to platysmal bands

There is considerable variety in the dosages of onabotulinumtoxinA used by various clinicians in treating platysmal bands. It has been suggested that no more than 30 to 40 IU onabotulinumtoxinA in total be injected in the cervical region at any particular treatment session, since doses exceeding this are associated with a higher risk of cervical weakness and deglutition difficulties [39]. The authors' own preference is to use a total of 15 IU onabotulinumtoxinA on the platysmal band on each side, this being made up of three injections, with the sites of injection placed 1–1.5 cm apart. It has been reported by some practitioners that a dose of abobotulinumtoxinA 30 IU to each platysmal band is also efficacious [40].

First the skin is prepared, then the patient clenches the platysma muscle, which reveals the full outline of the bands. A variety of different approaches are used for the injections, ranging from small numbers of injections to multiple. Electromyography is utilized for guidance by some clinicians. However, most cases do not require electromyographic guidance. A popular choice is to place injection sites 1–1.5 cm apart, starting at the anterior mandible and moving posteriorly. The dose usually ranges from 3 to 10 IU where onabotulinumtoxinA is used and is adjusted according to how bulky the platysmal band is [12].

A different method is to use three specific sites. Imagine a line connecting the horizontal under-chin and the vertical surface of the neck facing anteriorly. The sites are then defined as halfway between the forward limit of the platysmal band under the chin and the lowest extent of the band lying in front of the neck. The two most massive bands are each targeted with onabotulinumtoxinA 20 IU, whilst the small bands are injected with 5 IU each time [12].

14.5.5 Horizontally Oriented Cervical Rhytides

Horizontally oriented cervical rhytides result from the muscular contractions of the superficial musculoaponeurotic system (SMAS). The SMAS is a system of fibrous tissue and muscles that forms a layer enveloping the facial and cervical muscles. There are reports indicating that horizontally oriented cervical rhytides can be softened by injection of botulinum neurotoxin. The usual dose of onabotulinumtoxinA is between 10 and 20 IU. This dose is separated into numerous injections of around 1–2 IU, leaving a 2–3 cm gap between injections. Inject into the dermis. It is important not to inject at a deeper level than the dermis, since doing so entails a risk of hemorrhage from piercing a perforating vein and inadvertently denervating the deeper muscles, resulting in deglutition difficulties [33].

References

1. DasGupta BR. Structures of botulinum neurotoxin, its functional domains, and perspectives on the crystalline type A toxin. In: Jankovic J, Hallet M, editors. Therapy with botulinum toxin. Marcel Dekker; 1994. p. 15.
2. Schantz EJ, Johnson EA. Botulinum toxin: the story of its development for the treatment of human disease. Perspect Biol Med. 1997;40:317.
3. Burke GS. Notes on Bacillus botulinus. J Bacteriol. 1919;4:555.
4. Aoki KR, Guyer B. Botulinum toxin type A and other botulinum toxin serotypes: a comparative review of biochemical and pharmacological actions. Eur J Neurol. 2001;8(Suppl 5):21.
5. Dolly JO, Lisk G, Foran PG, et al. Insights into the extended duration of neuroparalysis by botulinum neurotoxin A relative to the other shorter-acting serotypes: differences between motor nerve terminals and cultured neurons. In: Brin MF, Jankovic J, Hallett M, editors. Scientific and therapeutic aspects of botulinum toxin. 1st ed. Philadelphia: Lippincott Williams & Wilkins; 2002. p. 91.
6. Scott AB. Botulinum toxin injection into extraocular muscles as an alternative to strabismus surgery. Ophthalmology. 1980;87:1044.
7. Wabbels B, Reichel G, Fulford-Smith A, et al. Double-blind, randomised, parallel group pilot study comparing two botulinum toxin type A products for the treatment of blepharospasm. J Neural Transm (Vienna). 2011;118:233.
8. Carruthers J, Stubbs HA. Botulinum toxin for benign essential blepharospasm, hemifacial spasm and age-related lower eyelid entropion. Can J Neurol Sci. 1987;14:42.
9. Borodic GE, Cheney M, McKenna M. Contralateral injections of botulinum A toxin for the treatment of hemifacial spasm to achieve increased facial symmetry. Plast Reconstr Surg. 1992;90:972.
10. Carruthers J. Overview of botulinum toxin for cosmetic indications. Dover JS, Ofori AO (Eds). UpToDate. Last updated: Jul 22, 2019.
11. Tsui JK, Eisen A, Mak E, et al. A pilot study on the use of botulinum toxin in spasmodic torticollis. Can J Neurol Sci. 1985;12:314.
12. Hauser RA. Botulinum toxin injections in plastic surgery. In: de la Torre JI (Ed). Medscape. Updated: Feb 08, 2019. https://emedicine.medscape.com/article/1271380-overview#a4. Accessed online at 15 April 15 2021.

13. Giordano CN, Matarasso SL, Ozog DM. Injectable and topical neurotoxins in dermatology: basic science, anatomy, and therapeutic agents. J Am Acad Dermatol. 2017;76:1013.
14. Meunier FA, Schiavo G, Molgó J. Botulinum neurotoxins: from paralysis to recovery of functional neuromuscular transmission. J Physiol Paris. 2002;96:105.
15. Carruthers J, Carruthers A. The evolution of botulinum neurotoxin type A for cosmetic applications. J Cosmet Laser Ther. 2007;9:186.
16. Jost WH, Blümel J, Grafe S. Botulinum neurotoxin type A free of complexing proteins (XEOMIN) in focal dystonia. Drugs. 2007;67:669.
17. Frevert J, Dressler D. Complexing proteins in botulinum toxin type A drugs: a help or a hindrance? Biologics. 2010;4:325.
18. Ramirez AL, Reeck J, Maas CS. Botulinum toxin type B (MyoBloc) in the management of hyperkinetic facial lines. Otolaryngol Head Neck Surg. 2002;126:459.
19. Alster TS, Lupton JR. Botulinum toxin type B for dynamic glabellar rhytides refractory to botulinum toxin type A. Dermatologic Surg. 2003;29:516.
20. Kim EJ, Ramirez AL, Reeck JB, Maas CS. The role of botulinum toxin type B (Myobloc) in the treatment of hyperkinetic facial lines. Plast Reconstr Surg. 2003;112:88S.
21. Sadick NS. Prospective open-label study of botulinum toxin type B (Myobloc) at doses of 2,400 and 3,000 U for the treatment of glabellar wrinkles. Dermatologic Surg. 2003;29:501.
22. Brandt F, O'Connell C, Cazzaniga A, Waugh JM. Efficacy and safety evaluation of a novel botulinum toxin topical gel for the treatment of moderate to severe lateral canthal lines. Dermatologic Surg. 2010;36(Suppl 4):2111.
23. Collins A, Nasir A. Topical botulinum toxin. J Clin Aesthet Dermatol. 2010;3:35.
24. Chajchir I, Modi P, Chajchir A. Novel topical BoNTA (CosmeTox, toxin type a) cream used to treat hyperfunctional wrinkles of the face, mouth, and neck. Aesth Plast Surg. 2008;32:715.
25. Atamoros FP. Botulinum toxin in the lower one third of the face. Clin Dermatol. 2003;21(6):505–12. https://doi.org/10.1016/j.clindermatol.2003.11.014.
26. Kane MA. Nonsurgical treatment of platysmal bands with injection of botulinum toxin A (published erratum appears in Plast Reconstr Surg 1999 Mar;103(3):following table of contents). Plast Reconstr Surg. 1999;103(2):656–63. discussion 664–5
27. Aston SJ. Platysma muscle in rhytidoplasty. Ann Plast Surg. 1979;3:529.
28. Brandt F, Bellman B. Cosmetic use of Botulinum toxin for the aging neck. Dermatologic Surg. 1998;24:1232–4.
29. Carruthers J, Carruthers A. Botox use in the mid and lower face and neck. Semin Cutan Med Surg. 2001;20:85–92.
30. Richard A, Ritz M, Donahue S, et al. Botox for contraction of pectoral muscles. Plast Reconstr Surg. 2001;108:270–1.
31. Becker-Wegerich PM, Rauch L, Ruzicka T. Botulinum toxin A: successful de'collete´ rejuvenation. Dermatologic Surg. 2002;28:168–71.
32. Moore KL, Dalley AF. Clinical oriented anatomy. In: Kelly PJ, editor. Muscles of the face. 4th ed. Baltimore: Lippincott Williams & Wilkins; 1999. p. 850–6. ch 7.
33. Carruthers J. Botulinum toxin for cosmetic indications: Treatment of specific sites. Dover JS, Ofori AO (Eds). UpToDate. Last updated: 07 June 2019.
34. Matarasso A, Matarasso SL, Brandt FS, Bellman B. Botulinum A exotoxin for the management of platysma bands. Plast Reconstr Surg. 1999;103:645.
35. Kane MA. Nonsurgical treatment of platysmal bands with injection of botulinum toxin A. Plast Reconstr Surg. 1999;103:656.
36. Brandt FS, Bellman B. Cosmetic use of botulinum A exotoxin for the aging neck. Dermatologic Surg. 1998;24:1232.
37. Brandt FS, Boker A. Botulinum toxin for the treatment of neck lines and neck bands. Dermatol Clin. 2004;22:159.
38. Carruthers J, Carruthers A. Botulinum toxin A in the mid and lower face and neck. Dermatol Clin. 2004;22:151.

39. Carruthers J, Carruthers A. Practical cosmetic Botox techniques. J Cutan Med Surg. 1999;3(Suppl 4):S49.
40. Kane M, Donofrio L, Ascher B, et al. Expanding the use of neurotoxins in facial aesthetics: a consensus panel's assessment and recommendations. J Drugs Dermatol. 2010;9:s7.

Botulinum Toxin Injections: Décolleté

15

Elif Kaya Çelik, Nuray Bayar Muluk, and Jarrod Keeler

15.1 Introduction

Amongst non-invasive procedures practised in aesthetic medicine, the use of injectable botulinum toxin of serotype A (BoNT-A) is one of the most frequent. This toxin can prevent cholinergic neurotransmission by preventing the release of acetylcholine from the presynaptic terminal of neurons at the muscle end-plate [1]. If rhytides form as a result of the contraction of particular muscles, injecting BoNT-A may weaken the muscle, resulting in softening of the wrinkles. This benefit may translate into a higher quality of life [2]. Clinicians have access to a number of different forms of BoNT-A for cosmetic applications. Dysport (Azzalure) and Botox (Vistabel) are the most popular preparations. Since their methods of preparation differ in terms of the bacterial strain used, method of purification and even the assay used to evaluate their potency, they are quite distinctly different and cannot simply be used interchangeably [3–6].

Dysport (Azzalure) doses are specified in Speywood units, abbreviated to s.U. It is contained in vials of either 500 s.U. or 300 s.U. It has been available for over two decades. During this time the product has demonstrated high levels of consistency and has been safe for both neuromuscular disorders and cosmetic applications [7–10].

E. K. Çelik
Tokat Gaziosmanpaşa University, Medical Faculty, Department of Otorhinolaryngology, Tokat, Turkey

N. Bayar Muluk (✉)
Faculty of Medicine, Department of Otorhinolaryngology, Kırıkkale University, Kırıkkale, Türkiye

J. Keeler
Otolaryngology & Facial Plastic and Reconstructive Surgery, Specialty Physician Associates, St. Luke's Medical Center, Bethlehem, PA, USA

C. Cingi et al. (eds.), *Minor Interventions, Major Outcomes on the Face*, Comprehensive ENT, https://doi.org/10.1007/978-3-032-01305-7_15

15.2 Décolleté Wrinkles

Both intrinsic and extrinsic factors affect how the chest ages. In most cases, a key factor is photoageing, and thus treatment commonly requires injectable fillers, skin peels and laser resurfacing in combination. There are specialists in treating décolleté wrinkles who have published recommendations [11].

In most individuals, the exposed upper portion of the chest, forming a V shape, sustains the effects of photoageing, which leads to the formation of rhytides, both superficial and deeper, together with alterations in the pigmentation of the skin and its texture. These changes may be felt to show a patient's age in an unwelcome way. This site, as elsewhere on the body, is one where static and dynamic wrinkles co-exist, with the former being a result of solar damage and the latter due to repeated muscular contractions [1].

15.3 Anatomical Considerations

The key muscles of interest in the upper chest region are the posterior portion of the platsyma and the fibres of the pectoralis major located medially. To be able to palpate these muscles, clinicians should get patients to cross their arms in front of them [11].

The origin of the platysma muscle is usually the second rib; however, it has been reported that in some individuals, the muscle originates at a more inferior site, i.e. the anterior portion of the fourth rib. The platysma overlies the pectoralis major muscle before reaching its insertion on the inferior aspect of the mandible [12–14].

15.4 Injection Site, Dosage and Method

Current recommendations [13] propose that Botox 100 IU as a single vial be reconstituted using between 1 and 5 mL of sterile saline. The pattern of injection sites chosen varies between practitioners, but all techniques aim to ensure even coverage of the whole upper chest. A V-shaped path may be followed, involving between 3 and 8 injection sites, or a curved shape is also suitable, which calls for between 4 and 10 injections. A further option is to form a triangle with the injections, in which case between 6 and 15 injections will be needed [1].

With Dysport, the total dosage advised is between 75 and 120 s.U. Each separate injection utilises between 7.5 and 10 s.U. The clinician should inject in a V pattern, with the number of injections dictated by how severe and numerous the rhytides are. At most, 12 injections of 10 s.U. each or 16 injections of 7.5 s.U. are appropriate. The needle should enter to a depth of 4 mm or more and should be at right angles to the skin. Those individuals in whom the rhytides have formed due to the way they sleep or the influence of gravity must not be treated, since there is no benefit in such cases. It may be prudent in some individuals to treat bands of platysma at the same time as the upper chest [11].

Treating décolleté in this way is associated with a very favourable safety profile. Where adverse events occur, they generally take the form of bruising, pain at the site injected or redness of the skin [11].

15.5 Areas of Controversy

The commercially available forms of botulinum toxin differ considerably from each other. It may not be possible to interchange different preparations. There are wide variations in the potency of the various serotypes, as well as in how long their effects last. This translates into different clinical results. There are even considerable differences in preparations based on the same serotype. For example, Botox 1 IU is equivalent in potency to around 4 IU of Dysport. In this case, one agent may replace another after adjusting for their different potencies. At present, the evidence base for different products is insufficient to state that one preparation is preferable to any other [15].

The two main preparations in use, Botox and Dysport, have both advantages and disadvantages. Botox has dominated the North American market for over 10 years and is known for being safe in clinical use. It does suffer from a disadvantage that, once reconstituted, it rapidly declines in potency. Some clinicians work around this issue by arranging to treat many patients at the same session, thereby eliminating waste. However, this may not fit the patients' preferred timing, and they may refuse [16].

In contrast, Myobloc (Elan) retains its potency for greater than a year following reconstitution. This feature is helpful to clinicians who need to treat multiple individuals from the same vial. Nonetheless, to produce a result similar to that of Botox, a higher volume of the preparation is potentially required. Moreover, since Myobloc contains a large amount of proteinaceous material, it may be more antigenic than other preparations [16].

15.6 Immunological Aspects

It has been calculated that between 5% and 15% of patients receiving serial injections with 79–11 Botox start to show a lack of response to the agent over time due to producing antibodies that deactivate the toxin. The likelihood of a patient developing secondary treatment resistance in this way increases if doses exceeding 200 IU are utilised at one time or if treatments are repeated more frequently than monthly. A newer form of Botox, BCB 2024, is likely to stimulate the production of neutralising immunoglobulins thanks to a lower level of protein. Animal studies using rabbits compared the novel preparation of Botox with the older 79–11 Botox preparation. About 100% of rabbits receiving the older preparation had developed neutralising immunoglobulins after 5 months, whereas no antibodies of this type occurred in the animals exposed to the novel preparation. Dressler et al. [17] report a significantly lower level of immunoglobulin-mediated treatment resistance in patients administered BSB 2024. Furthermore, results obtained by Jankovic [18] show that the frequency of neutralising immunoglobulins was six times lower with the newer preparation.

The fact remains that some individuals who receive botulinum toxin for a cosmetic indication develop immunoglobulin-mediated treatment resistance. If treatment resistance is noted, serological investigation may be undertaken, albeit this seldom occurs other than in research trials. An alternative approach is to observe the physiological effect of injecting Botox 15 IU unilaterally into the frontalis muscle. It has not been definitively established if immunoglobulin-mediated treatment resistance declines eventually, which might justify reattempting treatment. In the meantime, the most clinically judicious approach seems to aim for low doses and space treatments more than a month apart, with the rationale that this renders an immunological response less likely to occur [16].

References

1. Atamoros FP. Botulinum toxin in the lower one third of the face. Clin Dermatol. 2003;21(6):505–12. https://doi.org/10.1016/j.clindermatol.2003.11.014. PMID: 14759584.
2. Sadick NS. The impact of cosmetic interventions on quality of life. Dermatol Online J. 2008;14:2.
3. Huang W, Foster JA, Rogachefsky AS. Pharmacology of botulinum toxin. J Am Acad Dermatol. 2000;43:249–59.
4. Rzany B, Ascher B, Monheit GD. Treatment of glabellar lines with botulinum toxin type A (Speywood Unit): a clinical overview. J Eur Acad Dermatol Venereol. 2010;24:1–10.
5. Pickett AM, Hambleton P. Dose standardisation of botulinum toxin. Lancet. 1994;344:474–5.
6. Karsai S, Raulin C. Current evidence on the unit equivalence of different botulinum neurotoxin A formulations and recommendations for clinical practice in dermatology. Dermatologic Surg. 2008;34:1–8.
7. Rzany B, Dill-Muller D, Grablowitz D, Heckmann M, Carid D. Repeated botulinum toxin A injections for the treatment of lines in the upper face: a retrospective study of 4103 treatments in 945 patients. Dermatologic Surg. 2007;33:S18–25.
8. Markey AC. Dysport. Dermatol Clin. 2004;22:213–9.
9. Van den Bergh P, Francart J, Mourin S, Kollmann P, Laterre EC. Five-year experience in the treatment of focal movement disorders with low-dose Dysport botulinum toxin. Muscle Nerve. 1995;18:720–9.
10. Jitpimolmard S, Tiamkao S, Laopaiboon M. Long term results of botulinum toxin type A (Dysport) in the treatment of hemifacial spasm: a report of 175 cases. J Neurol Neurosurg Psychiatry. 1998;64:751–7.
11. Ascher B, Talarico S, Cassuto D, Escobar S, Hexsel D, Jaén P, Monheit GD, Rzany B, Viel M. International consensus recommendations on the aesthetic usage of botulinum toxin type A (Speywood Unit)—part II: wrinkles on the middle and lower face, neck and chest. J Eur Acad Dermatol Venereol. 2010;24(11):1285–95. https://doi.org/10.1111/j.1468-3083.2010.03728.x. PMID: 20569284.
12. Richard A, Ritz M, Donahue S, et al. Botox for contraction of pectoral muscles. Plast Reconstr Surg. 2001;108:270–1.
13. Becker-Wegerich PM, Rauch L, Ruzicka T. Botulinum toxin A: successful de'collete' rejuvenation. Dermatologic Surg. 2002;28:168–71.
14. Moore KL, Dalley AF. Clinical oriented anatomy. In: Kelly PJ, editor. Muscles of the face, Chapter 7. 4th ed. Baltimore: Lippincott Williams & Wilkins; 1999. p. 850–6.

15. Odergren T, Hjaltason H, Kaakkola S, et al. A double blind, randomised, parallel group study to investigate the dose equivalence of Dysport and Botox in the treatment of cervical dystonia. J Neurol Neurosurg Psychiatry. 1998;64(1):6–12.
16. Hauser RA. Botulinum toxin injections in plastic surgery. In: de la Torre JI, editor. Medscape. Updated: Feb 08, 2019. https://emedicine.medscape.com/article/1271380-overview#a6 (Accessed online at April 15, 2021).
17. Dressler D, Hallett M. Immunological aspects of Botox, Dysport and Myobloc/NeuroBloc. Eur J Neurol. 2006;13(Suppl 1):11–5.
18. Jankovic J, Vuong KD, Ahsan J. Comparison of efficacy and immunogenicity of original versus current botulinum toxin in cervical dystonia. Neurology. 2003;60(7):1186–8.

Botulinum Toxin as a Treatment for Functional Disorders

16

Mahmut Emre Gundogan, Cemal Cingi, and Hesham Negm

16.1 Blepharospasm

Blepharospasm refers to a condition where the blephara close involuntarily. It is a focal dystonic condition [1]. Typically, the orbicularis oculi muscles are involved bilaterally. It may become very disabling for patients. Blepharospasm may be an isolated condition or occur as part of other disorders involving abnormal muscular tone. Blepharospasm has frequently been noted in Parkinsonism, cerebral palsy with dystonia and tardive syndromes [2]. The condition often initially presents with excessive nictitation, and patients generally report their eyes feel dry and irritated. The next stage involves clonic contractions of the muscle, which ultimately becomes a tonic contraction, so the eye is permanently closed. This creates problems in performing daily activities [3]. Unless treatment is attempted, a patient with blepharospasm is effectively blind, i.e. a form of functional blindness. Whilst blepharospasm may initially affect only one eye, it virtually invariably ends up involving both orbicularis oculi muscles. The severity of the condition is not generally dependent on which task a patient is undertaking [4], but, as is common to other dystonic conditions, particular tasks may worsen or improve the symptoms. Blepharospasm is frequently more severe when patients face bright light, or try to read or watch TV [5]. And, just as with other dystonic conditions, there are certain "hacks" which may

M. E. Gundogan
Private Metrolife Hospital, Department of Otorhinolaryngology, Sanlıurfa, Turkey

C. Cingi (✉)
Eskisehir Osmangazi University, Medical Faculty, Department of Otorhinolaryngology, Eskisehir, Türkiye
e-mail: cemal@ogu.edu.tr

H. Negm
Cairo University, Faculty of Medicine, Department of Otorhinolaryngology, Cairo, Egypt

C. Cingi et al. (eds.), *Minor Interventions, Major Outcomes on the Face*, Comprehensive ENT, https://doi.org/10.1007/978-3-032-01305-7_16

improve symptoms, such as touching the eyes or the upper facial region, starting to talk or singing [6].

16.1.1 Pathophysiology

In common with many other diseases, the probable pathogenesis of dystonia depends on both inherited susceptibility and extrinsic factors. This is known as the dual hit hypothesis. A model of how dystonia is affecting the face and skull occur has been developed using rodents. These animals were rendered deficient in dopamine in the striatum by injecting oxidopamine (6-OHDA). In this state, when injury was induced peripherally, the rodents developed twitching of the face that resembled the picture seen in dystonic disorders of the skull [7]. Unless there was both malfunction of the striatum and peripheral injury, a dystonic lesion did not result [2].

The characteristic feature of a dystonic disorder is muscular hyperactivity. Thus, dystonia is a type of movement disorder featuring hyperkinesia. The hyperactivity is seen in contraction of both agonist and antagonist groups of muscles and a tendency for adjacent muscles to be stimulated. Electromyography reveals lengthy bursts of muscular activity in cases of dystonia [8]. The pathophysiological mechanisms common to dystonic disorders, including blepharospasm, include disinhibition, abnormal plasticity of the nervous system, and dysfunctional sensory input [2].

The clinically observable consequences of dystonia are due to disinhibition affecting multiple levels of the nervous system. Simultaneous contraction by groups of agonist and antagonist muscles occurs because the normal reciprocal inhibitory mechanism within the spinal cord is defective [1]. In blepharospasm, it has been shown that this reciprocal inhibitory mechanism is defective at the level of the brainstem, resulting in overly excitable nictitation [9]. It has also been demonstrated, through experiments involving transcranial magnetic stimulation (TMS) that the cortex also loses its ability to inhibit muscular contraction [10]. In healthy individuals, the contraction of other adjacent muscles is inhibited (surround inhibition) when precise movements are being executed, but this process has been demonstrated to be deficient in focal hand dystonia [11].

16.1.2 Management

At present, the majority of cases of blepharospasm are treated by injection of preparations containing botulinum neurotoxin. However, there are a range of other potential options, including drugs taken orally, physical treatments, topical medications, and surgery. Alongside these measures, it is essential to educate patients about the condition, avoid prescription of agents which may provoke dystonia (such as dopamine antagonists), ensure trauma does not occur to the cornea or eye generally, and provide general support [2].

The toxin which possesses the most potency in human subjects is botulinum neurotoxin (BoNT), which is synthesised by the bacterial organism, *Clostridium botulinum*. This toxin results in muscles becoming paralysed at the muscle end-plate. The affected muscle lacks tone and has absent reflexes [12]. The toxin occurs in seven forms, which can be distinguished on serological grounds and are labelled A to G. Serotypes A and B are marketed for clinical use. The seven serotypes all share a similar molecular mass of 150 kDa and consist of a heavy and light chain, which are bonded to each other by a disulphide linkage [12]. The light chain is the toxic component, whereas the heavy chain interacts with a cellular receptor prior to the entire toxin being endocytosed [2].

BoNT possesses a domain on the heavy chain which has a high affinity for a receptor on the neuronal surface. Receptor binding leads to BoNT being endocytosed within a vesicle. The acidic environment within the vesicle leads to dissociation of the disulphide bond, and this then leaves the light chain free. The light chain passes into the cytoplasm, where it attacks the SNARE (soluble N-ethyl-maleimide-sensitive factor attachment protein receptor) complex, rendering it incapable of its usual function of fusing acetylcholine-containing vesicles with the synaptic membrane and thus releasing neurotransmitter into the synaptic cleft. The light chain is, in fact, a metalloprotease [13].

Use of BoNT to treat dystonia has a very favourable safety profile and is usually efficacious for prolonged periods [14]. Although it is fairly frequent for adverse events to occur following injection around the eye, these events are typically of low severity and consist mostly of dry eye, diplopia, excess lacrimation, ptosis, and skin discolouration from bleeding. If ptosis occurs, this is generally due to BoNT diffusing into the ocular midline, thus weakening the levator palpebrae muscles. To avoid this adverse event, injections should not be placed close to the central portion of the superior orbicularis oculi muscle. Similarly, the injection site should not be too near to the inferior blepharon in the midline, as this makes entropion and sagging of the inferior blepharon more probable.

The possibility of systemic absorption of BoNT is amongst the key factors that limit how freely the toxin may be used. Botulism of iatrogenic origin, however, occurs very infrequently. Furthermore, the dose involved in treating blepharospasm is low. A systematic review which examined the evidence base on botulism of iatrogenic origin found no apparent complications associated with systemic absorption of BoNT if the dose given did not exceed the range 100–200 IU [15]. Thus, botulism would not be expected in patients treated for blepharospasm.

16.2 Treating Sialorrhoea with BoNT

Sialorrhoea refers to an excess of saliva, sometimes termed drooling. It is one of the most frequently occurring non-motor symptoms noted in patients with Parkinson's disease (PD), where its frequency is between 50% and 70% [16, 17]. Many factors probably contribute to sialorrhoea, which may result from excess saliva production or deficient mechanisms for clearing saliva [18]. Patients with swallowing difficulties cannot adequately clear pooled saliva, which is probably the main reason sialorrhoea is so common in patients with PD [17]. Another factor in PD patients with advanced disease is that the neck often remains flexed and the jaw is open. This anatomical position tends to produce sialorrhoea [17, 18]. Drooling is generally the cause of social discomfort and may contribute to depressed mood [19]. Furthermore, it may lead to unsatisfactory mouth and perioral hygiene and predispose patients to infections of the respiratory tract [17].

Recently, a number of trials have published results demonstrating that BoNT is efficacious in treating sialorrhoea [20–22]. A study dating from 2018 examined the use of incobotulinumtoxinA in treating sialorrhoea in children with cerebral palsy secondary to anoxia and found the treatment efficacious [21]. An older study which retrospectively examined a cohort of 45 paediatric patients suffering from various neurological disorders determined that BoNT could be used safely and effectively to treat sialorrhoea, when the technique involved injection of the salivary glands under ultrasound guidance. The benefit persisted for around 5 months on average [22] and was noticeable around 1 week after completion of the procedure [17]. A systematic review by Seppi et al. concluded that using botulinum toxin serotypes A and B was safe and effective in treating sialorrhoea. The evidence for this conclusion came from well-designed trials featuring randomisation and involving patients with PD. The clinicians performing the procedures had adequate training and guidance techniques, such as ultrasound, were available to them [20].

16.3 Use of BoNT to Treat Hyperhidrosis

Patients suffering from hyperhidrosis sweat profusely and excessively, especially from the palms of the hands, soles of the feet, and the armpits. No external factor is identifiable [23, 24]. Hyperhidrosis has negative effects on the sufferer's emotions and social function and leads to clothes becoming damaged through sweat staining and soaking of the material. If hyperhidrosis is of high severity, the skin may become macerated and infection may occur secondarily. It is a condition associated with social isolation and stigma [23–25].

Eccrine (sweat) glands fulfil a key role in keeping body temperature within normal bounds. These glands are normally responsive to a number of different signals. In hyperhidrosis, the microscopic architecture of the eccrine glands has normal appearances, but appears to have excessive sensitivity in situations where adrenaline release is expected, such as when the patient is anxious or under psychological stress [23, 24, 26].

A considerable number of different therapies are available for hyperhidrosis, but their benefit is usually short-lasting and does not produce high levels of patient satisfaction. Currently, the treatments in use include topically applied antiperspirant agents (based on aluminium salts), iontophoresis, and use of medications with a systemic anticholinergic action [27–29]. In most cases, the treatment is palliative in intent, rather than it addressing the underlying problem. Drugs, whether topical or systemic, are only effective for the period over which they are being utilised. Permanent use may be intolerable for patients with hyperhidrosis [25, 27–29]. There is also a risk that topically applied agents may be irritating to the skin. The surgical procedures used in this condition, e.g. sympathectomy or excision of sweat glands, are associated with a broad range of adverse effects and complications. These include haemorrhage, infection, scar formation, and pain [30–32].

It has been suggested that, given the lack of an ideal treatment for hyperhidrosis that would combine the features of being safe, effective and providing a durable benefit, BoNT serotype A may be suitable. Following injection into the dermis, BoNT has been shown potentially to offer benefit in hyperhidrosis. This benefit is because the toxin can interfere with cholinergic transmission within the autonomic system, just as it does at muscle end-plates [25, 32–35].

16.4 Botulinum Toxin in the Treatment of Masseter Muscle Hypertrophy

Masseter muscle hypertrophy causes an irregular contour of the angle of the face, which is unattractive. Common indications for masseter muscle reduction include asymmetric masseter muscle hypertrophy, changes in the mandibular angle, bruxism, and alterations in the square outline of the face, which can give a square, comprehensive look. In addition, reducing the bulk of the masseter muscle hypertrophy relieves muscle function and has aesthetic effects. Botulinum toxin muscle injection for masseter muscle hypertrophy was first performed by scientists, who demonstrated that substantial regression of the masseter muscle could occur, resulting in a slimming of the face (Fig. 16.1).

However, the present research is focused on the chewing and aesthetic effects after botulinum toxin A injection, and factors such as the dose, duration, and side effects associated with the botulinum toxin A injection have yet to be addressed. Therefore, this study adopted botulinum toxin preparations to implant the masseter muscles at varying degrees, evaluate the dose-effect relationship, and compare the clinical effects and situations after injection at different implantation sites. These changes from masseter atrophy not only reference the aesthetic outcomes and optimal dose but can also facilitate the development of new directions for botulin treatments and provide theoretical support for precise clinical implantation [36].

Masseter muscle hypertrophy (MMH) is an adaptive enlargement response to persistent excessive use of the muscles. The main factors contributing to MMH include excessive gum chewing, bruxism, stress, and genetics. Patients with MMH not only have an unattractive square lower face but also often suffer from masticatory muscle pain, temporomandibular joint disorders, and headaches. MMH is typically treated using cosmetic surgery, orthodontics, or pharmaceuticals. However, these methods are often associated with recurrence as well as surgical complications, long periods of orthodontic treatment, and various adverse effects. Accordingly, an alternative therapy for MMH is warranted [36, 37].

Botulinum toxin type A (BTXA) is a bacterial exotoxin that inhibits acetylcholine release from peripheral cholinergic nerves, resulting in temporary denervation, and inhibits the release of other neurotransmitters and attenuates inflammation. Notably, evidence has shown that BTXA not only effectively treats bruxism but also

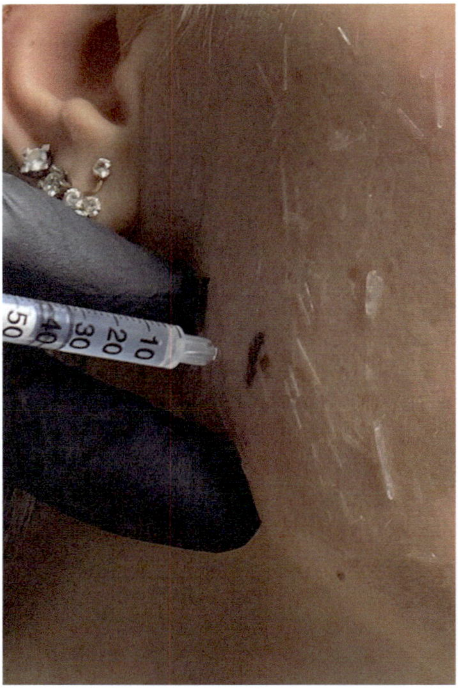

Fig. 16.1 Application of masseter botulinum toxin. (Courtesy of Murat Songu MD)

alleviates the symptoms of TMJD by paralysing the masseter muscles and preventing their excessive forceful functional movements. Therefore, BTXA injection has become a minimally invasive, effective, and safe technique for managing MMH. BTXA injections into hypertrophic masseter muscles have numerous advantages when compared with other treatment options: it is a fast procedure that is associated with few complications; there is no need for incision or suture; and the effect is stable, with no loss of the movement strength of the masseter muscle after ten weeks. In addition, given that BTXA resolves masseter muscle dysmorphia, recovery is relatively rapid compared with cosmetic surgery, making it very suitable for patients who seek rapid facial improvement [37, 38].

The development of the craniofacial areas is connected with the growth of the neurocranium and its bony facial part. The incisors are the first permanent teeth observed at around six years of age. By 12, the deciduous first molars have exfoliated, and the permanent first and second molars have erupted. From 12 to 17 years, during the growth of young adolescents, the masseter and temporal muscles increase in size and thickness. After 17 years of development, the masseter muscle continues to develop, and its hypertrophy can occur in some adults. As part of the muscles of mastication, the masseter muscle plays a vital role in mandibular deformation, and its physiological or pathological conditions directly and indirectly influence the mandible bones. The mandibles of mammals function in many activities, such as speech, facial expressions, chewing of food, and swallowing. Mastication, which results from the actions of the masseter, temporal, medial, and lateral pterygoid muscles, is one of the essential functions of the temporal muscle, crucial in promoting vertical growth. The behaviours that consume more time place more significant stress and require energy are related to larger muscle size and the frequency of particular behaviours. Different diets could involve the adjustment potential of masticatory muscle in the mandible, which is related to mandible growth [37, 38].

16.4.1 Masseter Muscle Hypertrophy: Etiology and Clinical Presentation

The phenotype of a hypertrophied masseter muscle can be multifactorial. Congenital masseter muscle hypertrophy has been reported, with masseter muscle hypertrophy beginning in early adolescence at a mean age of 14.2 years. The incidence is higher in females, but others have reported a male-to-female ratio of 7:4. In contrast, acquired masseter hypertrophy predominantly affects adult females, who attribute symptoms to changes in their lifestyles around the time of marriage and delivery. In short, a patient with masseter muscle hypertrophy who often chews gum has a history of bruxism, and a symptom of waking up with a tired masseter muscle, as well as a history of tooth grinding, habitual clenching, and biting hard foods. On physical examination, the muscle is tender, enlarged, and painful on palpation. The texture is firm or hard, and the facies ovina show a prominent or square shape of the face.

However, avascular necrosis, temporomandibular joint disorders, soft tissue and bone changes in the temporomandibular joint, local tumour invasion, and botulinum toxin muscle tropism have been reported as differential diagnoses. The treatment of masseter muscle hypertrophy varies depending on the situation, with botulinum toxin being a conservative, easy, and quick treatment method with minimal side effects despite current limitations such as multiple injections and relapses. Additionally, there is the unique characteristic of an increasing number of patients presenting with the symptoms of an enlarged masseter and requesting treatment of the masseter because of its small square face in the facial contouring state. Therefore, it is necessary to diagnose masseter muscle hypertrophy and perform the appropriate treatment accurately [38, 39].

16.4.2 Causes of Masseter Muscle Hypertrophy

There is no clear pathophysiological explanation of what causes idiopathic bilateral masseter muscle hypertrophy. Four different theories are mentioned, and some possible suggestions are proposed. Firstly, the most frequent explanation emphasises the excessive use of the masseter muscle. Depending on the shape and biting habit of the teeth placed on the molars, excessive function and force are found in the muscles. Compression and attrition affect the trigeminal nerve. Hyperplasia and hypertrophy follow as a response to the nerve [38, 39].

Further, under intermittent nerve inhibition, excessive forceful contraction of the masseter muscle is stimulated, and a chronic hypoxic state is created, which leads to the proliferation of fibrous tissue that may be due to hyperplasia. Other causes of masticatory muscle hypertrophy and muscle pain include bruxism, trauma, prolonged and excessive loading due to considerable malocclusion cusp interference, unilateral mastication, unbalanced prosthesis, chronic recurrent periodic pain, and lack of regular continuing periodical wounding of the muscle. Bruxism and mechanical stress are frequently mentioned among predisposing factors. There is no clear evidence for these claims. These are speculative possibilities [38, 39].

The second proposed explanation is that masseter muscle hypertrophy is frequently associated with bruxism or excessive spindly bursal activity. The emphasis is mainly on occlusal disorders. The clench level during physical examination is likely correlated with the propensity to develop masseter muscle hypertrophy. Increased topography of the masseter muscles is possibly associated with bruxism and other symptoms of temporomandibular dysfunction. Causation is possibly a hematoma during bruxism, which triggers myositis ossificans, and as healing occurs, it results in increased myofiber hypertrophy. Furthermore, masseter muscle enlargement is possibly facilitated by repetitive microtraumas during mastication. Bruxism causes the teeth to be otherwise arranged. As a result, coronal and buccal teeth protrude anteriorly, creating an improper bite and causing attrition, thus leading to constant activation of the masseter muscle. Therefore, idiopathic masticatory muscle hypertrophy is suggested if there is no proper orthodontic treatment. Decreased oral kinesthetic feedback significantly affects mandibular adaptation during maximum jaw opening [36–40].

The third possibility is that it may develop bilaterally based on a familial predisposition. A consecutive examination of three sisters by magnetic resonance imaging revealed no changes in muscle morphology due to treatment. This suggests that the shape of the face could be one of the genetic factors related to muscle growth. However, no genetic studies were found. Masseter muscle hypertrophy is also related to the components, which are part of the accommodating conditions associated with the crowding effect of the masseter muscle. Craniofacial growth hindered by masseter muscle hyperactivity may be an intrinsic part of masticatory muscle hypertrophy disorders. Increased and long-term activity sometimes stimulates muscle hypertrophy. Nevertheless, to fully explain an increased jaw elevator muscle mass, it is necessary to consider complex interactions ranging from the system's symmetry to signals routing from muscle to bone and vice versa. Information should be given about what might create the necessary increase in stimulatory activity [38, 39].

16.4.3 Botulinum Toxin Injection Technique for Treating Masseter Muscle Hypertrophy

Botulinum toxin can be used to treat hypertrophied masseter muscle. It can improve the appearance of the overlying soft tissue and produce significant aesthetic enhancement. Properly selecting appropriate injection sites is the key to achieving successful results with botulinum toxin for masseter hypertrophy reduction. The muscle may be thick and relatively tight in older women with hypertrophy, and the position and function of the inferior branch of the trigeminal nerve should be well understood. If the wrong injection site is chosen before treatment, it may cause dysesthesia and a reduction in the ability to chew hard food.

The masseter muscle is a powerful muscle located in the lower part of the face. Young women with a large volume will have a quadrate face shape; the masseter muscle will hypertrophy and become a specific health problem. Reduction of muscle hypertrophy with botulinum toxin type A has been shown to be safe and effective. There are two reasons for the injection of these muscles. The first is to improve the appearance of the overlying soft tissue and produce significant aesthetic enhancement. The second is the possibility of causing misuse of muscle activity, producing a calming effect on muscle hyperactive contraction and helping to prevent long-term dental problems. After reduction injection, attention should be paid to long-term maintenance. As a rule, the muscle autocorrects over time. The interval between treatments may then increase from approximately 4 to 6 months. It may then be extended to 8, 9, or 12 months. Finally, the massage muscle function will automatically reduce [38, 40].

16.4.4 Pre-Injection Assessment and Planning

Botulinum toxin injections in managing masseter muscle hypertrophy have become increasingly popular. Using botulinum toxin to reduce muscle hypertrophy can effectively reduce lower facial width, usually leading to a more aesthetically pleasing facial contour. It is crucial to perform a pre-injection clinical examination to assess masseter muscle bulk, shape, and function. A discussion is performed with the patient in terms of its maximal opening, pain in the temporal region, clicking noises during the mouth opening, and the existence of an axial deviation of jaw movement, especially at the opening phase. Although rare, trigeminal neuralgia is assessed. The presence of any generalised neuromuscular disorder, such as myasthenia gravis, is also discussed. The patient's history is significant, especially regarding headaches and bruxism. After the patient has read the Informed Consent Paper, it is signed.

Digital photographs, both frontal and lateral, are taken in the maximum intercuspal position. Since the maximal dentogliders opening is in the maximum intercuspal position, only the frontal and the lateral fixed reference points are used. Identical reference points for distances in the available gliding pathway will exist for the subsequent evaluation of changes in muscle size, or in the hypertrophy recovery process if/when the injections will be stopped. The level of consent to undergo treatment sessions and follow-ups should involve a precise methodology with fixed rules for decisions on a gummy smile, infra-positioned lip, and masseter clinical or electromyographic control. The level of consent to undergo injection treatment sessions should be specific. If different operational steps are required, specific consent is necessary. Screened protocols for active pathology should also be dealt with, in the prior clinical assessment. The patient must be informed that injection treatment cannot be performed when allergic skin reaction is present. The patient's expectations and treatment affordability should be in compliance with the protocol. No injection treatment should be offered if these criteria are not fulfilled. The patient should explicitly agree on the risk and expected success of the treatment before the protocol begins. For patients with temporomandibular disorders in one of the subgroups of the diagnostic taxonomy, a significant percentage of muscles in affiliated or unaffiliated centres recommend that the patient be offered some type of oral health care intervention. Finally, macro-prosthesis via other means, including the surgical insertion of absorbable screws or the fixed or removable extra-coronal framework, should be considered before injections are indicated. After the patient has been appropriately diagnosed, the clinician must inform the patient of masseter muscle hypertrophy (Fig. 16.1) [38, 39].

A transition phase is mandatory before tooth removal during the clinical examination of patients with terminal dentition. When temporomandibular disorders are diagnosed, orthodontic, occlusal, restorative therapy, and only in cases where the patient indicates a prone position and the relevant criteria, injection treatment, various medications, and the mucosal bone growth stimulator should all be assessed after rotating intraoral dental radiograph, scout identification. Also, panoramic imaging, including multislice coordinate associated technology, displaying a temporal ligament to evaluate the apex of the posterior condylar head, and open and close imaging with mandibular planning functions to see the joint space, will be informative. Distal imaging of the joint will not be informative in frontal/lateral open/closed position. Sonographic evaluation is essential in the presence of corned muscle, especially when uneasy about injections for balance preservation. Finally, the joint space and eminence in appropriate patient groups should be investigated by arthrography if the clinical examination is unreliable [38, 39, 40].

References

1. Stacy M. Handbook of dystonia. New York: Informa Healthcare USA, Inc; 2007.
2. Hellman A, Torres-Russotto D. Botulinum toxin in the management of blepharospasm: current evidence and recent developments. Ther Adv Neurol Disord. 2015;8(2):82–91. https://doi.org/10.1177/1756285614557475. PMID: 25922620; PMCID: PMC4356659.
3. Fahn S, Jankovic J, Hallet M. Principles and practice of movement disorders. Amsterdam: Elsevier Saunders; 2011.
4. Torres-Russotto D, Perlmutter J. Task-specific dystonias: a review. Ann N Y Acad Sci. 2008;1142:179–99.
5. Grandas F, Elston J, Quinn N, Marsden C. Blepharospasm: a review of 264 patients. J Neurol Neurosurg Psychiatry. 1988;51:767–72.
6. Weiner W, Nora L. "Trick" movements in facial dystonia. J Clin Psychiatry. 1984;45:519–21.
7. Schicatano E, Basso M, Evinger C. Animal model explains the origins of the cranial. J Neurophysiol. 1997;77:2842–6.
8. Cohen L, Hallett M. Hand cramps: clinical features and electromyographic patterns in a focal dystonia. Neurology. 1988;38:1005–12.
9. Berardeli A, Rothwell J, Day B, Marsden C. Pathophysiology of blepharospasm and oromandibular dystonia. Brain. 1985;108:593–608.

10. Ridding M, Sheean G, Rothwell J, Inzelberg R, Kujirai T. Changes in the balance between motor cortical excitation and inhibition in focal, task specific dystonia. J Neurol Neurosurg Psychiatry. 1995;59:493–8.
11. Sohn Y, Hallett M. Disturbed surround inhibition in focal hand dystonia. Ann Neurol. 2004;56:595–9.
12. Pellizzari R, Rossetto O, Schiavo G, Montecucco C. Tetanus and botulinum neurotoxins: mechanism of action and therapeutic uses. Phil Trans R Soc Lond B Biol Sci. 1999;354:259–68.
13. Montecucco C, Schiavo G. Mechanism of action of tetanus and botulinum neurotoxins. Mol Microbiol. 1994;13:1–8.
14. Ramirez-Castaneda J, Jankovic J. Long-term efficacy and safety of botulinum toxin injections in dystonia. Toxins. 2013;5(2):249–66.
15. Crowner B, Torres-Russotto D, Carter A, Racette B. Systemic weakness after therapeutic injections of botulinum toxin A: a case series and review of the literature. Clin Neuropharmacol. 2010;33(5):243–7.
16. Kulshreshtha D, Ganguly J, Jog M. Managing autonomic dysfunction in Parkinson's disease: a review of emerging drugs. Expert Opin Emerg Drugs. 2020;25:37–47.
17. Sławek J, Madaliński M. Botulinum toxin therapy for nonmotor aspects of Parkinson's disease. Int Rev Neurobiol. 2017;134:1111–42.
18. Shukla AW, Malaty IA. Botulinum toxin therapy for Parkinson's disease. Semin Neurol. 2017;37:193–204.
19. Quarracino C, Otero-Losada M, Capani F, Pérez-Lloret S. State-of-the-art pharmacotherapy for autonomic dysfunction in Parkinson's disease. Expert Opin Pharmacother. 2020;21:445–57.
20. Seppi K, Ray Chaudhuri K, Coelho M, Fox SH, Katzenschlager R, Perez Lloret S, Djamshidian-Tehrani A. Update on treatments for nonmotor symptoms of Parkinson's disease—an evidence-based medicine review. Mov Disord. 2019;34:180–98.
21. Foresti C, Stabile A. Botulinum toxin treatment of sialorrhea in children. Toxicon. 2018;156(Suppl. 1):S34–5.
22. Khan WU, Campisi P, Nadarajah S, Shakur YA, Khan N, Semenuk D, Connolly B. Botulinum toxin A for treatment of sialorrhea in children: an effective, minimally invasive approach. Arch Otolaryngol Head Neck Surg. 2011;137:339–44.
23. Sato K, Kang WH, Saga K, et al. Biology of sweat glands and their disorders. I. Normal sweat gland function. J Am Acad Dermatol. 1989;20:537–63. Sato K, Kang WH, Saga K, et al. Biology of sweat glands and their disorders. II. Disorders of sweat gland function. J Am Acad Dermatol. 1989;20:713–26.
24. Bushara KO, Park DM, Jones JC, et al. Botulinum toxin – a possible new treatment for axillary hyperhidrosis. Clin Exp Dermatol. 1996;21(4):276–8.
25. Shelley WB, Hurley HJ Jr. Studies on topical antiperspirant control of axillary hyperhidrosis. Acta Derm Venereol. 1975;55:241–60.
26. Galadari I, Alkaabi J. Botulinum Toxin in the Treatment of Axillary Hyperhidrosis. https://www.medscape.com/viewarticle/458335 (Accessed online April 15, 2021).
27. Reinauer S, Neusser A, Schauf G, Hölzle E. Iontophoresis with alternating current and direct current offset (AC/DC iontophoresis): a new approach for the treatment of hyperhidrosis. Br J Dermatol. 1993;129(2):166–9. https://doi.org/10.1111/j.1365-2133.1993.tb03521.x. PMID: 7654577.
28. Iontophoresis with alternating current and direct current offset (AC/DC iontophoresis): a new approach for the treatment of hyperhidrosis. Br J Dermatol. 1993;129:166–9.
29. Mack GW, Shannon LM, Nadel ER. Influence of beta-adrenergic blockade on the control of sweating in humans. J Appl Physiol. 1986;61:1701–5. Byrne J, Walsh TN, Hederman WP. Endoscopic transthoracic electrocautery of the sympathetic chain for palmar and axillary hyperhidrosis. Br J Surg. 1990;77:1046–9.
30. Lai YT, Yang LH, Chio CC, et al. Complications in patients with palmar hyperhidrosis treated with transthoracic endoscopic sympathectomy. Neurosurgery. 1997;41:110–3.
31. Heckmann M. Complications in patients with palmar hyperhidrosis treated with transthoracic endoscopic sympathectomy. Neurosurgery. 1998;42:1403–4.

32. Naumann M, Hofmann U, Bergmann I, et al. Focal hyperhidrosis: effective treatment with intracutaneous botulinum toxin. Arch Dermatol. 1998;134:301–4.
33. Side-controlled intradermal injection of botulinum toxin a in recalcitrant axillary hyperhidrosis. J Am Acad Dermatol. 1999;41:987–90.
34. Odderson IR. Axillary hyperhidrosis: treatment with botulinum toxin A. Arch Phys Med Rehabil. 1998;79(3):350–2.
35. Schnider P, Binder M, Kittler H, et al. A randomized, double-blind, placebo-controlled trial of botulinum A toxin for severe axillary hyperhidrosis. Br J Dermatol. 1999;140:677–80.
36. Kim NH, Park RH, Park JB. Botulinum toxin type A for the treatment of hypertrophy of the masseter muscle. Plast Reconstr Surg. 2010;125(6):1693–705. https://doi.org/10.1097/PRS.0b013e3181d0ad03. PMID: 20517093.
37. Peretta R, Melison M, Meneghello R, Comelli D, Guarda L, Galzignato PF, Concheri G, Ferronato G. Unilateral masseter muscle hypertrophy: morphofunctional analysis of the relapse after treatment with botulinum toxin. Cranio. 2009;27(3):200–10. https://doi.org/10.1179/crn.2009.030. PMID: 19697649.
38. Popescu MN, Beiu C, Iliescu CA, Racoviță A, Berteanu M, Iliescu MG, Stănescu AMA, Radaschin DS, Popa LG. Ultrasound-guided botulinum toxin-A injections into the masseter muscle for both medical and aesthetic purposes. Toxins (Basel). 2024;16(10):413. https://doi.org/10.3390/toxins16100413. PMID: 39453189; PMCID: PMC11511025.
39. Nishikawa A, Aikawa Y, Kono T. Treatment of masseter muscle hypertrophy with botulinum toxin type A injection: a review of adverse events. J Cosmet Dermatol. 2024;23(11):3544–50. https://doi.org/10.1111/jocd.16462. Epub 2024 Jul 12. PMID: 39001582.
40. Seok J, Koh YG, Hong JK, Yun SH, Kim DH, Son HS, Choi SY, Yoo KH, Lee YW, Kim BJ. Efficacy and safety of PrabotulinumtoxinA in subjects with benign masseteric hypertrophy: a double-blind, randomized, placebo-controlled, multicenter, phase 3 trial and open-label extension study. Dermatologic Surg. 2024;50(6):527–33. https://doi.org/10.1097/DSS.0000000000004146. Epub 2024 Mar 8. PMID: 38518110.

Part III

Volumizing the Face with Fillers

Filler Agents: Overview

17

Mehmet Akdag, Cemal Cingi, and Jan Plzak

17.1 Introduction

At the beginning of the 1970s, bovine collagen was the first injectable filler used to enhance the appearance of the face. Since then, several products have been produced for soft tissue augmentation. During the past 10 years, there has been a significant increase in the number of medications approved by the Food and Drug Administration (FDA) and the number of patients looking for these therapies. In 2012, the United States of America witnessed the completion of around two million soft tissue filler treatments, which both medical professionals and nurse injectors carried out [1–3]. Hyaluronic acid (HA) is the agent that is utilized the most commonly in the United States, accounting for 87% of all soft tissue filler treatments. Since 2004, there has been a 38% rise in the use of HA [2]. HA has emerged as the filler that is preferred the most worldwide. It is important to note that not all injectables are made equal, and no filler is perfect, nor is there a single filler that can fulfill the desires and aspirations of every single patient [4–6].

M. Akdag
Sanlıurfa Mehmet Akif İnan Training and Research Hospital, Department of Otorhinolaryngology, Sanlıurfa, Turkey

C. Cingi (✉)
Eskisehir Osmangazi University, Medical Faculty, Department of Otorhinolaryngology, Eskisehir, Türkiye
e-mail: cemal@ogu.edu.tr

J. Plzak
Department of Otorhinolaryngology, Head and Neck Surgery, Charles University, First Faculty of Medicine and University Hospital Motol, Prague, Czech Republic
e-mail: jan.plzak@fnmotol.cz

C. Cingi et al. (eds.), *Minor Interventions, Major Outcomes on the Face*, Comprehensive ENT, https://doi.org/10.1007/978-3-032-01305-7_17

17.2 Indications

Soft tissue fillers that are injectable are recommended for treating wrinkles, creases, and lines linked with aging. The forehead, the glabella, the nasolabial folds, and the lips are some of the areas of the face that are frequently treated. Several fillers are also utilized for the treatment of contour abnormalities that are caused by acne scarring or lipoatrophy that is linked with HIV. Practitioners have created a wide variety of off-label applications for each substance [7]:

According to the findings of a study conducted by Occhiogrosso and colleagues, the application of dermal fillers to patients who have facial paralysis not only improves facial symmetry but also improves the patients' psychosocial well-being. Using the FACE-Q Appearance-related Distress Screening Scale, it was discovered that there was a specific increase in self-confidence and emotional expression. Additionally, improvements in symmetry (self-reported) and psychosocial state were achieved after a single treatment of, on average, 2.3 mL of dermal filler, as observed at a follow-up period of 2 weeks [8].

17.3 Fillers

17.3.1 Hyaluronic Acid

Hyaluronic acid is the most prevalent glycosaminoglycan in the skin. When injected, it can powerfully bond to water and hydrate, soften, and volumize the skin. Hyaluronic acid has these advantages and contributes to cell proliferation, membrane receptor operation, and adhesion.

The production of the viscoelastic network that allows collagen and elastin fibers to bond together is facilitated by hyaluronic acid, which also serves to maintain intercellular structures. These linkages break down, forming disordered collagen and elastin clumps, as observed in the photoaging process. The combination of these advantages makes hyaluronic acid an ideal dermal filling agent. A cross-linked hyaluronic acid that does not come from an animal source was authorized by the FDA in February 2003. It was rapidly discovered that this dermal filler had a relatively long-lasting impact, had few side effects, was simple to use, was ready to use right out of the box, did not require refrigeration, was cost-efficient, and did not require skin testing before treatment [9–11].

The likelihood of an allergic reaction is relatively low because all species share hyaluronic acid. Because hyaluronic acid has an action similar to that of heparin, it causes more bruising than collagen fillers do [12, 13]. Before the year 2010, practically all of the hyaluronic acid products that the FDA authorized in the United States did not include lidocaine. As a result, the discomfort experienced with these dermal fillers was much higher than the discomfort experienced with the injection of bovine- and human-derived collagen fillers. Despite these drawbacks, hyaluronic acid fillers have nonetheless established themselves as the most popular dermal filling agents for soft tissue augmentation [11]. This is primarily because of the superior aesthetic outcomes that they consistently provide.

In the infrequent event that hyaluronic acid results in an unpleasant outcome, it is feasible to rectify the situation by administering an injection of hyaluronidase, which is a commercially available enzyme that degrades the unfavorable hyaluronic acid dermal filler. It is considered an off-label usage of hyaluronidase to use it for this reason because the FDA has not approved its use for this purpose. Many instances require only 10–30 units of unpreserved hyaluronidase to accomplish the necessary correction. Up to 25% of people may experience local site responses; however, these reactions are often fleeting and moderate. Initial therapy with as little as 5–10 units is generally suggested and frequently beneficial; however, some patients are treated with as many as 75 units with few ill effects. It is possible to make more modifications; however, it may take up to 4 weeks to thoroughly understand the whole fix. Additionally, skin testing is recommended before receiving treatment with these dermal fillers because specific preparations are made from bovines [14, 15].

The preparations of hyaluronidase are transparent and highly concentrated liquids, and they are kept in a chilled vial. Reconstitution of these dermal fillers often involves the addition of normal saline or lidocaine (with or without epinephrine) by the attending physician. Reconstitution with 3 milliliters of 1% lidocaine and one hundred thousand milliliters of epinephrine has been used frequently and proven effective when utilizing Amphadase. Following the mixing process, the vial is gently agitated. A skin test can be carried out before treatment by injecting 3–5 units (0.06–0.1 mL) of the reconstituted solution into the superficial dermis in the antecubital fossa. This is done until the medication is administered. A positive hypersensitive reaction is characterized by a wheal that appears within 5 min and continues for twenty to 30 min, along with itching in the affected area [14].

Hylaform (Genzyme) [9]

- *Composition*: Hyaluronic acid comes from the dermis of rooster combs, with a concentration of 5.5 mg/mL. The particles are 500 μm, and there is a 20% cross-linking.
- *Supply*: A disposable glass syringe with a needle measuring 30 gauge (ga).
- Skin testing: Tests on the skin are not required.
- *Duration*: 3–6 months.
- Depth of injection: The middle to the deep dermis is the depth of the injection.
- FDA indications: The FDA provides indications for moderate to severe creases and folds on the face, including nasolabial folds.
- *Off-label uses*: Among the off-label applications are the correction of facial depressions and rhytides caused by aging, surgery, and diseases, as well as volume augmentation at various body locations.
- *Contraindications*: hypersensitivity to proteins derived from humans or birds.

Restylane/Restylane-L (Galderma) [9]

- *Composition*: Hyaluronic acid obtained from Streptococcus equi has been chemically cross-linked using butanediol diglycidyl ether (BDDE). This hyaluronic acid has been stabilized and suspended in phosphate-buffered saline at 20 mg/mL. Additionally, the material contains non-animal stabilized hyaluronic acid (NASHA), 400 μm gel particles cross-linked by 1%. Restylane-L has a lidocaine concentration of 0.3%.
- *Supply*: Disposable glass syringes with a Luer-Lok fitting and a 30-gauge needle are the components provided.
- *Skin testing*: Tests on the skin are not required.
- *Duration*: The duration is 6 months.
- *Depth of injection*: The middle to the deep dermis is the depth of the injection.
- *FDA indications*: The FDA provides indications for moderate to severe creases and folds on the face, including nasolabial folds.
- *Off-label uses*: Among the off-label applications are the correction of facial depressions and rhytides caused by aging, surgery, and diseases, as well as volume augmentation at various body locations.
- *Contraindications*: Extreme allergies demonstrated by a history of anaphylaxis, allergies to proteins produced by gram-positive bacteria, and bleeding issues are all considered contraindications.

Perlane/Perlane-L (Galderma) [9]

- *Composition*: A material consisting of hyaluronic acid produced from S equi, which has been chemically cross-linked with BDDE, stabilized, and suspended in phosphate-buffered saline at a concentration of 20 mg/mL; NASHA; gel particles measuring 940–1090 μm in size. There is 0.3% lidocaine present in Perlane-L.
- *Supply*: Disposable glass syringes with a Luer-Lok fitting and a 27-gauge needle are included in the delivery method.
- *Skin testing*: Tests on the skin are not required.
- *Duration: 6–12 months.*
- Depth of injection: The injection depth is from the deep dermis to the superficial subcutis.
- FDA indications: The FDA provides indications for moderate to severe creases and folds on the face, including nasolabial folds.
- Off-label uses: The off-label applications include the correction of facial depressions and rhytids caused by aging, surgery, and diseases, as well as volume augmentation at various body locations.
- Contraindications: Extreme allergies demonstrated by a history of anaphylaxis, allergies to proteins produced by gram-positive bacteria, and bleeding issues are all considered contraindications.

Juvéderm XC (Allergan) [9]

- *Composition*: Hyaluronic acid produced from S equi that has been cross-linked with BDDE in a homogenized gel; concentration: 24 mg/mL.
- *Supply*: The syringe includes 0.8 milliliters of the substance, a Luer-Lok adapter, and a 30-gauge needle. The substance is suspended in a physiological buffer.
- *Skin testing*: Tests on the skin are not required.
- *Duration*: 3–6 months.
- *Depth of injection*: The middle to the deep dermis is the depth of the injection.
- *FDA indications*: The FDA provides indications for moderate to severe creases and facial folds, including nasolabial folds.
- *Off-label uses*: Off-label applications include correcting facial depressions and rhytids caused by aging, surgery, and diseases, as well as volume augmentation at various body locations.
- *Contraindications*: Contraindications include severe allergies characterized by a history of anaphylaxis and allergies to proteins produced by gram-positive bacteria.

Juvéderm Voluma XC (Allergan) [9]

- *Material*: Hyaluronic acid produced from S equi that has been cross-linked with BDDE in a homogenized gel; concentration of 24 mg/mL; increased proportion of cross-linked HA; includes lidocaine.
- *Supply*: The product is delivered in a physiological buffer suspension. The syringe has a Luer-Lok adapter and a 27-ga needle; its volume is 0.8 milliliters.
- *Skin testing*: Tests on the skin are not required.
- *Duration*: up to 24 months.
- *Depth of injection*: A deep subcutaneous injection is the depth of the injection.
- *FDA indications*: Deep injection in the cheek region to repair age-related volume loss in persons older than 21 years old is required by the FDA.
- *Off-label uses*: The off-label applications include the correction of facial depressions and rhytids caused by aging, surgery, and diseases, as well as volume augmentation at various body locations.
- *Contraindications*: Severe allergies, as demonstrated by a history of anaphylaxis, allergies to proteins produced by gram-positive bacteria, or allergies to lidocaine are also considered contraindications.

Prevelle Silk (Mentor) [9]

- *Composition*: The material is a homogenized gel and hyaluronic acid generated from S (equi).

- *Supply*: Hyaluronic acid gel that has been cross-linked with 0.3% lidocaine; the syringe has 0.9 milliliters of liquid, including a Luer-Lok adapter and 2 needles with a gauge of 30 grams each.
- *Skin testing*: Tests on the skin are not required.
- *Duration*: 2–3 months.
- *Depth of injection: The middle to the* deep dermis is the depth of the injection.
- *FDA indications: The FDA provides indications for* moderate to severe creases and folds on the face, including nasolabial folds.
- *Off-label uses*: Among the off-label applications are the correction of facial depressions and rhytides caused by aging, surgery, and diseases, as well as volume augmentation at various body locations.
- *Contraindications*: severe allergies, as demonstrated by a history of anaphylaxis; allergies to proteins produced by gram-positive bacteria; and hypersensitivity to lidocaine.

Belotero Balance (Merz) [9]

- *Composition*: The material is a homogenized gel and hyaluronic acid generated from S (equi).
- *Supply*: A monophasic hyaluronic acid gel that incorporates a variety of cross-linkages and is expected to reduce the danger of the Tyndall effect; a syringe that carries 0.9 milliliters and a Luer-Lok adapter, as well as two needles with a gauge of 30 grams each.
- *Skin testing*: Tests on the skin are not required.
- *Duration*: The duration is 6 months.
- *Depth of injection*: Injection depth ranges from the superficial to the middle dermis.
- *FDA indications*: Moderate to severe creases and folds on the face are the indications provided by the FDA.
- *Off-label uses*: The off-label applications include the correction of facial depressions and rhytids caused by aging, surgery, and diseases, as well as volume augmentation at various body locations.
- *Contraindications*: The following are examples of contraindications: severe allergies, as demonstrated by a history of anaphylaxis; allergies to proteins produced by gram-positive bacteria; and hypersensitivity to lidocaine.

17.3.2 Polymethylmethacrylate with Bovine Collagen

The FDA approved using Artefill, now known as Bellafill, in the United States in 2007. This dermal filler comprises non-resorbable polymethylmethacrylate (PMMA) microspheres with a 30–50 μm diameter. These microspheres are suspended in a water-based carrier gel composed of 3.5% bovine collagen, 92.6% buffered isotonic water, 0.3% lidocaine, 2.7% phosphate buffer, and 0.9% sodium chloride. Due to the presence of lidocaine in this dermal filler, the injection is significantly less painful when compared to other dermal fillers that do not include lidocaine. This dermal filler has been recommended for repairing the nasolabial folds; nevertheless, it has also been utilized to treat acne scars and furrows on the forehead. It is recommended that the injection of Bellafill be performed immediately under the skin fold into the deep dermis rather than into the subcutis, using a needle with a gauge of 26. Thread injection is the method that the majority of practitioners favor. In contrast to the other dermal fillers, this dermal filler should be regarded as a permanent dermal filler [16, 17].

Extreme caution

Due to the presence of bovine collagen in this product, skin testing is necessary before treatment. This is similar to what would be required with Zyderm or Zyplast (for more information, see collagen). Since the outcomes are long-lasting, it is typically recommended that one does not attempt to achieve complete correction in a single session but rather to get the desired result throughout many therapy sessions. Furthermore, lumpiness, prolonged swelling or redness, and enhanced sensitivity at the injection site are some unpleasant effects that may occur in addition to allergic reactions or reactions [18]. The product must be served cold.

Bellafill (Formerly, ArteFill) (Suneva Medical) [9]

- *Composition*: Microspheres made of polymethyl methacrylate, measuring between 30 and 50 micrometers in diameter.
- *Supply*: It is delivered by suspending it in a water-based carrier gel containing 3.5% bovine collagen, 92.6% isotonic buffer water for injection, 0.3% lidocaine, 2.7% phosphate buffer, and 0.9% sodium chloride.
- *Skin testing*: Skin testing is required.
- *Duration*: a certain amount of consistency across time.
- *Depth of injection*: subdermal.
- *FDA indications*: The correction of nasolabial folds and the therapy of acne scars are the indications provided by the FDA [10].
- *Off-label uses*: Uses that the manufacturer disapproves include deep wrinkles in other areas of the face and deficits or abnormalities in soft tissue contours.
- *Contraindications*: Positive response to required Bellafill skin test, severe allergies manifested by history of anaphylaxis or history or presence of multiple severe allergies, lidocaine hypersensitivity, allergy to any bovine collagen products, undergoing or planning to undergo desensitization injection to meat products, use in lip augmentation and injection into the vermillion or the wet mucosa of the lip, known susceptibility to keloid formation or hypertrophic scarring.

17.3.3 Poly-L-Lactic Acid

This innovative substance, Sculptra, is distinct from all previous agents in many critical respects. Poly-L-lactic acid is a biocompatible synthetic peptide polymer that is biodegradable and immunologically inert. It is believed to encourage fibroblasts to make more collagen, ultimately increasing face volume. Poly-L-lactic acid is exclusively licensed by the FDA for the treatment of HIV-associated lipoatrophy in the United States. Additionally, it is used to repair skin folds (nasolabial folds) and other cosmetic wrinkles in immunocompetent individuals [19].

Even though poly-L-lactic acid is almost always injected subdermally, dermal neocollagenesis nonetheless takes place. As a result, it is classified as a dermal stimulating agent rather than a genuine dermal filling agent. Several constraints have stopped poly-L-lactic acid from achieving the same level of popularity as other products. Since poly-lactic acid must be mixed before it can be used, quick therapy is not feasible. Unlike dermal fillers, the results are not noticeable for at least 4 weeks after the procedure. Most patients require two to three therapy sessions, with a minimum of 4–6 weeks between sessions [20].

Extreme Caution

The clinical effects of this drug are less predictable than those of natural dermal fillers. This is because poly-L-lactic acid is not an actual filler but relies on neocollagenesis to produce clinical improvement through medical treatment. The fact that it takes 4–6 weeks to see benefits should be appropriately communicated to patients. After therapy, there have been reports of the development of dermal nodules, which often take 7 months or even longer to manifest. When treating the face, these nodules are frequently felt but not visible to the naked eye. Additionally, it is considered that vigorous posttreatment massage, in conjunction with the reconstitution of the product with six milliliters or more of sterile water, might prevent nodule development [11].

Unfortunately, the frequency of nodules in this region may be as high as 10%, and the nodules are frequently noticeable, unattractive, and difficult to cure. Utilization of this product on the hands has grown; nevertheless, the incidence of nodules in this site may be as high as 10%. Therapy with Sculptra, which was reconstituted with as much as 10 milliliters of sterile water, has nonetheless resulted in the production of nodules in this particular site. It may take anywhere from one to 3 years for the nodules to arise following therapy [21, 22].

Sculptra (Galderma) [9]

- *Composition*: Poly-L-lactic acid, mannitol, and sodium carboxymethylcellulose are the components of the material.
- *Supply*: After being reconstituted with 5 milliliters of sterile water and lidocaine solution, the hydrocolloid suspension is delivered as a freeze-dried preparation for injection in a transparent glass vial.
- *Skin testing: Tests on the skin are not required:*

- *Duration*: The duration is 2 years.
- *Depth of injection*: The depth of the injection is subdermal.
- *FDA indications*: Lipoatrophy linked with HIV is one of the FDA's indications.
- *Off-label uses*: Cosmetic usage is an example of an off-label application.
- *Contraindications*: contraindications include hypersensitivity to any of the products.
- *Composition:*
- *Supply:*
- *Skin testing:*
- *Duration*: 2–3 months.
- *Depth of injection:*
- *FDA indications:*
- *Off-label uses:*
- *Contraindications:*

17.3.4 Calcium Hydroxylapatite

This innovative filler, known as Radiesse, was approved by the FDA in December 2006 for the treatment of facial creases and folds, as well as for the treatment of facial atrophy associated with HIV. Moreover, the FDA granted permission for its use as a cosmetic in people who did not have HIV in the year 2009. Calcium hydroxylapatite makes up 30% of the subdermal filler, while carrier gel makes up 70%. The clinical outcomes can persist for as long as 12 months or even longer; however, the carrier gel only lasts for a maximum of 6 months, frequently leading to a minor reduction in the correction achieved now.

The injection of Radiesse is typically performed subdermally at the dermis and subcutaneous tissue intersection or just above the periosteum; hence, this product is not considered a genuine dermal filler. The findings of studies conducted in 2008 indicate that calcium hydroxylapatite may be capable of inducing neocollagenesis; nevertheless, further study is required [23, 24]. The most typical applications for Radiesse include the treatment of nasolabial folds, atrophic cheeks, and temporal wasting. Radiesse is extensively utilized.

Some medical professionals added lidocaine to the syringe to alleviate the discomfort that is associated with injections; nevertheless, there was no discernible reduction in the effectiveness of the medication. Mariano Busso [25] has successfully treated a large number of patients by incorporating one drop of 10% lidocaine into the 1.3-mL syringe of Radiesse that was previously accessible. This was done to alleviate the discomfort that was associated with injections. Radiesse, which contains lidocaine, was introduced in 2010 to relieve pain with injections and does not require any pre-mixing.

The hands have been treated by adding 0.15–0.23 mL of 2% lidocaine to each 1.3-mL syringe of Radiesse. This has been successful in treating the hands. A nose-to-nose Luer-lock connector (female-to-female) may be utilized to achieve this task. This connector will connect the Radiesse syringe to a syringe containing lidocaine measuring 3 milliliters. It is advised that the product be passed between the two syringes a minimum of ten times to obtain an appropriate and even dispersion of the lidocaine. The Radiesse will have a little thinner consistency, making it more straightforward to distribute when utilizing a bolus injection strategy. Similarly, this combination is frequently used to treat the temples [11].

Extreme caution

Injections into the dermis should be avoided since they can potentially cause the development of nodules. A great deal of caution is required to prevent the injection from occurring while the needle is being removed from the skin. This is because the injection will deposit material into the dermis. The treatment administered to the lips has led to the creation of cysts holding the carrier gel [16]. Because of this, most cosmetic surgeons do not use Radiesse to treat the lips.

Radiesse (Merz) [9]

- *Composition*: Microspheres of calcium hydroxyapatite, measuring between 25 and 45 micrometers in size, are suspended in a gel carrier consisting of sterile water, glycerin, and sodium carboxymethylcellulose.
- *Supply*: The syringe is a one-milliliter kind.
- *Skin testing*: Tests on the skin are not required.
- *Duration*: one to 2 years.
- *Depth of injection*: The depth of the injection is subdermal.
- *FDA indications*: HIV-associated lipoatrophy, moderate to severe face creases and folds (such as nasolabial folds), and other indications from the Food and Drug Administration.
- *Off-label uses*: Marionette lines, glabella folds, prejowl sulcus, cheek volume loss, dorsal nasal abnormalities, and lip augmentation are treatment options that the FDA does not approve.
- *Contraindications*: Hypersensitivity to any of the components; severe allergies that have been demonstrated by a history of anaphylaxis or by the presence of numerous severe allergies; those who have a history of one or more severe allergies.

References

1. Chacon AH. Fillers in dermatology: from past to present. Cutis. 2015;96(5):E17–9. [Medline]. [Full Text].
2. ASAPS website. Available at http://www.surgery.org/sites/default/files/ASAPS-2012-Stats.pdf.
3. ASPS Website. Available at http://www.plasticsurgery.org/.
4. Buck DW 2nd, Alam M, Kim JY. Injectable fillers for facial rejuvenation: a review. J Plast Reconstr Aesthet Surg. 2009;62(1):11–8. [Medline].
5. Özdemir E, Bayar Muluk N, Sünnetci G, Arslanoğlu A, Yazir M, Kaya F, Cingi C. Investigation of the Effects of Minimally Invasive Facial Plastic Surgery Applications on Well-Being of

Individuals. J Craniofac Surg. 2025. https://doi.org/10.1097/SCS.0000000000011658. Epub ahead of print. PMID: 40663006.
6. Choi MS. Basic rheology of dermal filler. Arch Plast Surg. 2020;47(4):301–4. [Medline]. [Full Text].
7. Alam M, Gladstone H, Kramer EM, Murphy JP Jr, Nouri K, Neuhaus IM. ASDS guidelines of care: injectable fillers. Dermatologic Surg. 2008;34(Suppl 1):S115–48. [Medline].
8. Occhiogrosso J, Derakhshan A, Hadlock TA, Shanley KM, Lee LN. Dermal filler treatment improves psychosocial well-being in facial paralysis patients. Facial Plast Surg Aesthet Med. 2020;22:370. [Medline].
9. Injection Facial Fillers, Updated: 13 Aug 2020, Author: Andrew A Winkler, MD; Chief Editor: Arlen D Meyers, MD, MBA more. https://emedicine.medscape.com/article/1574158-overview17.1.Introduction.
10. Dilber M, Bayar Muluk N, Cingi C. A narrative-style review of non-surgical rhinoplasty: Indications, outcomes, and limitations. J Craniomaxillofac Surg. 2024;52(9):1012–18. https://doi.org/10.1016/j.jcms.2024.06.014. Epub 2024 Jun 10. PMID: 38876955.
11. Dermal fillers, Updated: 2 Apr 2018, Author: Robert S Bader, MD; Chief Editor: William D James, MD more. https://emedicine.medscape.com/article/1125066-overview#a7.
12. Sundaram H, Cassuto D. Biophysical characteristics of hyaluronic acid soft-tissue fillers and their relevance to aesthetic applications. Plast Reconstr Surg. 2013;132(4S-2 Clinical Introduction to the Hyaluronic Acid Dermal Filler Using Cohesive Polydensified Matrix Technology):5S–21S. [Medline].
13. Homicz MR, Watson D. Review of injectable materials for soft tissue augmentation. Facial Plast Surg. 2004;20(1):21–9.
14. Lambros V. The use of hyaluronidase to reverse the effects of hyaluronic acid filler. Plast Reconstr Surg. 2004;114(1):277. [Medline].
15. Cassuto D, Sundaram H. A Problem-oriented approach to nodular complications from hyaluronic acid and calcium hydroxylapatite fillers: classification and recommendations for treatment. Plast Reconstr Surg. 2013;132(4S-2 Clinical Introduction to the Hyaluronic Acid Dermal Filler Using Cohesive Polydensified Matrix Technology):48S–58S. [Medline].
16. Alam M, Gladstone H, Kramer EM, Murphy JP Jr, Nouri K, Neuhaus IM, et al. ASDS guidelines of care: injectable fillers. Dermatologic Surg. 2008;34(Suppl 1):S115–48. [Medline].
17. ArteFill – Instructions for use [package insert]. San Diego: Artes Medical, Inc; 2008. Available at [Full Text].
18. Lemperle G, Romano JJ, Busso M. Soft tissue augmentation with artecoll: 10-year history, indications, techniques, and complications. Dermatologic Surg. 2003;29(6):573–87. discussion 587. [Medline].
19. Butterwick K. Understanding injectable poly-L-lactic acid. Cosmet Dermatol. 2007;20:388–92.
20. Vleggaar D. Soft-tissue augmentation and the role of poly-L-lactic acid. Plast Reconstr Surg. 2006;118(3 Suppl):46S–54S. [Medline].
21. Narins RS, Brandt FS, Lorenc ZP, Maas CS, Monheit GD, Smith SR. Twelve-month persistency of a novel ribose-cross-linked collagen dermal filler. Dermatologic Surg. 2008;34(Suppl 1):S31–9. [Medline].
22. Cohen JL. Understanding, avoiding, and managing dermal filler complications. Dermatologic Surg. 2008;34(Suppl 1):S92–9.
23. Coleman KM, Voigts R, DeVore DP, Termin P, Coleman WP 3rd. Neocollagenesis after injection of calcium hydroxylapatite composition in a canine model. Dermatologic Surg. 2008;34(Suppl 1):S53–5. [Medline].
24. Berlin AL, Hussain M, Goldberg DJ. Calcium hydroxylapatite filler for facial rejuvenation: a histologic and immunohistochemical analysis. Dermatologic Surg. 2008;34(Suppl 1):S64–7. [Medline].
25. Busso M, Voigts R. An investigation of changes in physical properties of injectable calcium hydroxylapatite in a carrier gel when mixed with lidocaine and with lidocaine/epinephrine. Dermatol Surg. 2008;34(Suppl 1):S16–23. discussion S24.

Volumizing with Fillers: Forehead

18

Abdulbaki Sokmen, Nuray Bayar Muluk,
and Gabriela Kopacheva Barsova

18.1 Facial Rejuvenation with Fillers: Volume Restoration

In medical facial rejuvenation, volume restoration of the aged face has emerged as the most popular and widely used foundational technique. Sometimes, in the late 30 s, the face starts to experience fat loss. This results in a change in the form of the face, including a reduction in the prominence and width of the malar eminence, a loss of definition in the angle of the jaw, and a fall of the cheek fat pads. Additionally, fat pads in the face either decrease in volume or drop at varying rates, resulting in the visible segmentation of facial compartments that appear confluent in childhood [1]. This is in addition to the fact that the face is shedding fat. Folds and creases in the face gradually become more pronounced due to these changes, which also contribute to the loss of elasticity in the skin and the development of laxity in the skin. Injectable fillers are the principal treatment for such changes, particularly in the early stages of the aging process [2].

A. Sokmen
Sivas State Hospital, Department of Otorhinolaryngology, Sivas, Turkey

N. Bayar Muluk (✉)
Faculty of Medicine, Department of Otorhinolaryngology, Kırıkkale University, Kırıkkale, Türkiye

G. K. Barsova
Cyril and Methodius University of Skopje, Faculty of Medicine, Skopje, Republic of Macedonia

C. Cingi et al. (eds.), *Minor Interventions, Major Outcomes on the Face*, Comprehensive ENT, https://doi.org/10.1007/978-3-032-01305-7_18

18.2 Changing Facial Features with Filler

While injectable fillers can be used to make subtle to moderate changes to various facial features, these changes can be made in either the elderly patient or the younger patient. A change in facial shape can be achieved with filler injections in the cheeks, chin, nose, brows, and jaw angle. This is distinct from the restoration of a young appearance. This technique has the advantage of being able to be adjusted in very small increments, which allows for the creation of small alterations that cannot be done reliably using surgical techniques. Patients who are members of the acting, modeling, or comparable professions frequently require very few form alterations to enhance their symmetry or perfect the intricacies of their appearance. Solid face implants or osteotomies are the most effective treatment options when dealing with significant changes. There is also the possibility of using fillers to conceal the visible edge of an implant, which is particularly useful in cases where the patient is extremely thin or when the implant is quite large [2].

18.3 Dangerous Zones in the Upper Face

The forehead, temporal, and upper periorbital regions are all included in the domain of the upper face [3].

In the region of the forehead, the supraorbital and supratrochlear arterial branches of the ophthalmic artery and vein and their lesser branches are located. They leave their foramen on the orbital rim to go in a cephalic direction. In a short time, their deep origin splits into branches that move considerably more superficially, which means that vessels in the forehead region can be encountered at all injection planes [4, 5].

Skin, connective tissue, aponeurosis, loose areolar connective tissue, and periosteum are the anatomical layers that make up the forehead, and those layers are included in the standard mnemonic SCALP. These layers are arranged from superficial to deep, respectively. The loose areolar tissue is a relatively avascular plane connecting the galea aponeurosis with the periosteum underneath it. It is located deep in the forehead and scalp. It is common practice to do volumizing or reshaping of the forehead at this deeper level to reduce the likelihood of arterial blockage [4, 5].

In most instances, the horizontal lines produced by the dynamic activity of the frontalis muscle are intended to be concealed by injections of soft tissue fillers administered in the area associated with the forehead. The injector must remember that when one moves medially from the mid-pupillary line, they will come into contact with the supraorbital artery, the supratrochlear artery, and both branches. When this occurs, even superficial injections pose the potential risk of blockage of the distal branches, leading to cutaneous scalp and forehead necrosis. When enough pressure is applied during the injection process, a retrograde flow may occur toward the orbit and ophthalmic artery. This can lead to the closure of the retinal artery, which in turn causes vision loss [4, 5].

Located in the temple region, the temporal fossa is characterized by the superior temporal line (which is located anterosuperiorly), the frontal process of the zygomatic bone (which is located anteriorly), and the zygomatic arch (which is located inferiorly). A portion of the temporalis muscle, the superficial temporal artery and vein, and the auriculotemporal nerve are all located within the fossa. The anatomical layers arranged from superficial to deep are the skin, the subcutaneous layer, the superficial fascia, the loose areolar tissue, the deep temporal fascia, and the temporalis muscle.

The middle temporal vein, also known as the MTV, is a blood channel that receives various veins, including the sentinel vein, but also travels into the temporal fossa and ultimately reaches the superficial layer of the deep temporal fascia. It is a blood vessel that is both significant and relatively unknown. After that, it connects with the superficial temporal vein, located just above the level of the zygomatic arch [6]. When an injection is accidentally administered into the MTV, it can result in several problems, including a cavernous sinus embolism.

Casuaver's research has examined the size and location of the MTV [6]. The authors of this study proposed that the safest area for filler injection for temporal fossa augmentation is one finger width above the zygomatic arch [4, 5]. This conclusion was reached based on their measurements and the course of the MTV.

Additionally, the temporal (frontal) branch of the facial nerve, the superficial temporal artery and the arteries accompanying it, and the sentinel and middle temporal veins all go through the region of the temple augmentation [7]. There are a variety of planes at which injections for temporal fossa augmentation can be conducted successfully; each of these planes comes with its own set of benefits and vulnerabilities [8]. Notably, there have been cases of blindness that have been recorded as a result of temporal injection of soft tissue fillers [4, 5]:

One frequently selected plane is the immediate subcutaneous plane, even though medications can be injected into the more superficial branches of the temporal artery.

It might be challenging to precisely identify the loose areolar tissue plane, characterized by its relatively avascular nature and situated between the superficial and deep temporal fascia. On the other hand, this is a region in which the MTV system might be met.

The subperiosteal plane, situated deep to the temporalis muscle and above the periosteum, is another plane routinely selected using different procedures. One thing that should be considered is that the deep temporal veins and arteries are located directly beneath the temporalis muscle.

18.4 Upper Third of the Face

Subdermal or intradermal injections with low G′ products can be used cautiously to soften superficial forehead rhytids that are not sufficiently corrected via neuromodulation. The supratrochlear and supraorbital arteries provide a rich anastomotic network that begins intensely at the inferior aspect of the supraorbital rim and becomes more superficial as they approach the hairline. These arteries must refrain from being injected during injections. In the glabellar region, superficial injections that are medial to the vertical rhytids often avoid the supratrochlear artery, which passes under the crease in as many as 50 percent of patients, as well as the supraorbital artery, which runs more deeply and laterally [9–11]. Injections that are put laterally and deeply on the periosteum can elevate the lateral brow. In contrast, superficial injections can rectify the hollows in the upper lid and the medial brow [9, 12].

Cephalad movement causes the superficial temporal vessels to become more superficial as they move forward. Because of this, temporal augmentation necessitates injection in either a pre-periosteal (higher G′) or subdermal (lower G′) plane. Additionally, the injection should be positioned within a fingerbreadth of the arch or more than 25 mm above it in order to prevent harm to the middle temporal vein [10, 13, 14]. Visual examination is the most common method for avoiding the superficial temporal vessels; however, vascular imaging technologies may also be utilized in some circumstances. Although using a cannula can be useful in this region to avoid the vasculature, it is safe to inject the product with a needle into the pre-periosteal plane. This is because perpendicular injections that may contact vessels penetrate and transverse them before the product is placed on the periosteum.

In contrast to the female temple, which has a slight concavity to it, the male temple is flat or slightly convex. This is something that should be taken into consideration. In light of this, it is important to avoid overcorrecting the female temples [9]. In addition, the temple's shape should be filled so that the posterior aspect is broader or fuller than the anterior portion.

18.5 Forehead and Glabella

The glabella is responsible for forming rhytids, which are primarily dynamic and can be managed by administering botulinum toxin injections. A component of dermal alteration or contour depression, on the other hand, occurs as the aging process advances. Under these conditions, very little doses of HA applied intradermally have the potential to produce a more comprehensive repair. If subdermal injection is conducted, intravascular injection is possible; however, intradermal injection reduces the likelihood of this happening during the procedure. It is not the opinion of this author that the utilization of blunt cannulas completely prevents the possibility of intravascular injection. Because of the proximity of this region to the supraorbital and supratrochlear arteries, it is safer to use a dermal plane with consistent motion, threading, and no bleb implantation [2].

Injectable filler can be used to modify the contour of the forehead, particularly in the area of the forehead covering the supraorbital and lower regions. Threading is a procedure that can be used to fill small depressions that are located above the orbital rim. The injectable fillers that are currently accessible do not seem to be an effective means of correcting transverse forehead lines. When using low-viscosity and cohesive fillers, it is possible to execute superficial injections with caution; nonetheless, it is essential to exercise caution to prevent beading and obvious overcorrection.

Due to this particular cause, injections for this indication are not typically carried out [2].

18.6 Upper Eyelids and Brows

Anatomically speaking, the periocular region is quite dense. Suppose you want to inject the upper or lower lid. In that case, you need a solid understanding of this anatomy, a large acquaintance with the handling properties of the employed fillers, and a decent technical facility. These injections are not starter injections or the ones that are performed the most frequently. Despite these difficulties, the impact on facial appearance is typically significant. This is because the face's central region is the part that is most frequently exposed to eye contact during social interactions. In light of these factors, it is recommended that a provider who acts as an injector regularly should make an effort to become proficient in this field [2].

Even while upper lid treatments are less prevalent than lower lid treatments, they are, in some ways, less difficult and less harmful. This is even though upper lid treatments are less frequently indicated. Two of the most common procedures are to fill upper lid hollowing and boost the lateral brow. This hollowing can result from excessive surgical resection during blepharoplasty, proptosis, or the bone architecture of the orbit [2].

If the ptosis of the lateral brow is significant, the most effective treatment is a brow-raising procedure. Placing modest amounts of filler between the soft tissue of the brow and the bony orbital rim can, however, help decrease the appearance of early brow ptosis. This is similar to how minimal early laxity in the face can be controlled. The needle is inserted into the area just lateral to the brow to perform the injection procedure. Then, it is guided along the transition zone between the two structures under consideration. In withdrawing the needle, short threads or small blebs are positioned retroactively. One or two little blebs can be placed deep to superficial as a pillar, although this is a less typical occurrence. CaHa or a denser HA filler could be utilized in this situation. It is advisable to approach this treatment with reasonable expectations and self-control. Changes of a smaller magnitude are simple to achieve, but the effect does not increase linearly with the addition of filler [2].

Hollowing or skeletonization of the upper lid, with a visible orbital rim, and hollowing or depression inferior to this but above the pretarsal lid can be concealed with hyaluronate filler by employing a technique known as transverse threading. The material must be precisely positioned because it is difficult to move the substance after it has been injected using techniques such as manual massage, rolling, or any other method [2].

18.7 Temples

As people get older, their temples become deeper, most likely due to a decrease in the volume of the temporal fat pad, and, subsequently, the temporalis muscle itself falls less. It is common for the overlying skin to be relatively thin, and the vasculature beneath it may be easily discernible. This results in a significant increase in the likelihood of noticeable lumps and irregularities, and it also highlights the importance of avoiding overcorrection, which gives the appearance of an unnatural bulge in this region. The dilution of HA or CaHa fillers, which creates a thinner material that easily spreads throughout the tissue plane, makes it simpler to achieve an even result. Regarding this off-label method, there is some advice regarding the preferred dilutions.

In most cases, the dilution will add up to two times as much saline or local anesthesia as the original amount. The most typical method that this author employs is a dilution of one-to-one, which enables treatment of both temples with a single syringe of material, or occasionally even less if the depression is not particularly severe. The injection is administered as a bolus in one or two regions, and then the material is massaged into the skin to ensure that it is distributed evenly. Prior to the insertion of the needle, the skin is tensed up in order to facilitate implantation into the subcutaneous region or deep to the superficial temporal fascia, depending on the intention of the procedure. It is possible to execute accessory longitudinal threading along the medial sections of the temple in order to accentuate any depressions that extend into the supraorbital region [2].

In the process of rejuvenation of the temples, the objective is to achieve a youthful and aesthetic result that is suitable for each individual in a safe and effective manner. For instance, the temples of a person with bony structures of the face and thin skin should have a greater degree of concavity than those of a person with a rounder face and thicker skin. Among the obstacles that the injector must overcome in this region are the vascular architecture, the muscles of mastication, and the emissary and diploic veins of the skull. In persons who require treatment, the skin in this region may be thin; hence, the applied substance may become visible if it is not placed in a suitable position [15].

The skilled eye of the injecting physician is used to select an appropriate candidate for the injection. Many patients might need to be made aware of the hollowness in this region, and the treating physician needs to bring it to their attention by using a mirror or photographs [16]. In certain circumstances, the treatment of this aesthetic unit is necessary to achieve a more young and balanced result. The utilization of a superior oblique view is vital for taking photographs. Preparing the patient with an antiseptic solution needs to be done. Because infections have been reported to emerge in the face on occasion, frequently months after the procedure [17], this preparation has become more significant. One option for reducing the filler's viscosity is to use lidocaine. This dilution is ideal if there are any worries regarding the possibility of producing abnormalities in those with thin skin. During the injection, one must prepare to transition into the structures in the surrounding area. For instance, the temporal region transitions into the forehead at the temporal line. If there is a loss of volume medial to this, then a gradual injection medially beyond the temporal line may be required for an optimal aesthetic outcome [15]. This is because the transition from the temporal region to the forehead is soft.

18.7.1 Procedure

Because the temporal region is relatively stable and does not fluctuate or move considerably depending on the position of the head, the correct position is determined by how comfortable it is and how easy it is to inject. The midface and jawline, on the other hand, are different from this because they change based on the posture of the head, which can range from vertical to supine [15]. In this location, a few different injection strategies have been reported [18]. The authors favor subcutaneous injections because of their safe nature and the ease with which they can be augmented. The temporal hollowness grading method might be utilized to grade patients. This is followed by applying an anesthetic cream and preparing the skin with an antiseptic solution. The region that is going to be treated is first delineated. Within the immediate subcutaneous tissue, which is located between the skin and the superficial temporal fascia, the injections are administered (injections). Small aliquots of 0.1 milliliters or less are maintained so that the volume of each injection is kept at a minimum. A massage is performed on the skin following each injection [15].

It was determined that any undesirable or unanticipated sign, symptom, reaction, or disease connected in time with the utilization of an investigational drug was considered a complication or adverse event [15]. The evaluation of safety was carried out by analyzing all adverse events, both local and systemic, that occurred during each visit, as well as in the patient's diary. By the two-week follow-up, all of the adverse effects noted by the evaluator and through patient diaries were either mild or moderate in severity and had resolved. One of the patients wrote in her journal that she had experienced "hyperpigmentation." However, after 2 weeks, the mark had disappeared, and after questioning the patient, the investigator concluded that the adverse event was ecchymosis [15].

On two separate occasions, a community practitioner contacted one of the writers to discuss vascular necrosis in the temporal region. According to the reports, the filler was injected into the deeper tissues in both instances. In all instances, the primary symptoms consisted of a temporary blanching of the lateral forehead that progressed to a reticular pattern, severe pain that was delayed in onset and exacerbated after several hours of injection, and the emergence of vesicles that were interpreted as an outbreak of herpes simplex virus. There was a subsequent development of necrosis of the superficial dermis and scarring in these patients [15].

As soon as the treatment was finished, the patient was instructed to apply gentle pressure for around 5 minutes and then apply ice packs. Each participant was discussed the possibility of experiencing transient lumps, bruising, swelling, headaches, and soreness when chewing [15]. Immediately following the completion of the injection session, it is recommended that all patients resume their regular daily activities.

Finished now. To prevent the possibility of swelling and bruising, however, patients should be instructed to refrain from engaging in excessive physical activity for a period of 24 hours [15].

18.8 Complications

Due to the presence of the upper face vascular complex, filler injections in the forehead and glabellar region are at an especially high risk of causing intravascular occlusion. Therefore, it is strongly recommended that these injections be carefully placed either subdermally or intradermally 10. Injections that are suspected of being intraarterial in this region and others can result in the closure of the central retinal artery, which can lead to blindness. These injections require immediate assessment from an expert oculoplastic surgeon [19]. Changes in eyesight can become permanent in as little as 90 minutes if they are not corrected [13, 20, 21].

18.8.1 Vision Loss

Central retinal artery embolism resulting in blindness can occur as a result of retrograde flow of a filler into the central retinal artery after accidental injection of the supratrochlear or supraorbital arteries in the glabellar region, the dorsal nasal artery in the bridge of the nose, or branches of the facial artery in the cheek, nasolabial folds, or lips [22–27]. Between the years 2000 and 2018, there were 190 cases of filler-induced blindness documented, with autologous fat or hyaluronic acid fillers being the most common causes [27, 28]. This occurrence was discovered through a comprehensive analysis of the existing literature.

The following are some examples of measures that may help to reduce the risk of central retinal artery embolism: always aspirating before injection to detect accidental entry into a vessel; using needles, syringes, and cannulas of smaller sizes rather than larger ones when it is feasible; performing low-pressure injections that release a small amount of substance rather than bolus injections; and avoiding injection into traumatized tissues [24].

Due to a lack of data, it is impossible to validate the effectiveness of any therapy for acute vision loss, and it needs to be evident which therapeutic technique is the most effective. Injections of hyaluronidase, ocular massage, systemic glucocorticoids, hyperbaric oxygen, and other interventions are some examples of treatments that, according to case reports and case studies, have the potential to be beneficial [26]. In patients who have experienced vision loss due to the injection of hyaluronic acid fillers, it is common practice to administer an immediate injection of hyaluronidase into the injection site that caused the vision loss. Additionally, the incorporation of periocular injections of hyaluronidase has been proposed. This includes direct injections into the supratrochlear and supraorbital arteries, injections into the region of these vessels, and retrobulbar and peribulbar injections [26].

Although no treatment has been shown to be consistently effective, practitioners who inject soft tissue fillers should be prepared to manage this problem because the patient may experience irreversible and disabling eyesight loss. It is prudent to have immediate access to hyaluronidase and an ophthalmologist who is skilled in the acute therapy of pain caused by filler-induced vision loss. It is recommended that periocular hyaluronidase injections be carried out within 90 minutes [28].

18.8.2 Late and Delayed Onset Adverse Effects

They include the creation of nodules, granulomatous or other inflammatory reactions, persistent infections, and the consequences of filler migration [29–32]. Late and delayed onset reactions are characterized by the presence of unfavorable effects. Although there are specific adverse effects that improve over time, such as the injection of hyaluronidase in the case of hyaluronic acid fillers, corticosteroid injections, or the administration of systemic medications, there are others that may require surgical intervention or may be impossible to reverse [33].

References

1. Rohrich RJ, Pessa JE. The fat compartments of the face: anatomy and clinical implications for cosmetic surgery. Plast Reconstr Surg. 2007;119:2219–27.
2. Bass LS. Injectable filler techniques for facial rejuvenation, volumization, and augmentation. Facial Plast Surg Clin North Am. 2015;23(4):479–88.
3. Brennan C. Avoiding the “danger zones” when injecting dermal fillers and volume enhancers. Plast Surg Nurs. 2014;34:108.
4. Allen S. Anatomic danger zones for facial injection of soft tissue fillers. In: Dover JS, Corona R, editors. UpTodate. Last updated: 26 Aug 2019.
5. Sykes JM, Cotofana S, Trevidic P, et al. Upper face: clinical anatomy and regional approaches with injectable fillers. Plast Reconstr Surg. 2015;136:204S.
6. Jung W, Youn KH, Won SY, et al. Clinical implications of the middle temporal vein with regard to temporal fossa augmentation. Dermatologic Surg. 2014;40:618.
7. Trinei FA, Januszkiewicz J, Nahai F. The sentinel vein: an important reference point for surgery in the temporal region. Plast Reconstr Surg. 1998;101:27.
8. Moradi A, Shirazi A, Perez V. A guide to temporal fossa augmentation with small gel particle hyaluronic acid dermal filler. J Drugs Dermatol. 2011;10:673.
9. Mckee D, Remington K, Swift A, et al. Effective rejuvenation with hyaluronic acid fillers: current advanced concepts. Plast Reconstr Surg. 2019;143:1277e–89e.
10. Scheuer JF III, Sieber DA, Pezeshk RA, et al. Anatomy of the facial danger zones: maximizing safety during soft-tissue filler injections. Plast Reconstr Surg. 2017;139:50e–8e.
11. Scheuer JF III, Sieber DA, Pezeshk RA, et al. Facial danger zones: techniques to maximize safety during soft-tissue filler injections. Plast Reconstr Surg. 2017;139:1103–8.
12. Akinbiyi T, Othman S, Familusi O, Calvert C, Card EB, Percec I. Better results in facial rejuvenation with fillers. Plast Reconstr Surg Glob Open. 2020;8(10):e2763. https://doi.org/10.1097/GOX.0000000000002763. PMID: 33173655; PMCID: PMC7647625

13. Beer JI, Sieber DA, Scheuer JF III, et al. Three-dimensional facial anatomy: structure and function as it relates to injectable neuromodulators and soft tissue fillers. Plast Reconstr Surg Glob Open. 2016;4:e1175. 412 Suppl Anatomy and Safety in Cosmetic Medicine: Cosmetic Bootcampe 1175
14. de Maio M, DeBoulle K, Braz A, et al. Alliance for the future of aesthetics consensus committee. Facial assessment and injection guide for botulinum toxin and injectable hyaluronic acid fillers: focus on the midface. Plast Reconstr Surg. 2017;140:540e–50e.
15. Moradi A, Watson J. Current concepts in filler injection. Facial Plast Surg Clin North Am. 2015;23(4):489–94. https://doi.org/10.1016/j.fsc.2015.07.005. PMID: 26505545
16. Moradi A, Shirazi A, Perez V. A guide to temporal fossa augmentation with small gel particle hyaluronic acid dermal filler. J Drugs Dermatol. 2011;10(6):673–6.
17. Lowe NJ, Maxwell CA, Patnaik R. Adverse reactions to dermal fillers: review. Dermatologic Surg. 2005;31(s4):1626–33.
18. Moradi A, Shirazi A, Moradi J. A 12-month, prospective, evaluator-blinded study of small gel particle hyaluronic acid filler in the correction of temporal fossa volume loss. J Drugs Dermatol. 2013;12(4):470–5.
19. Signorini M, Liew S, Sundaram H, Global Aesthetics Consensus Group, et al. Global aesthetics consensus: avoidance and management of complications from hyaluronic acid fillers-evidence- and opinion-based review and consensus recommendations. Plast Reconstr Surg. 2016;137:961e–71e.
20. Lee SH, Ha TJ, Lee JS, et al. Topography of the central retinal artery relevant to retrobulbar reperfusion in filler complications. Plast Reconstr Surg. 2019;144:1295–300.
21. Ozturk CN, Li Y, Tung R, et al. Complications following injection of soft-tissue fillers. Aesthet Surg J. 2013;33:862–77.
22. McCleve DE, Goldstein JC. Blindness secondary to injections in the nose, mouth, and face: cause and prevention. Ear Nose Throat J. 1995;74:182.
23. Park SW, Woo SJ, Park KH, et al. Iatrogenic retinal artery occlusion caused by cosmetic facial filler injections. Am J Ophthalmol. 2012;154:653.
24. Lazzeri D, Agostini T, Figus M, et al. Blindness following cosmetic injections of the face. Plast Reconstr Surg. 2012;129:995.
25. Beleznay K, Carruthers JD, Humphrey S, Jones D. Avoiding and treating blindness from fillers: a review of the world literature. Dermatologic Surg. 2015;41:1097.
26. Beleznay K, Carruthers JDA, Humphrey S, et al. Update on avoiding and treating blindness from fillers: a recent review of the world literature. Aesthet Surg J. 2019;39:662.
27. Chatrath V, Banerjee PS, Goodman GJ, Rahman E. Soft-tissue filler-associated blindness: a systematic review of case reports and case series. Plast Reconstr Surg Glob Open. 2019;7:e2173.
28. Carruthers J, Humphrey S. Injectable soft tissue fillers: overview of clinical use. In: Dover JS, Butler CE, Ofori AO, editors. UpTodate. Last updated: 13 Nov 2019.
29. Gladstone HB, Cohen JL. Adverse effects when injecting facial fillers. Semin Cutan Med Surg. 2007;26:34.
30. Monheit GD, Rohrich RJ. The nature of long-term fillers and the risk of complications. Dermatologic Surg. 2009;35(Suppl 2):1598.
31. Christensen L. Normal and pathologic tissue reactions to soft tissue gel fillers. Dermatologic Surg. 2007;33(Suppl 2):S168.
32. Braun M, Braun S. Nodule formation following lip augmentation using porcine collagen-derived filler. J Drugs Dermatol. 2008;7:579.
33. Smith KC. Reversible vs. nonreversible fillers in facial aesthetics: concerns and considerations. Dermatol Online J. 2008;14:3.

19 Volumizing with Fillers: Middle Face

Fatih Yucedag, Cemal Cingi, and Alwyn D'Souza

19.1 Introduction

If you desire a more attractive appearance, midface rejuvenation is the ideal solution. By enhancing the upper cheeks with hyaluronic acid dermal fillers, you can make your cheekbones appear more prominent and achieve a more youthful appearance. Over the past two decades, hyaluronic acid fillers have undergone significant advancements, fulfilling various therapeutic needs, including enhanced projection and the ability to accommodate facial movements. As a result, individuals of all ages now choose them as their preferred midface rejuvenation procedure. They offer less invasive treatment options with quick results and minimal recovery time. Due to the crucial role the midface plays in shaping the human face, injecting this area can unintentionally accentuate other cosmetic concerns, such as nasolabial folds and infraorbital hollowness. The midface comprises five layers. To minimize procedural risks and achieve natural results, midface rejuvenation requires a customized treatment plan and a thorough understanding of anatomy. This chapter aims to provide a detailed anatomical overview of the midface, including its normal blood vessel pathways and depths. With this information, we can more accurately identify the treatment area and reduce the likelihood of complications during

F. Yucedag
Department of Otorhinolaryngology, Faculty of Medicine, Karamanoglu Mehmetbey University, Karaman, Turkey

C. Cingi (✉)
Eskisehir Osmangazi University, Medical Faculty, Department of Otorhinolaryngology, Eskisehir, Türkiye
e-mail: cemal@ogu.edu.tr

A. D'Souza
Private Practice, London Facial Surgery, London, UK
e-mail: ad@londonfacialsurgery.org

C. Cingi et al. (eds.), *Minor Interventions, Major Outcomes on the Face*, Comprehensive ENT, https://doi.org/10.1007/978-3-032-01305-7_19

procedures. We also propose a treatment strategy that considers the various mechanical constraints and levels of mobility present in the individual layers of the midface. By factoring in each patient's age, gender, skin type, and facial structure, this algorithm seeks to personalize the treatment plan.

19.2 Danger Zones

19.2.1 Periorbital Area

The area around the eyes contains several arteries, including the zygomaticotemporal, zygomaticofacial, middle palpebral, and lateral palpebral arteries [1]. These veins branch from the internal carotid artery system and connect to the ophthalmic branch.

The brow and upper eyelids undergo injections during periorbital augmentation. A common technique for creating the illusion of a higher brow involves injecting filler into the region of the retro-orbicularis oculi fat, located beneath the orbicularis oculi along the supraorbital rim. The depth of the fat compartment above the supratarsal fold is referred to as the retro-orbicularis oculi fat, responsible for the defined contour of the upper eyelid and brow [1, 2]. Superficial and supratrochlear neurovascular bundles emerge from their respective foramina, necessitating extreme care when medially injecting deeply.

Conversely, injections used to repair a skeletonized orbit by augmenting the superior sulcus of the upper eyelid are typically placed beneath the superior orbital rim, deep to the orbicularis oculi and superficial to the levator aponeurosis. The superior palpebral arteries tend to move horizontally, making it crucial to avoid them when operating in this area. Direct damage to the eye and vascular dysfunction pose two risks associated with injections [1].

19.2.2 The Area Around the Eyes

Angular, superior labial, and septal arteries, which branch from the maxillary artery in the orbit, pass through the areas of the nose, nasolabial fold, and lip injections, respectively. A tributary of the external carotid artery, the transverse facial artery crosses the mid-cheek and malar areas, ascends the zygomaticus and levator labii muscles, and eventually anastomoses with the angular artery [1].

With the exception of the region around the lower eyelid, the midface comprises the following anatomical layers: skin, subcutaneous fat, superficial musculoaponeurotic system (SMAS), deep areolar tissue, and mimetic muscles. When augmenting tissue volume, the infraorbital hollow just under the medial canthal area is a typical target. The facial vein (four to six millimeters medial to the mid-pupillary line) [3] and the facial artery (angular artery) are anatomically situated such that this area can be divided into a medial and a lateral component.

Observing the infraorbital depression from the side, you can see seven separate layers. The skin, orbicularis oculi, suborbicularis oculi, deep fascia, pre-periosteal fat, and periosteum comprise the layers that make up the eye. At this medial location [4], the only two layers that constitute the medial aspect of the eye are the skin and the orbicularis oculi muscle, which is attached to the bone. Since there is no subcutaneous fat layer to hold the filler, medial injections are often administered submuscularly [1].

Due to the anastomoses of numerous major arteries in these regions, the cheek and the infraorbital hollow are typically very vascularized. These vessels, along with their branches, include the angular, transverse facial, and infraorbital arteries [5]. It is possible to infuse the nasolabial folds and accidentally inject into the angular artery, which is related to the ophthalmic artery. This could block the retinal artery and induce blindness [6].

When treating the upper midface, which includes the upper cheek and tear trough, it is standard procedure to inject into the subperiosteal or deep subcutaneous plane. However, it is common practice to inject the dermis or subcutaneous area in the lower midface, encompassing the mid-cheek. Understanding the structures and pathways of specific blood vessels and their branches at these points allows for more precise and less risky injections [1].

19.3 The Center Third

Two common and often hereditary early signs of aging are a wide tear trough and an inconsistent lower lid-cheek junction. Therefore, individuals of all ages, from kids to grandmothers, seek fillers when needed [7]. The choice of filler and its administration method—subdermally or supraperiosteally—should depend on the patient's lower eyelid tone. One can limit the product's mobility during administration by placing a finger on the upper section of the infraorbital rim. When using hydrophilic materials, it is especially important to avoid injecting large volumes superficially to prevent surface irregularities and edema. Additionally, mixing high-G prime products with saline creates an injection that is homogeneous, smooth, and effectively corrects the issue at hand [8]. The tear trough and lower lid are suitable areas for cannula placement to minimize the risk of damaging blood vessels. Persistent lower lid edema may occur after using hyaluronic acid gels due to the risk of lymphatic blockage from water absorption. To prevent these potential problems, it is crucial to undertreat initially and use hyaluronic acid gels with low concentrations and medium particle sizes [9–11]. Furthermore, protecting the infraorbital nerve, which arises from the medial limbus about 11 mm below the infraorbital rim, must be prioritized [11–13].

The facial arteries continue as the angular arteries and branch out into the lateral nasal arteries. As they ascend, they become increasingly superficial as they pass inferiorly across the mandibular boundary. The angular artery runs laterally along the side of the nose, while the lateral nasal artery connects to the dorsal nasal artery through an anastomosis after wrapping over the top of the alae. The dorsal nasal artery is part of a complex anastomotic network that also includes arteries supplying the eyes and the center of the retina. Because the nasal vasculature is located superficially in the subcutaneous space, injecting deeply into the superficial musculoaponeurotic layer at the midline of the nasal dorsum is essential, just above the periosteum/perichondrium [9]. High-G′, low-concentration filler can be placed at the midline nasal tip and the columellar base at the anterior nasal spine to counteract under-rotation or nasal tip droop [10]. Extra caution should be exercised for patients with a history of rhinoplasty to avoid damaging any anatomical or vascular structures. For AR injections, a series of small, superficial injections are performed. To prevent targeting the lateral nasal artery, these needles should be inserted at least two or three millimeters above the alar groove [11, 14].

The cheek contains numerous fat pads and retaining ligaments at varying depths [15]. Uneven tissue movement, resulting from the age-related degradation of these structures, accentuates folds and creates undesirable outlines due to the differing rates at which they age. Enhancing the cheeks in the front, center, inner areas, and beneath the skin is common practice [16, 17]. The ideal shape of a female cheek, as observed in white and Asian women, features an apex that requires lateral or medial augmentation [10] and a smooth ogee curve [8] with increased volume above. Utilizing the depot approach and a high-G′ filler, small bolus injections can be made in the supraperiosteal plane to achieve the most effective correction of the medial and lateral malar eminences. There is also the possibility of employing a stacking technique to restore volume across multiple layers. These methods bolster the structural framework, thereby helping to elevate, enlarge, and sustain tissues that are drooping or atrophied [7]. To restore the full contour, subcutaneous filler—a flexible gel injected into the superficial tissues above—can be used to add volume to movable areas.

In most cases, three milliliters of product may be necessary for each side. Medial malar augmentation can provide lower eyelid support, especially for those with a negative vector. Given that the atrophic medial cheek exacerbates the tear trough, it is advisable to consider this approach first [8]. Fanning or cross-hatching techniques at the subcutaneous level with a low cohesivity, high flexibility filler, or a blended filler, if those are unavailable, can effectively treat isolated sub-malar deflation, which is uncommon but often seen in very thin patients with pan-facial atrophy or those who have previously undergone buccal fat pad removal [8]. Additionally, intraoral massage may offer further assistance in filler distribution [10].

Both age and surgical rejuvenation can contribute to preauricular atrophy and deflation. As the superficial fat compartment atrophies, preauricular volume diminishes [18]. Injections should be superficial to avoid penetrating the vital deep structures in the preauricular area. Injections can occur at the subcutaneous plane and into the mandible's inferior periosteum [13].

19.4 Complex of the Cheeks

Consider all the different areas of the cheek while planning an aesthetic strategy. The aging process can lead to changes such as volume loss and decline, which may result in certain zones appearing empty. These alterations occur at varying rates in different fat pads, shifting the face's dimensions and transforming the cheeks into disconnected regions that appear younger. Additional creases result from fibrous septae, often referred to as "ligaments," that connect fat pads. The objective of cheek augmentation is to restore the face's natural volume and proportions, making the lateral malar/zygomatic area appear wider than it actually is. It is preferable to diminish the visibility of crevices or depressions between fat pads. Even younger patients can achieve similar results with moderate to mild cheek augmentation. Injectable fillers, unlike surgically inserted implants, can be fine-tuned and tailored section by section within the cheeks. However, compared to the aforementioned cheek implants, the longevity of these fillers is lower [19]. Assess for wrinkles or depressions between the cheek's fat pads, submalar hollowing, the zygomaticomalar complex on the cheek's side, and the medial cheek. A dip superolateral to the nasolabial fold is a feature that characterizes facial lipoatrophy. Aged patients typically do not present this characteristic. The authors recommend enhancing the midface's width by sweeping slightly superior and lateral, augmenting the lateral region of the cheek (including the malar complex), and slightly improving the anterior projection for most patients as part of their aesthetic planning. The senior author generally avoids injecting the middle area of the cheek in older Caucasian individuals. This is based on the author's subjective observation that with age, the patient's inferior medial cheek (the area above the nasolabial fold) becomes broader and heavier. However, this rule is bent when addressing malar creasing. There is a significant volume difference between this area and others, except for the malar creases that run between fat pads or extend inferiorly from the tear trough. In contrast, procedures that enhance and convex this area may be more visually appealing for certain Asian patients and those with a wide and flat midfacial appearance [19]. It is standard practice to target the lateral sections by injecting one or two boluses of material deep into the malar fat pad or subperiosteum to elevate and emphasize the most pronounced region of the malar eminence. Due to their unique rheological properties, CaHA and high-cohesivity HA fillers effectively create lifting effects. The former can be easily shaped into the final form after injecting the bolus(es), including the final bolus along the zygomatic arch. High-cohesivity HA requires more time to mold, so it is recommended to inject it in smaller, deeper boluses or as little columns or pillars while withdrawing the needle retrogradely. Either of these injection techniques can be utilized. While this author typically threads CaHA into wrinkles, similar techniques work equally well with this substance during injections. However, emphasizing the relationship between the lid and the cheek may occur if the upper border of the malar region is overcorrected [19]. Evaluate the degree and severity of submalar hollowing. Neutral or slightly concave contours are very natural and, in some cases, even desirable. However, prominent hollowing can make the face appear older and more "worn-out" around the temples and cheeks.

Using a subcutaneous or cross-hatched fanning technique, submalar hollowing can be effectively addressed with a variety of materials. The aim is to create a noticeable hollowing out, achieving either a flat or slightly concave contour. Although it may be undesirable, convexity can give the appearance of "chipmunk" cheeks or, worse, a baby face. For a more youthful look, it may be better to smooth down the malar area instead of over-projecting the submalar region [19].

19.5 Lower Eyelids

Consider all the different parts of the cheek while planning an aesthetic strategy. The aging process can lead to changes such as volume loss and decline, which can result in some of these areas appearing noticeably absent. These alterations occur in various fat pads at different rates, changing the face's dimensions and transforming the cheeks into distinct regions that appear youthful. Additional creases are caused by fibrous septae, often referred to as "ligaments," that connect fat pads. The aim of cheek augmentation is to restore the face's natural volume and proportions; the lateral malar/zygomatic area is designed to appear wider than it actually is. It is preferable to minimize the visibility of crevices or depressions between fat pads.

Even younger patients can achieve similar results with moderate to mild cheek augmentation. Injectable fillers, unlike surgically inserted implants, can be fine-tuned and adjusted section by section within the cheeks. However, when compared to cheek implants, the durability of these fillers is lower [19].

Examine for wrinkles or depressions between the fat pads of the cheek, submalar hollowing, the zygomaticomalar complex on the side of the cheek, and the medial cheek. A dip superolateral to the nasolabial fold is a feature that identifies facial lipoatrophy. Typically, patients with aged faces do not exhibit this trait. The authors recommend enhancing the midface's width by sweeping slightly superior and lateral, augmenting the lateral area of the cheek (including the malar complex), and slightly enhancing the anterior projection for most patients as part of their aesthetic planning. The senior author often avoids injecting the middle portion of the cheek in older Caucasian individuals. This is due to the author's subjective observation that, with age, the inferior medial cheek area (above the nasolabial fold) tends to become broader and heavier. However, this guideline is adjusted when addressing malar creasing. There is a significant volume difference between this area and others, except for malar creases that run between fat pads or extend inferiorly from the tear trough. Conversely, procedures that enhance and convex this area may be more visually pleasing to certain Asian patients and others with a wide and flat midfacial structure [19].

It is common practice to address the lateral sections by injecting one or two boluses of material deep into the malar fat pad or subperiosteum to elevate and highlight the most prominent part of the malar eminence. Due to their unique rheological properties, CaHA and high-cohesivity HA fillers effectively produce lifting effects. After injecting the bolus(es), the former can be easily shaped into the final form, including the last bolus along the zygomatic arch. High-cohesivity HA requires more time to mold, so it is best injected in smaller, deeper boluses or as small columns or pillars while withdrawing the needle retrogradely. You can employ either of these injection techniques. While this author typically threads CaHA into wrinkles, similar methods are equally effective for this substance during injection. However, if the upper border of the malar region is overly corrected, it may accentuate the relationship between the lid and the cheek [19].

Consider the extent and severity of submalar hollowing. Neutral or slightly concave contours appear quite natural and, in some cases, even desirable. However, prominent hollowing can make the face look older and more "worn-out" around the temples and cheeks. Various materials can effectively fill submalar hollowing using a subcutaneous or cross-hatched fanning technique. The objective is to achieve a contour that is either flat or slightly concave, creating a noticeable hollowing effect. Although undesirable, convexity can result in a "chipmunk" cheek appearance or, worse, a baby face. To achieve a more youthful look, it may be better to smooth the malar area rather than over-project the submalar area [19].

19.6 The Lower Eyelids

Various therapeutic techniques can effectively address the changes that occur in the lower eyelid due to aging. Surgery is an option for those looking to correct a developing tear trough or a noticeable distinction at the lid-cheek junction, but HA filler injections are quick, reliable, and tend to last for some time. If you want to avoid visible lumps and unintended overcorrection, opt for HA fillers. They are smooth, supple, fully hydrated, and spread easily through tissues due to their low viscosity and cohesiveness. The thin skin in this area is the reason for this. In other words, if you can access something gentler and silkier, it would be ideal for the eyelids [19].

When treating the lower eyelid, the tear trough is the most reliable, fastest, and easiest area to focus treatment on. To determine if the tear trough is an age-related issue that could benefit from aesthetic treatment, it is helpful to review the patient's photographs from their younger years and conduct a thorough consultation. Addressing the tear trough, which may have become deeper over time, can create the appearance of more relaxed skin. For mechanical dispersion, the author recommends using a cotton applicator to roll the material upward after linear threading or supraperiosteal bleb implantation has occurred. Threading must always avoid the angular artery, located at the trough's tip at the medial canthus. Another concern is the risk of embolization from vascular cannulation, which can happen after a bleb is implanted. Applying a large amount of HA filler in this delicate skin area may also lead to a Tyndall effect. To prevent a bulge in the upper malar area a week or two later, it is essential to place the material in the obvious depression rather than just below it [19].

While correcting the junction of the cheek and the lid, there is a significant risk of ecchymosis, although it remains possible. The middle region often contains many superficial arteries; at times, these vessels are visible on the surface, but more frequently, they arise from a recessed section of the junction that requires correction.

This writer favors the suborbicularis threading method, which requires the use of very small amounts of filler. If ecchymosis does occur, stopping the therapy for a few minutes to apply gentle, continuous pressure is advised. Although ecchymosis is a possible side effect of this treatment, it can be minimized with a careful, gradual injection technique. This is also likely to happen in the lateral canthal area and the third of the lid-cheek junction on the left side. When the upper malar region is overly augmented, the step-off in this area becomes even more pronounced, despite already being noticeable.

Despite the importance of this consideration, it is rare for the skin to show the branches of the zygomaticofacial vessels. This author performs tear trough repair and cautions about potential ecchymosis without excessive concern. Patients should also be prepared for ecchymosis in the remaining lower lid tissue, according to the author. It is common to observe a crease in the pretarsal segment or at the junction of the pretarsal and orbital parts. Suborbicular fill with fine threads of injectable HA filler or a combination of the two can moderately address this issue. Although the volumes injected are barely noticeable, it is possible to achieve significant improvement in crepey skin and wrinkles after the injected filler has settled and integrated. By incorporating vertical threads for cross-hatching, the correction can be enhanced in the lid and at the junction of the lid and cheek [19].

19.7 Midface and Malar Region Augmentation

A number of surgical options for rejuvenating the midface have been considered [20–22]. More doctors are increasingly using fillers to reshape the midface by adding volume and enhancing the area's overall appearance, thanks to the rising popularity of these cosmetic enhancements. According to the authors, one of the most important considerations when injecting facial fillers for cosmetic rejuvenation is the midface. This area is more amenable to treatment than the temples, which have more defined limits of augmentation due to their anatomical boundaries. At the request of the Food and Drug Administration (FDA), specifications were made for the facial subregions that could be used to gather data on therapy, safety, and effectiveness. The three independent subregions that comprise the midface are the zygomaticomalar region, the anteromedial cheek, and the submalar region. This research primarily focuses on the findings related to the total midface volume deficit [23, 24], as all results were consistent across facial subregions.

The injection site can alter the midface prominence and focal point [23] (Figs. 19.1, 19.2, and 19.3):

1. The lateral zygoma shifts the focus laterally, bringing it closer to the midface width; it is placed lateral to a line drawn from the lateral canthus to the oral commissure.
2. A line between the lateral canthus and the oral commissure, which is positioned above Hinderer's line [25], passes medially through the mid-cheek. The focal

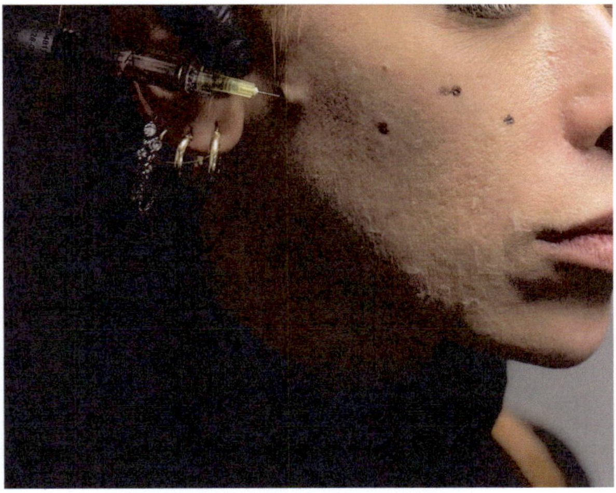

Fig. 19.1 Application to midface and malar region

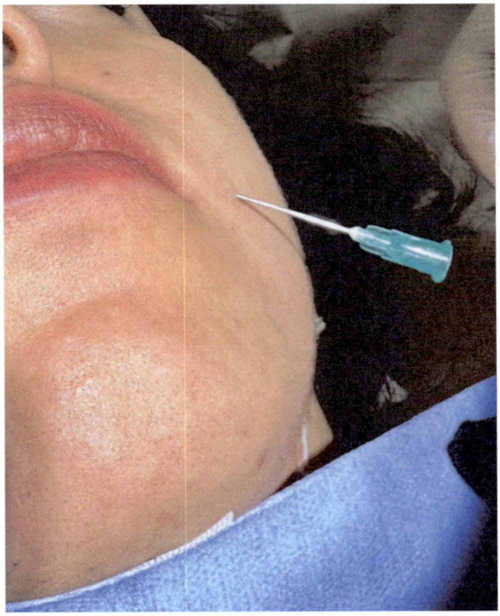

Fig. 19.2 Application to midface and nasolabial sulcus

point could shift to the middle of the screen due to the frontal projection of the midface.

3. We direct the focus to the submalar region, which is located beneath Hinderer's line and across from the oral commissure and lateral to a line connecting the lateral canthus.

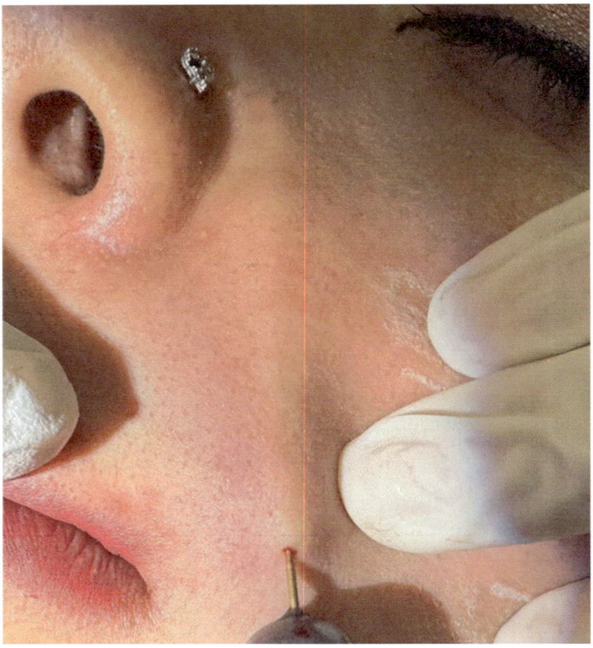

Fig. 19.3 Application to midface and nasolabial sulcus

19.7.1 Treatment Goals and Anticipated Results

The purpose of midface augmentation can vary from simply replacing lost volume to dramatically altering the shape of the midface by injecting fillers into areas that may appear unnatural. Because every person's face is unique and one side often looks younger than the other, it is crucial to discuss with the patient their goals and consider their facial shape. In such instances, informing the individual about the potential results is important. Furthermore, the authors believe that the initial step in face filler augmentation is to inject the opposite side of the face to achieve symmetry, using the younger-looking side as a template.

When the face is nearly symmetrical, additional injections may be administered on either side to enhance attractiveness. After the patient and doctor agree on the desired outcome, at least three views of the patient's face should be taken into account, including frontal and bilateral oblique perspectives, as these viewpoints are essential. The authors have sought details such as differences in zygoma height and width and minor asymmetries in the malar prominence through extensive examination of printed photographs. By capturing images of the midface and its surrounding aesthetic components, one can observe their variations. Additionally, these visuals may help the patient recognize subtle details they might have overlooked [23].

To maximize the diagnostic and therapeutic procedures, the patient should maintain an upright head position, as the midface soft tissue structures are quite malleable. A complex geometric architecture characterizes the three-dimensional face. Subtle changes can significantly impact appearance. The doctor requires unrestricted mobility to navigate around the treatment table and assess the results from various angles for a better three-dimensional effect [23].

The periosteum of the zygoma is typically the starting point for injections. Most practitioners employ this technique. When lifting the midface in a supralateral direction, the authors believe the zygoma provides a reliable and stable foundation. For a smooth transition to adjacent facial aesthetic units, the injector must maintain a comprehensive view of the face and be capable of working in three dimensions. Swelling and bruising are the most common side effects, yet they typically resolve within a week. Furthermore, this procedure can result in asymmetrical deformities, infections, skin necrosis, and even blindness [23].

19.7.2 Care Following the Procedure

In this treatment, the patient will receive a full massage of the affected area and then be advised to use a cold compress. The patient should also promptly notify the medical team if they experience any unusual discomfort or changes in skin color, in addition to the typical pain, swelling, or bruising. Patients are generally able to return to their regular routines the day after treatment. A more attractive and youthful appearance is the desired result of this therapy [23].

19.8 Complications

To prevent vasculature, visible surface abnormalities, and the Tyndall effect—a bluish-gray discoloration that occurs due to the thinness of the lower lid skin—injections into the tear trough should be performed deep on the periosteum [26, 27]. Asymmetry, chronic edema, and ecchymosis are also common in this area, particularly in patients with reduced lower lid tone, a history of allergies or hypersensitivity, or both [26, 27].

References

1. Allen S. Anatomic danger zones for facial injection of soft tissue fillers. In: Dover JS, Corona R, editors. UpTodate. Last updated: 26 Aug 2019.
2. Goldberg RA, Wu JC, Jesmanowicz A, Hyde JS, Eyelid anatomy revisited. Dynamic high-resolution magnetic resonance images of Whitnall's ligament and upper eyelid structures with the use of a surface coil. Arch Ophthalmol. 1992;110:1598.
3. Cotofana S, Schenck TL, Trevidic P, et al. Midface: clinical anatomy and regional approaches with injectable fillers. Plast Reconstr Surg. 2015;136:219S.
4. Tong J, Lopez MJ, Fakoya AO, Patel BC. Anatomy, head and neck: orbicularis oculi muscle. 2024. In: StatPearls [Internet]. Treasure Island (FL): StatPearls Publishing; 2024 Jan–.
5. Kim YS, Choi DY, Gil YC, et al. The anatomical origin and course of the angular artery with regard to its clinical implications. Dermatologic Surg. 2014;40:1070.
6. Park SW, Woo SJ, Park KH, et al. Iatrogenic retinal artery occlusion caused by cosmetic facial filler injections. Am J Ophthalmol. 2012;154:653.

7. Sundaram H, Liew S, Signorini M, Global Aesthetics Consensus Group, et al. Global aesthetics consensus: hyaluronic acid fillers and botulinum toxin type A-recommendations for combined treatment and optimizing outcomes in diverse patient populations. Plast Reconstr Surg. 2016;137:1410–23.
8. Mckee D, Remington K, Swift A, et al. Effective rejuvenation with hyaluronic acid fillers: current advanced concepts. Plast Reconstr Surg. 2019;143:1277e–89e.
9. Beer JI, Sieber DA, Scheuer JF III, et al. Three-dimensional facial anatomy: structure and function as it relates to injectable neuromodulators and soft tissue fillers. Plast Reconstr Surg Glob Open. 2016;4:e1175. 412 Suppl Anatomy and Safety in Cosmetic Medicine: Cosmetic Bootcampe 1175
10. de Maio M, DeBoulle K, Braz A, et al. Alliance for the future of aesthetics consensus Committee. Facial assessment and injection guide for botulinum toxin and injectable hyaluronic acid fillers: focus on the midface. Plast Reconstr Surg. 2017;140:540e–50e.
11. Scheuer JF III, Sieber DA, Pezeshk RA, et al. Anatomy of the facial danger zones: maximizing safety during soft-tissue filler injections. Plast Reconstr Surg. 2017;139:50e–8e.
12. Scheuer JF III, Sieber DA, Pezeshk RA, et al. Facial danger zones: techniques to maximize safety during soft-tissue filler injections. Plast Reconstr Surg. 2017;139:1103–8.
13. Akinbiyi T, Othman S, Familusi O, Calvert C, Card EB, Percec I. Better results in facial rejuvenation with fillers. Plast Reconstr Surg Glob Open. 2020;8(10):e2763. https://doi.org/10.1097/GOX.0000000000002763. PMID: 33173655; PMCID: PMC7647625
14. Rohrich RJ, Gunter JP, Friedman RM. Nasal tip blood supply: an anatomic study validating the safety of the transcolumellar incision in rhinoplasty. Plast Reconstr Surg. 1995;95:795–9. discussion 800
15. Rohrich RJ, Pessa JE. The retaining system of the face: histologic evaluation of the septal boundaries of the subcutaneous fat compartments. Plast Reconstr Surg. 2008;121:1804–9.
16. Wilson AJ, Taglienti AJ, Chang CS, et al. Current applications of facial volumization with fillers. Plast Reconstr Surg. 2016;137:872e–89e. (PubMed) (Google Scholar)
17. de Maio M, Swift A, Signorini M, Committee ALiFAC, et al. Facial assessment and injection guide for botulinum toxin and injectable hyaluronic acid fillers: focus on the upper face. Plast Reconstr Surg. 2017;140:265e–76e.
18. Salti G, Rauso R. Facial rejuvenation with fillers: the dual plane technique (published correction appears). J Cutan Aesthet Surg. 2015;8:127–33. In J Cutan Aesthet Surg. 2016 Jul-Sep;9(3):211
19. Bass LS. Injectable filler techniques for facial rejuvenation, Volumization, and augmentation. Facial Plast Surg Clin North Am. 2015;23(4):479–88.
20. Ramirez OM. Three-dimensional endoscopic midface enhancement: a personal quest for the ideal cheek rejuvenation. Plast Reconstr Surg. 2002;109(1):329–40.
21. Hamra ST. The zygorbicular dissection in composite rhytidectomy: an ideal midface plane. Plast Reconstr Surg. 1998;102(5):1646–57.
22. Terino EO, Edward M. The magic of mid-face threedimensional contour alterations combining alloplastic and soft tissue suspension technologies. Clin Plast Surg. 2008;35(3):419–50.
23. Moradi A, Watson J. Current concepts in filler injection. Facial Plast Surg Clin North Am. 2015;23(4):489–94. https://doi.org/10.1016/j.fsc.2015.07.005.
24. Jones D, Murphy DK. Volumizing hyaluronic acid filler for midface volume deficit: 2-year results from a pivotal single-blind randomized controlled study. Dermatologic Surg. 2013;39:1–11.
25. Jung W, Youn KH, Won SY, et al. Clinical implications of the middle temporal vein with regard to temporal fossa augmentation. Dermatologic Surg. 2014;40:618.
26. Urdiales-Gálvez F, Delgado NE, Figueiredo V, et al. Treatment of soft tissue filler complications: expert consensus recommendations. Aesth Plast Surg. 2018;42:498–510.
27. Signorini M, Liew S, Sundaram H, Global Aesthetics Consensus Group, et al. Global aesthetics consensus: avoidance and management of complications from hyaluronic acid fillers-evidence- and opinion-based review and consensus recommendations. Plast Reconstr Surg. 2016;137:961e–71e.

Volumizing with Fillers: Nose

20

Ali Seyed Resuli, Felicia Manole, and Alireza Mesbahi

20.1 Introduction

Malar elevation should be considered a first line of treatment for nasolabial folds if the malars are insufficient in volume. This is because malars can potentially alter the malformation of the nasolabial folds [1, 2]. When it comes to injection, the linear or fanning approaches and the superomedial advancement of the needle are both effective. To achieve the desired outcomes and to prevent artery injury, the product should ideally be applied in the deep-dermal plane for superficial rhytids along the medial aspect of the fold [3]. This will allow for the most effective application possible. It is recommended that depot insertion be performed at the periosteum of the alar base before proceeding with deep folds with a significant superior component. This is because it has the potential to reduce the quantity of superficial products that are required. A second method that can assist in correcting noticeable folds is applying the cross-hatching technique to the cutaneous upper lip. Injections that are administered laterally to the fold in the nasolabial mound should be avoided at all costs since they have the potential to exaggerate the look of the fold. To prevent vascular harm, using a cannula in this region may be beneficial [4, 5, 6].

A. S. Resuli (✉)
İstanbul Yeni Yüzyıl University, Faculty of Medicine, Department of Otorhinolaryngology, Istanbul, Turkey

F. Manole
Faculty of Medicine, Department of ENT, University of Oradea, Oradea, Romania

A. Mesbahi
Facial Plastic Surgery Clinic, Fars Province, Shiraz, Iran

C. Cingi et al. (eds.), *Minor Interventions, Major Outcomes on the Face*, Comprehensive ENT, https://doi.org/10.1007/978-3-032-01305-7_20

20.2 Danger Zones

Because the vascularization of the nose is so dense, any injections in any plane pose a more significant risk of necrosis than injections in other parts of the face compared to the danger of necrosis. It is common practice to inject the nasal dorsum in the supraperiosteal or supraperichondrial plane because these planes are typically comparatively devoid of blood vessels [7]. Before or after rhinoplasty, nose-shaping injections may be used to get the desired results. Because of the presence of scar tissue, the restructured vascular pattern in the area, and the diminished pliability that occurs with volume injection, injections administered after rhinoplasty may have a higher risk of necrosis from arterial occlusion [8, 9].

Accidental injection into the dorsal nasal, lateral nasal, and external nasal arteries, as well as their arcades, might result in skin necrosis and deformity. Additionally, retrograde flow and retinal artery obstruction can lead to blindness [8, 10].

20.3 The Nose

When injectable fillers are used, it is possible to make slight adjustments to the form of the dorsum or the tip. Patients with cosmetic abnormalities that are too tiny to be reliably refined through surgical correction or patients who refuse to undergo surgical therapy are frequently good candidates for this particular procedure. An additional benefit of experimenting with a potential surgical outcome or appearance is that it can help certain patients feel more confident in undergoing surgical correction. However, it is important to note that there is no assurance that an identical appearance can be achieved through surgical means [11].

Even though the benefits of nonoperative nasal shaping appear enticing, it is important to exercise caution. The nasal cavity is a highly vascular structure that contains thin tissues subjected to some pressure and tension against the osseocartilaginous framework beneath it. There are several potential risks associated with intravascular injection, including the possibility of tissue loss in the nose, stroke, blindness, vascular compromise due to compression with tissue loss, erosion or ulceration of the skin due to inflammation, and induration or skin atrophy due to inflammation or compression. When a patient has received several injections or has a big scar or vascular compromise as a result of multiple nose surgeries in the past, these risks become much more pronounced. When doing future surgery on a patient who has received many injections, the surgeon should be aware that this may present additional technical obstacles and hazards [11].

A deep dermis injection, a subcutaneous injection at the tip, and a subcutaneous injection in the dorsum are all possible injection sites. To minimize the temptation of placing big boluses of material with the needle in a fixed position, it is recommended that small amounts be utilized with short linear threads. Small amounts of molding or rolling can smooth the injected material into the required form (Figs. 20.1 and 20.2) [11].

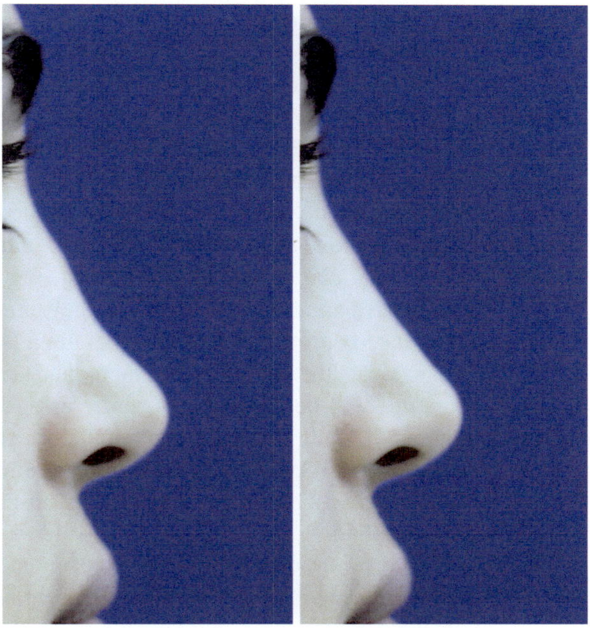

Fig. 20.1 Filler on the dorsum of a female patient

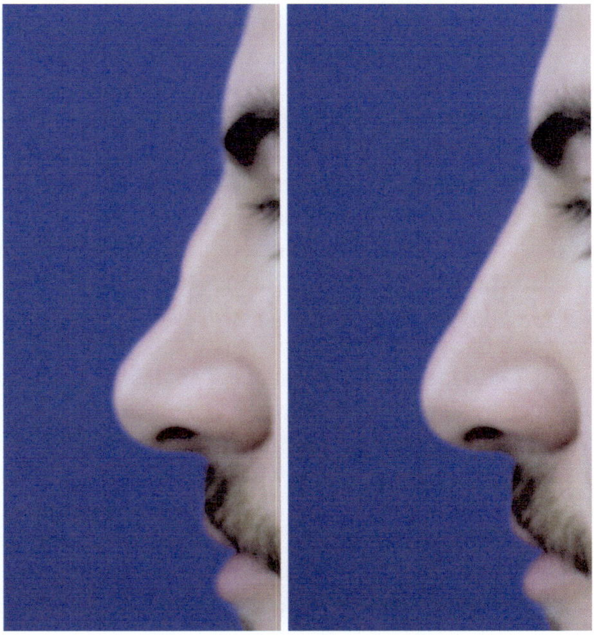

Fig. 20.2 Post-surgical correction of the dorsum with filler

20.4 Nasolabial Fold

This particular treatment area, which served as the testing ground for most of the research conducted on FDA-approved fillers, continues to be an essential component of clinical treatment. Because it is not a conspicuous aging feature and may be better rectified with filler cheek augmentation, it is included in most of this author's treatment plans for patients who are relatively unskilled or who are naïve. However, some people have come to disapprove of it. Proper correction of the nasolabial fold is nearly always beneficial for patients in their late 30s and early 40s or older [11].

Most patients have an increase in depth as they age; however, other characteristics must be evaluated during the treatment planning. Before beginning treatment, it is necessary to evaluate the patient's asymmetry and show them how it affects them. These asymmetries will be reduced in severity using filler augmentation, but they will seldom be eradicated. The degree of depth correction must be natural-looking and not overly dramatic. At no point can the nasolabial fold be entirely effaced or bulging with convexity [11]. This is because the nasolabial fold is a typical facial feature in young people.

Not only should the nasolabial depth be considered, but the presence of any dermal rhytids along the length of the fold has to be examined. An HA filler that can be injected in the deep dermis or dermal-subcutaneous junction, and mid-dermis is the one that this author chooses to use on patients who have a rhytid. This allows for a more comprehensive repair of the rhytid and the fold depth. Alternatively, CaHa may be chosen for deep correction at the dermal-subcutaneous junction, followed by rectification of the rhytid at the mid-dermal level. This bilayer treatment can be performed in a single sitting or in a manner that alternates between phases. Some patients strongly tend to focus on rectifying the rhytid rather than the depth or the other way around [11]. Patients need to be questioned about which aspect of the fold they believe to be the most disagreeable.

The final evaluation will determine whether or not there is overhanging inferomedial cheek skin, as well as the severity of the condition. This will also determine how the injection technique is performed. The most effective method for correcting severe skin overhang is a facialplasty or a middle facelift to resuspend the cheek. If you have moderate skin redundancy in this area, consider getting some filler cheek augmentation and cross-hatching transversely across the fold. This will help you flatten and structure the skin surface conformation more effectively. It is typically possible to cross-hatch only when dealing with mild redundancy. An excellent situation for a fold-only volume fill using a fanning approach is one with no discernible degree of skin redundancy. The treatment can continue without adhering to this protocol; however, the patient should be warned about the compromise due to this compromise and the inadequate correction of the overhanging skin that will result [11].

Fanning is the technique that is utilized for basic fold filling. This technique involves putting the needle inferiorly on the fold and then advancing it superiorly till it reaches the apex at the base of the nose. The injection is performed retroactively, with 0.05–0.1 mL of material being injected in each pass until the desired correction level is achieved. CaHa and HA are both effective in this region; however, they are recommended to be used with 0.2–0.3 mL of 1% lidocaine and epinephrine to reduce the risk of ecchymosis. Subdermal placement of filler, as opposed to intradermal implantation, makes it more difficult to achieve an overfilled appearance or create an unnatural surface feature [11].

It is possible to adjust the residual depth at the superior region of the fold by employing cross-hatching with a needle introduced laterally to the fold and then further advanced toward the midline. Following this, a retrograde injection is performed as the needle is removed. Additionally, this is utilized to treat mild to moderate excess cheek skin located just above or next to the fold. It is possible to fill in the depth of the fold with subcutaneous tissue; however, the cross-hatched threads should be at the dermal-subcutaneous junction or deep dermis and very thin at the lateral edge of the fold and lateral to the fold. Using this lateral cross-hatching technique, the surface structure of the skin is supposed to be altered, resulting in a flatter appearance [11].

20.5 Complications

Necrosis of the nasal tip, especially in patients who have had open rhinoplasty in the past, or blindness as a result of intravascular filler placement, are two examples of the disastrous outcomes that can result from nasal injections administered improperly and with a high volume [1].

The trademark sign of intra-arterial injection is immediate and acute pain and blanching throughout a vascular trajectory. The tissue loss in the distal vasculature due to the injection begins 24 and 48 h after. Subsequent cutaneous necrosis, which is often referred to as Nicolau syndrome [12], has the potential to be a catastrophic consequence. Loss of vision, blindness, and stroke are the intravascular problems that are the most serious. Filler injections can cause these complications.

Additionally, the administration of aspirin and maybe acetazolamide is included in the standard of care therapy for vascular impairment. These treatments include the recurrent washing of the injection trajectory with hyaluronidase, nitroglycerin paste, topical corticosteroids, and warm compresses [13, 14]. It is possible to inject hyaluronidase on an hourly basis, as needed, in doses ranging from 500 to 1500 international units, depending on the severity of the problem and the extent of tissue involvement [15].

References

1. Mckee D, Remington K, Swift A, et al. Effective rejuvenation with hyaluronic acid fillers: current advanced concepts. Plast Reconstr Surg. 2019;143:1277e–89e.
2. de Maio M, Swift A, Signorini M, et al. Committee ALiFAC. Facial assessment and injection guide for botulinum toxin and injectable hyaluronic acid fillers: focus on the upper face. Plast Reconstr Surg. 2017;140:265e–76e.

3. de Maio M, DeBoulle K, Braz A, et al. Alliance for the Future of Aesthetics Consensus Committee. Facial assessment and injection guide for botulinum toxin and injectable hyaluronic acid fillers: focus on the midface. Plast Reconstr Surg. 2017;140:540e–50e.
4. Moradi A, Watson J. Current concepts in filler injection. Facial Plast Surg Clin North Am. 2015;23:489–94.
5. Scheuer JF III, Sieber DA, Pezeshk RA, et al. Facial danger zones: techniques to maximize safety during soft-tissue filler injections. Plast Reconstr Surg. 2017;139:1103–8.
6. Akinbiyi T, Othman S, Familusi O, Calvert C, Card EB, Percec I. Better results in facial rejuvenation with fillers. Plast Reconstr Surg Glob Open. 2020;8(10):e2763. https://doi.org/10.1097/GOX.0000000000002763. PMID: 33173655; PMCID: PMC7647625.
7. Saban Y, Andretto Amodeo C, Bouaziz D, Polselli R. Nasal arterial vasculature: medical and surgical applications. Arch Facial Plast Surg. 2012;14:429.
8. Ozturk CN, Li Y, Tung R, et al. Complications following injection of soft-tissue fillers. Aesthet Surg J. 2013;33:862.
9. Allen S. Anatomic danger zones for facial injection of soft tissue fillers. In: Dover JS, Corona R, editors. UpTodate. Last updated: 26 Aug 2019.
10. DeLorenzi C. Complications of injectable fillers, part I. Aesthet Surg J. 2013;33:561.
11. Bass LS. Injectable filler techniques for facial rejuvenation, volumization, and augmentation. Facial Plast Surg Clin North Am. 2015;23(4):479–88.
12. Andre P, Haneke E. Nicolau syndrome due to hyaluronic acid injections. J Cosmet Laser Ther. 2016;18:239–44.
13. Salti G, Rauso R. Facial rejuvenation with fillers: the dual plane technique (published correction appears). J Cutan Aesthet Surg. 2015;8:127–33. in J Cutan Aesthet Surg. 2016 Jul–Sep;9(3):211.
14. Signorini M, Liew S, Sundaram H, et al. Global Aesthetics Consensus Group. Global aesthetics consensus: avoidance and management of complications from hyaluronic acid fillers-evidence- and opinion-based review and consensus recommendations. Plast Reconstr Surg. 2016;137:961e–71e.
15. DeLorenzi C. New high dose pulsed hyaluronidase protocol for hyaluronic acid filler vascular adverse events. Aesthet Surg J. 2017;37:814–25.

21 Volumizing with Fillers: Lips

Bilal Sizer, Zeliha Kapusuz Gencer, and Cemal Cingi

21.1 Danger Zones

It is possible to reliably feel the facial artery throbbing at the anterior edge of the clenched masseter muscle. The facial artery is typically placed around three centimeters anterior to the angle of the jaw. At the lateral aspect of the nose, where it becomes the angular artery and anastomoses with the infraorbital and dorsal nasal arteries, this is the primary arterial supply of the lower face. It also gives off the inferior and superior labial arteries as it travels toward the lateral part of the nose. Through the anastomoses that are located in this region around the nose, communication can take place between the internal carotid system and the external carotid system. This connection occurs through the angular and ophthalmic artery branches [1].

Avoiding the superior labial artery when performing lip augmentation, effacement of vertical lip rhytides, and augmentation of the nasolabial area. This artery is located deep within the lip mucosa and supplies the septal branch to the nasal area and the columellar branch of the nose simultaneously [2].

B. Sizer
Istanbul Arel University Faculty of Medicine Department of Otorhinolaryngology, Istanbul, Turkey

Z. K. Gencer
Department of Otorhinolaryngology, University of Health Sciences, Basaksehir Cam and Sakura City Hospital, Istanbul, Turkey

C. Cingi (✉)
Eskisehir Osmangazi University, Medical Faculty, Department of Otorhinolaryngology, Eskisehir, Türkiye
e-mail: cemal@ogu.edu.tr

C. Cingi et al. (eds.), *Minor Interventions, Major Outcomes on the Face*, Comprehensive ENT, https://doi.org/10.1007/978-3-032-01305-7_21

When injecting the lower perioral region, it is essential to avoid injecting the mental artery and the labii inferioris branch of the facial artery. These are the two major vessels that should be avoided [1].

21.2 Lower Third

The perioral and platysmal musculature control the lower part of the face, which is the most dynamic and intricate region. These muscles are responsible for defining the grin and other important facial emotions. The facial artery travels in a deep, bony plane over the mandibular border. Then, it changes to a more intermediate subcutaneous plane when it passes lateral to the angle of the mouth under the modiolus [3, 4]. This occurs so that the facial artery can serve its function. As it gets closer to the nose, the facial artery travels deeper until it reaches the nasolabial fold, where it becomes more superficial. To avoid vasculature, it is recommended that injections be administered in the nasal base either superficially or deeply on the periosteum [5] for optimal results. Following its origin from the facial artery, which is located approximately 15 millimeters superiorly and laterally of the oral commissure [6], the superior labial artery subsequently travels in a plane between the orbicularis oris and the labial mucosa [4, 7]. In rare instances, the labial artery runs between the orbicularis oris and the deep cutaneous dermis [8]. This is a more superficial path of the artery.

Therefore, considering the normal vasculature (Fig. 21.1), it is possible to increase the volume of the lips by placing filler at the vermillion-cutaneous boundary at a depth of three millimeters or less [7, 9]. Injections that target the vermillion border improve the structural aspects of the lips; nevertheless, if full volumetric correction is required, additional injections must be administered to the mucosal or cutaneous lip. In the beginning, these synergistic injections should be positioned between the epidermis and the orbicularis oris to reestablish the subcutaneous fat

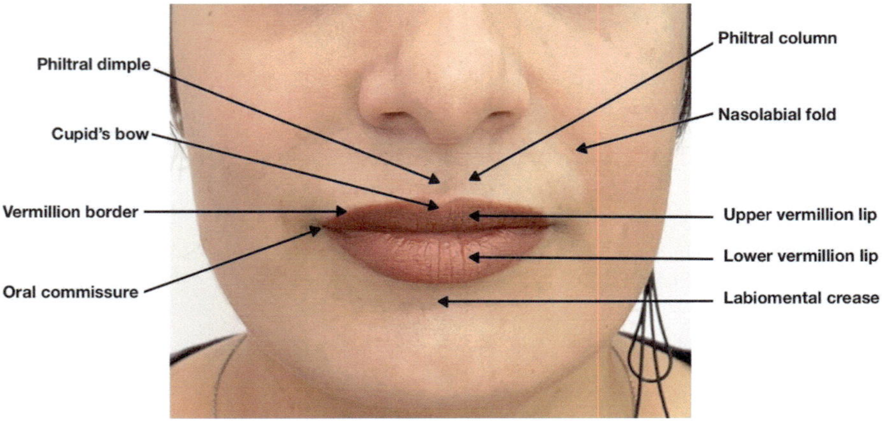

Fig. 21.1 Lip anatomy

pads in the upper and lower cutaneous lips [6]. By supporting the orbicularis oris muscle, restoring these fat pads that are not widely recognized can facilitate the production of natural lip volumization. If you want to avoid lumps that are visible and can be felt, you should use a product that is softer and more flexible for this area [3]. Maintaining the proportion of the top lip to the lower lip is essential to oral hygiene. Among Caucasians, the ratio is 1.618:1, whereas among Asians, it is closer to 1:1 [10]. This indicates that the injection technique used for lip enhancement with filler is appropriate. When filler is injected into the perioral region in the subcutaneous plane, it can further enhance the perioral area by treating marionette lines, mental creases, vertical cutaneous rhytids, and overall volumizing the cutaneous lip and chin [11]. This technique demonstrates a proper method for perioral enhancement, which includes treating marionette lines, mental creases, and augmentation of the cutaneous lip [8].

21.3 Lips

Since they have witnessed some of the more dramatic therapies being administered to younger patients, many patients who are part of the aging population are reluctant to consider this repair. Filler injections in the lip of elderly patients often concentrate on restoring or accentuating the natural curves of the lip, reflating the lip to decrease vermillion creasing, and repairing rhytids in the white lip skin. These procedures are performed to improve the appearance of the patient's lips. As people get older, they often have a lip that is flatter and thinner, which reduces the natural curves seen in a youthful lip. Accentuation of the natural curves of the lip, including the tubercle and Cupid's bow peaks, is the primary focus of correction. If the patient desires and it is necessary, a minimal accent of the white roll may also be included. Vermillion is only augmented to the level required to fill the deflated contour or partially if full correction would result in the patient's other face shapes being out of proportion (Fig. 21.2) [12].

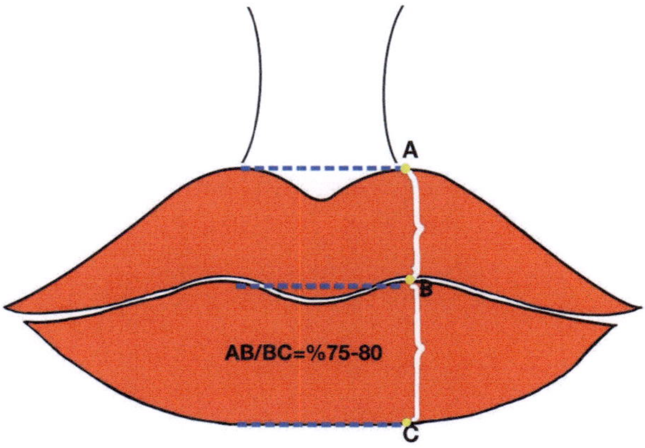

Fig. 21.2 Ideal lip

These modifications are achieved by administering injections into the white roll or the vermillion-cutaneous junction. The injections should run along the entire roll in the appropriate plane. This characteristic is well accentuated by a little bleb of material located at the peak of the Cupid's bow itself and has a somewhat more rigid HA. The philtrum columns will also be injected with minimal fluid on rare occasions. Any excessive injection of the white roll will result in an unnatural "duck bill" lip, a telltale sign of a lip that has been treated. There is also the possibility of producing this by applying a significant amount of vermillion, which causes the white roll to be pushed upward [12].

Vermillion adjustments, including the tubercle, are performed at the vermillion-muscosal junction in the submuscular plane. A small secondary injection is administered halfway across the vermillion breadth if necessary. This is done to provide a more thorough reflation. The youthful and beautiful vermillion shape is usually seen as being most prominent at the tubercle in the upper lip, with an adjacent area of relative emptiness and then relative fullness or convexity that tapers medially to laterally. This is the most famous representation of the vermillion form. An additional telltale sign of an unnaturally treated lip is the "puffy" lip, characterized by an excessive filling of the latter. To a similar extent, the upper lip that is filled equally across its entire length or each side of the lip from the commissure to the tubercle is unnatural. Ideally, the lip's border at the oral opening should be curved rather than straight. This indicates the filler must continuously vary throughout the lip to get a natural shape [12].

In younger patients, lip augmentation is performed using the injection techniques outlined, but with increased volumes, particularly in the vermillion, to enhance the size and shape of the lips more noticeably. As opposed to developing a lip or perioral contour that is disproportionately large about the rest of the face, this should still be maintained in proportion to the basic facial features present [12].

In patients, the goal was to correct the asymmetry and enhance the upper and lower lips using a hyaluronic acid filler. The procedure involved linear threading on the vermillion border, followed by creating a bolus depot. Linear threading refers to the process of injecting the filler along the border, while a bolus depot is a technique where a concentrated amount of filler is delivered at a specific point. After the linear threading and bolus depot, the injected filler must be gently massaged to be placed properly (Figs. 21.3, 21.4, 21.5, 21.6, 21.7, 21.8, 21.9, 21.10, 21.11, 21.12, and 21.13).

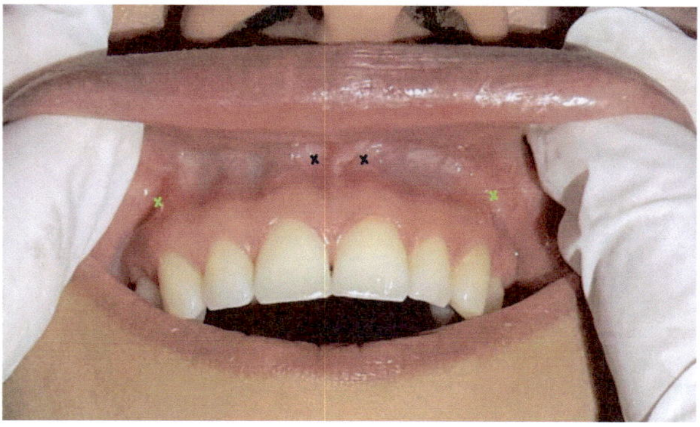

Fig. 21.3 Application points of infiltration anesthesia for the upper lip

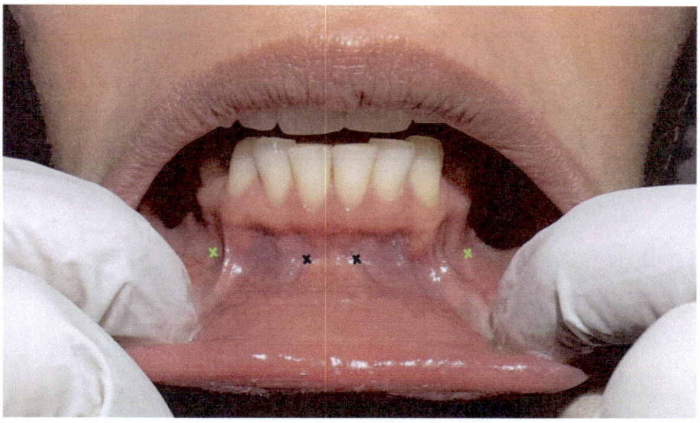

Fig. 21.4 Application points of infiltration anesthesia for the lower lip

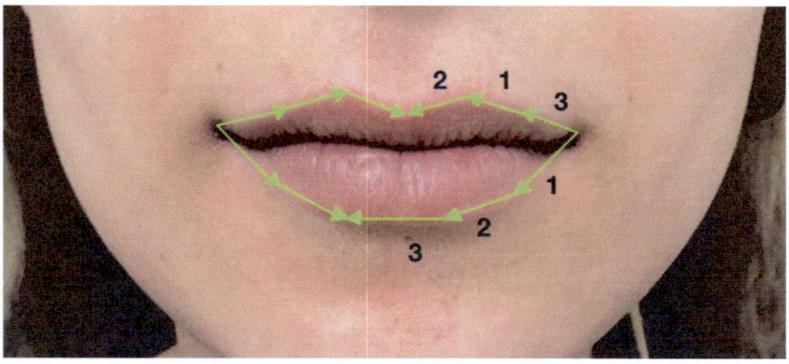

Fig. 21.5 Application diagram for lip contour

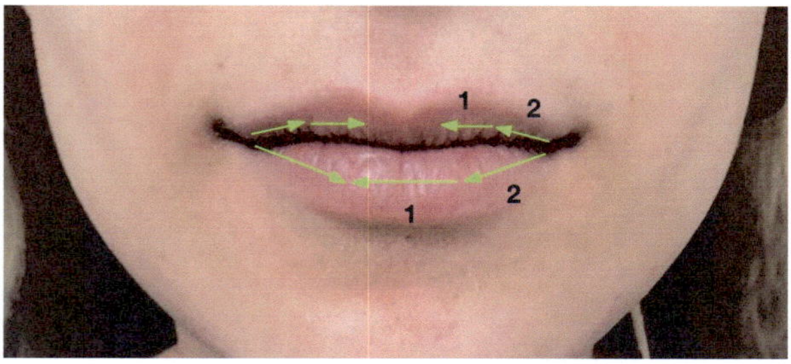

Fig. 21.6 Application diagram for lip unit

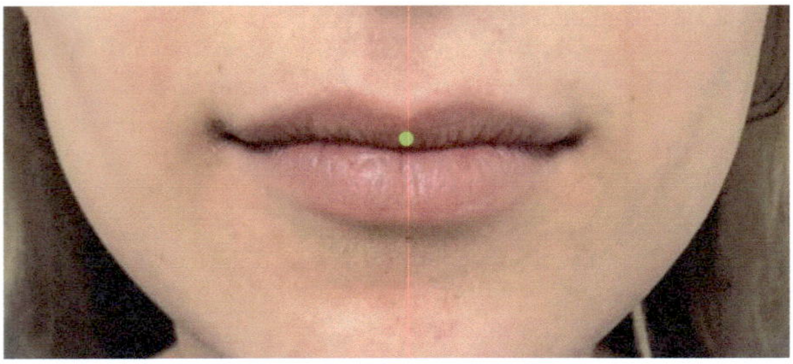

Fig. 21.7 Application point for lip tubercle

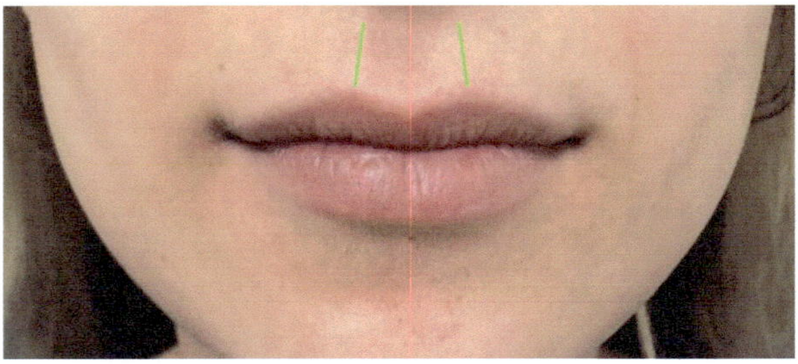

Fig. 21.8 Application diagram for philtrum columns

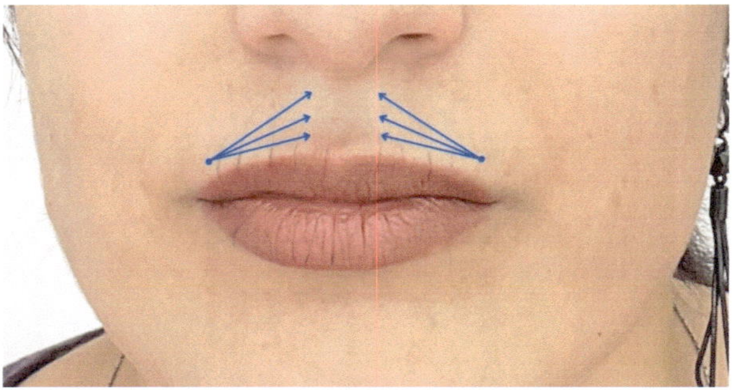

Fig. 21.9 Application scheme for perioral upper lip lines

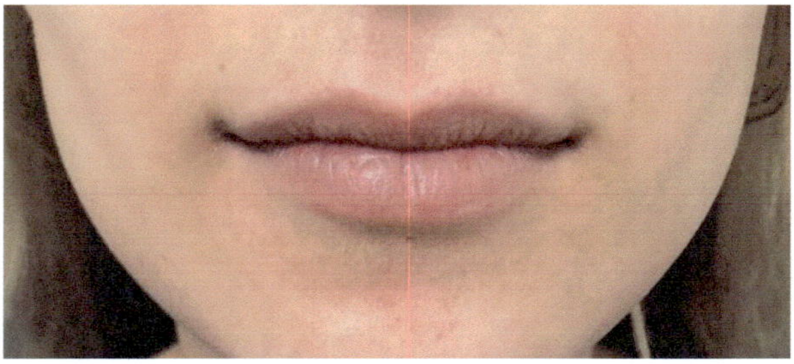

Fig. 21.10 Front view before application

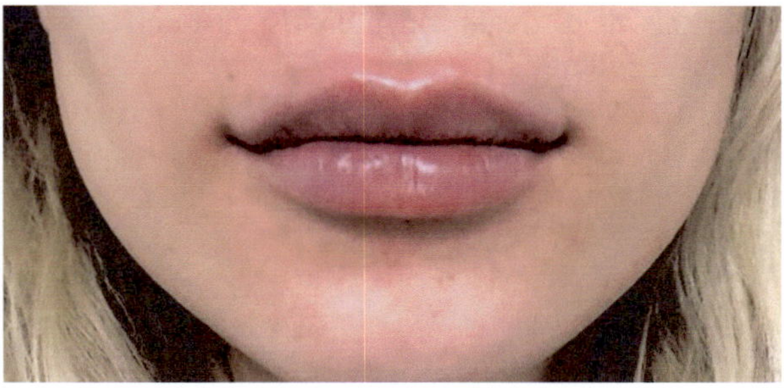

Fig. 21.11 Front view after application

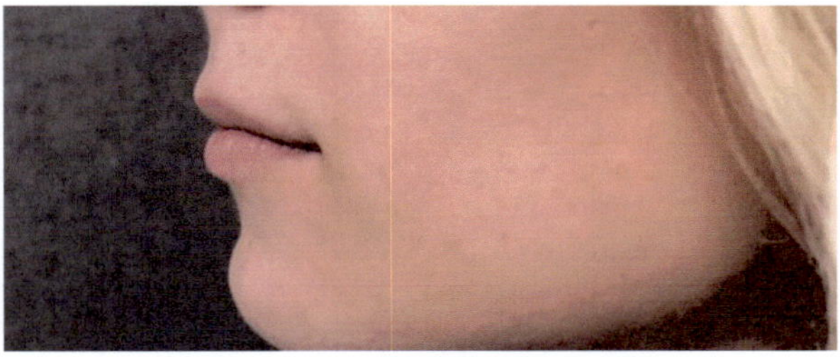

Fig. 21.12 Side view before application

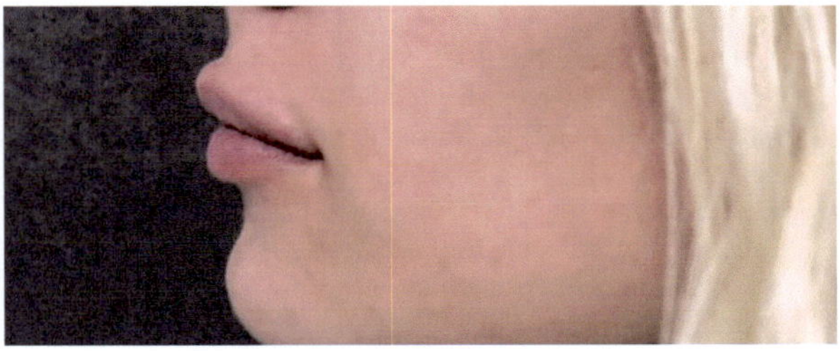

Fig. 21.13 Side view after application

21.4 Marionette Lines

In contrast to the nasolabial fold, typical of young people, the marionette line is a characteristic only seen in older people's faces. In light of this, total effacement is a desirable goal, but it is never accomplished in practice. The fibrous septae (also known as "ligaments") that divide fat compartments in this region of the face, in addition to dermal attachments to muscle fascia, are among the factors that contribute to this phenomenon. Despite this, there is room for significant development. Using an HA filler that can be lined (threaded superficially—mid dermis) into the crease and then infiltrated in small amounts throughout the entire patch of skin in the corner of the mouth to structure or flatten these tissues is the most effective method for correcting surface creases in the oral commissure. Due to the presence of fibrous septae between the skin and deeper tissues, which segment fat compartments in this region, it is unavoidable that there would be certain limitations in the corrective process. When performed in the dermis and subcutaneously, biplanar correction can give a more comprehensive correction [12].

In this field, treatment is highly customized and determined by each unique patient's findings. It is virtually always necessary to support the corners of the mouth, which gradually sink in and lose support, resulting in a frown. It is also typical to build this skin flat by directly filling the marionette line and cross-hatching across the area. Depending on the variation, contour depressions in the labiomental groove might be considered. Just to the side of this, a triangular depression is frequently observed, which either did not exist when the individual was younger or has become more pronounced as they have gotten older. Using subcutaneous fanning is an effective method for correcting this characteristic [12].

References

1. Altin F, Muluk NB, Isci Dt KD, Cingi C. The Relationship Between Lip Augmentation and Teeth Visibility: A Cosmetic Perspective. J Craniofac Surg. 2025. https://doi.org/10.1097/SCS.0000000000011567. Epub ahead of print. PMID: 40576706.
2. Saban Y, Andretto Amodeo C, Bouaziz D, Polselli R. Nasal arterial vasculature: medical and surgical applications. Arch Facial Plast Surg. 2012;14:429.
3. Mckee D, Remington K, Swift A, et al. Effective rejuvenation with hyaluronic acid fillers: current advanced concepts. Plast Reconstr Surg. 2019;143:1277e–89e.
4. Tansatit T, Apinuntrum P, Phetudom T. A typical pattern of the labial arteries with implication for lip augmentation with injectable fillers. Aesth Plast Surg. 2014;38:1083–9.
5. Sieber DA, Scheuer JF III, Villanueva NL, et al. Review of 3-dimensional facial anatomy: injecting fillers and neuromodulators. Plast Reconstr Surg Glob Open. 2016;4(12 Suppl Anatomy and Safety in Cosmetic Medicine: Cosmetic Bootcamp):e1166.
6. Lee SH, Gil YC, Choi YJ, et al. Topographic anatomy of the superior labial artery for dermal filler injection. Plast Reconstr Surg. 2015;135:445–50.
7. Scheuer JF III, Sieber DA, Pezeshk RA, et al. Anatomy of the facial danger zones: maximizing safety during soft-tissue filler injections. Plast Reconstr Surg. 2017;139:50e–8e.
8. Akinbiyi T, Othman S, Familusi O, Calvert C, Card EB, Percec I. Better results in facial rejuvenation with fillers. Plast Reconstr Surg Glob Open. 2020;8(10):e2763. https://doi.org/10.1097/GOX.0000000000002763.
9. Scheuer JF III, Sieber DA, Pezeshk RA, et al. Facial danger zones: techniques to maximize safety during soft-tissue filler injections. Plast Reconstr Surg. 2017;139:1103–8.
10. Swift A, Remington K. Beautiphication: a global approach to facial beauty. Clin Plast Surg. 2011;38:347–77.
11. Rohrich RJ, Pessa JE. The retaining system of the face: histologic evaluation of the septal boundaries of the subcutaneous fat compartments. Plast Reconstr Surg. 2008;121:1804–9.
12. Bass LS. Injectable filler techniques for facial rejuvenation, volumization, and augmentation. Facial Plast Surg Clin North Am. 2015;23(4):479–88.

Volumizing with Fillers: Lower Face and Mandibular Definition

22

Emin Ozturk, Zeliha Kapusuz Gencer, and Cemal Cingi

22.1 Introduction

The chin and jawline can be augmented with the use of a high G′ filler placed using the bolus technique in the preperiosteal plane posteriorly (mandibular angle) and anteriorly (Menton) [1], which displays proper injection and augmentation of the lateral jawline, which shows an augmentation of the chin and mental crease in a female patient. We recommend administering injections in the subcutaneous plane to specific regions of the mandibular ramus or body to avoid damaging vital underlying structures. Furthermore, this method optimizes facial features while providing structural support [2].

22.2 Danger Zones

For jowl correction, we typically administer injections to the mandibular region. We usually administer these injections deep along the mandibular line's periosteum and at the mandibular ramus. The massive, square-shaped masseter muscle has deep and superficial components and is located in the mandibular region. Recognizing and avoiding the facial artery located at the anterior border of the masseter muscle is

E. Ozturk
Doruk Yildirim Hospital, Department of Otorhinolaryngology, Bursa, Turkey

Z. K. Gencer
Department of Otorhinolaryngology, University of Health Sciences, Basaksehir Cam and Sakura City Hospital, Istanbul, Turkey

C. Cingi (✉)
Eskisehir Osmangazi University, Medical Faculty, Department of Otorhinolaryngology, Eskisehir, Türkiye
e-mail: cemal@ogu.edu.tr

C. Cingi et al. (eds.), *Minor Interventions, Major Outcomes on the Face*, Comprehensive ENT, https://doi.org/10.1007/978-3-032-01305-7_22

essential. When you clench your jaw, you can feel the facial artery throbbing near the anterior border of the masseter [3]. It is located approximately three centimeters in front of the mandibular angle.

Additionally, you can find the parotid gland along the posterior margin of the masseter muscle, and the anterior border may include a portion of the buccinator muscle. The Tensen duct, or the parotid gland duct, enters the buccinator muscle and emerges from the gland's front part and the front edge of the masseter muscle. This allows it to reach the mouth. Lacerations made with a needle can cause damage to the Stensen duct, which can result in the formation of a sialocele, with or without the establishment of a cutaneous fistula. We regularly inject the prejowl sulcus along the mandibular line, the region along the bony edge of the mandible between the angle of the jaw and the chin. Such injections are conducted frequently. Several layers make up this region, including the skin, the surface fat compartment, the fibers of the platysma muscle, the deep fat compartment, the periosteum, and the bone tissue [4]. Typically, we administer subcutaneous injections anteriorly to the mandibular ligament and in the ligament's area. The jowl is located posterior to the mandibular ligament. Even though the deep supraperiosteal plane might offer some protection against inadvertent arterial penetration, the clinician ought to be aware of the high vascularity of this region. This is because the inferior labial artery, the mental and submental arteries, and their anastomoses [3] all run through this region.

Over time, the jawline undergoes a variety of transformations. These alterations, as is the case in other regions of the face, are the result of changes in both the soft tissue and the bone tissue. Throughout the course of the aging process, these regions often become more noticeable at various decades after birth as the aging process progresses. It is helpful to get it right by restoring the patient's youthful shape or achieving the correct balance, as evidenced by old images of the patient when they were in their 30s. An excessive expansion of the jaw in order to accommodate skin laxity can result in a hideous and disproportionately large face, which is especially unattractive in females [5]. The mandibular angle follows the prejowl sulcus in the list of jawline shapes most frequently corrected. The migration of soft tissue over the angle and the loss of soft tissue reduce the facial breadth in this region. When skin laxity is present, the inferior border of the mandible becomes vague, and it frequently blends in with the neck contour or comes very close to doing so. It is necessary to project this form to blend in superiorly and anteriorly with the tissues surrounding it, leaving a clearly defined marginal border inferiorly. Cross-hatching with vertical filler threads along the ramus and horizontal threads along the body, with a two-centimeter space of overlap at the angle, is an excellent starting point for constructing the desired shape. There are times when depressions can be visible along the body posterior to the jowl. These depressions react to linear threading or, on occasion, multiple small superficial-deep pillars or blebs of filler. When combined with appropriate cheek contouring, jawline correction can dramatically enhance the beauty of the youthful face and significantly contribute to the regeneration of the aging face [5].

22.2.1 Treatment Goals and Planned Outcomes

The right evaluation and treatment plan are paramount when forming a more natural, youthful, and appealing appearance. This concept applies to every facial region. The number of structural variables involved in this region of the face makes it more challenging to evaluate and treat. Some examples of these variables include the following [6]:

1. The position of the mandibular angle and its amount of prominence (Figs. 22.1 and 22.2).
2. The circumference of the mandible.
3. The skin's thickness and the tissue beneath it.
4. The chin's height, protrusion, and width (Fig. 22.2).
5. The cervical spine's angle.
6. Among the many aspects that may be considered in a full review are the thickness of the skin and the subcutaneous tissues, the inherent asymmetries of the face, the bony structures, and the history of facial operations and surgeries. The injector needs to thoroughly understand the anatomical features that are located near the injection sites, including the parotid gland, the masseter muscle, blood vessels, and nerves [6].

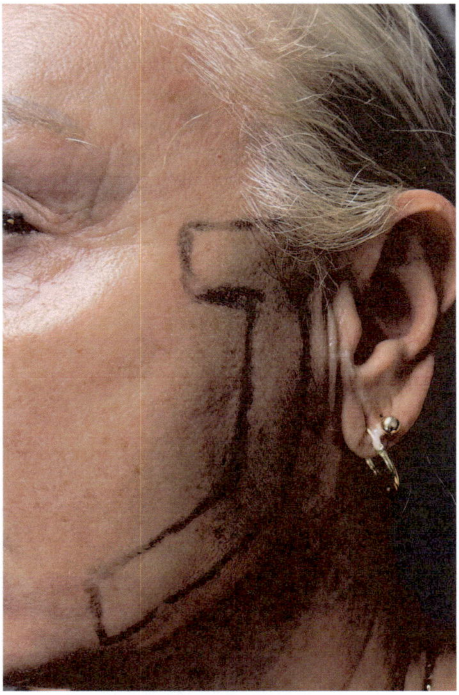

Fig. 22.1 Marking for injections. (Courtesy of Murat Songu MD)

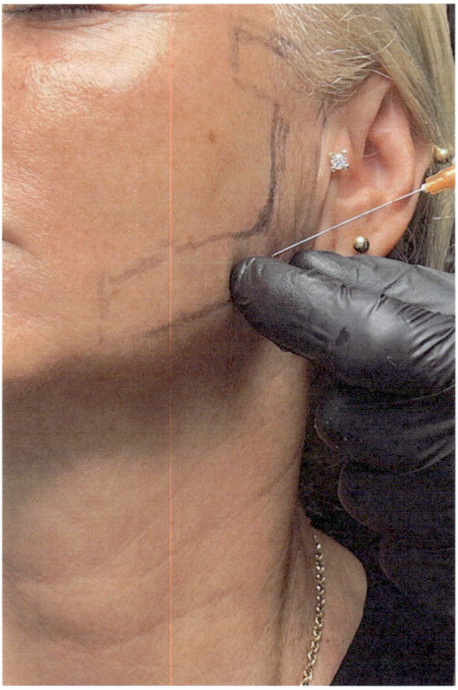

Fig. 22.2 Injection of HArmonyCa™ with Lidocaine (Allergan) on the lower face. (Courtesy of Murat Songu MD)

22.2.2 Procedure

This facial aesthetic unit can shift depending on the head and neck position. During the diagnostic and treatment processes, the patient must remain upright. The injector must be able to move about the treatment chair to see the face from various perspectives. Furthermore, the injector must be able to see the inferior mandible boundary [6]. In most cases, a youthful jawline is characterized by a smooth transition from the mentum to an imaginary line parallel to the angle of the auricle next to the tragus. Patients with a non-defined bony outline can achieve a visually acceptable jawline by using this topographic guide [6]. The procedure aims to achieve the optimal aesthetic outcome by using the safest and most effective process and product. The first author would like to use the current product, which meets the requirements for achieving a particular individual's most desirable aesthetic result. Based on the past 10 years, future fillers may become even more specific to their target structural tissues. Products such as Juvederm Voluma XC (Allergan), Perlane (Galderma), and solid particles of calcium hydroxylapatite (Radiesse, Merz) are considered the most suitable for use at the time of this article's publication. Another option is to use a hybrid blend of Radiesse and hyaluronic acid, adjusting the mixture's concentration to achieve the desired aesthetic result. The attraction for these items stems from the fact that they offer a hard and sculpted enlargement of the bone structure. This decision is based on the physical properties of the products. While both treatments can rejuvenate the jawline, in most cases, there are instances where either Juvederm Voluma XC, Perlane, or Radiesse provides the most desirable aesthetic result [6] (Figs. 22.3, 22.4, and 22.5).

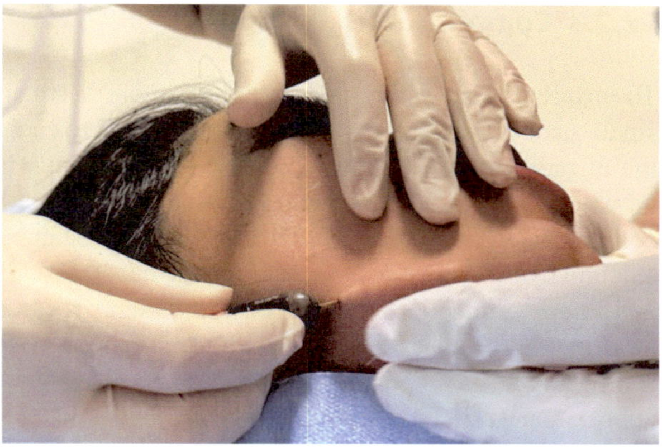

Fig. 22.3 Volumizing and highlighting the jawline. (Courtesy of Zeliha Kapusuz MD)

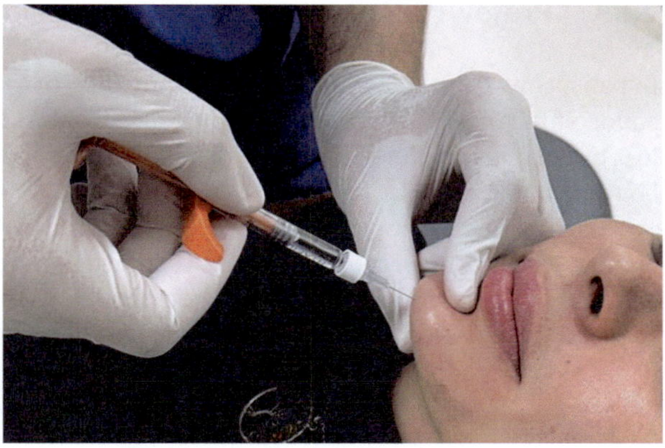

Fig. 22.4 Contouring the mentum with a harder softer superficially. (Courtesy of Zeliha Kapusuz MD)

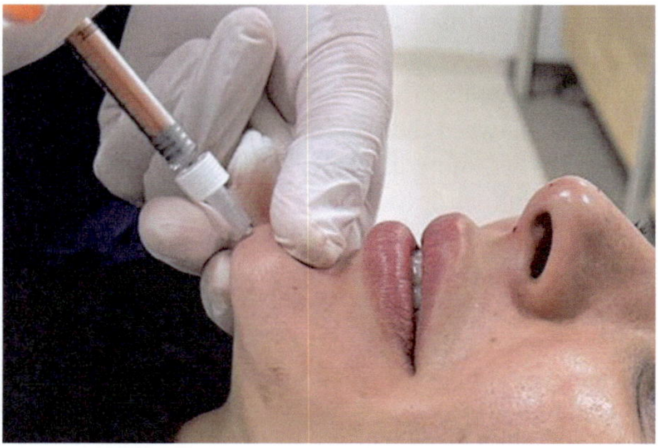

Fig. 22.5 Augmenting the mentum with a harder filler just above the bone. (Courtesy of Zeliha Kapusuz MD)

22.2.3 Complications

To ensure patient safety and achieve a more aesthetically pleasing result, apply small quantities of less than 0.1 milliliters (mL) to each injection spot and rub. With the introduction of the new Radiesse formulation, which contains lidocaine, it is now possible to inject the product using a needle with a gauge setting of 27. We combined 0.26 milliliters of either 1% or 2% lidocaine (plain) with 1.5 milliliters of calcium hydroxylapatite using a 29-gauge needle. We did this to reduce the flow rate and improve injection volume control. Patients receive counseling about the pain, swelling, and bruises that come with mastication. Before discharge, each patient receives a cold compress. We advise patients to massage the area twice daily for approximately 2–3 min over 3 days [6].

22.3 Prejowl Sulcus

In patients who are becoming older, the formation of the jowl is caused by a combination of factors, including the gradual decline and loss of fat pads in the face and the loss of flexibility in the skin. A depression or a minor notch between the jowl and the bony mentum, with an underlying fat pad, may also result from bone loss, often occurring as the aging process proceeds. We treat minor jowling by injecting the prejowl sulcus. The purpose of this procedure is to hide the depression between the jowl and the mentum. We achieve this by creating a smooth ramp or graded transition between the two areas instead of a relative concavity or depression. Surgical lifting is the recommended treatment for moderate or worse jowl development and laxity; however, filler injection, as a compromise strategy, can reduce the appearance of the jowls to some extent [5]. It is feasible to use various injection techniques, such as deep dermal or dermal-subcutaneous junction injection between the two locations, employing a fanning or cross-hatching approach appropriate for the approximate height of the visible jowl. A different approach can also enhance the surface contour by inserting “pillars” of material into small bleb or bolus injections deep under the soft tissues, either supraperiosteally or in a deep-to-superficial column [5]. One of the primary goals of the correction procedure is to restore the inferior border of the mandible between the two locations by subcutaneous injection in a linear threading pattern. When more advanced age changes are evident in the area, it is possible to execute minimal threading or cross-hatching for the approximate vertical height of the jowl. This is appropriate in cases where generalized depression is present in the area. We introduce the needle into the skin of the jowl and/or the mentum, then thread it into the prejowl sulcus along the inferior border of the mandible. This procedure begins with the needle’s insertion. As we withdraw the needle, we inject to create a smooth surface contour that slopes smoothly from the jowl to the chin section. Avoiding the facial artery and vein, along with their side branches, is crucial due to the potential for significant ecchymosis, which can take up to 2 weeks or longer to clear up completely. Patients should be warned that there is a higher likelihood of bruising in this region, just as with injections into the eyelids [5].

References

1. Schaverien MV, Pessa JE, Rohrich RJ. Vascularized membranes determine the anatomical boundaries of the subcutaneous fat compartments. Plast Reconstr Surg. 2009;123:695–700.
2. Akinbiyi T, Othman S, Familusi O, Calvert C, Card EB, Percec I. Better results in facial rejuvenation with fillers. Plast Reconstr Surg Glob Open. 2020;8(10):e2763. https://doi.org/10.1097/GOX.0000000000002763. PMID: 33173655; PMCID: PMC7647625.
3. Dilber M, Bayar Muluk N, Cingi C. A narrative-style review of non-surgical rhinoplasty: Indications, outcomes, and limitations. J Craniomaxillofac Surg. 2024;52(9):1012–8. https://doi.org/10.1016/j.jcms.2024.06.014. Epub 2024 Jun 10. PMID: 38876955.
4. Braz A, Humphrey S, Weinkle S, et al. Lower face: clinical anatomy and regional approaches with injectable fillers. Plast Reconstr Surg. 2015;136:235S.
5. Bass LS. Injectable filler techniques for facial rejuvenation, volumization, and augmentation. Facial Plast Surg Clin North Am. 2015;23(4):479–88.
6. Moradi A, Watson J. Current concepts in filler injection. Facial Plast Surg Clin North Am. 2015;23(4):489–94. https://doi.org/10.1016/j.fsc.2015.07.005.

Volumizing with Fillers: Neck and Décolleté

23

Mehtap Koparal, Heather Yeakel, and Jarrod Keeler

23.1 Introduction

Nowadays, injectable fillers are a common component of face rejuvenation procedures. Thanks to the development of several long-lasting and biocompatible filler materials, especially hyaluronic acid (HA) fillers, many unfulfilled demands can now be handled in a repeatable and predictable way, contributing to their rising popularity. Most of these procedures are used to treat aging-related volume loss in the face, which can lead to several changes early and late in life. These no-downtime treatments are preferred in most therapeutic situations due to their immediacy, predictability, and safety. The aging face can be more effectively corrected with the addition of volume or shape restoration, energy-based treatments (such as radiofrequency or lasers) for changes to the skin's surface (such as wrinkles or pigmentation), and surgical lifting for laxity of the skin [1].

M. Koparal (✉)
Adiyaman Training and Research Hospital, Department of Otorhinolaryngology, Adiyaman, Turkey

H. Yeakel
Department of Otolaryngology-Head and Neck Surgery, St. Luke's University Health Network, Bethlehem, PA, USA
e-mail: heather.yeakel@sluhn.org

J. Keeler
Otolaryngology & Facial Plastic and Reconstructive Surgery, Specialty Physician Associates, St. Luke's Medical Center, Bethlehem, PA, USA

C. Cingi et al. (eds.), *Minor Interventions, Major Outcomes on the Face*, Comprehensive ENT, https://doi.org/10.1007/978-3-032-01305-7_23

23.2 Age

As we age, our skin's dermal and epidermal layers get thinner, collagen production drops, dermal elastosis decreases, and actinic damage causes laxity, rhytids, and pigment abnormalities [2]. Additional causes of skin laxity include fat and bone volume loss [3] and facial retaining ligament attenuation. Deterioration of the skeletal skeleton occurs in predictable patterns as we age [4]. The bony orbit enlarges due to resorption of the orbital margin along superomedial and inferolateral vectors. As a result, the contents of the orbit fall and retrude, leading to cosmetic issues such as an elongated and accentuated lid-cheek junction and an elevated medial fat pad [5]. As we age, our faces go through several changes. These include the maxilla resorption and posterior rotation, which includes retrusion of the medial infraorbital area [6], expansion of the pyriform aperture [7], recession of the jaw, chin, and cheeks, and changes in the skin and soft tissue, such as nasolabial folds and jowls [3]. These abnormalities are believed to be made worse because facial strain increases with age [8].

23.3 Overarching Strategy

Aesthetic design, an in-depth understanding of facial anatomy, and familiarity with regular aging changes are all necessary for artistic, balanced, and natural-looking outcomes. The technique of injecting filler is crucial. A three-dimensional latticework of injectable material is inserted beneath the skin's surface to essentially thicken skin or subcutaneous tissues, fill a rhytid, alter surface conformation, or add volume. A person's face can change due to any of these sculpture-like practices. The injection technique employed has a significant impact on the amount of correction and volume needed for any certain outcome. The same holds true for therapies; exceeding their reasonable limitations will lead to unnatural-looking outcomes, or even worse, tissue damage and problems. Although these therapies are usually harmless, they can nonetheless cause problems if administered too frequently or in too large a volume [1].

Each facial anatomy has its own unique set of requirements for treatment. Having said that, a few general rules do apply across the board. First, depending on the situation, you cannot always rely on a single filler. Second, in everyday clinical practice, there is not a single filler that works best everywhere. Every supplier has to choose a handful of fillers to have on hand and master the subtleties and characteristics of those fillers [1].

23.4 Filler Selection

No filler is ideal for every situation, as previously mentioned; for example, picking out a golf club for a particular shot, certain clubs may be playable by an expert. Of course, there are times when specific options would not cut it; for instance, you cannot expect a soft, spreadable filler to give your cheeks a defined contour. In this author's hands, the expected depth of placement is the starting point for filler choices. Weight, in the form of increased viscosity and cohesivity, is a common characteristic of heavier subcutaneous or subperiosteal (orbital) fillers. This filler class includes high-viscosity, high-cohesivity HA, and calcium hydroxylapatite (CaHa). Deep dermal tissue planes and the dermal/subcutaneous junction are ideal for initial, lower-viscosity HA fillers. To inject into the middle dermis, use a thinner filler with a lower viscosity and elastic modulus, like monophasic, poly-densified HA. The specific anatomical applications addressed in this chapter [1] provide a detailed illustration of the circumstances most suitable for a given injection depth.

The list of fillers approved for aesthetic use by the US Food and Drug Administration (FDA) is currently quite small. Changes to filler selection are inevitable, given the proliferation of novel fillers on the market. The community of clinical practitioners evaluates the new product's performance after several years of use and considers the filler alternatives available at that time, in addition to clinical experience and the general principles outlined below, when making this selection. These methods and choices are the authors' favorites or standard operating procedures; nonetheless, they are by no means exhaustive or optimal. Every doctor has to do what's best for their patients based on their expertise [1].

While research has shown that HA filler injection can cause neocollagenesis—a process that produces new collagen by fibroblasts in response to a pressure phenomenon—the exact amount of collagen that this process can replace remains unknown [9]. However, these results may have practical relevance because repeated HA filler treatments appear to generate longer intervals and decreased volumes [1].

Keeping a complete inventory of HA fillers is unnecessary. Although several fillers can be used interchangeably, the authors think that some procedures benefit more from the subtle correction that each one offers due to its unique characteristics. A different filler may be more appealing to other injectors [1].

23.5 Fillers for the Neck

Vines and creepiness are visible on parts of the skin that are thin and sun-damaged, such as the hands, chest, and neck. A diluted injection of an active dermal response filler—which stimulates the body to generate collagen in large quantities—can gradually thicken the skin, making creepy changes less noticeable [10]. The optimal medium for this is polylactic acid or calcium hydroxide. A standard dilution ratio for CaHa is 1.5–3 times the initial volume in the syringe [1].

Linear furrows or depressions covering the neck's front part are known as horizontal wrinkles [11]. Unlike other wrinkles on the face, their origin is unrelated to skin aging [12–14]. While sagging skin around the neck is a common symptom of aging, horizontal wrinkles can also appear in younger people [15, 16]. Wrinkles might be accentuated by skin laxity that comes with aging [15, 17, 18]. Wrinkles may also appear on young people's faces due to their habit of bending their necks to glance down at electronic devices [19].

Rejuvenating the neck can be achieved by various interventions [20, 21]. To improve skin texture and neck laxity, you can try ablative or nonablative laser treatments, micro-focused ultrasound with visualization, radiofrequency, or plasma resurfacing [20–24]. Despite their skin-tightening capabilities, they do little to diminish rhytides. Platysmal bands can be effectively reduced by botulinum toxin type A injections [25, 26]; however, horizontal necklines are only somewhat improved. Again, horizontal necklines may not respond well to liposuction, platysma plication, or skin excision for contour improvement [27–29]. Nevertheless, there is a lack of effective treatments for horizontal neck wrinkles [16, 30, 31].

For several years, hyaluronic acid (HA) fillers have been successfully used to address horizontal neck creases. When treating horizontal neck wrinkles, you can use HA fillers of various brands; however, not all of these types are equally lumpy or have the same amount of Tyndall effect. Esthelis Basic, an alternative HA filler, is a cohesive poly-densified matrix HA (CPM-HA) filler with a low viscous modulus, a high tan delta, and a low elastic modulus [32, 33]. This filler is ideal for superficial subdermal or intradermal injection [32–34] when tissue integration is desired. Its rheological properties make it soft and spreadable while still being elastic and having a high fluidity component. This makes it easy to shape after implantation, reducing the likelihood of lumpiness or irregularities.

Additional research with Esthelis Basic corroborated this finding by showing that no patients experienced the bluish appearance known as the Tyndall effect [35, 36] following superficial HA filler implantation [34, 37]. As shown in previous histologic studies [38, 39], the lack of concentration in discrete or optically-isolated pools is responsible for this. As a result, blue light is not scattered [35, 40], and the Tyndall effect is minimized, thanks to CPM-HA. The periorbital region, fine lines and wrinkles, and the neck are good areas to apply filler superficially beneath thin skin [19].

References

1. Bass LS. Injectable filler techniques for facial rejuvenation, volumization, and augmentation. Facial Plast Surg Clin North Am. 2015;23(4):479–88.
2. Wong CH, Mendelson B. Newer understanding of specific anatomic targets in the aging face as applied to injectables: aging changes in the craniofacial skeleton and facial ligaments. Plast Reconstr Surg. 2015;136(5 suppl):44S–8S.
3. Mckee D, Remington K, Swift A, et al. Effective rejuvenation with hyaluronic acid fillers: current advanced concepts. Plast Reconstr Surg. 2019;143:1277e–89e.
4. Beer JI, Sieber DA, Scheuer JF III, et al. Three-dimensional facial anatomy: structure and function as it relates to injectable neuromodulators and soft tissue fillers. Plast Reconstr Surg Glob Open. 2016;4(12 Suppl Anatomy and Safety in Cosmetic Medicine: Cosmetic Bootcamp):e1175.
5. Mendelson B, Wong CH. Changes in the facial skeleton with aging: implications and clinical applications in facial rejuvenation. Aesth Plast Surg. 2012;36:753–60.
6. Mendelson BC, Hartley W, Scott M, et al. Age-related changes of the orbit and midcheek and the implications for facial rejuvenation. Aesth Plast Surg. 2007;31:419–23.

7. Shaw RB Jr, Kahn DM. Aging of the midface bony elements: a three-dimensional computed tomographic study. Plast Reconstr Surg. 2007;119:675–81. discussion 682.
8. Akinbiyi T, Othman S, Familusi O, Calvert C, Card EB, Percec I. Better results in facial rejuvenation with fillers. Plast Reconstr Surg Glob Open. 2020;8(10):e2763. https://doi.org/10.1097/GOX.0000000000002763. PMID: 33173655; PMCID: PMC7647625.
9. Wang F, Garza LA, Kang S, et. al. In vivo stimulation of de novo collagen production caused by cross-linked hyaluronic acid dermal filler injections in photodamaged human skin. Arch Dermatol. 2007;143:155–63.
10. Van Loghem J, Yutskovskaya YA, Werschler WP. Clacium hydroxylapatite: over a decade of clinical experience. J Clin Aesthetic Derm. 2015;8:38–49.
11. Dibernardo BE. The aging neck: a diagnostic approach to surgical and nonsurgical options. J Cosmet Laser Ther. 2013;15:56–64.
12. Silva SAM, Michniak-Kohn B, Leonardi GR. An overview about oxidation in clinical practice of skin aging. An Bras Dermatol. 2017;92:367–72.
13. Vashi NA, de Castro Maymone MB, Kundu RV. Aging differences in ethnic skin. J Clin Aesthet Dermatol. 2016;9:31–8.
14. Puri P, Nandar SK, Kathuria S, et al. Effects of air pollution on the skin: a review. Indian J Dermatol Venereol Leprol. 2017;83:415–23.
15. Jones D, Carruthers A, Hardas B, et al. Development and validation of a photonumeric scale for evaluation of transverse neck lines. Dermatologic Surg. 2016;42(Suppl 1):S235–42.
16. Lee SK, Kim HS. Correction of horizontal neck lines: our preliminary experience with hyaluronic acid fillers. J Cosmet Dermatol. 2018;17:590–5.
17. Shadfar S, Perkins SW. Anatomy and physiology of the aging neck. Facial Plast Surg Clin North Am. 2014;22:161–70.
18. Lemperle G, Holmes RE, Cohen SR, et al. A classification of facial wrinkles. Plast Reconstr Surg. 2001;108:1735–50. discussion 1751
19. Tseng F, Yu H. Treatment of horizontal neck wrinkles with hyaluronic acid filler: a retrospective case series. Plast Reconstr Surg Glob Open. 2019;7(8):e2366. https://doi.org/10.1097/GOX.0000000000002366. PMID: 31592383; PMCID: PMC6756638.
20. Duplechain JK. Neck skin rejuvenation. Facial Plast Surg Clin N Am. 2014;22:203–16.
21. Oni G, Hoxworth R, Teotia S, et al. Evaluation of a microfocused ultrasound system for improving skin laxity and tightening in the lower face. Aesthet Surg J. 2014;34:1099–110.
22. Oram Y, Akkaya AD. Neck rejuvenation with fractional CO2 laser: long-term results. J Clin Aesthet Dermatol. 2014;7:23–9.
23. Alster TS, Konda S. Plasma skin resurfacing for regeneration of neck, chest, and hands: investigation of a novel device. Dermatologic Surg. 2007;33:1315–21.
24. Sadick NS, Trelles MA. Nonablative wrinkle treatment of the face and neck using a combined diode laser and radiofrequency technology. Dermatologic Surg. 2005;31:1695–9.
25. Brandt FS, Boker A. Botulinum toxin for the treatment of neck lines and neck bands. Dermatol Clin. 2004;22:159–66.
26. Brandt FS, Bellman B. Cosmetic use of botulinum A exotoxin for the aging neck. Dermatologic Surg. 1998;24:1232–4.
27. Adamson PA, Litner JA. Surgical management of the aging neck. Facial Plast Surg. 2005;21:11–20.
28. Knize DM. Limited incision submental lipectomy and platysmaplasty. Plast Reconstr Surg. 1998;101:473–81.
29. Feldman JJ. Corset platysmaplasty. Plast Reconstr Surg. 1990;85:333–43.
30. Chao YY, Chiu HH, Howell DJ. A novel injection technique for horizontal neck lines correction using calcium hydroxylapatite. Dermatologic Surg. 2011;37:1542–5.
31. Han TY, Lee JW, Lee JH, et al. Subdermal minimal surgery with hyaluronic acid as an effective treatment for neck wrinkles. Dermatologic Surg. 2011;37:1291–6.
32. Santoro S, Russo L, Argenzio V, et al. Rheological properties of cross-linked hyaluronic acid dermal fillers. J Appl Biomater Biomech. 2011;9:127–36.

33. Kablik J, Monheit GD, Yu L, et al. Comparative physical properties of hyaluronic acid dermal fillers. Dermatologic Surg. 2009;35(Suppl 1):302–12.
34. Sundaram H, Rohrich RJ, Liew S, et al. Cohesivity of hyaluronic acid fillers: development and clinical implications of a novel assay, pilot validation with a five-point grading scale, and evaluation of six U.S. Food and drug administration-approved fillers. Plast Reconstr Surg. 2015;136:678–86.
35. Sundaram H, Cassuto D. Biophysical characteristics of hyaluronic acid soft-tissue fillers and their relevance to aesthetic applications. Plast Reconstr Surg. 2013;132(4 Suppl 2):5S–21S.
36. Funt D, Pavicic T. Dermal fillers in aesthetics: an overview of adverse events and treatment approaches. Clin Cosmet Investig Dermatol. 2013;6:295–316.
37. Kühne U, Imhof M, Kirchmeir M, et al. Five-year retrospective review of safety, injected volumes, and longevity of the hyaluronic acid belotero basic for facial treatments in 317 patients. J Drugs Dermatol. 2012;11:1032–5.
38. Flynn TC, Sarazin D, Bezzola A, et al. Comparative histology of intradermal implantation of mono and biphasic hyaluronic acid fillers. Dermatologic Surg. 2011;37:637–43.
39. Tran C, Carraux P, Micheels P, et al. *In vivo* bio-integration of three hyaluronic acid fillers in human skin: a histological study. Dermatology. 2014;228:47–54.
40. Micheels P, Sarazin D, Besse S, et al. A blanching technique for intradermal injection of the hyaluronic acid belotero. Plast Reconstr Surg. 2013;132(4 Suppl 2):59S–68S.

Part IV

Liposculpture of the Face

Fat-Harvesting Techniques

24

Mehmet Arici, Nuray Bayar Muluk,
and Sergei Karpischenko

24.1 Introduction

The biocompatible, natural, and cost-effective autologous fat grafting technique has been extensively used in reconstructive and cosmetic surgery to augment and replace soft tissues. The use of wetting solutions, the identification of fatty tissue donor sites, and the methods for harvesting, processing, and placement are only a few of the many recent developments in this field. Despite considerable breakthroughs in this topic, the lack of procedure uniformity and the unpredictability of graft resorption present a severe barrier to graft preservation and subsequent filling [1].

Even though autologous fat grafting has been around for a while, a big problem is that the resorption after the transplant is unpredictable, which means you might have to inject yourself more often and still not get the results you want [2, 3]. To reduce fat graft loss to a minimum, it is crucial to optimize fat grafting procedures [1].

Mature adipocytes, extracellular matrix, and a stromal vascular fraction (SVF) made up of various cell types, including ADSCs, endothelial cells, fibroblasts, erythrocytes, vascular smooth muscle cells, hematopoietic cells, and immune cells, make up harvested adipose tissue [4–6]. Importantly, new studies have shown that

M. Arici
Department of Otorhinolaryngology, Adıyaman University, Faculty of Medicine, Adiyaman, Turkey

N. Bayar Muluk (✉)
Faculty of Medicine, Department of Otorhinolaryngology, Kırıkkale University, Kırıkkale, Türkiye

S. Karpischenko
The First Pavlov State Medical University of Saint Petersburg, Department of Otorhinolaryngology, Saint Petersburg, Russia

C. Cingi et al. (eds.), *Minor Interventions, Major Outcomes on the Face*, Comprehensive ENT, https://doi.org/10.1007/978-3-032-01305-7_24

adult stem cells are most concentrated in adipose tissue [7, 8]. Fat graft take may depend on these ADSCs, which can undergo multilineage differentiation [8–16]. This is because mature adipocytes that make it through harvesting processes cannot reproduce and will perish, leading to detrimental inflammatory reactions [17]. Transplant success and graft viability are both improved when cell-assisted lipotransfer (CAL) results in ADSC-enriched grafts [6, 18]. However, there is still some disagreement on this. Some clinical studies have found that SVF-enriched fat grafting has a higher risk of postoperative complications, while others have found no difference in the transplanted fat's survival rate between conventional and SVF-enriched fat grafting [19]. Regardless of the injection site (breast or face), CAL had a considerably higher fat survival rate compared to conventional procedures, according to a recent meta-analysis by Laloze et al., which compared 16 studies. However, this was only true for small injection volumes (below 100 mL). Similar research found that CAL increases the risk of complications and does not reduce the frequency of subsequent surgical procedures required following the first fat graft [19].

24.2 Background Information

The use of fat grafts to repair complex traumatic wounds and congenital malformations following severe cancer surgery was first suggested in 1893 by Neuber, followed by Hollander in 1921, Neuhof in 1921, and Josef in 1931 [20]. The development of the lipofilling technique was sped up by the introduction of the tumescent technique by Klein in 1985 and the liposuction technique by Fisher in 1974. With the tumescent approach, patients might receive local anesthesia through tiny cannulas during liposuction [21]. To lessen the trauma of liposuction, Coleman unveiled a new method in 1987. Manual lipoaspiration under low pressure, centrifugation for 3 min at 3400 rpm, and 3D reinjection were the three procedures that made up his method. Despite certain technical advancements, this method is still considered the best for lipo filling and liposuction [21, 22]. One of the most common operations carried out by plastic surgeons since the 1980s is autologous fat transplantation [23]. Fat grafting accounted for 5.9% of non-surgical cosmetic procedures in 2009 [24, 25].

24.3 Harvesting Fat

Numerous studies have shown that less invasive fat-harvesting techniques improve adipocyte viability and graft survival [26]. The literature has continued to discuss which fat-harvesting procedures produce more live and functional adipocytes. The three primary methods include surgical excision, syringe, and vacuum aspiration. Direct fat excision, instead of aspiration, has recently gained support in experimental and clinical investigations. The "fat cylinder graft" was first described by Fagrell et al. [26, 28], which involves punching out fat cores using a punching device.

On the other hand, the core graft was advocated for block grafting by Qin et al. [26, 29], who argued that it preserves the structure and viability of the harvested fat by avoiding damage to the adipocytes. Pu et al. [26, 30] discovered that conventional liposuction aspirates had substantially decreased adipocyte function when contrasted with fresh fatty tissue samples and fat that was aspirated using a syringe. Low negative-pressure lipo aspiration can be utilized for situations requiring a significant volume of fat, such as breast surgery. It has the potential to produce fat more quickly than syringe aspiration. Up to 90% of adipocytes may have their structures disrupted by the high vacuum pressures used in traditional liposuction [26, 27]. The cannula size could impact the fat viability extracted [31]. Preservation of original tissue architecture and reduction of cellular rupture are achieved using large-bore cannulas and the excisional approach of fat harvesting. The diameter of the fat-extracting device was found to have an inverse correlation with cellular damage, according to research by Campbell et al. [32]. Compared to lipoaspirates collected with 4-mm or 2-mm cannulas, Erdim et al. [33] found that 6-mm cannulas resulted in greater graft viability.

A method for fat extraction that caused minimal damage to adipocytes was detailed by Coleman et al. [34]. To manually suction fat, one uses a 10-milliliter syringe attached to a 3-millimeter blunt-edged, 2-hole cannula. Surgeons employ digital manipulation to pull back the syringe plunger and provide a moderate negative pressure while pushing the cannula into the harvest site [34]. A parcel of fat can be introduced into the syringe barrel via the Luer-Lok hole and the cannula using slight negative pressure and the cutting action of the cannula through the tissues [34]. At the end of the filling process, the syringe is sealed at the Luer-Lok end by replacing the plug initially on the cannula [34]. The syringe is prepared for centrifugation by removing the plunger [34] (Figs. 24.1, 24.2, 24.3, 24.4, 24.5, and 24.6).

After a thorough evaluation of the patient, surgeons should determine the best location for the procedure by analyzing the patient's natural fat deposits. Most fat-harvesting procedures include the abdominal region, the trochanteric area (saddlebags), inner thighs, and knees [35, 36]. Fat grafts can be harvested using either a "wet" or a "dry" technique. The "wet" approach was first published in 1993 by

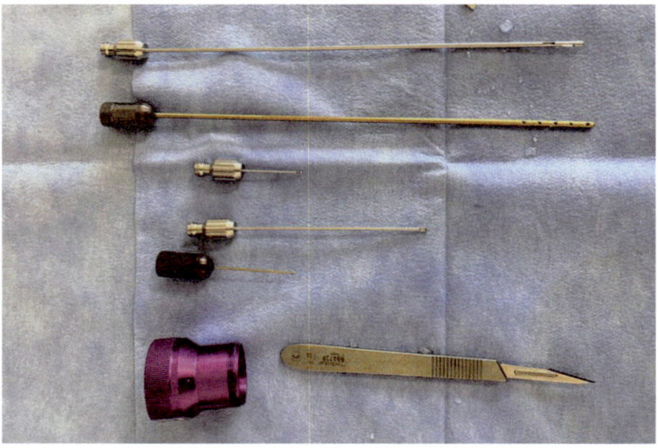

Fig. 24.1 Cannulas for fat collection. (Courtesy of Zeliha Kapusuz Gencer)

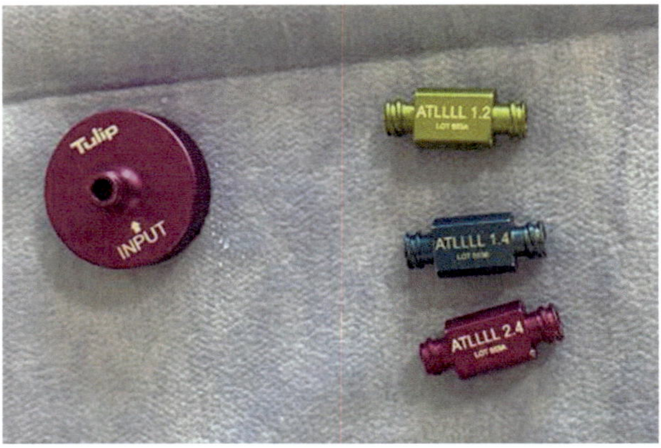

Fig. 24.2 Filters that will be used in fat injection preparation. (Courtesy of Zeliha Kapusuz Gencer)

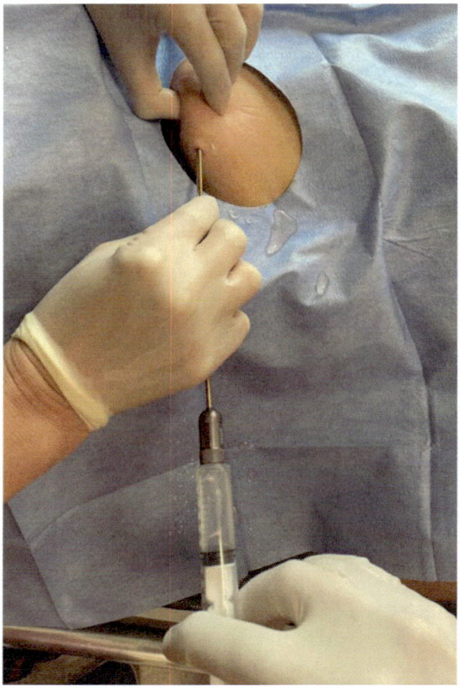

Fig. 24.3 Local anesthesia with the tumescent approach. (Courtesy of Zeliha Kapusuz Gencer)

Klein et al. [26, 37]. Injecting a fluid (Klein's) solution containing 0.9% NaCl, epinephrine, and a local anesthetic into the donor site. The wet approach promotes hydrodissection and enlarges the target fat layer, which facilitates the subsequent aspiration with decreased pain and ecchymosis, as pointed out by Illouz and de Villers [26, 38]. The shear stress applied to harvested fat is shown to alter the viability of adipocytes, and it has been found that low shear stress leads to graft survival [39]. A "dry" technique, which does not use the tumescent fluid, is another

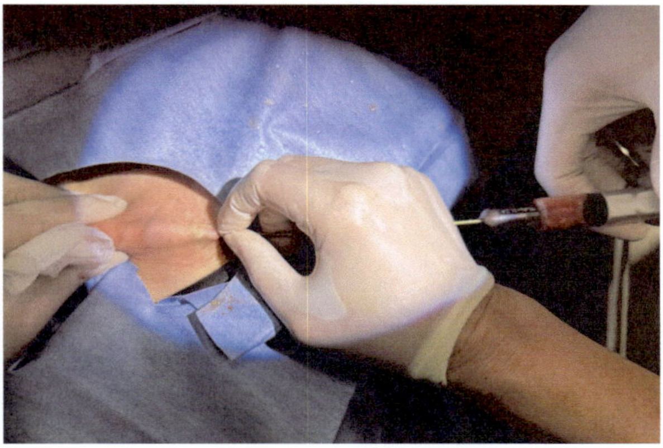

Fig. 24.4 Fat tissue collection through the cannula. (Courtesy of Zeliha Kapusuz Gencer)

possibility. On the other hand, more analgesics may be needed after using the "dry" method [25, 37].

Fragile eyelids and lips can be treated with micro- and nano-fat grafts, usually extracted using cannulas as small as 0.7 mm in diameter [40, 41]. Tonnard et al. [32] emphasized the latter's potential clinical utility when comparing macro fat grafts with micro- and nano-fat grafts. Micro-fat particles were extracted from the abdominal cavity using a cannula with a diameter of 1 mm. A Luer-to-Luer connector with two 10-mL syringes was used to shear a portion of the micro-fat into smaller particles [42, 43]. After that, the nanoparticles were gathered after filtering. A conventional 3-mm cannula was also used to extract macro fat particles to serve as a control [42, 43]. The micrographs obtained by the investigation demonstrated that the macro- and micro-fat particles had typical cellular architecture with sparse, nonviable cells [42, 43]. No adipocytes existed in the nano-fat grafts, and the native structure was broken [42, 43]. Nanografts, on the other hand, kept a lot of ASCs, and these ASCs proliferated and differentiated just like the macro- and micro-fat samples [42, 43]. By 6 months after surgery, the skin quality of several patients treated with nano-fat grafts had improved [42, 43]. Nanografts lack functional adipocytes,

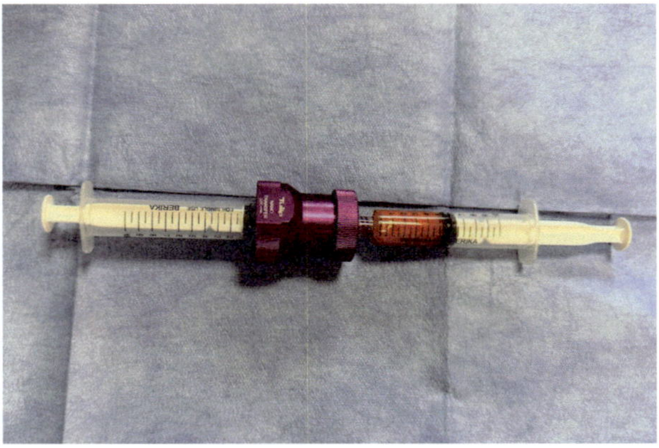

Fig. 24.5 Final preparations of fat tissue for injection. (Courtesy of Zeliha Kapusuz Gencer)

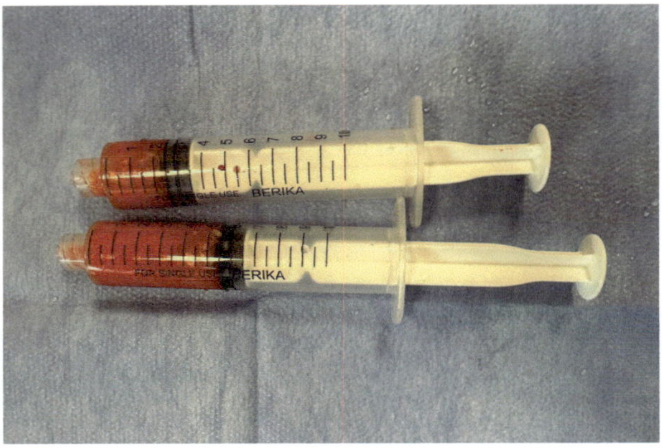

Fig. 24.6 Fat tissue ready to implant. (Courtesy of Zeliha Kapusuz Gencer)

but the author posits that their high stem cell content would make them therapeutically beneficial for skin rejuvenation [42, 43].

24.4 What Is the Best Donor Site?

The most common donor sites for choosing a region on the body to harvest from are the flank, belly, thigh, and knee. Six women and several donor sites (flank, upper and lower abdomen, and lateral and inner thigh) were compared in a study by Li et al. Subcutaneously implanted adipose tissue into naked mice was followed by graft harvest and analysis at 12 weeks. Weight, volume, and histological characteristics (such as integrity, cysts, inflammation, fibrosis, and neovascularization) were not significantly different across grafts from different donor sites, according to the authors. Additionally, SVF and cell surface markers were not different in their quantities. So, when choosing a donor site, the authors argued that convenience and patient preference should take precedence [44]. Fat from three different donor sites—a woman's thigh, abdomen, and breast—implanted into a nude mouse model did not differ in volume, weight, or histological characteristics like vascularization and fibrosis, according to research by Ullmann et al. [45]. Retroactive analysis of 73 breast reconstruction patients by Small et al. [1, 46] revealed no difference in volume retention between thigh and abdominal fat.

24.5 What Is the Best Cannula?

The cannula's diameter and number of holes are the most important variables determining the success of fat graft surgeries. In their study, Campbell et al. found that the diameter of the fat-extracting tool had an inverse connection with cellular damage [47].

The obtained samples are less likely to be damaged when using multi-perforated cannulas since the pressure on each hole is reduced [48]. With a 170 mm length and a rounded tip, Trivisonno et al. compared cannulas with a diameter of 2 mm and a diameter of 3 mm. The 2 mm cannula included five 1 mm diameter ports arranged in a spiral pattern, whereas the 3 mm cannula featured a single 3 × 9 mm port on one side. Concurrently, the 2 mm cannula eased patient pain and stress while allowing harvesting from more profound, more vascularized layers of fat. More ADSCs could be isolated with this 2 mm cannula, which had a greater propensity to create capillary-like structures than the 3 mm cannula. Still, the two cannulas had no discernible difference in ADSC proliferation capability, morphology, or survivability [49]. In their study, Alharbi et al. contrasted a standard 3 mm single-hole blunt tip cannula with a micro-harvesting 2 mm cannula with four 600 μm gauged orifices and a blunt tip, finding that the former achieved far better viability and migration of isolated ADSCs [50]. But, according to Rubino et al., 3 mm cannula-harvested fat had a higher adipocyte density than 2 mm cannula-harvested fat [51]. When comparing grafts acquired with 4 mm and 2 mm cannulas to those obtained with a 6 mm cannula after liposuction, Erdim et al. found that the latter had higher graft viability in ten female patients [52]. In a prospective study, Ozsoy et al. found that a 4 mm diameter cannula yielded more viable adipocytes than 2 or 3 mm cannulas [1, 72].

24.6 Processing of Fats

Fat graft preparation methods include sedimentation, filtration, washing, and centrifugation. Adipocytes, collagen fibers, blood, and residue are all components of lipoaspirate, making fat processing essential. Inflammation at the recipient location, brought on by these factors, can be harmful to the fat graft [53]. Blood extraction is necessary because blood speeds up the breakdown of the donated fat [54]. In addition, because the debris will be removed after a few hours, injecting it produces an inaccurate impression of the extent of correction [53]. The weight and architecture of fat grafts prepared by centrifugation, filtration, or sedimentation have not been found to differ significantly in animal tests [55–59]. The results of patient trials using centrifugation instead of gravity separation were more favorable, albeit [55]. Research comparing centrifugation, washing, and filtration as fat processing methods found no statistically significant differences in fat retention; nevertheless, nodule formation was observed with filtration but not centrifugation [60, 61]. The structural integrity of adipose tissue was damaged, cell necrosis and apoptosis were enhanced, and adipogenic differentiation capability and tubule formation were diminished, according to Ferraro et al. [62], who showed that centrifugation with a force greater than 50 g caused these effects. Ultimately, the fat graft is sustained for long-term retention by the tubules formed during angiogenesis, which provide nutrients and blood to the adipose tissue [55, 63, 64]. In addition to damaging adipocytes, higher centrifugation speeds have been linked to an increase in fluid part, a decrease in injectable tissue volume, and a rise in oil portion [55, 65].

24.7 Is There a Difference in Wet or Dry Aspiration Outcomes?

Various liposuction procedures are available depending on the amount of solution injected into the fat donor location. A significant amount of blood might be lost during the aspiration process, which makes the dry approach, which involves direct aspiration without injecting any preparation fluid, obsolete [2, 66–68]. Surgical pioneers Clayton and Hetter developed the wet technique, which consists of injecting a wetting solution—which could include saline, anesthetics, and other substances—into the fat donor site before aspiration. This is done following a volume-to-volume ratio of infiltrate to aspirate that is less than 1:1, leading to a blood loss of 4–30% of the aspirated volume [68–70]. Afterward, Fodor et al.'s super-wet technique involved using a 1:1 infiltrate-to-total aspirate ratio, which resulted in a 1–2% reduction in blood loss relative to the aspirated volume [45, 68–70].

In conclusion, Klein's tumescent approach produced a high volume of infiltrate, with an infiltrate volume to total aspirate volume ratio of 2–3:1. This method is seen as the safest option for bigger aspirations, with better cosmetic outcomes and less blood loss (around 1% of the aspirated volume). It also does not require general anesthesia. To guarantee hydro dissection and bloodless collection, tumescent anesthesia must be administered 45 min before harvesting [1, 67, 68].

Moore et al. discovered short-lived alterations to lipolysis and glucose transport in the presence of local anesthetic, suggesting that lidocaine alone may reduce adipocyte function. These levels were restored to normal after washing harvested lipoaspirate to remove lidocaine [71]. Additionally, tumescent anesthesia can transport drugs that have a specific impact on the target fatty tissue. In contrast to Moore et al.'s theory that lidocaine hindered the proliferation of adipocytes [71, 72], it was discovered that local anesthetics, with or without vasoconstrictor drugs, did not significantly impact the long-term survival of grafted fat. When comparing dry and wet harvesting liposuction, Agostini et al. found no significant differences in histomorphometric features (such as cell viability, cytoplasmic swelling/disruption, apoptosis/necrosis, connective tissue, amorphous ground substance, vacuoles, and cross-sectional profile) [1, 66].

24.8 Conclusion

There has been a recent uptick in the utilization of autologous fat grafting for various volume-filling procedures. Standardized harvesting, processing, and implantation protocols still need to be improved, which is a significant roadblock to their broad clinical usage [73]. Numerous writers have acknowledged the lack of a generally agreed-upon technique for fat grafting [1, 74, 75].

Extreme caution is required when working with fat because of its fragility and the importance of preserving it [76]. There has been a lot of recent interest in the optimal methods for autologous fat grafting; however, when planning a study, it is essential also to include patient-related aspects [1].

One potential downside of adipose tissue transplant is donor-site morbidity, which might include bleeding or, more commonly, local deformities created by liposuction. On the other hand, recipient-site problems can consist of infections and, although highly improbable, pulmonary embolism, cardiac arrest, or deep venous thrombosis. However, there have been reports of autologous fat grafting being a highly safe operation with minimal morbidity [77].

References

1. Fontes T, Brandão I, Negrão R, Martins MJ, Monteiro R. Autologous fat grafting: harvesting techniques. Ann Med Surg (Lond). 2018;36:212–8.
2. Strong AL, Cederna PS, Rubin JP, Coleman SR, Levi B. The current state of fat grafting. Plast Reconstr Surg. 2015;136(4):897–912.
3. Laloze J, Varin A, Bertheuil N. Cell-assisted lipotransfer: current concepts. Ann Chir Plast Esthet. 2017;62(6):609–16.
4. Tabit CJ, Slack GC, Fan K, Wan DC, Bradley JP. Fat grafting versus adipose-derived stem cell therapy: distinguishing indications, techniques, and outcomes. Aesthet Plast Surg. 2012;36(3):704–13.
5. Bourin P, Bunnell BA, Casteilla L. Stromal cells from the adipose tissue-derived stromal vascular fraction and culture expanded adipose tissue-derived stromal/stem cells: a joint statement of the International Federation for Adipose Therapeutics and Science (IFATS) and the International Society for Cellular Therapy (ISCT). Cytotherapy. 2013;15(6):641–8.
6. Tocco I, Widgerow AD, Lalezari S. Lipotransfer: the potential from bench to bedside. Ann Plast Surg. 2014;72(5):599–609.
7. Bellini E, Grieco MP, Raposio E. The science behind autologous fat grafting. Ann Med Surg. 2017;24:65–73.
8. Baer PC, Geiger H. Adipose-derived mesenchymal stromal/stem cells: tissue localization, characterization, and heterogeneity. Stem Cell Int. 2012;2012:1–11.
9. Zuk PA, Zhu M, Mizuno H. Multilineage cells from human adipose tissue: implications for cell-based therapies. Tissue Eng. 2001;7(2):211–28.
10. Zuk PA, Zhu M, Ashjian P. Human adipose tissue is a source of multipotent stem cells. Mol Biol Cell. 2002;13(12):4279–95.
11. Gimble JM, Guilak F. Adipose-derived adult stem cells: isolation, characterization, and differentiation potential. Cytotherapy. 2003;5(5):362–9.
12. Strem BM, Hicok KC, Zhu M. Multipotential differentiation of adipose tissue-derived stem cells. Keio J Med. 2005;54(3):132–41.
13. Fraser JK, Schreiber R, Strem B. Plasticity of human adipose stem cells toward endothelial cells and cardiomyocytes. Nat Clin Pract Cardiovasc Med. 2006;3:S33–7.
14. Jack GS, Almeida FG, Zhang R. Processed lipoaspirate cells for tissue engineering of the lower urinary tract: implications for the treatment of stress urinary incontinence and bladder reconstruction. J Urol. 2005;174(5):2041–5.
15. Rodríguez LV, Alfonso Z, Zhang R. Clonogenic multipotent stem cells in human adipose tissue differentiate into functional smooth muscle cells. Proc Natl Acad Sci USA. 2006;103(32):12167–72.
16. Lee J-H, Kemp DM. Human adipose-derived stem cells display myogenic potential and perturbed function in hypoxic conditions. Biochem Biophys Res Commun. 2006;341(3):882–8.
17. Huss FRM, Kratz G. Adipose tissue processed for lipoinjection shows increased cellular survival in vitro when tissue engineering principles are applied. Scand J Plast Reconstr Surg Hand Surg. 2002;36(3):166–71.
18. Matsumoto D, Sato K, Gonda K. Cell-assisted lipotransfer: supportive use of human adipose-derived cells for soft tissue augmentation with lipoinjection. Tissue Eng. 2006;12(12):3375–82.

19. Laloze J, Varin A, Gilhodes J. Cell-assisted lipotransfer: friend or foe in fat grafting? Systematic review and meta-analysis. J Tissue Eng Regen Med. 2018;12(2):e1237–50.
20. Billings E Jr, May JW Jr. Historical review and present status of free fat graft auto transplantation in plastic and reconstructive surgery. Plast Reconstr Surg. 1989;83:368–81.
21. Coleman SR. Structural fat grafting. Aesthet Surg J. 1998;18:386–8.
22. Coleman SR. Long-term survival of fat transplants: controlled demonstrations. Aesthet Plast Surg. 1995;19:421–5.
23. Li BW, Liao WC, Wu SH, Ma H. Cryopreservation of fat tissue and application in autologous fat graft: in vitro and in vivo study. Aesthet Plast Surg. 2012;36:714–22.
24. Gir P, Brown SA, Oni G, Kashefi N, Mojallal A, Rohrich RJ. Fat grafting: evidence-based review on autologous fat harvesting, processing, reinjection, and storage. Plast Reconstr Surg. 2012;130:249–58.
25. Simonacci F, Bertozzi N, Grieco MP, Grignaffini E, Raposio E. Procedure, applications, and outcomes of autologous fat grafting. Ann Med Surg (Lond). 2017;20:49–60.
26. Kakagia D, Pallua N. Autologous fat grafting: in search of the optimal technique. Surg Innov. 2014;21:327–36.
27. Pu LL, Coleman SR, Cui X, Ferguson RE Jr, Vasconez HC. Autologous fat grafts harvested and refined by the Coleman technique: a comparative study. Plast Reconstr Surg. 2008;122:932–7.
28. Fagrell D, Eneström S, Berggren A, Kniola B. Fat cylinder transplantation: an experimental comparative study of three different kinds of fat transplants. Plast Reconstr Surg. 1996;98:90.
29. Qin W, Xu Y, Liu X, Xu S. Experimental and primary clinical research of core fat graft. Zhongguo Xiu Fu Chong Jian Wai Ke Za Zhi. 2012;26:576–82.
30. Pu LL, Cui X, Fink BF, Cibull ML, Gao D. The viability of fatty tissues within adipose aspirates after conventional liposuction: a comprehensive study. Ann Plast Surg. 2005;54:288–92.
31. Ozsoy Z, Kul Z, Bilir A. The role of cannula diameter in improved adipocyte viability: a quantitative analysis. Aesthet Surg J. 2006;26:287–9.
32. Campbell G-L, Laudenslager N, Newman J. The effect of mechanical stress on adipocyte morphology and metabolism. Am J Cosmet Surg. 1987;4:89–94.
33. Erdim M, Tezel E, Numanoglu A, Sav A. The effects of the size of liposuction cannula on adipocyte survival and the optimum temperature for fat graft storage: an experimental study. J Plast Reconstr Aesthet Surg. 2009;62:1210–4.
34. Coleman SR. Structural fat grafting: more than a permanent filler. Plast Reconstr Surg. 2006;118:108S–20S.
35. Crawford JL, Hubbard BA, Colbert SH, Puckett CL. Fine tuning lipoaspirate viability for fat grafting. Plast Reconstr Surg. 2010;126:1342–8.
36. Hamza A, Lohsiriwat V, Rietjens M. Lipofilling in breast cancer surgery. Gland Surg. 2013;2:7–14.
37. Klein JA. Tumescent technique for local anesthesia improves safety in large-volume liposuction. Plast Reconstr Surg. 1993;92:1085–98.
38. Illouz YG, de Villers YT. Body sculpturing by lipoplasty. New York: Churchill Livingstone; 1989. p. 120–6.
39. Kasem A, Wazir U, Headon H, Mokbel K. Breast lipofilling: a review of current practice. Arch Plast Surg. 2015;42:126–30.
40. Dasiou-Plakida D. Fat injections for facial rejuvenation: 17 years experience in 1720 patients. J Cosmet Dermatol. 2003;2:119–25.
41. Mazzola RF. Fat injection: from filling to regeneration. St. Louis: Quality Medical Publishing; 2009. p. 373–422.
42. Tonnard P, Verpaele A, Peeters G, Hamdi M, Cornelissen M, Declercq H. Nanofat grafting: basic research and clinical applications. Plast Reconstr Surg. 2013;132:1017–26.
43. Gause TM, Kling RE, Sivak WN, Marra KG, Rubin JP, Kokai LE. Particle size in fat graft retention: a review on the impact of harvesting technique in lipofilling surgical outcomes. Adipocytes. 2014;3:273–9.
44. Li K, Gao J, Zhang Z. Selection of donor site for fat grafting and cell isolation. Aesthet Plast Surg. 2013;37(1):153–8.

45. Ullmann Y, Shoshani O, Fodor A. Searching for the favorable donor site for fat injection: in vivo study using the nude mice model. Dermatologic Surg. 2005;31(10):1304–7.
46. Small K, Choi M, Petruolo O, Lee C, Karp N. Is there an ideal donor site of fat for secondary breast reconstruction? Aesthet Surg J. 2014;34(4):545–50.
47. Campbell GL, Laudenslager N, Newman J. The effect of mechanical stress on adipocyte morphology and metabolism. Am J Cosmet Surg. 1987;4(2):89–94.
48. Hivernaud V, Lefourn B, Guicheux J. Autologous fat grafting in the breast: critical points and technique improvements. Aesthet Plast Surg. 2015;39(4):547–61.
49. Trivisonno A, Di Rocco G, Cannistra C. Harvest of superficial layers of fat with a microcannula and isolation of adipose tissue-derived stromal and vascular cells. Aesthet Surg J. 2014;34(4):601–13.
50. Alharbi Z, Opländer C, Almakadi S, Fritz A, Vogt M, Pallua N. Conventional vs. micro-fat harvesting: how fat harvesting technique affects tissue-engineering approaches using adipose tissue-derived stem/stromal cells. J Plast Reconstr Aesthet Surg. 2013;66:1271–8.
51. Rubino C, Mazzarello V, Faenza M. A scanning electron microscope study and statistical analysis of adipocyte morphology in lipofilling. Ann Plast Surg. 2015;74(6):718–21.
52. Erdim M, Tezel E, Numanoglu A, Sav A. The effects of the size of liposuction cannula on adipocyte survival and the optimum temperature for fat graft storage: an experimental study. J Plast Reconstr Aesthet Surg. 2009;62(9):1210–4.
53. Mojallal A, Foyatier JL. The effect of different factors on the survival of transplanted adipocytes. Ann Chir Plast Esthet. 2004;49:426–36.
54. Sommer B, Sattler G. Current concepts of fat graft survival: histology of aspirated adipose tissue and review of the literature. Dermatologic Surg. 2000;26:1159–566.
55. Strong AL, Cederna PS, Rubin JP, Coleman SR, Levi B. The current state of fat grafting: a review of harvesting, processing, and injection techniques. Plast Reconstr Surg. 2015;136:897–912.
56. Condé-Green A, Wu I, Graham I, Chae JJ, Drachenberg CB, Singh DP, Holton L 3rd, Slezak S, Elisseeff J. Comparison of 3 techniques of fat grafting and cell-supplemented lipotransfer in athymic rats: a pilot study. Aesthet Surg J. 2013;33:713–21.
57. P1Smith AWP Jr, Lipschitz AH, Chau B, Sorokin E, Rohrich RJ, Brown SA. Autologous human fat grafting: effect of harvesting and preparation techniques on adipocyte graft survival. Plast Reconstr Surg. 2006;117:1836–44.
58. Minn KW, Min KH, Chang H, Kim S, Heo EJ. Effects of fat preparation methods on the viabilities of autologous fat grafts. Aesthet Plast Surg. 2010;34:626–31.
59. Ramon Y, Shoshani O, Peled IJ, Gilhar A, Carmi N, Fodor L, Risin Y, Ullmann Y. Enhancing the take of injected adipose tissue by a simple method for concentrating fat cells. Plast Reconstr Surg. 2005;115:197–201.
60. Botti G, Pascali M, Botti C, Bodog F, Cervelli V. A clinical trial in facial fat grafting: filtered and washed versus centrifuged fat. Plast Reconstr Surg. 2011;127:2464–73.
61. Khater R, Atanassova P, Anastassov Y, Pellerin P, MartinotDuquennoy V. Clinical and experimental study of autologous fat grafting after processing by centrifugation and serum lavage. Aesthet Plast Surg. 2009;33:37–43.
62. Ferraro GA, De Francesco F, Tirino V, Cataldo C, Rossano F, Nicoletti G, D'Andrea F. Effects of a new centrifugation method on adipose cell viability for autologous fat grafting. Aesthet Plast Surg. 2011;35:341–8.
63. Pfaff M, Wu W, Zellner E, Steinbacher DM. Processing technique for lipofilling influences adipose-derived stem cell concentration and cell viability in lipoaspirate. Aesthet Plast Surg. 2014;38:224–9.
64. Kurita M, Matsumoto D, Shigeura T, Sato K, Gonda K, Harii K, Yoshimura K. Influences of centrifugation on cells and tissues in liposuction aspirates: optimized centrifugation for lipotransfer and cell isolation. Plast Reconstr Surg. 2008;121:1033–41.
65. Hoareau L, Bencharif K, Girard AC, Gence L, Delarue P, Hulard O, Festy F, Roche R. Effect of centrifugation and washing on adipose graft viability: a new method to improve graft efficiency. J Plast Reconstr Aesthet Surg. 2013;66:712–9.

66. Agostini T, Lazzeri D, Pini A. Wet and dry techniques for structural fat graft harvesting. Plast Reconstr Surg. 2012;130(2):331e–9e.
67. Rusciani SA, Rusciani SL, Troccola A. Autologous fat transfer for face rejuvenation with tumescent technique fat harvesting and saline washing: a report of 215 cases. Dermatology. 2012;224(3):244–50.
68. Trott SA, Beran SJ, Rohrich RJ. Safety considerations and fluid resuscitation in liposuction: an analysis of 53 consecutive patients. Plast Reconstr Surg. 1998;102(6):2220–9.
69. Rohrich RJ, Beran SJ, Fodor PB. The role of subcutaneous infiltration in suction-assisted lipoplasty: a review. Plast Reconstr Surg. 1997;99(2):514–9.
70. Clayton DN, Clayton JN, Lindley TS, Clayton JL. Large volume lipoplasty. Clin Plast Surg. 1989;16(2):305–12.
71. Moore JH, Kolaczynski JW, Morales LM. Viability of fat obtained by syringe suction lipectomy: effects of local anesthesia with lidocaine. Aesthet Plast Surg. 1995;19(4):335–9.
72. Weichman KE, Warren SM. Effects of lidocaine plus epinephrine and prilocaine on autologous fat graft survival. J Craniofac Surg. 2012;23(4):1019.
73. Yuan Y, Zhang S, Gao J, Lu F. Spatial structural integrity is important for adipose regeneration after transplantation. Arch Dermatol Res. 2015;307(8):693–704.
74. Özkaya Ö, Egemen O, Barutça SA, Akan M. Long-term clinical outcomes of fat grafting by low-pressure aspiration and slow centrifugation (Lopasce technique) for different indications. J Plast Surg Hand Surg. 2013;47(5):394–8.
75. Philips BJ, Marra KG, Rubin JP. Adipose stem cell-based soft tissue regeneration. Expert Opin Biol Ther. 2012;12(2):155–63.
76. Coleman SR, Saboeiro AP. Primary breast augmentation with fat grafting. Clin Plast Surg. 2015;42(3):301–6.
77. Maione L, Vinci V, Klinger M, Klinger FM, Caviggioli F. Autologous fat graft by needle. Ann Plast Surg. 2015;74(3):277–80.

Fat Injections as Volumizer on the Face: Overview

25

Çiğdem Fırat Koca, Cemal Cingi, and Codrut Sarafoleanu

25.1 Introduction

By injecting extracted adipose tissue under the skin, a technique called fat grafting can restore traumatic, oncologic, or congenital defects. You can also utilize this approach to renew your lips and face for cosmetic purposes. "Autologous fat grafting" describes the identical procedure that is used when the recipient's own fat is harvested. There is no more common clinical case than this. For facial rejuvenation, many people think autologous fat is the best filler material. Why? Because it is supposedly a permanent intervention, it is soft and natural, and it is totally biocompatible. The article highlights the advantages of this method for face rejuvenation [1, 2].

25.2 History of the Procedure

Though fat transfer as an idea has been around for a while, fat transplantation's rise to prominence in the field of plastic surgery is more recent. As early as 1893, soft tissue defects were filled with free-fat autografts. In a 1909 article, the use of autogenous abdominal fat to fix malar and chin deficits is detailed. Modern fat grafting did

The original version of the chapter has been revised. A correction to this chapter can be found at https://doi.org/10.1007/978-3-032-01305-7_51

C. Fırat Koca
Malatya Inonu University, Medical Faculty, Department of Otorhinolaryngology, Malatya, Turkey

C. Cingi (✉)
Eskisehir Osmangazi University, Medical Faculty, Department of Otorhinolaryngology, Eskisehir, Türkiye
e-mail: cemal@ogu.edu.tr

C. Sarafoleanu
University of Medicine and Pharmacy "Carol Davila", Sfanta Maria Clinical Hospital ENT & HNS Department, Bucharest, Romania

C. Cingi et al. (eds.), *Minor Interventions, Major Outcomes on the Face*, Comprehensive ENT, https://doi.org/10.1007/978-3-032-01305-7_25

not happen until the early 1980s, when liposuction became more fashionable [3]. Efforts to cure additional disorders, such as hemifacial atrophy and breast anomalies, continued throughout the early 1900s.

When it came to liposuction aspirate fat transfer, Illouz published a paper in 1984. Free pearl fat autografts were used to treat a variety of atrophic and post-traumatic facial abnormalities, according to a study published by Ellenbogen in 1986 [4]. Modern techniques have made fat grafting the go-to for a variety of cosmetic concerns, including lip enhancement, facial rhytids (which encompass a number of areas that are notoriously hard to treat, like the nasolabial fold and glabellar furrows), and scarring on the face [3].

25.3 Anatomy and Physiology

The face changes a great deal as a person grows older. The nasolabial folds, tear troughs, marionette lines, and other unsightly folds and shadows that contribute to the appearance of aging are caused by the descent of the face's soft tissues, which is caused by gravity. Furthermore, as a result of skin thinning, muscle atrophy, fat volume loss, and a decrease in bone thickness, facial volume decreases with age [5]. Although resuspension procedures like face, brow, midface, and neck lifts are the usual go-to for dealing with gravity-related changes, there are a number of filler materials that can reverse the effects of volume loss and, in certain instances, even outperform surgical lifting. The use of dermal fillers and fat grafting to augment face rejuvenation operations has grown so much in favor in recent years. A thorough understanding of the face and its anatomy, as well as the connections between different tissues and fascial planes, is essential for successful fat grafting and the prevention of problems [6]. Following careful preparation, the targeted areas are injected with the harvested fat, which is often taken from the inner thigh, flank, or belly. Before fat compartments may receive grafts, it is crucial to determine their proper location and depth. Of the face's fat compartments, the two most important are the superficial and deep spaces. What divides these areas is the superficial musculoaponeurotic system [7]. There are subspaces within each of these places, and picking the right recipient sites is an experience-only affair. Deep within the surface fat layer are a number of fat pads. Nasal, orbital, frontal, medial, and lateral fat pads; jowl, fad, and cheek fat pads; and temporal and frontal fat pads are also part of this group. The deep fat space is composed of the following structures: the buccal fat pad, the medial and lateral sub-orbicularis oculi fat pads, the sub-orbicularis oris fat pad, the deep medial and lateral cheek fat pads, and the buccal fat pad. The tenth By mastering these units, injectors can choose the best locations for fat transfer, calculate the volume needed, and use the best injection technique and equipment.

25.4 Problem

Several methods exist for removing rhytidosis, including surgical excision, redraping of excess skin, and skin resurfacing procedures such as chemical peels, laser ablation, and dermabrasion. The following are some of the drawbacks of these methods [3].

Inserting a filler component into a deficient area is another option. Face resurfacing is like leveling mountains; using an implanted material fills valleys. To remedy defects and irregularities in soft tissue, numerous materials have been studied. Most of these substances, however, have a number of negative attributes, including being fleeting, reacting to foreign bodies, having an unusual texture, and perhaps transmitting diseases [3].

If there were an ideal material, it would be one that met all of the following criteria: it would be cheap, durable, feel natural, and not cause any negative immune reactions. Autologous tissue has the ability to meet these requirements. Transplantation is possible with many different types of tissue. Longer scars on the dermis and fascia are necessary for harvesting. An ideal situation would be to prevent the development of a new donor site defect by harvesting dermal tissue from the location of an existing incision, such as a scar from a previous abdominal operation or a cesarean delivery. While these tissues can help larger areas and deeper flaws, they lack the pliability of a semi-liquid or liquid material. It is possible to slice these tissues into narrow strips. To achieve fat harvesting, discreet access incisions are used.

Furthermore, fat removal is usually a good idea, and there are no flaws in the harvesting procedure. Liquid fat feels natural and is quite malleable. It is safe to use for treating a wide range of deficiencies, readily available, cheap, and does not have any immunogenic characteristics [3].

Using autologous fat transfer, scarring on the face, such as acne scars, can be eliminated. Patients with cosmetic problems, such as those seeking lip augmentation, or those experiencing disease processes, like hemifacial atrophy, might also benefit from the enhancement of facial volume. Slowing down the aging process of the face is within reach. Rhytides that are too deep to be treated by resurfacing treatments or areas that are not properly addressed by standard lifting procedures (such as nasolabial folds, glabellar wrinkles, or tear troughs) can also be treated with transplanted fat [3].

25.5 Etiology

As we become older, our skin loses some of its elasticity, thickness, and adherence to the deeper layers of our body. The amount of melanocytes and Langerhans cells in the epidermis is decreased. This enhances the skin's susceptibility to shear pressures by flattening the rete pegs that link the dermis to the epidermis. Loss of dermal ground substance, elastic fibers, and collagen causes the dermis to progressively degrade. Sunburn is an inevitable consequence of spending too much time outside.

When sun damage occurs, the dermis experiences elastosis, which is the buildup of thicker, irregular, and partially deteriorated elastic fibers [3].

Cigarette smoking is also associated with changes in skin features. Results are predicted due to the histologic modifications caused by post-traumatic scarring, acne, and the repeated action of the underlying muscle. Wrinkles can be accentuated by frequent changes in weight. A depressed scar could result from improperly everting the skin's corners as the wound is being closed. As an added bonus, there is proof of a genetic component [3].

25.6 Presentation

Patients who are a bit older may seek out procedures that rejuvenate their entire face or target particular areas for improvement. For procedures like classic rhytidectomy, facial resurfacing, and auxiliary suspensory treatments that don't target specific areas of the body, fat grafting is often thought of as the gold standard. Patients of any age can undergo facial cosmetic improvement procedures; the most common of these is lip augmentation. To a large extent, patients learn about their conditions through word of mouth and numerous web resources. It is crucial to educate and understand the patient in order to attain the highest potential results [3].

Under the influence of a local anesthetic, this procedure can be performed as an outpatient procedure. It is crucial to have a consultation before surgery. A thorough discussion outlining the areas that will be treated is, by far, the most important part of the preoperative workup. Further clarification of therapy details, post-operative care, expectations, and possible adverse effects is required [3].

Photographic documentation is essential for the planning and evaluation of this surgical procedure. For proper detail delineation and adequate comparison of pre- and post-operative views, it is necessary to standardize lighting, angle, and expression. To guarantee reliable photographic documentation before and after surgery, the patient should refrain from wearing cosmetics. It can be helpful for the patient to bring digital images of any trouble spots to show the doctor during the consultation. In addition, images are useful for post-op comparisons [3].

25.7 Indications

Not only can autologous fat grafting for facial rejuvenation restore volume to the face, but it also has the potential to renew the skin by improving its tone and texture. Although fat grafting is typically used for cosmetic purposes, it is also a crucial minimally invasive method for several reconstructive indications [2].

Several age-related alterations in the face can be corrected using autologous fat grafting, including the following conditions [2]:

- Hollowing of the forehead
- Deep rhytides, especially those in the forehead and glabellar regions

- Hollowing of the temporal region
- Hollowing of the supraorbital disk
- An increase in the size of the lower lid's vertical length
- Deformation of the tear trough and a deep nasojugal groove on the nose
- Bags and malars
- The creases below the nose
- The lines of a marionette
- Jowls or a lack of a defined jawline contour
- Thin lips
- Chin that retracts

Not only can autologous fat grafting assist in treating the aging face, but it also helps address many other issues. It can be performed on its own or in conjunction with facial rejuvenation [8]. Some of the indications for this procedure include the following:

Inconsistencies in the nasal contour zone

- Scars
- Causes fires

Dermatitis is caused by radiation.
The lipodystrophy that is associated with the human immunodeficiency virus.
Facial abnormalities, whether they be congenital, acquired, or the result of trauma

- Disparities in the face

The enhancement of the flap

25.8 Contrindications

There are several scenarios in which fat grafting could not be the most effective form of rejuvenation and might even be risky, particularly if general anesthesia is going to be used. If there is a significant likelihood of instability in the volume of the fat, such as in cases of targeted weight loss or continuous weight gain, or if the patient has a previous history of complete or subtotal resorption of earlier transplanted fat, then autologous fat grafting may not be an appropriate treatment option. Patients receiving fat injections for breast reconstruction or recontouring should also be informed that injected fat may produce nodules or calcifications, which may subsequently appear suspicious for cancer on subsequent imaging [2]. This is something that patients should be aware of.

In addition, patients who have illnesses that are local, regional, or systemic and that have the potential to impair blood flow or wound healing are at an increased risk of developing complications or having outcomes that are less than ideal. There are several examples, such as a history of significant burn scarring, radiation therapy, keloid scarring, coagulopathies, the requirement for immunosuppressive drugs, and other metabolic or chronic disorders [2].

25.9 Consideration of Facial Aesthetic Units

The patient's goals and the injector's experience level are considered when determining the amount of fat injected and the facial components into which it is injected. When injecting each facial subunit, the method and technique used are specific to that subunit, with subtle variations in the techniques and instruments used. The following is a list of general points that pertain to the areas of the face that are injected more frequently [2, 9]:

- Injections are administered subcutaneously, intramuscularly, or submuscularly to the forehead, brow, and temple. These injections are typically accessed by stab incisions made in the hairline or lateral edge of the brow. After the injection, any apparent ridging should be rubbed until it becomes smooth. Eight to fifteen milliliters of fat may be needed in hollow temples.

- *Glabella and nose:*

The most common problems that need to be addressed in this region are the glabellar vertical rhytids (also known as "frown lines" or "number 11s") or a deep radix to conceal a dorsal hump. However, any imperfection in the nose's contours can be rectified by this procedure. The cannula can enter the body through the upper cutaneous lip, the forehead, the medial eyebrow, the cheek, the alar base, or the nasal tip. Even though several different cannulas may be used, the 19 ga Coleman type 3 cannula is the most frequently utilized to layer the fat from the periosteum to the intradermal layers. It is possible to inject fat posterior to the nasal cartilage to expand the internal valve, fill concavities in the radix or within a saddle deformity, or smooth contour irregularities that have occurred due to rhinoplasty or trauma [10]. When it comes to the glabella, it is essential to avoid intravascular injection and to remain superficial. Some people advocate intradermal injection. An intravascular injection is not recommended.

- *The periorbital region:*

Because this region presents specific technical challenges, rookie fat grafters should be cautious when working in this area. Before beginning, it is essential to continue cautiously by injecting small aliquots of fat. It is important to avoid placing an excessive number of fat parcels at the same time. The initial infiltration should be deep around the orbital rim, and then immediately after that, another layer should be applied just superficially to it. Injections should be administered deep to the orbicularis oculi muscle to prevent the formation of palpable or visible nodules. This is because the skin that covers the eyelid is so thin.

- *Lips*

To prevent damaging the orbicularis oris muscle and the labial arteries, which are branches of the facial artery, fat injections should be put superficially (just beneath the mucosa) in this area. The injector's preference determines cannula selection; however, smaller cannulas, such as the Coleman cannula with a gauge of 22, are recommended when injecting into the lips.

- *Malar, zygomatic, and infraorbital regions*

Fat placement in the malar, zygomatic, and infraorbital regions superior to a ptotic cheek can assist in lifting the soft tissue back into a more youthful posture. This is accomplished by placing fat on the cheek. In many cases, it is necessary to make two stab incisions, one lateral to the mid-nasolabial fold and the other to the zygomatic arch. To prevent nerve damage, it is essential to mark the location of the infraorbital nerve, which is approximately one centimeter below the orbital rim in the middle of the pupillary line. To prevent the face from seeming overly full due to injections that are put more medially, consider filling the area anterior to the auricle, the lateral cheek compartment.

This region is reached by making stab incisions in the lateral chin or the vicinity of the oral commissures. The nasolabial fold includes this region. Grafting can be performed deep (periosteal) or superficially (subcutaneous). Despite this, it should be kept in the middle of the nasolabial fold to prevent damage to the facial artery or excessive depth of the nasolabial fold.

Fat grafting to the mandible and chin can treat a retruded chin, jowls, or poor jawline definition. This region is also a potential target for fat grafting. It is possible to insert stab incisions along the border of the mandible, in the submental area, and in the pre-jowl sulcus to access this region. Fat placement is accomplished by fanning the injections laterally and inferiorly, avoiding damage to the facial artery when it crosses over the jaw at the gonial notch, anterior to the masseter [1, 2].

25.10 Harvest

- The method is intended to harvest the fat in pieces of an easily transportable size. The periumbilical, lumbar, and trochanteric regions and the knee and arm's thigh and medial locations are frequently used as donor surgical sites.
- Use a local anesthetic to anesthetize the area where a minor access incision will be made. Once this incision has been made, a long syringe should be used to provide tumescent fluid to induce anesthesia in the area. All of the harvesting access points are located in the exact location.

It is possible to select a different tumescent fluid. To make a standard solution, one milligram of epinephrine, 200 milligrams of lidocaine, and five milliequivalents of sodium bicarbonate are combined in one liter of normal saline. For the tumescent approach, dosages of lidocaine as high as 35 mg/kg are possible; however, a far lower amount is required for the straightforward fat-harvesting technique.

The use of an aspiration cannula (such as a Mercedes) that is attached to a syringe should be performed after the region that is to be harvested has been infiltrated. Another option is to use a needle with a 14-gauge, which does not result in any loss in the survival of the fat taken. Use either a hand vacuum or a mechanical vacuum to suction. Aspiration should be performed with a smooth passing motion. It is advisable to use small syringes to prevent the production of negative pressures in more than one atmosphere. It has been established through experimentation that increasing the power suction from −0.5 to −0.95 atm causes fat cells to be broken up and vaporized, destroying their capacity to be properly transplanted [3–17].

25.10.1 Transfer and Purification

Following the harvesting process, the aspirate is transferred sterilely through several syringes, utilizing the tulip connections to tuberculin syringes containing one milliliter. With this transfer, the liquid portion of the graft is rinsed gently to remove any oil, lidocaine, and blood that may be present.

Using the centrifuge is an alternative to gently tipping the container with your hand. Even though Chajchir discovered that the fatty cells were destroyed when the centrifugal machine was used at a high or moderate speed [18, 19], other groups reported positive outcomes using the centrifuge. The aspirate is composed of three distinct layers. The top layer is composed of oil released from ruptured fat cells. Gently blotting or decanting this layer is now being done. The bottom layer is drained and retains varying levels of blood and tumescent fluid throughout its entirety. In the intermediate layer, fat cells suitable for grafting are found. The fragile cells may be damaged by more rigorous washing or squeezing, which will further reduce the viability of the transplant [3].

During autologous face fat grafting, the long-term retention of fat processed by closed-membrane filtration is much higher than that of fat processed through centrifuges, according to Gerth and colleagues' study. The study, which included 26 patients who had undergone grafting with closed-membrane filtration fat, discovered that the mean retention rate for these patients was over 41% at a mean follow-up time of 17 months. This was in contrast to the 31.8% retention rate observed for patients who had undergone grafting with centrifuge-processed fat [20].

Recently, Kuran was successful in transferring aspirated fat to a sterile cup that was dressed in gauze. This particular approach was inspired by a yogurt concentration process utilized in Anatolia [21]. The following five washes were done with lactated Ringer solution, the local anesthetic solution, and blood removed from the fat. The aspirate and the concentrated product are transferred to tiny syringes after the aspirate dries. Regarding sterility concerns, most organizations advocate for a closed approach, yet there is no documented evidence that open procedures pose a higher risk of infections. The open approach allows the surgeon to manipulate fat to make a graft easier to inject [3]. This is one of the advantages of open procedure.

Controversial is the choice of fluid for fat suspension. Most of the time, regular saline or lactated Ringer solution is used. However, a serum-free culture medium is also an option, although the cost is higher. Additionally, some organizations support using supplements like heparin, insulin, vitamin E, and nonsteroidal anabolic hormones. Additionally, the contribution of lidocaine is a contentious issue [3].

Adipocytes can be frozen at −30 °C and reused in preparation for future lipografts. After defrosting, a significant percentage of viable cells remain. To preserve the greatest possible number of living cells, the method of choice is to slowly freeze and thaw the material [3].

25.10.2 Placement

Regional nerve blocks can be used to administer sufficient anesthesia, which is the most beneficial since they do not obscure the problem being addressed [3].

The objective of any grafting operation is to gently place the graft into a well-vascularized bed to get the highest possible graft take. Every transplant component must be within 1.5 millimeters of live vascularized tissue. It is likely that the center region, which is the most isolated from the blood supply, will not survive if a substantial part is removed and grafted. Despite this, some clinical evidence indicates that lip grafting is booming in specific tissues that are not well vascularized, such as hemifacial hemiatrophy and post-traumatic scars [3].

Maintaining the transplanted fat adherent to the recipient location is helpful by creating little tracks for the grafts once they have been placed. It is essential to keep the tracks independent to prevent the fat from escaping via the tunnel. Also, make sure that the track is balanced with passengers. The unfavorable effects of overfilling can be seen in both the survival of the graft and its placement [3].

You can use a bevel-tipped needle or a No. 11 blade scalpel to make an access incision between one and two millimeters to insert the cannula. When the patient withdraws, the needle or cannula should be guided superficially under the rhytid or scar, and fat should be injected using a gentle, regulated approach. Because there is some absorption of the liquid carrier, it is essential to ensure a slight overcorrection. Some groups recommend a 30% overcorrection [3].

The amount of fat grafted varies depending on the structure being supplemented. A fat graft is performed, moving from the deeper layer to the more superficial layer [3].

To address the malar, buccal, and mental regions, the technique developed by Kuran requires injections to be administered in parallel and crossing directions and at subcutaneous, intramuscular, and subperiosteal levels. When correcting rhytids and prominent nasolabial folds, injections are only administered parallel to the line [21].

Lip augmentation involves grafting along the mucosa, increasing the amount of visible vermilion. The perioral rhytids seem tighter after grafting close to the white roll. Although far more significant amounts have been observed, Gatti recounts injecting three milliliters into the top lip and four milliliters into the lower lip simultaneously [22].

Serial injections can be administered at 3-month intervals. In most cases, three different procedures are to be anticipated. Noteworthy is the fact that the infusion is distributed evenly. As a result of having excessive bulk in a particular place, the fat in the central region may be cut off from the new blood supply [3].

According to a study by Lin and colleagues, the microautologous fat transplantation (MAFT) technique was an efficient method for precisely grafting small fat packages. One hundred sixty-eight patients participated in the trial and received the operation for sunken upper eyelids. The procedure results were satisfactory, suggesting that MAFT can be utilized to avoid the potential difficulties associated with fat grafting surgical procedures [23].

References

1. Bohluli B, Bagheri SC, Consky EK. Fat grafting as an adjunct to facial rejuvenation procedures. Atlas Oral Maxillofac Surg Clin North Am. 2018;26(1):51–7.
2. Vasavada A, Raggio BS. Autologous fat grafting for facial rejuvenation. [Updated 2023 Feb 14]. In: StatPearls [Internet]. Treasure Island: StatPearls Publishing; 2023. Available from: https://www.ncbi.nlm.nih.gov/books/NBK557860/. Accessed online at 10 June 2023.
3. Gampper TJ. Facial fat grafting treatment & management. In: Granick MS, editor. Medscape. Updated: 11 Feb 2021. https://emedicine.medscape.com/article/1283020-treatment#d12. Accessed online at 10 June 2023.
4. Ellenbogen R. Free autogenous pearl fat grafts in the face–a preliminary report of a rediscovered technique. Ann Plast Surg. 1986;16(3):179–94.
5. Cotofana S, Fratila AA, Schenck TL, Redka-Swoboda W, Zilinsky I, Pavicic T. The anatomy of the aging face: a review. Facial Plast Surg. 2016;32(3):253–60.
6. Coleman SR, Katzel EB. Fat grafting for facial filling and regeneration. Clin Plast Surg. 2015;42(3):289–300. vii.
7. Rohrich RJ, Pessa JE. The fat compartments of the face: anatomy and clinical implications for cosmetic surgery. Plast Reconstr Surg. 2007;119(7):2219–27.
8. Diepenbrock RM, Green JM. Autologous fat transfer for maxillofacial reconstruction. Atlas Oral Maxillofac Surg Clin North Am. 2018;26(1):59–68.
9. Khan HA, Keyhan SO. Fat grafting in facial aesthetic units. Atlas Oral Maxillofac Surg Clin North Am. 2018;26(1):15–23.
10. Raggio BS, Asaria J. StatPearls [Internet]. Treasure Island: StatPearls Publishing; 2022. Filler Rhinoplasty.
11. Illouz YG. L'avenir de la reutilization de la graisse apres liposuccion. Rev Chir Esthet Lang Franc. 1984;9:36.
12. Frame JD. The past, present, and future of facial fat grafting. Atlas Oral Maxillofac Surg Clin North Am. 2018;26(1):1–6.
13. Ramanadham SR, Rohrich RJ. Newer understanding of specific anatomic targets in the aging face as applied to injectables: superficial and deep facial fat compartments–an evolving target for site-specific facial augmentation. Plast Reconstr Surg. 2015;136(5 Suppl):49S–55S.
14. Warren RJ, Aston SJ, Mendelson BC. Face lift. Plast Reconstr Surg. 2011;128(6):747e–64e.

15. Winters R, Moulthrop T. Is autologous fat grafting superior to other fillers for facial rejuvenation? Laryngoscope. 2013;123(5):1068–9.
16. Clauser LC, Tieghi R, Galiè M, Carinci F. Structural fat grafting: facial volumetric restoration in complex reconstructive surgery. J Craniofac Surg. 2011;22(5):1695–701.
17. Niechajev I, Sevcuk O. Long-term results of fat transplantation: clinical and histologic studies. Plast Reconstr Surg. 1994;94(3):496–506.
18. Chajchir A, Benzaquen I, Moretti E. Comparative experimental study of autologous adipose tissue processed by different techniques. Aesth Plast Surg. 1993;17(2):113–5.
19. Botti G, Pascali M, Botti C, Bodog F, Cervelli V. A clinical trial in facial fat grafting: filtered and washed versus centrifuged fat. Plast Reconstr Surg. 2011;127(6):2464–73.
20. Gerth DJ, King B, Rabach L, et al. Long-term volumetric retention of autologous fat grafting processed with closed-membrane filtration. Aesthet Surg J. 2014;34(7):985–94.
21. Kuran I, Tumerdem B. A new simple method used to prepare fat for injection. Aesthetic Plast Surg. 2005;29(1):18–22. discussion 23.
22. Gatti JE. Permanent lip augmentation with serial fat grafting. Ann Plast Surg. 1999;42(4):376–80.
23. Lin TM, Lin TY, Chou CK, et al. Application of microautologous fat transplantation in the correction of sunken upper eyelid. Plast Reconstr Surg Glob Open. 2014;2(11):e259.

26 Fat Injections as Volumizer on the Face: Forehead

Halil Erdoğan, Saime Sagiroglu, and Gheorghe Muhlfay

26.1 Introduction

Contrary to the chin, the forehead has been largely overlooked or disregarded in its connection to the nose. Ousterhout [1] states that the primary role of the forehead is to communicate beauty, strength, intelligence, and a range of emotions. Techniques for modifying its shape include bony advancement, bone transplants, Silastic implants (Dow Corning, Midland, Mich.), and methyl methacrylate, the preferred approach at the time of publishing. A search on the internet for "forehead augmentation" produced a limited number of outcomes related to forehead augmentation using fat or methyl methacrylate. These results were only from Asian cosmetic websites [2–4], and none discussed the impact of the forehead on the nose. The review of forehead rejuvenation discussed the inclusion of forehead contouring in addition to conventional procedures [5, 6, 7].

H. Erdoğan (✉)
Private Practice, Aydın, Turkey

S. Sagiroglu
Department of Otolaryngology, Faculty of Medicine, Kahramanmaras Sutcu İmam University, Kahramanmaras, Turkey

G. Muhlfay
Department of Otolaryngology, University of Medicine and Pharmacy of Tirgu Mures, Tirgu Mures, Romania

C. Cingi et al. (eds.), *Minor Interventions, Major Outcomes on the Face*, Comprehensive ENT, https://doi.org/10.1007/978-3-032-01305-7_26

26.2 Anatomy

The process of aesthetic facial analysis commences by partitioning the face into several anatomic zones. Four hypothetical horizontal lines are marked: [1] at the front hairline [2], at the eyebrows [3], at the junction between the columella and the upper lip, and [4] at the border of the chin. It is ideal for equal vertical distances between lines 1 and 2, 2 and 3, and lines 3 and 4. This is frequently referred to as "the rule of thirds." Thus, the forehead encompasses the largest portion of the upper third of the face. However, it is surprisingly overlooked when it comes to improving aesthetics and reducing signs of aging. The forehead comprises four lamellar components: bone, muscle, fat pads, and skin [6]. Thus far, the modifications have primarily targeted the muscle and skin layers through neurotoxic injections, resurfacing techniques, and foreheadplasty. To achieve a balanced and enhanced facial appearance, it is crucial to focus on the bone and fat pads and consider the natural changes that occur with aging. While bone is challenging to replace and shape, autologous fat grafting and temporary dermal fillers can be used to address congenital deformities and the effects of aging. These procedures have been shown to directly impact the position and shape of various facial structures, such as the brow, glabella, and radix, resulting in a restoration of more natural anatomy [6].

The forehead is anatomically composed of the upper forehead and the supraorbital bar. These components play a role in determining the nasofrontal angle [1]. The forehead, glabella, and radix are three important components in aesthetic rhinoplasty that create the nasofrontal angle together. The relationship in question resembles the interaction between the upper lip, the columella, and the nasal tip, which indicates the nasolabial angle [6].

26.2.1 Forehead

The forehead is the uppermost area of the face. The outermost layer of the forehead consists of the epidermis. The fat pads are located in the deeper layers of the forehead. The central forehead fat pad is located precisely in the middle of the forehead. The intermediate forehead fat pad is situated laterally to the central forehead pad. The middle forehead fat pad is positioned above the orbits. The lateral temporal fat pad is the primary component of the upper face's outermost portion. The lateral temporal fat pad is located over the temporal regions and extends downward to the angle of the jaw [8].

The upper face's muscle layer is located beneath the fat pads. The procerus muscle, occipitofrontalis muscle, depressor supercilii muscle, and corrugator supercilii muscle comprise most of the forehead, while the temporal section houses the temporalis muscle. The procerus muscle has a pyramidal structure and extends from the nasal bone's lower portion to the forehead's middle portion. The procerus muscle is located in the region between the eyebrows and is connected to the frontalis muscle. The procerus muscle contracts to raise the eyebrows. The occipitofrontalis muscle extends across the entirety of the forehead. The occipitofrontalis muscle originates from the galea aponeurosis at the top and connects and merges with the orbicularis oculi muscle. The contraction of the occipitofrontalis muscle results in the elevation of the eyebrows and the formation of wrinkles on the forehead. The depressor supercilii muscle arises from the medial orbital border and inserts at the medial aspect of the bony orbit. The primary function of the depressor supercilii muscle is to lower or depress the position of the eyebrows. The corrugator supercilii muscle is a diminutive muscle that originates from the supraorbital ridge and attaches to the skin of the forehead close to the eyebrows. Contraction of the corrugator supercilii muscle causes the forehead to wrinkle. The temporalis muscle has its genesis at the parietal and sphenoidal bones. The temporalis muscle attaches to the coronoid process and the retromolar fossa. The temporalis muscle contracts, causing the jaw to move upward and backward [8].

The frontal bone primarily comprises the skeletal structure of the forehead, whereas the temporal and sphenoid bones contribute to the lateral region of the top face, specifically the temporal section [8].

26.2.2 Anatomic Descriptions of the Distinct Subcutaneous Facial Fat Compartments for the Forehead

1. *Central compartment*
   Depth: Superficial.
   Anatomical landmarks: The middle line of the forehead, bordered below by the nasal dorsum [9].
2. *Middle temporal fat compartments*
   Depth: Superficial.
   Anatomical landmarks: Bordered medially/laterally by central forehead fat and inferiorly by the orbicularis retaining ligament [9].
3. *Lateral temporal malar fat compartment*

   Depth: Superficial.
   Anatomical landmarks: Immediately superficial to the parotid gland, it connects the temporal fat to cervical fat [9].

26.3 Autologous Fat Transfer

Facial aging is a multifaceted and ever-changing process due to facial skin, bones, and subcutaneous soft tissue alterations. Comprehending these alterations is crucial for effectively reinstating the innate, appealing, and youthful face attributes in facial rejuvenation techniques. As a person ages, the bones in their face rotate in a clockwise direction concerning the base of the skull. This rotation causes the midface to move forward and upward while the maxilla (upper jaw) becomes larger and moves backward. Additionally, the opening of the eye socket becomes bigger, and the mandible (lower jaw) becomes smaller horizontally and vertically [10]. These modifications efficiently move the holding ligaments and soft tissue that covers the face, resulting in the reduction of specific facial fat compartments and the emergence of sagging skin and noticeable creases in the areas around the nose and mouth, eyes, and jawline [9, 11, 12].

Autologous fat grafting to the face is becoming increasingly common and is currently considered a dependable and effective treatment [13, 14]. It is widely used to restore volume to the aging face, either as a standalone treatment or combined with surgical treatments like facelifts and rhinoplasties. Facial atrophy, which involves the loss of soft tissues and changes in the facial bones' structure, directly impacts both the nasofrontal and the nasolabial angles [15–17]. Effective adipose tissue transplantation can address the aesthetic concerns related to aging and manage the progressive loss of facial volume [18, 19]. The senior author suggests that a gradual decrease in blood flow causes age-related bone atrophy. The vascular growth factors in fat cells that have been properly transplanted can slow down the continuous loss of bone [6].

Adipose tissue is vital in providing essential structural support to the facial region [9]. The lift-and-fill facelift has transformed how aesthetic surgery addresses the aging face according to these principles [20–22]. This approach involves fat transplantation to the deep and superficial layers of fat compartments, followed by modification of the superficial musculoaponeurotic system (SMAS) and platysma. Additional superficial fat grafting can be done on the forehead, temples, tear trough, oral commissure, chin, and other areas that need more volume. Unlike injectables not derived from the patient's body, fat grafting to these areas combines with facial tissues to produce a smoother, more natural-looking, and enduring enhancement in facial shape. Adipose-derived stem cells (ADSCs) can regenerate and enhance the quality of face tissue, leading to improvements in scars and sun damage over some time [9, 22, 23].

26.4 Evaluation and Planning

Modifications in the muscles of the forehead and glabellar region can be characterized as dynamic, exhibiting either an increase in size (hypertrophy) or a decrease in size (atrophy), typically due to regular use of neurotoxins. These changes can either enhance or reduce the volume of the soft tissues that cover them [24]. Collectively, these characteristics have a direct impact on the nasofrontal angle, which in turn directly affects the perceived length of the nose and its forward projection. Nevertheless, efforts to decrease a substantial radix by surgically removing bone and/or soft tissue have been shown to be less effective. Sheen and Sheen [25] and Daniel et al. [26] have reported that the response rate is 25%, meaning that for every 4 mm of resection, there is a 1 mm deepening. This is likely caused by inadequate repositioning of the skin on the glabellar area, which makes it challenging to enhance the depth of the radix.

Fat grafting can effectively impact the appearance of the nose when viewed from the front. Replenishing face volume, particularly in the malar area and the lateral facial fat pad, promptly and significantly diminishes the perceived size of the nose and enhances the balance among facial features [6].

An assessment of facial volume will determine the specific locations that need to be treated with fat grafting. An effective approach to achieve this is to divide the face into anatomical thirds and methodically evaluate crucial characteristics. The interface between the subcutaneous and deep fat compartments will become apparent as noticeable creases in the aging face and regions of excess soft tissue. It is crucial to distinguish aging characteristics that can be treated alone with fat grafting from those that necessitate additional surgical methods [9].

26.4.1 Upper Third

The key facial elements in the top third that experience notable transformations due to aging include the eyebrows, upper eyelids, and temples [11]. A young person's brow and top eyelid area are plump and curved, with a slight outward curve seamlessly blending into the temple region. The aging process is linked to the development of empty areas on the sides of the forehead and the drooping of the outer part of the eyebrows due to the loss of fat in the temporal region. Fat grafting on the temples and forehead can rejuvenate the temporal contour and elevate the lateral brow. This results in a more authentic look than a surgical brow lift, which primarily raises the inner brow [27]. Upper lid blepharoplasty is solely recommended for patients who have brow ptosis. Injecting fractionated fat after blepharoplasty can enhance the volume of the upper eyelid and promote skin regeneration [28].

26.5 The Process of Collecting Adipose Tissue from the Body

When selecting a donor site for fat grafting, it is important to consider the aesthetics of the donor site, the patient's desire, the surgical setting, the amount of fat required, and the amount of accessible fat. The lower belly and inner thighs, which have a significant abundance of adipose-derived stem cells (ADSCs), are the preferred areas for obtaining tissue for facial augmentation treatments. Around 30 mL of fat is typically needed for most facial rejuvenation and contouring procedures [29, 30].

The preferred method for extracting fat is syringe aspiration, which involves using a 10-mL Luer-Lok syringe connected to a harvesting cannula. The harvesting efficiency is enhanced by using a modified multihole Coleman cannula, which generates negative pressure when the syringe plunger is retracted [11, 23]. To achieve the extraction of fat lobules of the correct size, it is important to utilize a small cannula (12 gauge) with small holes (1 × 1 mm) when working on the face, since it is a region that is sensitive to volume changes [31]. The locations for cannula insertion should be chosen carefully in inconspicuous places, such as the umbilicus (for obtaining tissue from the lower abdomen) or the inguinal line (for obtaining tissue from the medial thigh). To prevent injury to the rectus fascia and provide a smooth post-procedure contour, it is important to avoid inserting the cannula too deeply and to collect fat uniformly [9, 11].

26.6 Fat Refinement and Purification

Centrifugation is commonly the favored technique for refining fat [11]. Centrifugation enables the segregation and consolidation of broken fat cells (the oil component) and blood and local anesthetic (the water component) from undamaged fat cells. The centrifuge is used to spin unprocessed fat for no more than 1 min at a speed of 2250 rpm. The water and oil fractions containing traces of blood are removed, and a Telfa strip or Codman neuropad is inserted into the barrel to absorb any remaining oil [23]. After centrifugation, fractionated fat needs to undergo mechanical emulsification by forcing the fat between two syringes that are joined by a Luer-Lok connector [32, 33]. Refined fat can then be put into 1-mL syringes for accurate injection. Fat with a higher density has been shown to have a higher success rate when grafting than fat with a lower density. Therefore, it is recommended to prioritize using higher density fat [9, 32, 34]. The aging process leads to changes in soft tissues that require increasing the volume, lifting sagging tissues, and removing excess tissue [35].

26.7 Fat Placement

Optimizing the precision of fat distribution and reducing the risk of problems such as fibrosis, calcification, infections, or oil cyst formation requires infusing a small amount of fat with each injection [30]. During each injection, injecting no more than 0.5 to 1 mL of fat per second is recommended. Injections should be done in several tissue planes and in various orientations while always being mindful of the cannula tip [35–37]. Furthermore, it is important to exercise caution to prevent any potential harm to neighboring veins and nerves. When administering injections to smaller areas of the face, such as the periorbital region, it is advisable to use a smaller cannula to control the amount of volume injected [30]. The injection of fat will result in immediate and noticeable face enlargement. If factors limit the volume, such as fibrotic adhesions or a tight skin envelope, it may be necessary to perform dissection using an 18-gauge needle or a forked tip cannula [30]. The deep compartments can be reached by moving to the side of the alar-cheek junction [9, 38].

26.8 Conclusion

Autologous fat grafting can be consistently and reliably employed to change the nasofrontal and nasolabial angles by targeting the forehead/glabellar/radix complex and pyriform aperture, respectively [6].

References

1. Ousterhout DK. Aesthetic contouring of the craniofacial skeleton. 1st ed. San Francisco: Little, Brown and Co; 1991.
2. Park DK, Song I, Lee JH, et al. Forehead augmentation with a methyl methacrylate onlay implant using an injection-molding technique. Arch Plast Surg. 2013;40:597–602.
3. Grand Plastic Surgery. Forehead augmentation through fat grafting GRAND plastic surgery. Available at: http://eng.grandsurgery.com/forehead-augmentation-through-fat-grafting/. Accessed 12 June 2014.
4. ID Hospital. Forehead augmentation. Available at: http://eng.idhospital.com/face/face0601.php. Accessed 12 June 2014.
5. Guyuron B, Lee M. A reappraisal of surgical techniques and efficacy in forehead rejuvenation. Plast Reconstr Surg. 2014;134:426–35.
6. Kornstein AN, Nikfarjam JS. Fat grafting to the forehead/glabella/radix complex and pyriform aperture: aesthetic and anti-aging implications. Plast Reconstr Surg Glob Open. 2015;3(8):e500.
7. Guyuron B. Patient assessment. In: Guyuron B, Eriksson E, Persing JA, editors. Plastic surgery: indications and practice. 1st ed. Philadelphia: Saunders Elsevier; 2009. p. 1341–51.
8. Nguyen JD, Duong H. Anatomy, head and neck: face. [Updated 2022 Jun 11]. In: StatPearls [Internet]. Treasure Island: StatPearls Publishing; 2023. Available from: https://www.ncbi.nlm.nih.gov/books/NBK551530/.
9. Schultz KP, Raghuram A, Davis MJ, Abu-Ghname A, Chamata E, Rohrich RJ. Fat grafting for facial rejuvenation. Semin Plast Surg. 2020;34(1):30–7.
10. Farkas JP, Pessa JE, Hubbard B, Rohrich RJ. The science and theory behind facial aging. Plast Reconstr Surg Glob Open. 2013;1(01):e8–e15.
11. Glasgold R, Glasgold M, Lam S. Complementary fat grafting. Berlin, Heidelberg: Springer; 2018. p. 321–32.
12. Rohrich RJPJ, Pessa JE. The fat compartments of the face: anatomy and clinical implications for cosmetic surgery. Plast Reconstr Surg. 2007;119(07):2219–27. discussion 2228–2231.
13. Monreal J. Fat grafting to the nose: personal experience with 36 patients. Aesth Plast Surg. 2011;35:916–22.
14. Baptista C, Nguyen PS, Desouches C, et al. Correction of sequelae of rhinoplasty by lipofilling. J Plast Reconstr Aesthet Surg. 2013;66:805–11.
15. Moody M, Ross AT. Rhinoplasty in the aging patient. Facial Plast Surg. 2006;22:112–9.
16. Pessa JE, Desvigne LD, Zadoo VP. The effect of skeletal remodeling on the nasal profile: considerations for rhinoplasty in the older patient. Aesth Plast Surg. 1999;23:239–42.
17. Pessa JE, Peterson ML, Thompson JW, et al. Pyriform augmentation as an ancillary procedure in facial rejuvenation surgery. Plast Reconstr Surg. 1999;103:683–6.
18. Kornstein A, Nikfarjam JS. Facial rejuvenation with fat cells. In: Herman CK, Strauch B, editors. Encyclopedia of aesthetic rejuvenation through, vol. Enhancement. 1st ed. New York: Thieme; 2014. p. 52–9.
19. McArdle A, Senarath-Yapa K, Walmsley GG, et al. The role of stem cells in aesthetic surgery: fact or fiction? Plast Reconstr Surg. 2014;134:193–200.
20. Rohrich RJ, Ghavami A, Constantine FC, Unger J, Mojallal A. Lift-and-fill face lift: integrating the fat compartments. Plast Reconstr Surg. 2014;133(06):756e–67e.
21. DeFatta RJ, Williams EF III. Fat transfer in conjunction with facial rejuvenation procedures. Facial Plast Surg Clin North Am. 2008;1604:383–90.
22. Marten TJ, Elyassnia D. Fat grafting in facial rejuvenation. Clin Plast Surg. 2015;42(02):219–52.
23. Coleman SR, Katzel EB. Fat grafting for facial filling and regeneration. Clin Plast Surg. 2015;42(03):289–300.
24. Rohrich RJ, Hollier LH Jr, Janis JE, et al. Rhinoplasty with advancing age. Plast Reconstr Surg. 2004;114:1936–44.

25. Sheen J, Sheen A. Aesthetic Rhinoplasty, vol. 1. 2nd ed. St Louis: Mosby; 1987.
26. Daniel RK, Kosins A, Sajjadian A, et al. Rhinoplasty and brow modification: a powerful combination. Aesthet Surg J. 2013;10:1–12.
27. Chiu CH. Objective evaluation of eyebrow position after autologous fat grafting to the temple and forehead. Aesth Plast Surg. 2017;41(06):1342–50.
28. Rohrich RJ, Villanueva NL, Afrooz PN. Refinements in upper blepharoplasty: the five-step technique. Plast Reconstr Surg. 2018;141(05):1144–6.
29. Khan HA, Keyhan SO. Fat grafting in facial aesthetic units. Atlas Oral Maxillofac Surg Clin North Am. 2018;26(01):15–23.
30. Pu LLQ. Fat grafting for facial rejuvenation and contouring: a rationalized approach. Ann Plast Surg. 2018;81(6S, Suppl 1):S102–8.
31. Del Vecchio D, Rohrich RJ. A classification of clinical fat grafting: different problems, different solutions. Plast Reconstr Surg. 2012;130(03):511–22.
32. Rohrich RJ, Durand PD, Dayan E. The lift-and-fill facelift: superficial musculoaponeurotic system manipulation with fat compartment augmentation. Clin Plast Surg. 2019;46(04):515–22.
33. Rohrich RJ, Mahedia M, Shah N, Afrooz P, Vishvanath L, Gupta RK. Role of fractionated fat in blending the lid-cheek junction. Plast Reconstr Surg. 2018;142(01):56–65.
34. Allen RJ, Canizares O Jr, Scharf C, et al. Grading lipoaspirate: is there an optimal density for fat grafting? Plast Reconstr Surg. 2013;131(01):38–45.
35. Coleman SR. Structural fat grafting: more than a permanent filler. Plast Reconstr Surg. 2006;118(3, Suppl):108S–20S.
36. Lee JH, Kirkham JC, McCormack MC, Nicholls AM, Randolph MA, Austen WG Jr. The effect of pressure and shear on autologous fat grafting. Plast Reconstr Surg. 2013;131(05):1125–36.
37. Xie Y, Zheng DN, Li QF, et al. An integrated fat grafting technique for cosmetic facial contouring. J Plast Reconstr Aesthet Surg. 2010;63(02):270–6.
38. Rohrich RJ, Afrooz PN. Finesse in facial lifting: the role of facial fat compartment augmentation in facial rejuvenation. Plast Reconstr Surg. 2019;143(01):98–101.

Fat Injections as Volumizer on the Face: Periorbital Region

27

Fatma Ceyda Akın Öcal, Mumtaz Taner Torun, and Murat Songu

27.1 Introduction

Fat grafting is a procedure that involves injecting collected fatty tissue beneath the skin to repair or reconstruct deformities caused by trauma, cancer, or birth abnormalities. The method can also be employed for aesthetic reasons, specifically facial revitalization. Autologous fat grafting (AFG) is a process in which fat is taken from the recipient's body and then used for transplantation. This is the most typical scenario in clinical practice. Autologous fat is often regarded as the optimal substance for face rejuvenation due to its complete biocompatibility, ability to provide a soft and natural outcome, and potential for permanent effects. This activity examines the effectiveness of this treatment for rejuvenating the face. It emphasizes the importance of a team of professionals in maintaining and enhancing the care of patients with autologous fat grafting [1].

27.2 Anatomy of the Orbital Region: Correlation with Risky Areas

The glabella and nasal root region provide a significant risk when administering cutaneous filler injections on the face. Although it has a rich blood supply, this region is distinct from other facial parts because it exhibits two different

F. C. A. Öcal (✉)
Gulhane Faculty of Medicine, Department of Otorhinolaryngology, University of Health Sciences, Ankara, Turkey

M. T. Torun
Bandırma 17 Eylül University, Department of Otorhinolaryngology, Bandirma, Turkey

M. Songu
Songu Private Clinic, Izmir, Turkey

C. Cingi et al. (eds.), *Minor Interventions, Major Outcomes on the Face*, Comprehensive ENT, https://doi.org/10.1007/978-3-032-01305-7_27

occurrences. Despite a complex network of blood arteries, many of the vessels in the area are located close to the surface and have smaller branches at their ends. This increases susceptibility to necrosis, which can occur due to the movement of emboli toward the forehead and the blood flow restriction caused by external compression. The supraorbital artery exits the orbit by the supraorbital foramen, whereas the supratrochlear artery emerges through the upper and medial part of the orbit. Both arteries appear in the glabella region, in front of the corrugator supercilii muscle and behind the orbicularis oculi muscle. Afterward, both arteries travel briefly toward the frontal muscle and emerge closer to the surface [2].

Another significant occurrence involves the anastomoses network seen in the glabellar and periorbital regions, particularly in the medial portion. This finally raises the likelihood of embolism in the central retinal artery. Topical administration in this area may access blood vessels connected to the internal carotid system, ultimately reaching the ocular artery in a reverse direction and, subsequently, the central retinal artery. The autonomic nervous system regulates blood flow in the ophthalmic artery. When the cervical sympathetic receptors are stimulated, the blood flow in the ophthalmic artery decreases.

Conversely, sympathectomy leads to an increase in blood flow. On the other hand, the central retinal artery is a final blood vessel that possesses a distinct method of self-regulation and is not influenced by the autonomic nervous system. Therefore, changes in the ophthalmic artery's blood flow directly impact the central retinal artery. The anastomoses between the systems assist in controlling and sustaining the blood supply to the central nervous system [3].

However, the secondary vascular axis is triggered when the flow is decreased. When the internal carotid artery is narrowing, the blood flow can change direction. This means that even if the patient has no symptoms, there is a higher risk of an embolism that could travel to the central retinal artery—dangers associated with dermal filler procedures in the orbital area. Cutaneous fillings often lead to consequences primarily related to circulation problems. The locations that are more commonly damaged and pose a higher risk of ischemia or embolization in the orbital-palpebral region, leading to blindness, include: The nasojugal sulcus is a region where blood circulation occurs in the eyelid through an anastomosis of the branches of the ophthalmic artery. Specifically, it is supplied laterally by the lacrimal artery, which originates from the lateral palpebral branches, and medially by the branches of the medial palpebral artery, which originates from the upper and lower eyelid arteries. The medial and lateral palpebral arteries connect, creating two marginal and peripheral arches. The marginal arch is located 3 mm away from the palpebral edge, directly across from the tarsus. The peripheral arch is located in the upper eyelid, between the aponeurosis of the eyelid levator muscle and the Müller muscle. It is situated above the superior border of the tarsus. The location of the lower eyelid may vary. This lower and middle region is consequently one of the locations that provide a risk for embolization after the application of cutaneous filling in the nasojugal sulcus [2].

Glabella

The supraorbital and supratrochlear arteries are located close to the surface in the glabella region. Additionally, the glabellar area has little blood vessel formation due to its primarily terminal circulation. Consequently, the tiny arteries can be easily blocked when injecting exterior and interior filling materials. The superficial course of these arteries is the most susceptible area, posing a significant risk of intravascular injection [2].

The medial portion of the orbit

The medial portion of the orbit is the area adjacent to the nasojugal sulcus's upper part and the nasal root's lateral part. In this region, the angular artery, a branch of the facial artery (a branch of the external carotid artery), passes. The angular artery connects with the dorsal nasal artery, the final branch of the ophthalmic artery. Currently, in individuals with thin skin, it is feasible to observe the angular vein, which is positioned significantly closer to the center than the angular artery. The angular artery and vein intersect the medial canthal tendon and connect with branches of the ophthalmic arteries above the superior edge of the tendon. These sites have one of the connections to the carotid system, which allows clots to go backward and reach the central artery of the retina. Due to its connection with the ophthalmic artery, if clots from the injected filling product are released, they can travel in the opposite direction and reach the central retinal artery. This can result in a disruption of the normal blood flow in the ophthalmic artery. Several studies indicate that the secondary vascular axis of anastomosis between the internal carotid artery (ICA) and external carotid artery (ECA), which causes the ophthalmic artery to flow in the opposite direction, becomes active in cases of hemodynamically significant stenosis of the ICA. This is supported by Doppler records showing retrograde flow in the ophthalmic arteries [3].

Consequently, this raises doubts about whether certain people, including those without symptoms, may have a constantly active reverse flow, leading to a higher likelihood of issues associated with fillings in the skin in this area, which can impact the central retinal artery. Hence, knowing the initial indications of embolic or ischemic consequences is crucial, such as pain and localized paleness, increased blood flow or discoloration, visual distortion, and vision loss. As mentioned before, the thickness of the skin on the eyelid and its relationship with the orbicularis muscle, along with the lack of subcutaneous tissue, increase the possibility of less significant but unwanted issues in the area, such as the implant being easily visible in the eyelid region [2].

27.3 Periorbital Fat Grafting (Injection)

The periorbital area presents technical challenges. Hence, inexperienced fat grafters should adopt a cautious approach. It is essential to avoid placing many fat parcels at once. It is crucial to go slowly by injecting small amounts of fat. The initial infiltration should be performed intensely along the orbital rim, followed by the placement of the second layer only superficially to it. To prevent the formation of noticeable or obvious lumps, injections should be administered beneath the orbicularis oculi muscle, as the skin of the eyelid is fragile [2].

Autologous fat grafting (AFG) has become increasingly recognized in plastic, reconstructive, and aesthetic eyelid surgeries due to its significant advantages over traditional treatments. AFG offers a minimally invasive approach that results in less pain and fewer complications [4, 5]. Lipofilling is a surgical technique involving adipose tissue harvested from the hip, abdomen, or inner thigh to reconstruct and augment a sunken eyelid. The Coleman approach was the most widely utilized method. However, not all investigations were exclusively focused on this technique; they implemented a few specific alterations. Pelle-Ceravolo Mario and Angelini Matteo mixed 70% fat with saline and infranatant fluid to enhance the compatibility of fat with the texture of the periocular location [6]. A recent study conducted by Rohrich et al. showed that the lipoaspirate should be placed in a centrifuge for a maximum of 1 min (at 2250 rpm) and low pressure. This process helps to enhance the amount and viability of adipose-derived mesenchymal stem cells, improving skin quality [7]. Gennai et al. [8] suggested that using a cannula with a tiny port size of 0.5 mm resulted in improved effectiveness and viability of collected fat compared to using a cannula with an even smaller side-port size of 0.3 mm for correcting aging/thin skin in the periocular region.

The strong demand has been reduced primarily due to ambiguity regarding anatomical safety resulting from its unique placement, which has limited its use in recent years. Prior research on this subject did not use randomized controlled trials (RCTs) due to practical and ethical considerations. In 2016, Boudreaux et al. conducted a comprehensive study that examined the indications, operational methods, and complications associated with eyelid fat grafting [9]. The study included data from 16 studies that documented the use of AFG in individuals with eyelid issues. The majority of the publications included in the study were case series, whereas only five studies were case reports. Therefore, we have revised the evidence. The survival of adipocytes partially relies on the nutrients supplied to the outside regions of the fat graft. If the central graft is too far from the blood vessels, it will perish [10]. The present study is centered on tissue regeneration, explicitly using additive agents, enhancers, or scaffolds for adipose tissue. For instance, the pairing of adipose stem cells (ASCs) with vascular endothelial growth factor (VEGF) can stimulate the formation of new blood vessels while also decreasing inflammation and the development of scar tissue in the surrounding area [11]. In nanofat injection, the procedure involves removing the nonliving portion of fat cells and injecting only the pure stromal vascular fraction to revitalize the skin around the eyes [12].

Furthermore, Stromal Vascular Fraction-gel (SVF) exhibits a greater density of ASC and other SVF cells than Coleman fat [13]. Therefore, it can serve as a viable option. However, additional in vitro studies are required to fully understand the underlying fat grafting process.

The atraumatic transfer of fat is the critical principle in surgical management. The viability of the graft is influenced by damage to the fatty tissue during the fat harvesting or transplantation procedure. Although an initially unsuccessful graft may have resolved the issue, the subsequent tissue absorption nullifies the outcome. The presence of any blood in the collected fat further accelerates the breakdown of the implanted lipograft. The procedure consists of three main stages: graft harvesting, transfer, and placement [14].

Equipment

The procedure of autologous fat grafting necessitates the utilization of the subsequent equipment [1]:

The wetting or tumescent solution consists of 500 mL of normal saline, 25 mL of lidocaine with a concentration of 1–2%, and 0.5 mL of epinephrine with a ratio of 1:100,000 or 1:200,000.

- Topical analgesic (lidocaine or bupivacaine).
- An infiltration needle or cannula is utilized to deliver local anesthetic to the cannula's entry sites and supply the wetting/tumescent solution to the locations where grafts are harvested.
- Fat harvesting and donor cannulas—the Coleman type 2 (side-port cannula) is the most often utilized injection cannula. The optimal length for face injections is between 5 and 9 cm. The cannula selection, which includes the gauge and size, primarily relies on the location where the graft will be placed, as well as the injector's expertise and personal preferences.
- Luer-lock syringes: These are giant syringes, often 10 mL or 20 mL in size, used for harvesting. Additionally, multiple 1 mL syringes are used for injecting. A closed suction machine can be utilized as a substitute for syringes when collecting substantial quantities of fat. However, it is essential to note that using low-strength suction for harvesting enormous amounts of fat may cause stress and compromise the integrity of the collected fat.
- The following items are required for the fat injection procedure:
  - A plug to seal the Luer-lock while loading fat into the syringes.
  - A #11 or #15 blade scalpel to create an entry site for the harvest cannulas.
  - An 18 ga needle to create an entry site for the fat injection.
  - Sterile skin markers.
  - Gauze.
  - A compression garment.
  - A Luer-to-Luer connector specifically for micro-fat and nanofat is used for skin regeneration.

Analyzing

The choice of fat processing method (such as sedimentation, filtering, washing, and centrifugation) may necessitate the following steps [1]:

- 1 mL syringes equipped with absorbent material such as non-adherent gauze to soak up excess oil.

- Commercial kit for preparing fat grafts.
- Strainer and saline solution.
- Use a centrifuge at 3000 revolutions per minute for 3 min to separate the fat and reduce damage [1].

27.4 Clinical Significance

The face plays a crucial role in defining a person's identity, and an appealing face enhances self-confidence, credibility, friendliness, and even individual achievements. Autologous fat grafting is a highly effective technique reconstructive surgeons use to rejuvenate the face. Autologous facial fat is the preferred filler for facial rejuvenation because of its long-lasting effects, cost-effectiveness, compatibility with the body, low risk, and high satisfaction rates compared to alternative materials [15–17].

Autologous fat grafting is a complex procedure that involves assessing the places where the fat will be transferred and the areas from which the fat will be taken. The fat is then collected, treated, and injected into the recipient area. Any mistakes, inaccuracies, or exclusions throughout these stages could hurt the final result. Due to the individuality of each patient and treatment, the physician must convey the specific equipment requirements, such as cannulae and apparatus for harvesting, processing, and transfer, to the surgical team before the procedure. Nurses and other team members must be able to proficiently convey their expectations regarding the surgery and any consequences to the patient. Before the treatment, it is essential to address and clarify any misunderstandings or confusion the patient may have [18].

If imaging is acquired, it should be reviewed with a radiologist to clarify any anatomical abnormalities. Collaboration is crucial for people who have experienced facial trauma or other medical conditions. When fat grafting is included in a complex surgical procedure such as face reconstruction, it may be required to collaborate with maxillofacial surgeons, orthopedic surgeons, orthodontists, and interventional radiologists [1].

References

1. Vasavada A, Raggio BS. Autologous fat grafting for facial rejuvenation. [Updated 2023 Feb 14]. In: StatPearls [Internet]. Treasure Island: StatPearls Publishing; 2023. Available from: https://www.ncbi.nlm.nih.gov/books/NBK557860/. Accessed online at 10 June 2023.
2. Palermo EC. Anatomy of the periorbital region. Surg Cosmet Dermatol. 2013;5(3):24556.
3. Diniz ALD, Moron AF, Santos MC, Sass N. Dopplervelocimetria colorida dos vasos orbitais: técnica de exame e anatomia vascular normal. Radiol Bras. 2004;37(4):287–90.
4. Yang F, Ji Z, Peng L, Fu T, Liu K, Dou W, Li J, Li Y, Long Y, Zhang W. Efficacy, safety and complications of autologous fat grafting to the eyelids and periorbital area: a systematic review and meta-analysis. PLoS One. 2021;16(4):e0248505.
5. Cetinkaya A, Devoto MH. Periocular fat grafting: indications and techniques. Curr Opin Ophthalmol. 2013;24(5):494–9. Epub 2013/08/09. pmid:23925063.

6. Pelle-Ceravolo M, Angelini M. Properly diluted fat (PDF): an easy and safe approach to periocular fat grafting. Aesthet Surg J. 2020;40(1):19–33. Epub 2019/02/13. pmid:30753276.
7. Rohrich RJ, Mahedia M, Shah N, Afrooz P, Vishvanath L, Gupta RK. Role of fractionated fat in blending the lid-cheek junction. Plast Reconstr Surg. 2018;142(1):56–65. Epub 2018/06/08. pmid:29878987.
8. Gennai A, Zambelli A, Repaci E, Quarto R, Baldelli I, Fraternali G, et al. Skin rejuvenation and volume enhancement with the micro superficial enhanced fluid fat injection (M-SEFFI) for skin aging of the periocular and perioral regions. Aesthet Surg J. 2017;37(1):14–23. Epub 2016/06/01. pmid:27241362.
9. Boureaux E, Chaput B, Bannani S, Herlin C, De Runz A, Carloni R, et al. Eyelid fat grafting: indications, operative technique and complications; a systematic review. J Craniomaxillofac Surg. 2016;44(4):374–80. Epub 2016/02/18.
10. Hsu VM, Stransky CA, Bucky LP, Percec I. Fat grafting's past, present, and future: why adipose tissue is emerging as a critical link to the advancement of regenerative medicine. Aesthet Surg J. 2012;32(7):892–9. Epub 2012/09/04. pmid:22942117.
11. Behr B, Tang C, Germann G, Longaker MT, Quarto N. Locally applied vascular endothelial growth factor A increases the osteogenic healing capacity of human adipose-derived stem cells by promoting osteogenic and endothelial differentiation. Stem Cells. 2011;29(2):286–96. Epub 2011/07/07. pmid:21732486.
12. Tonnard P, Verpaele A, Peeters G, Hamdi M, Cornelissen M, Declercq H. Nanofat grafting: basic research and clinical applications. Plast Reconstr Surg. 2013;132(4):1017–26. Epub 2013/06/21. pmid:23783059.
13. Jiang S, Quan Y, Wang J, Cai J, Lu F. Fat grafting for facial rejuvenation using stromal vascular fraction gel injection. Clin Plast Surg. 2020;47(1):73–9. Epub 2019/11/20. pmid:31739900.
14. Gampper TJ. Facial fat grafting treatment & management. In: Granick MS, editor. Medscape. Updated: Feb 11, 2021. https://emedicine.medscape.com/article/1283020-treatment#d10. Accessed online at 10 June 2023.
15. Obagi S, Willis C. Autologous fat augmentation of the face. Atlas Oral Maxillofac Surg Clin North Am. 2018;26(1):41–50.
16. Groen JW, Krastev TK, Hommes J, Wilschut JA, Ritt MJPF, van der Hulst RRJW. Autologous fat transfer for facial rejuvenation: a systematic review on technique, efficacy, and satisfaction. Plast Reconstr Surg Glob Open. 2017;5(12):e1606.
17. Krastev TK, Beugels J, Hommes J, Piatkowski A, Mathijssen I, van der Hulst R. Efficacy and safety of autologous fat transfer in facial reconstructive surgery: a systematic review and meta-analysis. JAMA Facial Plast Surg. 2018;20(5):351–60. [PMC free article].
18. Coleman SR, Lam S, Cohen SR, Bohluli B, Nahai F. Fat grafting: challenges and debates. Atlas Oral Maxillofac Surg Clin North Am. 2018;26(1):81–4.

Fat Injections as Volumizer on the Face: Middle Third of the Face

28

Mustafa Yazir, Murat Songu, and İbrahim Cukurova

28.1 Introduction

One of the most popular uses for dermal fillers made of hyaluronic acid is rejuvenating the midface. This is because full upper cheeks and a prominent extension of the malar arch play significant roles in conveying an impression of freshness. Over the last 20 years, hyaluronic acid fillers have advanced significantly, addressing specific therapeutic needs such as adaptability to facial dynamics and strong projection capabilities. Their potential for noninvasive treatment, rapid results, and minimal downtime has made them the preferred choice for midface rejuvenation treatments for individuals of all ages. This noninvasive treatment potential is a significant factor in their popularity. Injecting the midface region may also indirectly address infraorbital hollowing and nasolabial folds, among other cosmetic concerns, due to the crucial role of the five-layered structure in the human face. This is particularly important as the midface attracts the most attention. Nevertheless, an in-depth understanding of anatomy and a personalized treatment plan are crucial for achieving natural results in midface rejuvenation while minimizing risks [1].

M. Yazir (✉)
Yazir Private Clinic, Izmir, Turkey

M. Songu
Songu Private Clinic, Izmir, Turkey

İ. Cukurova
İzmir University of Health Sciences, Tepecik Training and Research Hospital, Department of Otorhinolaryngology, Izmir, Turkey

C. Cingi et al. (eds.), *Minor Interventions, Major Outcomes on the Face*, Comprehensive ENT, https://doi.org/10.1007/978-3-032-01305-7_28

28.2 Multilayer Anatomy of the Midface and Changes Due to Aging

28.2.1 Superficial Fat Compartments

The midface's superficial adipose compartments form a living, breathing soft tissue layer that moves in harmony with the deeper muscles. This layer lies just beneath the dermis. The skin is firmly attached to the muscles via surface fat pads [2–5]. The connective tissue fibers extending to the dermis support this connection. Due to changes in volume distribution, four superficial fat pads significantly impact the signs of midface aging. The nasolabial fat compartment (NLF), middle cheek fat compartment (MiCF), infraorbital fat compartment (IOF), and medial cheek fat compartment (MCF) represent various fat pads [1]. The inferior orbital follicles (IOF) and the superficial extension of the orbicularis retention ligament (ORL), along with the inferior eyelid, define the superior limits of the connection between the medial cheek fat compartment (MCF) and IOF. As we age, the IOF atrophies, giving the orbital rim a bony appearance and potentially worsening tear trough deformities [6, 7].

Overlying the lateral portion of the deep medial cheek fat (DMCF), the middle cheek fat (MCF) occupies the central region of the cheek. In contrast to the fullening of the nasolabial fat, the mid-cheek concavity and groove may deepen and become more noticeable with time due to MCF atrophy [8].

The medial direction of the MiCF is closely connected to the MCF. In contrast, the lateral direction relates to the temporal cheek fat, while the superior direction is associated with the superficial extension of the zygomatic cutaneous ligament (ZCL). Volume loss in the MiCF due to aging typically exacerbates MCF depression in most cases [1]. Finally, in the midface, you will find the NLF, which is the most superficial fat compartment. On the side facing the medial aspect of this fat pad are the nasal wall, the nasolabial septum, and the levator labii superior alaeque nasi muscle. On the opposite side, it connects to the medial cheek septum, the IOF, and the MCF when viewed from the side. The NLF widens and compresses less than the adjacent fat compartments over time. In older patients, this more noticeably accentuates the nasolabial folds and nasojugal grooves [1, 7–9].

28.2.2 Facial Muscles and Superficial Musculoaponeurotic System

The superficial musculoaponeurotic system (SMAS) transmits muscle contractions to the skin, which is crucial for facial expression. Given that the superficial fat pads are tightly connected to the underlying muscle layer, it is essential to thoroughly understand the dynamic nature of this region when filling the superficial fat. This understanding is necessary to prevent any unpleasant lumpy appearance when the muscles are activated, such as when smiling [1]. This layer of soft tissue lies just below the superficial fat compartments and consists of facial muscles and tissue resembling ligaments. The aponeurosis is made up of three laminae: [1] a very thin fascia on the surface of the muscles [2], the mimetic muscles, and [3] a thicker fascia at the bottom of the muscles. When no muscles are present, fascias 1 and 3 fuse together [8, 10]. The superficial layer of facial muscles includes the orbicularis oculi muscle (OOM), the levator labii superioris, the levator labii superior alaeque nasi, the zygomaticus minor, and notably, the depressor anguli oris, the platysma, and the risorius. All of these muscles are located in the midface region. The deeper layer consists of the levator anguli oris and the buccinator [11].

28.2.3 Deep Fat Compartments

Three deep fat compartments are attached to the bone in the middle of the face, providing structural support to the soft tissue layers above them (SMAS and superficial fat). The deflation of the upper cheeks that occurs due to the atrophy of these compartments is thus a consequence of aging [12]. In recent anatomical research, it was discovered that the fat in the deep sub-orbicularis oculi is systematically divided into two distinct compartments: the medial compartment and the lateral compartment [8, 13]. The medial sub-orbicularis oculi fat, also known as mSOOF, is a triangular fat compartment that extends from the lateral canthal line to the maxillary bone. A vertical septum separates it from the lateral superior orbital fossa, while the orbital ossicles (ORL) delineate it from the pre-septal region of the inferior eyelid. Additionally, the medial ZCL connects to the mSOOF, which is located inferiorly. In conclusion, the deep fascia of the OOM creates a "hermetic" cover by fusing with the ligaments surrounding the mSOOF, ultimately encompassing the mSOOF. The lateral sub-orbicularis oculi fat, also known as lSOOF, is situated laterally to the vertical septum and covers the prominence of the zygomatic bone. It also meets the temporal fat laterally. Its inferior boundary consists of the buccal fat pad and the lateral zone of the lumbar region [8]. Besides the authors' observations, published anatomical evidence primarily supports the concept that the SOOF directly adheres to the bone [8, 14, 15]. This is despite specific interpretations of the periorbital architecture differentiating the SOOF from a deeper pre-periosteal fat. Lastly, the triangular-shaped DMCF directly overlies the maxillary bone beneath the superficial MCF and the SMAS. Occasionally, the DMCF is depicted as two distinct compartments, namely the medial and lateral DMCF, which are separated by the levator anguli oris [16].

28.3 Ligaments and Septa

As they extend from the facial skeleton, the orofacial ligaments (ORL), tear trough ligament, zona occludens (ZCL), buccal-maxillary ligaments, and mandibular ligaments penetrate the submaxillary artery (SMAS) and subsequently insert into and disperse within the dermis [17–20]. Currently, these ligaments are referred to by medical professionals as "true" retaining ligaments. The age-related loosening of this ligamentous system may contribute to the gravitational descent of surface tissues [17]. The tear trough deformity and the palpebromalar groove are most often caused by a weak orofacial ligament (ORL) [1, 6]. This is true, even though not enough is understood about the role ligaments play in facial aging.

28.4 Anatomical Dangers

To reduce the likelihood of issues related to vascular injuries, it is essential to have a comprehensive understanding of the anatomy of the blood vessels running through or near the midface area, including their depth and course. We recommend using two anatomical lines: the mid-cheek safety line, which stretches from the medial canthus to the mandibular angle, and the lateral safety line, which travels vertically from the center of the zygomatic arch [1]. This aligns with the typical path of critical neurovascular structures. The facial structure is significantly improved by the presence of fat. Therefore, volume augmentation, resuspending ptotic tissue, and removing excess tissue are necessary due to age-related changes in soft tissue [21].

Facial Artery

The face receives most of its blood flow from the facial artery (FA). Beginning in the submaxillary area, it descends from the external carotid artery until it reaches the face. The route it takes as it swoops up on you is truly unique from one person to the next [22–25].

According to current anatomical studies, the majority of FAs end their journeys at the angular artery (36.6% of the population), lateral nasal artery (48.6% of the population), or superior labial artery (8.5%). The FA travels along the nasolabial fold. Conversely, 6.8% of patients with a hypoplastic FA have it terminating at the inferior labial artery. Additionally, about 30% of individuals have an FA that splits into an infraorbital trunk and a nasolabial trunk; the infraorbital trunk then flows vertically toward the nasojugal groove [23, 24].

Infraorbital Artery

Two or three main branches—the palpebral, nasal, and labial—emerge from the infraorbital foramen after the emergence of the infraorbital artery. The next two branches also originate in the DMCF; they serve the superior labial and lateral nasal areas, respectively, but their circulation mainly occurs below the mid-cheek safety line [26].

Specifically, the opening of the infraorbital foramen angles downward in relation to the maxilla. Therefore, to avoid cutting the artery, this area should not be approached from below at an angle [27].

Superficial Temporal Artery (STA)

A major artery that provides blood flow to the parietal and temporal areas originates in the parotid gland. It ascends superficially along the auriculotemporal nerve and the accompanying vein from the tragus of the ear to the posterior root of the zygomatic arch. The frontal and parietal lobes emerge from it afterward [28]. As long as the injector remains within the lateral safety line, these neurons and blood vessels pose no threat [1].

Transverse Facial Artery (TFA)

One of the main blood supplies to the cheeks is the transverse FA (TFA), in addition to the FA [29]. Anatomical studies indicate that, in most individuals, the superficial temporal artery gives rise to a single TFA, which divides into a superior emerging branch and a deep emerging branch. The latter supplies the masseter, parotid duct, and parotid gland [30]. Caution is essential when injecting subcutaneous fat into the lateral cheek's superficial fat [31], due to the location of the superior emerging branch.

Zygomaticofacial Artery (ZFA)

An offshoot of the lacrimal artery, the zygomaticofacial foramen is located in the SOOF and serves as the origin point for the zygomaticofacial artery (ZFA). Research indicates that this opening is positioned approximately 12–15 mm below the lateral canthus and 5–9 mm laterally. Investigations have identified its exact location, although accounts of its foramen are limited. Some patients were reported to lack a ZFA, or foramen, according to a couple of writers [14, 32–34].

28.5 Middle Third Fat Grafting

Areas requiring fat grafting will be identified through an examination of facial fullness. One method to achieve this is by anatomically dividing the face into thirds and carefully analyzing its distinctive features. Facial wrinkles and areas of excess soft tissue reveal the junctions between the subcutaneous and deep fat compartments. It is crucial to determine which signs of aging can be addressed with fat grafting alone and which may necessitate additional surgical treatments [35].

When considering midface features, the lower eyelid, tear trough, and malar region are most prominent [35]. Aging leads to a hollowing of the infraorbital region, which creates a significant tear trough deformity, a slack orbital holding ligament, and a loss of volume in the front cheek. Patients who experience fat herniation at the inferior orbital rim may need to undergo blepharoplasty before fat transfer procedures [36]. This approach facilitates a smooth transition from the lower eyelid to the cheek. In treating orbital hollowing and enhancing the lid-cheek interface, fractionated fat grafting stands as the gold standard [37].

To increase the volume of the malar region, four distinct types of fat must be addressed. Each area serves a specific purpose: the deep nasolabial malar, middle superficial, high lateral, and deep malar (medial) compartments. It is advisable to start with the superficial high and middle malar compartments before moving on to the deep malar compartment, which is considered the "workhorse" of midface volume restoration [38]. Compared to implant insertion, fat grafting to the cheek enhances malar shape, although to a lesser degree. Furthermore, it is quite straightforward to rectify any noticeable malar asymmetries. While the buccal fat pad is often overlooked in youth, it plays a crucial role in the midface. To avoid the appearance of hollowness, it is recommended to reconstruct the buccal fat pad in a complementary manner after malar augmentation [36, 39].

28.6 Complications

The most common problem that arises after fat grafting is slight unevenness or irregularity in the treated area. When fat tissue is placed too superficially or in large aliquots, it can lead to necrosis and, eventually, the formation of palpable lumps. Three procedures are available for addressing these issues: suction lipectomy, direct open excision, and the administration of Lipodissolve [40]. The procedure is relatively straightforward. Subcutaneous nodules that develop due to fat necrosis after surgery are easily excisable if the patient desires [41].

Aside from these concerns, other potential side effects include infection, fatty embolism, hematoma, and nerve damage. Although infections are rare, it is still important to take precautions to reduce the chances of developing one. Areas like the lips, which can be contaminated with oral flora, are injected last. Additionally, acyclovir should be administered to individuals who have previously experienced cold sores as a preventive measure [40]. To minimize the risk of an intravascular fat injection and subsequent embolic event, it is recommended to pre-inject 1% lidocaine and 1:200,000 epinephrine into the anticipated recipient sites [41] (Figs. 28.1, 28.2, and 28.3).

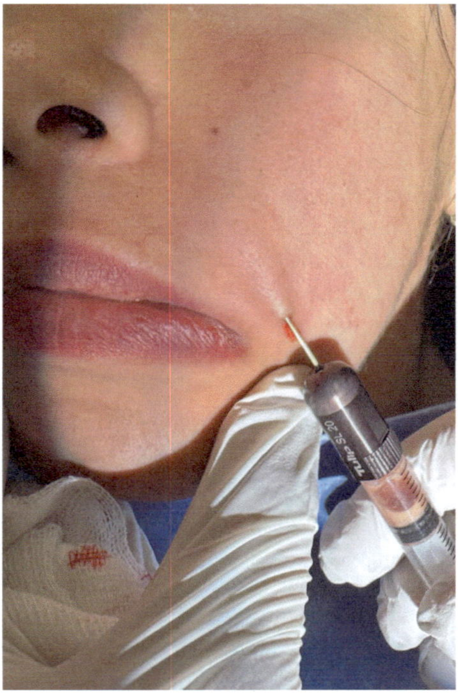

Fig. 28.1 Fat injection to nasolabial sulcus. (Courtesy of Zeliha Kapusuz Gencer MD)

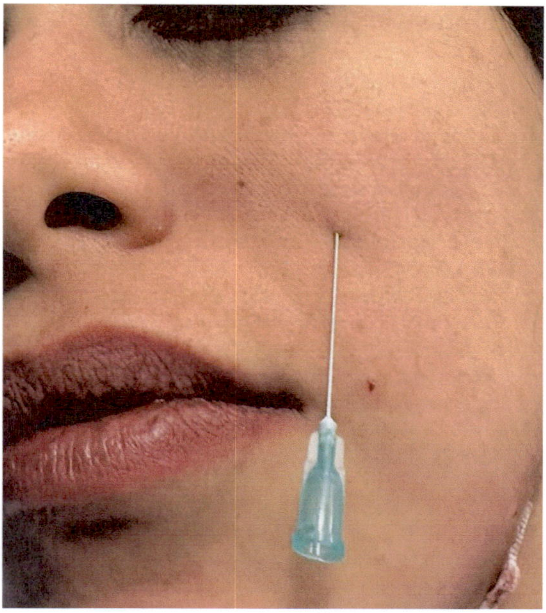

Fig. 28.2 Skin puncture before the fat injection to zygoma. (Courtesy of Zeliha Kapusuz Gencer MD)

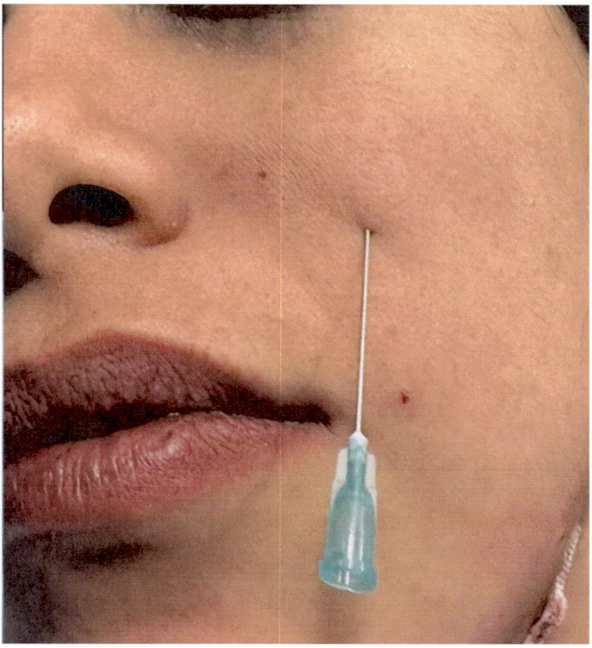

Fig. 28.3 Fat injection to zygoma. (Courtesy of Zeliha Kapusuz Gencer MD)

References

1. Trévidic P, Kaufman-Janette J, Weinkle S, Wu R, Dhillon B, Antunes S, Macé E, Maffert P. Injection guidelines for treating midface volume deficiency with hyaluronic acid fillers: the ATP approach (anatomy, techniques, products). Aesthet Surg J. 2022;42(8):920–34.
2. Rohrich RJ, Pessa JE, Ristow B. The youthful cheek and the deep medial fat compartment. Plast Reconstr Surg. 2008;121(6):2107–12.
3. Rohrich RJ, Pessa JE. The fat compartments of the face: anatomy and clinical implications for cosmetic surgery. Plast Reconstr Surg. 2007;119(7):2219–27.
4. Gierloff M, Stöhring C, Buder T, Gassling V, Açil Y, Wiltfang J. Aging changes of the midfacial fat compartments: a computed tomographic study. Plast Reconstr Surg. 2012;129(1):263–73.
5. Rohrich RJ, Pessa JE. The retaining system of the face: histologic evaluation of the septal boundaries of the subcutaneous fat compartments. Plast Reconstr Surg. 2008;121(5):1804–9.
6. Lee JH, Hong G. Definitions of groove and hollowness of the infraorbital region and clinical treatment using soft-tissue filler. Arch Plast Surg. 2018;45(3):214–21.
7. Cevik Cenkeri H, Sarigul Guduk S, Derin CE. Aging changes of the superficial fat compartments of the midface over time: a magnetic resonance imaging study. Dermatologic Surg. 2020;46(12):1600–5.
8. Özdemir E, Bayar Muluk N, Sünnetci G, Arslanoğlu A, Yazir M, Kaya F, Cingi C. Investigation of the Effects of Minimally Invasive Facial Plastic Surgery Applications on Well-Being of Individuals. J Craniofac Surg. 2025. https://doi.org/10.1097/SCS.0000000000011658. Epub ahead of print. PMID: 40663006.
9. Gierloff M, Stöhring C, Buder T, Wiltfang J. The subcutaneous fat compartments in relation to aesthetically important facial folds and rhytides. J Plast Reconstr Aesthet Surg. 2012;65(10):1292–7.
10. Pirayesh A, Bertossi D, Heydenrych I. Aesthetic facial anatomy essentials for injections. CRC Press; 2020.
11. Pilsl U, Anderhuber F, Rzany B. Anatomy of the cheek: implications for soft tissue augmentation. Dermatologic Surg. 2012;38(7 Pt 2):1254–62.
12. Lambros V. Observations on periorbital and midface aging. Plast Reconstr Surg. 2007;120(5):1367–76.
13. Cotofana S, Gotkin RH, Frank K, et al. The functional anatomy of the deep facial fat compartments: a detailed imaging-based investigation. Plast Reconstr Surg. 2019;143(1):53–63.
14. Alghoul MS, Vaca EE, Bricker JT, Mioton LM. Enhancing the lateral orbital "C-angle" with calcium hydroxylapatite: an anatomic and clinical study. Aesthet Surg J. 2021;41(8):952–66.
15. Cotofana S, Schenck TL, Trévidic P, et al. Midface: clinical anatomy and regional approaches with injectable fillers. Plast Reconstr Surg. 2015;136(5 Suppl):219s–34s.
16. Lamb JP, Chase SC. Chapter 1: The midface. In: Thieme, editor. Facial volumization. Georg Thieme Verlag; 2018.
17. Stuzin JM, Baker TJ, Gordon HL. The relationship of the superficial and deep facial fascias: relevance to rhytidectomy and aging. Plast Reconstr Surg. 1992;89(3):441–9.
18. Moss CJ, Mendelson BC, Taylor GI. Surgical anatomy of the ligamentous attachments in the temple and periorbital regions. Plast Reconstr Surg. 2000;105(4):1475–90.
19. Alghoul M, Codner MA. Retaining ligaments of the face: review of anatomy and clinical applications. Aesthet Surg J. 2013;33(6):769–82.
20. Wong CH, Hsieh MKH, Mendelson B. The tear trough ligament: anatomical basis for the tear trough deformity. Plast Reconstr Surg. 2012;129(6):1392–402.
21. Coleman SR. Structural fat grafting: more than a permanent filler. Plast Reconstr Surg. 2006;118(3 Suppl):108S–20S.
22. Hong SJ, Park SE, Jo JW, et al. Variant facial artery anatomy revisited: conventional angiography performed in 284 cases. Medicine. 2020;99(28):e21048.
23. Lee HJ, Won SY, Jehoon O, et al. The facial artery: a comprehensive anatomical review. Clin Anat. 2018;31(1):99–108.

24. Lee JG, Yang HM, Choi YJ, et al. Facial arterial depth and relationship with the facial musculature layer. Plast Reconstr Surg. 2015;135(2):437–44.
25. Scheuer JF 3rd, Sieber DA, Pezeshk RA, Campbell CF, Gassman AA, Rohrich RJ. Anatomy of the facial danger zones: maximizing safety during soft-tissue filler injections. Plast Reconstr Surg. 2017;139(1):50e–8e.
26. Kim HS, Lee KL, Gil YC, Hu KS, Tansatit T, Kim HJ. Topographic anatomy of the infraorbital artery and its clinical implications for nasolabial fold augmentation. Plast Reconstr Surg. 2018;142(3):273e–80e.
27. Galadari H. Middle third. In: Galadari H, editor. Soft tissue augmentation: principles and practice. Berlin: Springer Berlin Heidelberg; 2018. p. 39–65.
28. Lee J-G, Yang H-M, Hu K-S, et al. Frontal branch of the superficial temporal artery: anatomical study and clinical implications regarding injectable treatments. Surg Radiol Anat. 2015;37(1):61–8.
29. von Arx T, Tamura K, Yukiya O, Lozanoff S. The face – a vascular perspective. A literature review. Swiss Dent J. 2018;128(5):382–92.
30. Yang H-J, Gil Y-C, Lee H-Y. Topographical anatomy of the transverse facial artery. Clin Anat. 2010;23(2):168–78.
31. DeLorenzi C, Karpova E, Rzany B, Trévidic P, Lamilla GC. Anatomy and filler complications. E2e Medical Publishing; 2017.
32. Beheiry EE, Abdel-Hamid FAM. An anatomical study of the temporal fascia and related temporal pads of fat. Plast Reconstr Surg. 2007;119(1):136–44.
33. Bozikov K, Shaw-Dunn J, Soutar DS, Arnez ZM. Arterial anatomy of the lateral orbital and cheek region and arterial supply to the "peri-zygomatic perforator arteries" flap. Surg Radiol Anat. 2008;30(1):17–22.
34. Nakajima H, Imanishi N, Minabe T. The arterial anatomy of the temporal region and the vascular basis of various temporal flaps. Br J Plast Surg. 1995;48(7):439–50.
35. Schultz KP, Raghuram A, Davis MJ, Abu-Ghname A, Chamata E, Rohrich RJ. Fat grafting for facial rejuvenation. Semin Plast Surg. 2020;34(1):30–7.
36. Glasgold M, Glasgold R, Lam S. Autologous fat grafting for midface rejuvenation. Clin Plast Surg. 2015;42(01):115–21.
37. Rohrich RJ, Mahedia M, Shah N, Afrooz P, Vishvanath L, Gupta RK. Role of fractionated fat in blending the lid-cheek junction. Plast Reconstr Surg. 2018;142(01):56–65.
38. Rohrich RJ, Ghavami A, Constantine FC, Unger J, Mojallal A. Lift-and-fill face lift: integrating the fat compartments. Plast Reconstr Surg. 2014;133(06):756e–67e.
39. Cohen SR, Fireman E, Hewett S, Saad A. Buccal fat pad augmentation for facial rejuvenation. Plast Reconstr Surg. 2017;139(06):1273e–6e.
40. Coleman SR, Katzel EB. Fat grafting for facial filling and regeneration. Clin Plast Surg. 2015;42(3):289–300.
41. Pu LLQ. Fat grafting for facial rejuvenation and contouring: a rationalized approach. Ann Plast Surg. 2018;81(6S, Suppl 1):S102–8.

29 Fat Injections as Volumizer on the Face: Lips

Umit Yılmaz, Zeliha Kapusuz Gencer, and Cemal Cingi

29.1 Anatomy

The lip components serve as the primary focus of attention in the bottom portion of the face. The cutaneous regions of the upper lip are located below the nose, in the area of the mustache. These regions are separated from the cheek by the nasolabial fold. The central dip below the nose, referred to as the philtrum, is an essential anatomic component. This is because even a slight shift of this structure can result in substantial deformity. Lips are the components that make up the vermilion subunit. It is below the vermillion [1] that the cutaneous lower lip is located. This lower lip borders the chin in an inferior direction and is later confined by the nasolabial fold (Figs. 29.1, 29.2, 29.3, and 29.4).

29.1.1 Muscles of the Mouth

One of the most extensive networks of facial muscles is found in the mouth, which is also responsible for a significant portion of an individual's capacity for facial expression. The tongue, also known as the orbicularis oris, is the primary

U. Yılmaz
Department of Otorhinolaryngology, Selahattin Eyyubi State Hospital, Diyarbakır, Diyarbakır, Turkey

Z. K. Gencer
Department of Otorhinolaryngology, University of Health Sciences, Basaksehir Cam and Sakura City Hospital, Istanbul, Turkey

C. Cingi (✉)
Eskisehir Osmangazi University, Medical Faculty, Department of Otorhinolaryngology, Eskisehir, Türkiye
e-mail: cemal@ogu.edu.tr

C. Cingi et al. (eds.), *Minor Interventions, Major Outcomes on the Face*, Comprehensive ENT, https://doi.org/10.1007/978-3-032-01305-7_29

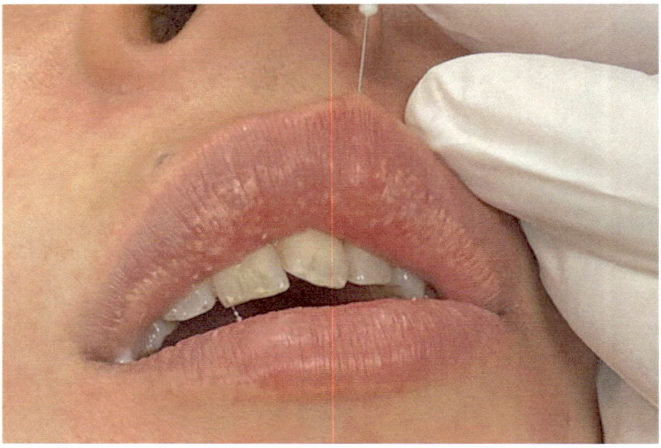

Fig. 29.1 Volumizing upper lip with injection

component of the lips and surrounds the mouth. For the most part, the orbicularis oris muscle is responsible for pulling the lips against the teeth, drawing the lips together, pulling the corners of the mouth together, and puckering the mouth. These are the primary tasks of the muscle. This muscle is also particularly crucial for phonation sounds that depend on the lips, such as pronouncing M, V, F, and P [1]. It ensures that the sounds are spoken correctly.

A collection of six muscles generally called the quadratus labii superioris muscle is responsible for manipulating the upper jaw. The following is a list of the six muscles: [1].

- Zygomaticus major muscle—Starts from the posterolateral zygomatic bone and travels medially to insert on the top portion of the orbicularis oris muscle; the zygomaticus major muscle helps in producing the lower nasolabial fold and is principally responsible for smiling.
- The zygomaticus minor muscle is located just medially to the zygomaticus major muscle and contributes to its functions.

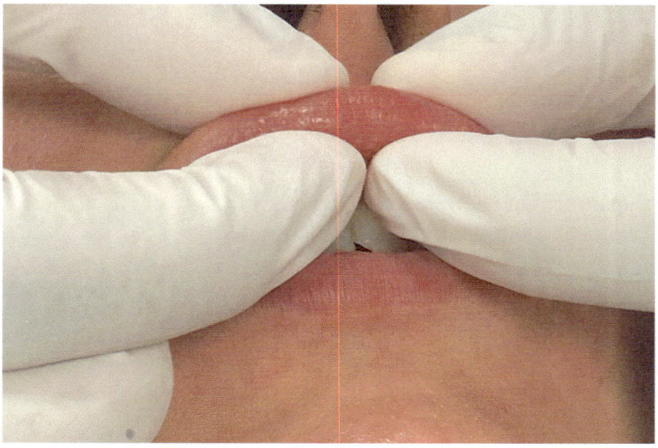

Fig. 29.2 Equally distribution and retouching of the injected fat tissue

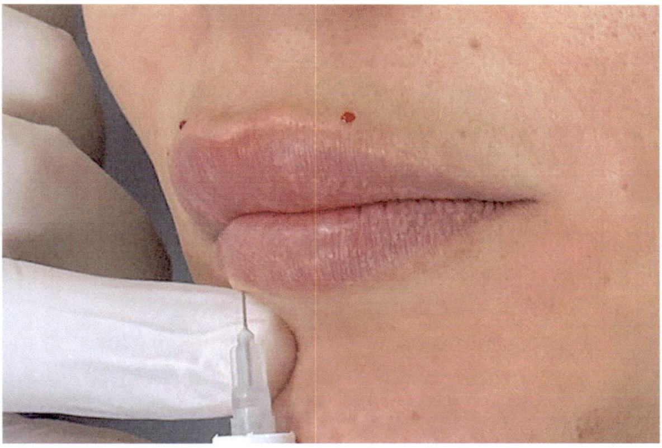

Fig. 29.3 Volumizing lower lip with injection

- Levator labii superioris muscle—Arises from the inferior portion of the maxilla and inserts on the upper lip, more medially than the zygomaticus muscles; the levator labii superioris muscle helps to elevate the medial part of the upper lip and assists the zygomatic muscles with open smiling (the levator and zygomaticus muscles form the nasolabial fold).
- Levator anguli oris is the most profoundly positioned lip elevator muscle; it inserts on the upper corner of the mouth to assist with lip elevation.
- The risorius muscle helps with smiling. It is located over the parotid gland and enters the skin and mucosa of the lateral corner of the mouth. However, the risorius muscle is not always present.
- The buccinator muscle is neither an elevator nor a depressor of the lip; it originates just posterior and medial to the final molar tooth and continues forward to become continuous with the orbicularis oris muscle. In other words, it is responsible for lifting and lowering the lip.

For example, the buccinator muscle is the primary component of the cheek musculature when playing a wind instrument. Its primary function is to prevent the

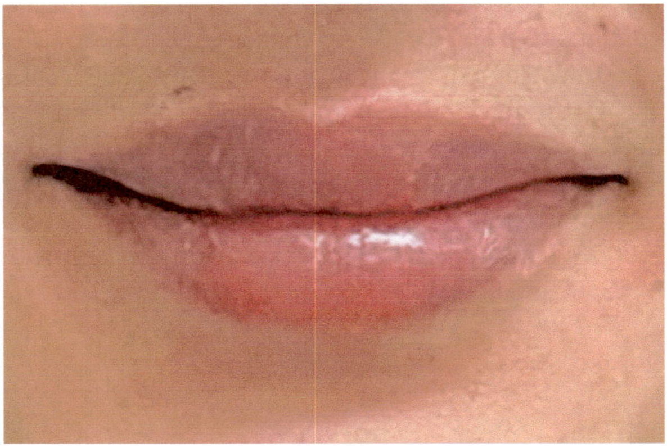

Fig. 29.4 Frontal view after application

cheek from becoming overly stretched out. When whistling, this muscle assists the orbicularis oris muscle by [1].

The following is a list of the depressors of the lip, which are innervated by the facial nerve along the marginal mandibular branch [1]:

- The depressor anguli oris muscles originate from the lateral region of the mandible and move superomedially to insert, together with the orbicularis oris muscle, in the corners of the mouth. Their primary purpose is to depress and retract the corners of the mouth.
- The depressor labii inferioris muscles are located more medially on the mandible and travel superiorly to enter, together with the orbicularis oris muscle, the lower and medial region of the lip. These muscles, identical to the depressor anguli oris muscle, help retract and depress the lower lip.
- The mentalis muscle is deep in the depressor anguli oris and labii inferioris muscles. It originates from the mandible and lower lateral incisor and travels inferiorly until it reaches the skin that covers the chin. The mentalis muscle elevates and wrinkles the chin and contributes to the protrusion of the lower lip.

29.1.2 Superficial Musculoaponeurotic System

The facial muscles must cooperate to enable as diverse face expressions as possible. A discrete fibromuscular layer that envelops and interlinks the muscles to create these synergies is referred to as the superficial musculoaponeurotic system (SMAS). It is important to do extensive undermining in facial rejuvenation operations [1], and the SMAS is responsible for delineating the dissection planes for this.

Additionally, the SMAS is a helpful marker that can be utilized to determine the location of critical blood arteries and nerves. In most cases, the axial blood vessels and sensory nerves are located in the superficial segment of the superficial muscular artery (SMAS). At the same time, the deeper levels of the SMAS are home to the more important motor neurons [1].

In most cases, the subcutaneous muscle adipose tissue (SMAS) is situated beneath the subcutaneous fat and is found atop the muscles. A freely movable and continuous plane, the SMAS connects the temporalis, frontalis, occipitalis, and procerus muscles to the subgaleal space. This plane is located above the zygoma and is superior to the zygoma. On the other hand, the fascial architecture could be more obvious; however, the SMAS is responsible for connecting the platysma, risorius, and depressor anguli oris muscles located inferior to the zygoma [1].

An interconnected structural muscular attachment system does not protect the muscles located on the medial portion of the face, such as the orbicularis oculi, lip elevator, and nasal muscles [1].

29.2 Adipose Tissue Biology

Types

Thermogenically active brown adipose tissue (BAT) and energy-storing white adipose tissue (WAT) are the two forms of adipose tissue that are typically distinguished from one another [2]. It was traditionally believed that BAT was only found in infants and tiny mammals; however, over the last 10 years, investigations have demonstrated that metabolically active BAT may also be found in children and adults [2]. In humans, brown fat can be found in various locations, including the cervical, supraclavicular, axillary, paravertebral, mediastinal, and upper abdominal regions [3]. On the other hand, the most common type of fat found in humans is called adipose tissue (WAT), which can be found viscerally or subcutaneously [4, 5]. This review focuses primarily on subcutaneous WAT, the type of fat employed for autologous fat grafting in cosmetic and reconstructive surgeries [2].

Surviving the Graft

Three hypotheses have been proposed to explain how fat grafts can survive after being implanted by avascular surgical procedures. Studies have shown that each of these hypotheses may play a role in the survival process [26]. The graft survival hypothesis, the graft replacement theory, and the host cell replacement theory are the names of the three ideas that have been investigated [6].

The Theory of Graft Survival

Peer et al. [7] were the first to describe this idea, arguing that after surgical transfer, fat grafts initially survive through nutrition diffusion from the plasma until neovascularization from the recipient location occurs [8]. This theory was also the first to describe the concept. Only those fat cells that receive an adequate amount of fresh blood supply can survive [9]. Consequently, grafts with lower volumes may survive better than larger ones. Smaller volumes are better suited for complete diffusion and perfusion [6].

The Theory of Graft Replacement

The transplanted adipocytes are primarily replaced by the donor adipocyte stem cells (ASCs) that are concurrently transmitted in the graft, according to this idea, which argues that relatively few donor adipocytes survive the process of grafting. Adipogenesis and angiogenesis are processes attributed to the donor stem cell transplant (SVF) [8]. Multiple studies have been conducted to explore the enrichment of fat grafts with stem cells (SVC) and adipose stem cells (ASCs), and these studies have revealed significant increases in graft retention [10]. It has also been demonstrated that fat grafts with a higher density possess higher concentrations of adipose stem cells (ASCs). As a result, they have higher survival rates when compared to grafts with a lower density [11].

Theory of the Replacement of Host Cells

This idea proposes that neither the grafted cells nor the recipient cells survive and that all cells are replaced by the recipient cells [8]. Cells that have been grafted undergo necrosis and are subsequently replaced by fibrous tissue, new fat cells, and the ingrowth of blood vessels from the recipient tissue [8]. Therefore, the integrity of the recipient site and the environment are key factors that determine the life of the graft. Over the last few decades, several different approaches of preparing the recipient site have been developed. Consequently, the outcomes of fat grafting surgical procedures have shown signs of improvement [12].

29.3 Fat Injections on the Lower Third of the Face

The nasolabial fold, the labio-mandibular fold (also known as marionette lines), the pre-jowl sulcus (also known as the craniomandibular groove), the labio-dental sulcus, the lips, and the chin are the primary features that are prominent in the lower third of the face. The deflation of the cheek causes the nasolabial fold to become more pronounced. Therefore, to prevent overcorrection, it is recommended that the malar fat compartments be filled to lift the nasolabial fold adequately. This procedure should be undertaken before any nasolabial extensions.

Dentate mandible expansion and relative pre-jowl concavity are the two factors that lead to the development of jowls [14–16]. Even though fat grafting along the lateral mandible posterior to the jowl can generate a young and angular jaw shape, considerable jowling necessitates surgical cervicofacial rhytidectomy [17]. However, surgical lift of the jowl cannot address the geniomandibular groove. To achieve a smooth transition from the chin to the posterior mandible, fat grafting is required in this particular location [18].

The lips become more delicate and lose their sharpness along the philtral columns as their age increases. Perioral rhytids are a manifestation of these alterations, which, when combined with subcutaneous fat atrophy, make it impossible for surgical rhytidectomy to be the sole treatment for the condition. Although resurfacing procedures are helpful, they are insufficient to correct perioral pucker lines independently. Instead, fat grafting to superficial compartments close to the vermillion-cutaneous interface is required to achieve volume augmentation of a perioral region that has been atrophied [19]. On the other hand, the white roll and vermillion should be filled with injectables since the extent to which fat grafts are taken up in these places is not always predicted [13, 19].

Loss of chin projection, vertical height, and a deepening of the labio-mental crease are all aspects of the chin associated with volume depletion that occurs with advancing age. Fat grafting is a viable method for restoring a youthful lower lip contour and refined chin in individuals with soft tissue descent and tiny asymmetries or flaws, such as a bifid chin or microgenia [20]. Chin implants may benefit patients who require more than three milliliters of augmentation on each side [18]. This is because chin implants prevent a spherical appearance.

29.4 Fat Harvesting

When selecting a donor site for fat grafting, it is essential to consider the aesthetics of the donor site, the patient's preferences, the surgical positioning, the amount of fat required, and the amount available [21]. Harvesting sites for facial augmentation procedures are typically the lower belly and the inner thighs since these areas contain a high concentration of adipose-derived stem cells (ADSCs). In most cases involving face rejuvenation and contouring, an average of thirty milliliters of fat is required [22].

Syringe aspiration, which involves attaching a 10-mL Luer-Lok syringe to a harvesting cannula, is the method that is currently considered to be the most effective for fat harvesting. When the syringe plunger is drawn back, a modified multihole Coleman cannula generates negative pressure, increasing the harvesting process's efficiency [17, 23]. Because the face is a recipient site sensitive to volume, it is recommended to use a small cannula with a gauge of 12 and small holes 1 mm in diameter. This will guarantee that the harvested fat lobules are of the right size [24]. For cannula insertion, entry sites should be created in discrete regions such as the umbilicus (for harvesting from the lower abdomen) or the inguinal line (for harvesting from the medial thigh). To avoid causing damage to the rectus fascia and to harvest fat uniformly, it is essential to avoid deep passage of the cannula [17]. This will ensure that the body's shape is smooth after the treatment.

29.5 Fat Placement

With each injection, a small amount of fat should be provided to achieve the highest possible control over fat distribution and reduce the risk of problems such as fibrosis, calcification, infections, or the formation of oil cysts [22]. Injections should be performed within multiple tissue planes and in various orientations, with awareness of the cannula tip at all times [25–27]. The maximum amount of fat injected per second is between 0.5 and 1 milliliter, and each pass should not exceed that amount. Additionally, it is essential to avoid veins and nerves near the area. When injecting smaller facial locations, such as the periorbital region, it is recommended to use a smaller cannula to have greater control over the volume that is placed [22]. Facial augmentation will become immediately apparent once fat is injected into the desired area. When it is hypothesized that volume-restrictive factors are present, such as fibrotic adhesions or a tight skin envelope, it may be necessary to perform dissection using a needle with an 18-gauge gauge or a cannula and forked tip [22]. Access to deep compartments can be gained only laterally next to the junction of the alar and cheek [28].

The fat injection process should begin at the deepest level and go up to the superficial level. The depth of fat insertion should be adjusted to reach the desired outcomes for the patient. The application of the product in the intradermal or subdermal layers has the potential to enhance the appearance of wrinkles, the overall facial complexion, and the skin quality [29]. When placing superficial fat, extreme caution is required because abnormalities are more readily apparent. A more profound placement of fat in the intermediate subcutaneous layers could renew facial proportions.

Additionally, positioning fat against the bony periosteum can alter how the overlying soft tissue envelope encases the facial bony structure [23]. It is possible to reduce the risk of fat necrosis and resorption by ensuring that no shaping of fat has been deposited. There is the possibility of using interrupted sutures to close the infusion sites after grafting. To facilitate the healing process of the incisions, it is possible to implant small, concentrated quantities of roughly 0.2 to 0.3 milliliters into the closed incisions [23].

Because intercompartmental membranes are elastic and can accept the graft volume, unnecessary overcorrection should not be conducted in the face. Excessive correction can quickly result in an unsightly and excessively overfilled face shape [30].

29.5.1 Procedure and Technique

When injecting fat into the lips, the treated area must be masked appropriately to allow a precise injection technique over the predefined line. Local anesthetic can be administered just before or after encasing if the patient agrees, since office-based lip augmentation is typically more comfortable than in other areas, with the localized nature of the procedure and the more avascular tissues allowing for less anesthetic use than in different situations. The materials for adipose processing should be available at all times. Before the procedure, the physical examination results and personal objectives should be discussed and recorded—pre-injection care. Care for the treatment area involves a full assessment of the lip and facial muscles. Medical photographs of the front, sides, and 45° angles are essential. The treatment must be performed aseptically during the clinical procedure. Technique. The technology and the patterns displayed here are utterly personal and are influenced by the knowledge and results. Layering is the technique employed. With the deposition of a microinjection volume, no greater than 0.2 mL, tunnels of injected fat are created here and should be roughly arranged. The use of a cannula, although dissuaded from the injection of the facelift, aids in dealing with injection-free zones. The width of the auricular needles used for injection is 0.4 mm. The second layer, again consisting of microinjection tunnels of not more than 0.2 mL, is positioned laterally. Extraction during management needs a surgical procedure with the tunnel release of tiny clots as clinically indicated and a tincture of the test area. Discontinue utilizing the suction cannula and use it in its place for trials that do not demonstrate blood or a graft [21–24].

29.6 Comparative Analysis of Fillers and Fat Injections

Patients looking to volumize and enhance their lips have options, with fillers representing one choice and fat representing the other. Effects produced by injectable fillers can be seen immediately, and the procedure requires no downtime. They are, by and large, the most popular means of volumizing lips and are also completely reversible. The biggest downside to fillers is the fact that volume restoration is necessary. Generally, hyaluronic acid-based fillers last 3 to 6 months, while others can remain for 2 to 5 years. Volumizing lips using fat is meant to be a long-term reconstructive option. When fat transplants are used, they can last for many years, sometimes permanently. They cost a bit more at first, depending on how much fat must be used to make them. However, they can save individuals considerable money in the long run. Patients undergoing fat transplants generally require no downtime [21–24].

Slight bruising and some tenderness may appear at injection sites. Some patients will swell, but to what extent is difficult to say, as is when such symptoms will decrease. Fat transplant patients should take it easy after surgery, but a fat transplant is far less invasive than one might imagine. Volumizing lips using injectable fillers is an option as well, and it has been around longer than fat injection therapy. Because insurance generally does not cover fillers to enhance the lip, some argue that the cost comes out in the wash in the long run. Complications do occur with both, and the satisfaction rate is high. The time for results and satisfaction should guide you when choosing which suits you. It should be noted that all people are different, and some people prefer a more temporary approach. It is one of the oldest methods of reducing the signs of aging [21–24].

29.7 Postoperative Care

Patients who have undergone facial fat grafting should be informed by their surgeons that they should anticipate experiencing some bruising and swelling for up to 6 weeks after the procedure [23, 31]. The pigment of the lower eyelids, sometimes known as "tea staining," can last from a few months to a year until the skin that overlays the affected area becomes thicker [23]. Cool compresses may be provided to the patient after face fat grafting to reduce the likelihood of bruising, edema, and discomfort. To minimize fat migration or necrosis, you should avoid deep massage. Additionally, any shear stress or damage to the area could potentially impair the survival of the graft [23].

Before the initial fat grafting procedure, patients should be educated that subsequent surgeries are nearly always required to attain the desired outcome. The grafted volume will frequently drop by 50 to 90% [23]. It is recommended that subsequent facial fat grafting procedures be carried out at least 6 months to 1 year following the initial procedure. This will allow for the resolution of the inflammatory response and the accurate evaluation of the surgical outcome [23, 31]. Furthermore, it is anticipated that the volume loss resulting from face aging will persist, and additional augmentation will probably be wanted regardless of the graft taken [13, 31].

In addition, counseling should provide an approximate schedule of the anticipated outcomes. In the operation's immediate aftermath, facial volume restoration is readily apparent. The thickening and softening of the skin on top, the improvement of scars, and the decrease of wrinkles are all progressive processes that become more noticeable over a few months. It is possible that, after a year, the complexion of sun-damaged or aging skin will have improved [23].

References

1. Orengo I. Facial anatomy in cutaneous surgery. In: Elston DM, editor. Medscape. Updated: Jul 21, 2015. https://emedicine.medscape.com/article/1127307-overview#a9. Accessed online on 10 June 2023.
2. Hoppela E, Grönroos TJ, Saarikko AM, et al. Fat grafting can induce browning of white adipose tissue. Plast Reconstr Surg Glob Open. 2018;6(06):e1804.
3. Saely CH, Geiger K, Drexel H. Brown versus white adipose tissue: a mini-review. Gerontology. 2012;58(01):15–23.
4. Stanford KI, Middelbeek RJW, Goodyear LJ. Exercise effects on white adipose tissue: beiging and metabolic adaptations. Diabetes. 2015;64(07):2361–8.
5. Bucky LP, Percec I. The science of autologous fat grafting: views on current and future approaches to neo adipogenesis. Aesthet Surg J. 2008;28(03):313–21. quiz 322–324
6. Shih L, Davis MJ, Winocour SJ. The science of fat grafting. Semin Plast Surg. 2020;34(1):5–10.
7. Peer LA. Loss of weight and volume in human fat grafts with postulation of a "cell survival theory". Plast Reconstr Surg. 1950;5:217–30.
8. Doornaert M, Colle J, De Maere E, Declercq H, Blondeel P. Autologous fat grafting: latest insights. Ann Med Surg (Lond). 2018;37(37):47–53.
9. Pu LLQ. Mechanisms of fat graft survival. Ann Plast Surg. 2016;77(01):S84–6.
10. Rasmussen BS, Lykke Sørensen C, Vester-Glowinski PV, et al. Effect, feasibility, and clinical relevance of cell enrichment in large volume fat grafting: a systematic review. Aesthet Surg J. 2017;37(suppl_3):S46–58.
11. Allen RJ Jr, Canizares O Jr, Scharf C, et al. Grading lipoaspirate: is there an optimal density for fat grafting? Plast Reconstr Surg. 2013;131(01):38–45.
12. Oranges CM, Striebel J, Tremp M, et al. The preparation of the recipient site in fat grafting: a comprehensive review of the preclinical evidence. Plast Reconstr Surg. 2019;143(04):1099–107.
13. Schultz KP, Raghuram A, Davis MJ, Abu-Ghname A, Chamata E, Rohrich RJ. Fat grafting for facial rejuvenation. Semin Plast Surg. 2020 Feb;34(1):30–7.
14. Mendelson B, Wong CH. Changes in the facial skeleton with aging: implications and clinical applications in facial rejuvenation. Aesth Plast Surg. 2012;36(04):753–60.
15. Pecora NG, Baccetti T, McNamara JA Jr. The aging craniofacial complex: a longitudinal cephalometric study from late adolescence to late adulthood. Am J Orthod Dentofacial Orthop. 2008;134(04):496–505.
16. Shaw RB, Katzel EB Jr, Koltz PF, Kahn DM, Girotto JA, Langstein HN. Aging of the mandible and its aesthetic implications. Plast Reconstr Surg. 2010;125(01):332–42.
17. Glasgold R, Glasgold M, Lam S. Complementary fat grafting. Berlin, Heidelberg: Springer; 2018. p. 321–32.
18. Marten TJ, Elyassnia D. Fat grafting in facial rejuvenation. Clin Plast Surg. 2015;42(02):219–52.
19. Pezeshk RA, Stark RY, Small KH, Unger JG, Rohrich RJ. Role of autologous fat transfer to the superficial fat compartments for perioral rejuvenation. Plast Reconstr Surg. 2015;136(03):301e–9e. [PubMed] [Google Scholar]

20. Rohrich RJ, Sanniec K, Afrooz PN. Autologous fat grafting to the chin: a useful adjunct in complete aesthetic facial rejuvenation. Plast Reconstr Surg. 2018;142(04):921–5.
21. Khan HA, Keyhan SO. Fat grafting in facial aesthetic units. Atlas Oral Maxillofac Surg Clin North Am. 2018;26(01):15–23.
22. Pu LLQ. Fat grafting for facial rejuvenation and contouring: a rationalized approach. Ann Plast Surg. 2018;81(6S, Suppl 1):S102–8.
23. Coleman SR, Katzel EB. Fat grafting for facial filling and regeneration. Clin Plast Surg. 2015 Jul;42(3):289–300.
24. Del Vecchio D, Rohrich RJ. A classification of clinical fat grafting: different problems, different solutions. Plast Reconstr Surg. 2012;130(03):511–22.
25. Coleman SR. Structural fat grafting: more than a permanent filler. Plast Reconstr Surg. 2006;118(3, Suppl):108S–20S.
26. Lee JH, Kirkham JC, McCormack MC, Nicholls AM, Randolph MA, Austen WG. Jr the effect of pressure and shear on autologous fat grafting. Plast Reconstr Surg. 2013;131(05):1125–36.
27. Xie Y, Zheng DN, Li QF, et al. An integrated fat grafting technique for cosmetic facial contouring. J Plast Reconstr Aesthet Surg. 2010;63(02):270–6.
28. Rohrich RJ, Afrooz PN. Finesse in facial lifting: the role of facial fat compartment augmentation in facial rejuvenation. Plast Reconstr Surg. 2019;143(01):98–101.
29. Mojallal A, Lequeux C, Shipkov C, et al. Improvement of skin quality after fat grafting: clinical observation and an animal study. Plast Reconstr Surg. 2009;124(03):765–74.
30. Rohrich RJ, Ghavami A, Constantine FC, Unger J, Mojallal A. Lift-and-fill face lift: integrating the fat compartments. Plast Reconstr Surg. 2014;133(06):756e–67e.
31. Glasgold M, Glasgold R, Lam S. sAutologous fat grafting for midface rejuvenation. Clin Plast Surg. 2015;42(01):115–21.

30 Fat Injections as Volumizer on the Face: Lower Third of the Face

Mehmet Akif Abakay, İbrahim Sayin, and Cemal Cingi

30.1 Introduction

The aesthetic appearance of the face has been of interest to man since ancient Greek times. Da Vinci defined the ideal face as one having three equal horizontal and five equal vertical portions [1]. The lower third was defined into three separate divisions: subnasale station, storming-labiodental, and labiodental-gnathion. Furthermore, the golden ratio is also important in analyzing subunits of the face [1].

Several procedures can be performed on the face to establish the ideal appearance, to counter either aging, a malignant process, or accidents. Depending on the patients' needs, these procedures may involve localized injections, facelifts, or more complex surgeries.

Loss of facial volume and skin sagging may cause an unhealthy and unwanted appearance. To restore facial volume, several biomaterials, such as hyaluronic acid, autologous fat (AF) tissue, and silicone [1], can be used.

Autologous fat transfer (AFT) for facial rejuvenation is a safe procedure with nearly 80% patient satisfaction and a low complication rate of approximately 6% [2]. Autologous fat is a biocompatible material with easy harvesting, easy application, low cost, and the ability to achieve long-lasting effects [3]. Besides the volumizing effect, it also improves nearby skin appearance, and with injected stem cells, it improves healing [4, 5]. However, the absence of vascular connection and volume depletion till the postoperative third month limits its clinical success [4].

M. A. Abakay (✉) · İ. Sayin
Department of Otorhinolaryngology, Bakirkoy Dr. Sadi Konuk Research and Training Hospital, İstanbul, Türkiye

C. Cingi
Eskisehir Osmangazi University, Medical Faculty, Department of Otorhinolaryngology, Eskisehir, Türkiye
e-mail: cemal@ogu.edu.tr

C. Cingi et al. (eds.), *Minor Interventions, Major Outcomes on the Face*, Comprehensive ENT, https://doi.org/10.1007/978-3-032-01305-7_30

30.2 General Principles

To establish satisfactory results, besides detecting pathologies, patient age, health status, medications, smoking status, and expectations must be investigated carefully [5]. Skin quality, facial asymmetries, and body mass index must be analyzed [5]. It would be better to analyze young photos of patients preoperatively. As is known, sagging may be secondary to fat atrophy or hypertrophy. While evaluating a patient's face, fat status must be defined properly to decide whether an additional liposuction procedure is needed [6]. Moreover, when skin laxity is evident, additional lifting procedures may be appropriate [7].

AFT can be used successfully with either general or local anesthesia [2]. Donor side selection can be performed according to the patient's characteristics because one side has no relevant advantages over another [8]. We prefer the Coleman technique to harvest fat, described more than 20 years ago [9]. We eliminate nonviable products but do not prefer to wash the harvested fat to avoid eliminating beneficial biological materials. After harvesting, a centrifuge or filter-wash can be used; they have no significant difference [10, 11]. Fat grafts larger than 3 mm are unsuitable for injection because of the high regression rate due to insufficient blood supply and microcyst formation. Millifat is between 2 and 2.5 mm, microfat is approximately 1 mm, and nanofat is less than 0.5 mm. Millifat is preferred for deep fat compartments, whereas nanofat and microfat are usually preferred for superficial layers [12].

The injection plane of harvested AF mainly depends on the placement of facial fat layers and the purpose of the injection. There are superficial and deep fat layers in the face. The superficial layers comprise nasolabial fat, medial and middle cheek fat, and lateral temporal cheek fat, and the deep layers include Ristow's space and deep medial cheek fat [5]. Superficial fat is tightly organized under the skin, and injections to superficial layers will heal wrinkles [5, 12]. Deep fat is loosely organized under the skin and decreases in deep layers because of pseudoptosis of skin envelopment; therefore, injections to deep layers provide lifting and contour restoration [5, 12, 13]. Recently, injections to deeper fat planes have caused anterior projection rather than inferior displacement [14]. Butterwick et al., in their 100-patient series, showed that fat could be injected into facial muscles [15]. They demonstrated that injected fat survived longer when injected near muscles.

The amount of fat that should be injected mainly depends on the patient's needs [16]. Dasiou-Plakida presented 1720 patients with 17 years of experience, reporting that resorption of 20–30% of volume occurred in the first 3 months, and from the 12th to the 24th months, approximately 40–60% of implanted fat was resorped. Also, the author emphasized that small amounts of implanted fat tissue were more easily vascularized compared to large amounts, recommending injecting small amounts of fat with fine needles (21–23 g) instead of performing overcorrection [8, 15, 17–19]. The researcher mentioned that fat stored at −30 °C was usable for up to 24 months for re-injection [17], and also debated the results presented in the current literature [15]. In a recent review, it was stated that volume loss could be between 13% and 68% and varied at different sites of the face [2]. We prefer to perform re-injection and not to deal with the transient, unpleasant appearance of overcorrection. Adding platelet-rich plasma (PRP) to injected material improves recovery time, but patient satisfaction is not affected [20].

30.3 Special Subsites

30.3.1 Nasolabial Folds

Fat injections to nasolabial folds have been performed safely for several years. Although cosmetic results are very acceptable, the duration of the result is still being determined, and repeat injections may be required. In the literature, very different recurrence rates exist with variable follow-up periods, but most authors accept that multiple procedures are needed [21]. Malar injections should be planned before the nasolabial folds because injections to the malar region also improve the nasolabial folds [22].

Maxillary resorption secondary to aging is managed by deep injection to Ristow's space, and to treat nasolabial creases, subcutaneous injections are performed along the crease line; patients usually need both injections [23, 24]. For most patients, 2- to 3-mm injections are usually sufficient. In the literature, the average volume per side is 2.8 (range, 1–7.5) mm [7, 16]. The entrance at the lateral and slightly superior to the oral commissure enables performing injections to the nasolabial sulcus and upper lip with the same entrance point [7]. Before injecting, dermofacial detachment should be performed [25]. Injections should be performed in a fan-shaped manner along four to five tunnel lines. Canulas (0.7–0.9 mm) are suitable for injecting [24, 26]. Although different criteria were accepted, in different studies, the satisfaction rates for 6, 12, and 24 months were 100%, 97.4%, and 66.7%, respectively [25, 26].

30.3.2 Lips/Marionette Lines

Lips are a special area, playing a role in aesthetic facial appearance and expressing feelings and emotions. Ideal lips have special attractive contours, impressive volume, and a nice Cupid's bow. Aging lips have decreased volume, increased length, sagging, and usually rhytids. Autologous fat can increase lip volume, enhance lip definition, and smooth vertical rhytides.

More than 20 years ago, it was shown that permanent lip augmentation could be achieved with serial injections [27]. Colić presented a series of more than 400 patients treated with intramuscular fat injections for the lips and the perioral region. It was observed that after a 2-year follow-up period, the resorption rate was not more than 20% [28]. It is recommended to inject at 3- to6-month intervals. Churukian et al. claimed that long-lasting results could be obtained after five injections [21, 29]. However, AFT to the lip is harder to predict because more swelling occurs in the lips than in other facial regions [21, 24, 30]. Therefore, we prefer to apply AFT to the lip only if we plan to use it in the other facial regions. That is, we usually choose other augmentation products if the lips are the only planned injected region.

To increase volume, injections of 1–2 mm of microfat with an 18- to 22-mm gauge needle to all three layers are recommended [4, 9, 24]. Injections are performed along the vermilion border, wet-dry junction, and the inner aspect of the lip [24, 31]. To improve lip definition, injections of 1 mm of microfat subdermally, and for rhytids, subdermal injections can be performed using a 23-mm gauge needle [7, 23]. To increase vermillion show, injections are performed approximately 2 mm near the junction [21, 27]. Minor irregularities can be corrected through digital massage [32]. Although fat injections provide excellent results for volume restoration, at the vermilion border, their effectiveness is decreased because of enhanced resorption or the inability to inject the correct space [20].

Autologous fat injections to the perioral area are one of the options to correct marionette lines; excellent results can be obtained by grafting near lines. Injections to the depressor labii muscle and subcutaneous plane usually improve appearance. This region should be correctly corrected to avoid the enlargement of grooves [33].

30.3.3 Chin

Chin augmentation can be achieved with fat injections. Usually, 3- to 5-mm injections via a 21- to 22-mm gauge cannula to subcutaneous, submuscular, and supraparsonal layers are performed via a single entry point at the midline [34–36]. Overinjection may cause a bulky and sagging of the chin. However, it should be kept in mind that correction of chin abnormalities with only fat injections is usually insufficient if additional mandibular pathologies exist; the best method must be determined based on the patient's deformity [37]. If the lip–chin distance is below 7 mm, fat injections alone are usually enough, and if it is more than 7 mm, additional procedures should be added [38].

30.3.4 Mandibular Angle

Another target for a young appearance on patients' faces is an uninterrupted and slightly curving natural appearance from the chin to the posterior mandible. AFT can be applied through this line, but it is usually insufficient to correct alone; a facelift procedure is usually needed.

Entrance lateral to the base of the nasolabial fold and mid-portion of the mandible enables injections to all mandibular lines. Gauge needles of 18 or 22 mm can be used, and 3–6 mm material is usually injected into all three layers [24]. Besides injecting the mandibular line, injecting inferior to the mandibular line causes some borrow of the neck skin, which improves the mandibular line appearance (Fig. 30.1) [33].

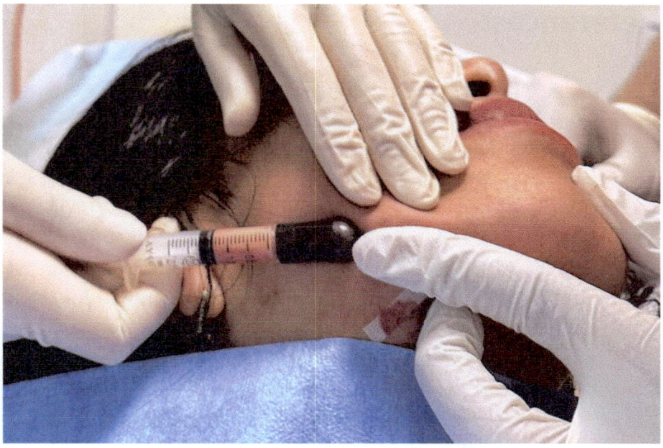

Fig. 30.1 Fat application to the mandibular angle

30.4 Complications

A recent systematic review found that asymmetry was the most common complication of AFT, followed by irregularity, hypertrophy, edema, fat necrosis, and infection [30]. Overall, the complication rate was only 2.23% [30].

To avoid complications and obtain satisfactory results, injections should be performed slowly and retrogradely with blind-fine cannulas [2, 8, 39]. Before injection, needle aspiration is performed to understand whether the injector is inside the vascular structure [18]. Coleman et al. advised injecting 0.1-mL fat per pass with a blind cannula [8]. After injecting, a digital examination is necessary to check the deposit and smoothen contours [21]. Injections should be performed with multiple crisscrossing to increase the injection surface and avoid bulky fat deposits, which may cause swelling, excessive resorption, and microcysts [24]. As recommended, we hold the syringe in the palm to improve control while injecting [24]. Ecchymosis and edema are seen in most patients and usually resolve spontaneously within 10 days.

Lip injections should not be performed deeper than 3 mm to avoid the superior or inferior labial artery [39]. The facial artery should be medial/lateral to or cross the nasolabial fold [39]. The artery becomes more superficial at the upper one-third of the nasolabial fold; therefore, injections should be performed either intradermally or supraperiostally [39]. High-pressure injections to the arterial system may cause localized necrosis, blindness, and even cerebrovascular events [39–41].

30.5 Conclusion

Autologous fat injection is well-tolerated, cheap, reapplicable, and has long-lasting effects. Although AFT is not considered the first choice for some subareas, the lower third of the face is a moderately appropriate zone for AFT. After an easily achievable learning curve and well-determined patient needs and desires, patients and physicians can obtain long-lasting, satisfactory results.

References

1. Ding A. The ideal lips: lessons learnt from the literature. Aesth Plast Surg. 2021;45(4):1520–30. https://doi.org/10.1007/s00266-021-02190-x. Epub 2021 Mar 1
2. Groen JW, Krastev TK, Hommes J, Wilschut JA, Ritt MJPF, van der Hulst RRJW. Autologous fat transfer for facial rejuvenation: a systematic review on technique, efficacy, and satisfaction. Plast Reconstr Surg Glob Open. 2017;5(12):e1606. https://doi.org/10.1097/GOX.0000000000001606. PMID: 29632784; PMCID: PMC5889440
3. Xiong S, Yi C, Pu LLQ. An overview of principles and new techniques for facial fat grafting. Clin Plast Surg. 2020;47(1):7–17. https://doi.org/10.1016/j.cps.2019.08.001. Epub 2019 Oct 21
4. Piombino P, Marenzi G, Dell'Aversana Orabona G, Califano L, Sammartino G. Autologous fat grafting in facial volumetric restoration. J Craniofac Surg. 2015;26(3):756–9. https://doi.org/10.1097/SCS.0000000000001663. Erratum in: J Craniofac Surg 2016 Jan;27(1):274. Pasquale, Piombino [corrected to Piombino, Pasquale]; Gaetano, Marenzi [corrected to Marenzi, Gaetano]; Giovanni, Dell'Aversana Orabona [corrected to Dell'Aversana Orabona, Giovanni]; Luigi, Califano [corrected to Califano, Luigi]; Gilberto, Sammartino [co. PMID: 25974786; PMCID: PMC4568901
5. Obagi S, Willis C. Autologous fat augmentation of the face. Atlas Oral Maxillofac Surg Clin North Am. 2018;26(1):41–50. https://doi.org/10.1016/j.cxom.2017.10.004. Epub 2017 Dec 8
6. Donofrio LM. Fat distribution: a morphologic study of the aging face. Dermatologic Surg. 2000 Dec;26(12):1107–12.
7. Buckingham ED, Glasgold R, Kontis T, Smith SP Jr, Dolev Y, Fitzgerald R, Lam SM, Williams EF, Pollei TR. Volume rejuvenation of the lower third, perioral, and jawline. Facial Plast Surg. 2015;31(1):70–9. https://doi.org/10.1055/s-0035-1544945. Epub 2015 Mar 12
8. Coleman SR, Katzel EB. Fat grafting for facial filling and regeneration. Clin Plast Surg. 2015;42(3):289–300, vii. https://doi.org/10.1016/j.cps.2015.04.001.
9. Coleman SR. Facial recontouring with lipostructure. Clin Plast Surg. 1997;24:347–67.
10. Kuran I, Tumerdem B. A new simple method used to prepare fat for injection. Aesth Plast Surg. 2005;29:18–22.
11. Botti G, Pascali M, Botti C, Bodog F, Cervelli V. A clinical trial in facial fat grafting: filtered and washed versus centrifuged fat. Plast Reconstr Surg. 2011;127(6):2464–73. https://doi.org/10.1097/PRS.0b013e3182131d5d.
12. Cohen SR, Womack H, Ghanem A. Fat grafting for facial rejuvenation through injectable tissue replacement and regeneration: a differential, standardized, anatomic approach. Clin Plast Surg. 2020;47(1):31–41. https://doi.org/10.1016/j.cps.2019.08.005. Epub 2019 Oct 28
13. Ramanadham SR, Rohrich RJ. Newer understanding of specific anatomic targets in the aging face as applied to injectables: superficial and deep facial fat compartments – an evolving target for site-specific facial augmentation. Plast Reconstr Surg. 2015;136(5 Suppl):49S–55S. https://doi.org/10.1097/PRS.0000000000001730.
14. Cotofana S, Gotkin RH, Frank K, Koban KC, Targosinski S, Sykes JM, Schlager M, Schlattau A, Schenck TL. The functional anatomy of the deep facial fat compartments: a detailed imaging-based investigation. Plast Reconstr Surg. 2019 Jan;143(1):53–63. https://doi.org/10.1097/PRS.0000000000005080.
15. Butterwick KJ, Lack EA. Facial volume restoration with the fat autograft muscle injection technique. Dermatologic Surg. 2003 Oct;29(10):1019–26. https://doi.org/10.1046/j.1524-4725.2003.29294.x.
16. Shue S, Kurlander DE, Guyuron B. Fat injection: a systematic review of injection volumes by facial subunit. Aesth Plast Surg. 2018;42(5):1261–70. https://doi.org/10.1007/s00266-017-0936-6. Epub 2017 Aug 8
17. Dasiou-Plakida D. Fat injections for facial rejuvenation: 17 years experience in 1720 patients. J Cosmet Dermatol. 2003 Jul;2(3–4):119–25. https://doi.org/10.1111/j.1473-2130.2004.00060.x.

18. Wilson AJ, Taglienti AJ, Chang CS, Low DW, Percec I. Current applications of facial volumization with fillers. Plast Reconstr Surg. 2016 May;137(5):872e–89e. https://doi.org/10.1097/PRS.0000000000002238.
19. Clauser L, Zavan B, Galiè M, Di Vittorio L, Gardin C, Bianchi AE. Autologous fat transfer for facial augmentation: surgery and regeneration. J Craniofac Surg. 2019;30(3):682–5. https://doi.org/10.1097/SCS.0000000000005257.
20. Willemsen JC, Van Dongen J, Spiekman M, Vermeulen KM, Harmsen MC, van der Lei B, Stevens HP. The addition of platelet-rich plasma to facial lipofilling: a double-blind, placebo-controlled, randomized trial. Plast Reconstr Surg. 2018;141(2):331–43.
21. Metzinger S, Parrish J, Guerra A, Zeph R. Autologous fat grafting to the lower one-third of the face. Facial Plast Surg. 2012;28(1):21–33. https://doi.org/10.1055/s-0032-1305787. Epub 2012 Mar 14. Erratum in: Facial Plast Surg 2012 Aug;28(4):467–9
22. Schultz KP, Raghuram A, Davis MJ, Abu-Ghname A, Chamata E, Rohrich RJ. Fat grafting for facial rejuvenation. Semin Plast Surg. 2020;34(1):30–7. https://doi.org/10.1055/s-0039-3402767. Epub 2020 Feb 15. PMID: 32071577; PMCID: PMC7023965
23. Tonnard PL, Verpaele AM, Ramaut LE, Blondeel PN. Aging of the upper lip: part II. Evidence-based rejuvenation of the upper lip-a review of 500 consecutive cases. Plast Reconstr Surg. 2019 May;143(5):1333–42. https://doi.org/10.1097/PRS.0000000000005589.
24. Marten TJ, Elyassina D. Fat grafting in facial rejuvenation. Clin Plast Surg. 2015;42:219–52. https://doi.org/10.1016/j.cps.2014.12.003.
25. Tsai FC, Liao CK. Clinical outcomes of patients with prominent nasolabial folds corrected by the technique: dermo-fascial detachment and fat grafting. J Plast Reconstr Aesthet Surg. 2011;64(3):307–12. https://doi.org/10.1016/j.bjps.2010.05.022. Epub 2010 Jun 29
26. Favarin GJ, Favarin E, Koseki FY, Koseki IAY, Rocha LPS, Horner C. Treatment of nasolabial fold with lipofilling. Adv Plast Reconstr Surg. 2017;1(2):35–8.
27. Gatti JE. Permanent lip augmentation with serial fat grafting. Ann Plast Surg. 1999 Apr;42(4):376–80. https://doi.org/10.1097/00000637-199904000-00005.
28. Colić MM. Lip and perioral enhancement by direct intramuscular fat autografting. Aesth Plast Surg. 1999;23(1):36–40. https://doi.org/10.1007/s002669900240.
29. Churukian M. Red lip augmentation using fat injections. Facial Plast Surg Clin North Am. 1977;5:61–4.
30. Gornitsky J, Viezel-Mathieu A, Alnaif N, Azzi AJ, Gilardino MS. A systematic review of the effectiveness and complications of fat grafting in the facial region. JPRAS Open. 2018;19:87–97. https://doi.org/10.1016/j.jpra.2018.12.004. PMID: 32158860; PMCID: PMC7061561
31. Braz A, Humphrey S, Weinkle S, Yee GJ, Remington BK, Lorenc ZP, Yoelin S, Waldorf HA, Azizzadeh B, Butterwick KJ, de Maio M, Sadick N, Trevidic P, Criollo-Lamilla G, Garcia P. Lower face: clinical anatomy and regional approaches with injectable fillers. Plast Reconstr Surg. 2015;136(5 Suppl):235S–57S. https://doi.org/10.1097/PRS.0000000000001836.
32. Pezeshk RA, Stark RY, Small KH, Unger JG, Rohrich RJ. Role of autologous fat transfer to the superficial fat compartments for perioral rejuvenation. Plast Reconstr Surg. 2015 Sep;136(3):301e–9e. https://doi.org/10.1097/PRS.0000000000001506.
33. Khan HA, Keyhan SO. Fat grafting in facial aesthetic units. Atlas Oral Maxillofac Surg Clin North Am. 2018;26(1):15–23. https://doi.org/10.1016/j.cxom.2017.10.001.
34. Wang Q, Guo X, Wang J. Autogenous fat grafting for chin augmentation: a preliminarily clinical study of cosmetic outcome. J Craniofac Surg. 2015;26(7):e625–7.
35. Rohrich RJ, Mohan R. Role of ancillary procedures in facial rejuvenation. Plast Reconstr Surg Glob Open. 2019;7(6):e2075. https://doi.org/10.1097/GOX.0000000000002075. PMID: 31624657; PMCID: PMC6635208
36. Sahan A, Karaosmanoglu N, Ozdemir CP. Chin augmentation with the use of cannula from a single, midline entry point: evaluation of 50 patients. J Cosmet Dermatol. 2020;19(6):1301–6. https://doi.org/10.1111/jocd.13411. Epub 2020 Apr 12

37. Sykes JM, Fitzgerald R. Choosing the best procedure to augment the chin: is anything better than an implant? Facial Plast Surg. 2016;32(5):507–12. https://doi.org/10.1055/s-0036-1592162. Epub 2016 Sep 28
38. Rohrich RJ, Sanniec K, Afrooz PN. Autologous fat grafting to the chin: a useful adjunct in complete aesthetic facial rejuvenation. Plast Reconstr Surg. 2018;142(4):921–5. https://doi.org/10.1097/PRS.0000000000004817.
39. Scheuer JF 3rd, Sieber DA, Pezeshk RA, Gassman AA, Campbell CF, Rohrich RJ. Facial danger zones: techniques to maximize safety during soft-tissue filler injections. Plast Reconstr Surg. 2017;139(5):1103–8. https://doi.org/10.1097/PRS.0000000000003309.
40. Yoon SS, Chang DI, Chung KC. Acute fatal stroke immediately following autologous fat injection into the face. Neurology. 2003;61(8):1151–2. https://doi.org/10.1212/wnl.61.8.1151.
41. Yoshimura K, Coleman SR. Complications of fat grafting: how they occur and how to find, avoid, and treat them. Clin Plast Surg 2015;42(3):383–388, ix. https://doi.org/10.1016/j.cps.2015.04.002. Epub 2015 May 16.

Part V

Transcutaneous Suture Lifts and Suspention

Transcutaneous Suture Lifts: Overview 31

Furkan Kaya, Zerrin Ozergin Coskun,
and Nuray Bayar Muluk

31.1 Introduction

Recently, there has been a spike in interest in minimally invasive treatments for facial rejuvenation, which has led to an increase in the popularity of thread-lifting. Thread-lifting is a procedure that has various advantages over the typical facelift [1]. It involves the placement of barbed sutures along specified trajectories to lift the superficial musculoaponeurotic system to treat facial ptosis.

Many people opt for minimally invasive procedures as scientists have gained a better knowledge of the mechanisms behind the aging process and the mechanical factors that contribute to it. Even though noninvasive neurotoxins, injectable dermal fillers, radiofrequency, and ablative resurfacing tools all play a crucial role in face rejuvenation, these treatments do not address the requirement to lift the laxity of the underlying ptotic tissues [2].

31.2 Anatomy

To achieve the best possible outcomes with the fewest possible difficulties, it is necessary to have a comprehensive grasp and knowledge of the anatomy of the facial region. A popular method involves making a temporal incision that continues

F. Kaya
Department of Otorhinolaryngology, Eskisehir Yunus Emre State Hospital, Eskisehir, Türkiye

Z. O. Coskun
Faculty of Medicine, Department of Otorhinolaryngology, Recep Tayyip Erdoğan University, Rize, Türkiye

N. Bayar Muluk (✉)
Faculty of Medicine, Department of Otorhinolaryngology, Kırıkkale University, Kırıkkale, Türkiye

C. Cingi et al. (eds.), *Minor Interventions, Major Outcomes on the Face*, Comprehensive ENT, https://doi.org/10.1007/978-3-032-01305-7_31

inferiorly to a preauricular incision, which then becomes postauricular as it bends around the ear and the hairline's edge. Although there are numerous variations, this method is the most frequent. After carrying the incision horizontally along the sideburn/cheek junction, the next step is to have it vertically along or just posterior to the anterior hairline. This is an alternative method for doing the temporal section of the incision.

Consequently, the superficial temporal arteries are spared from the temporal dissection that would otherwise be performed along the deep temporal fascia. The majority of surgeons perform a post-tragal incision in front of the ear, although some surgeons opt to perform a pre-tragal incision for male patients or patients who smoke. There is no need to disrupt the underlying SMAS layer while performing a skin-only facelift because all that is necessary is a subcutaneous dissection [3].

In 1889, Manchot described the vascular supply to the face [4]. The research was improved by Whetzel and Mathes, who also provided a more detailed description of the vascular regions of the face and scalp [5]. Musculocutaneous perforators are the primary ones responsible for supplying the facelift flap. These perforators originate from three primary artery trunks: the facial, superficial temporal, and ophthalmic arteries. There are abundant anastomotic networks present in the central face region, where the majority of blood flow originates. Because of this, skin flaps can survive after being undermined. Ischemia in the flaps is a concern that grows as the extent of the dissection that is performed medially becomes more extensive. The blood supply is kept to a more significant degree with other deeper plane procedures, such as composite facelifts, which makes ischemia less likely even with tremendous stress that a subcutaneous facelift would not allow [6, 7]. Composite facelifts are one example of these types of treatments.

The subcutaneous muscle of the face (SMAS) [3] is located under the dissection plane and covers the underlying facial musculature.

31.3 What Is a Thread-Lifting?

Through thread-lifting, a facelift has been transformed into a less invasive treatment that does not leave scars and has fewer consequences. On the other hand, absorbable PDO sutures, which are widely used by cosmetologists and have received a lot of publicity, have yet to win over surgeons' acceptance. This is because they are not durable, do not provide genuine fixation, and are applied to the skin rather than the subcutaneous muscle adhesions (SMAS). It is challenging to find thread strategies that combine the utilization of permanent threads, the utilization of a stable fixation point, and the utilization of work on the SMAS layer. However, these methods necessitate utilizing costly suture materials or devices specifically constructed and the completion of specialized training courses. As a result, their application is restricted in modern society, which is a highly cost-conscious market [8].

It was claimed that the applications of polydioxanone (PDS) and polylactic acid (PLA) barbed sutures for the closed suspension technique known as thread lift 1 [9, 10] could not only be used for robust and dramatic tissue suspension but also for facial rejuvenation. However, this technique needed to be improved due to the absence of long-term aesthetic outcomes, high costs, and complications [2, 9, 11, 12].

31.4 Tissue Suspension with Suture

Since the beginning of time, the repositioning and stabilizing of subcutaneous tissues has been accomplished by utilizing absorbable or non-absorbable sutures [13, 14]. Regarding facial rejuvenation, suspension techniques in conjunction with classic rhytidectomy incisions are typically used for superior results. The procedure known as skin and SMAS suspension, also known as deep subperiosteal suspension, can be carried out using either autologous tissue, such as tendons or fascia, or prosthetic materials, such as sutures, slings, or mesh [15, 16]. Several different kinds of suture material have been utilized for this purpose, the most common of which being polytetrafluoroethylene (Gore-TexTM), polyglactin (VicrylTM), and polypropylene [16]. Two general principles of facial rejuvenation are now being developed [17], and they are among the various suspending techniques currently available. The first method uses SMAS as the fixation basis, which involves subcutaneous suspension. Tissue elevation is achieved through the use of posterolateral vectors. The second method is based on the subperiosteal separation and en-bloc repositioning of all structures using exclusively vertical vectors [17].

Additionally, suspension techniques have been applied to minimally invasive operations involving the middle and lower face thirds. These procedures are performed using the endoscope. Therefore, it is conceivable to reposition and anchor the face's soft tissues to the temporal fascia or the periosteum by making minor incisions [13, 18]. This can be accomplished effectively.

Elevating the eyebrows or the center part of the face with minimal morbidity can be accomplished with the simple transfixion of silky threads through the skin [19, 20]. Several approaches have been described to produce mild facial lifting. These techniques involve the insertion of suture threads that hold the portion of the face that is to be suspended, ultimately anchoring it to the scalp (Curl Lift, Arch Lift) [21]. Unpredictability may be associated with the outcomes of various operations. The threads tend to cut the tissues easily, and the wrinkles and creases of the skin tend to fade along with the results [19, 20].

31.5 Barbed Sutures

There was a significant increase in the sutures' capacity to tolerate loads after the introduction of polypropylene barbed sutures [16]. Barbed sutures were initially mentioned by Alcamo in 1964 [19], then by Fukuda in 1984, and finally by Ruff in 1994 [22]. Alcamo was the first person to suggest the idea. These pioneers did not need to tie knots to seal wounds because they employed barbed sutures. On the other hand, the aesthetic applications differed from what they had anticipated [19].

They described a suture containing barbs arranged sequentially along its length. There was a place in the thread close to the center when the barbs changed direction, which resulted in the creation of a mirror copy of the barbs in the opposite direction. When one extremity was wrapped around the tissues, it either healed the wound. It anchored the other extremity or brought the tissues closer to the thread's center, creating new gradients of tension and compression [22, 23].

In the late 1980s, Russian scholars Sulamanidze et al. [24, 25] were the first to disclose the use of barbed sutures for tissue suspension. The subcutaneous tissue is where the sutures are put, and there is very little or no soft tissue dissection [25, 26]. Since they were first introduced, modifications have been made to the design and the placement of the items. The initial Anti-Ptosis Suture (APTOS) was a multi-toothed thread later modified to become bidirectional. The barbs were positioned so that they attached the tissues to the core portion of the thread, eliminating the necessity for anchoring at the extremities. Afterward, it was altered to provide traction and suspension in only one direction [25]. An additional modification was made to the fastening procedures to accommodate the one-way barbs [25, 26]. Even though numerous methods have been utilized over time, they all entail the interposition of the soft tissues to the suture barbs, which in turn triggers the inflammatory response and the formation of fibrosis around the suture barbs [27].

Numerous lengths and various inlay needles are available for the most recent generation of barbed sutures for soft tissue support [26]. These sutures are available in non-absorbable and absorbable materials, depending on the type of material. A variety of applications are possible as a result of the numerous current presentations, which include self-fixation, curved passages that envelop the ptotic tissue, loops, and fixation of the two extremities of the thread at a single site, with anchoring at the temporal fascia or other deep points [13, 19, 21, 27].

The FDA does not have approval for the mono-filament, double-convergence polypropylene threads that are used in Brazil. These threads are known as Beramendi or Russian threads. However, ANVISA has given its approval for them [25, 28]. In general, permanent strands are permitted to treat facial and cervical ptosis, whereas absorbable threads are only allowed for the approach of soft tissue and the suturing of wounds [23]. Polydioxanone (PDO), a polymer that undergoes slow hydrolysis, is the absorbent substance utilized most frequently in producing threads [22].

Both the forehead and the middle and lower thirds of the face, in addition to the neck, are excellent candidates for the application of barbed sutures. It does not matter where the threads are utilized on the face; incisions should be made where they can be concealed, regardless of how little they are. This should be followed by the subcutaneous tissue's dissection, the threads' passage, and their proximal anchoring. Last but not least, the soft tissues ought to be molded in such a way that a contour that is both smooth and harmonious is achieved [13–20].

31.6 Transcutaneous Suture Lifts: Nose

The nasal aesthetic difficulties are one of the few areas in which we are unable to provide our patients with a suitable option that is less invasive. This is even though "less is more" is becoming increasingly popular today. To address their issues, not every patient needs all of the essential components in a conventional rhinoplasty procedure; a sizable minority of patients do not require all of these components. Furthermore, we have patients who are unable to adjust their daily routines to allow the necessary recovery period or who do not wish to undertake such a large operation due to the health issues that are involved with it or the fear that they feel about the irreversible change that will occur in their facial characteristics. The primary purpose of the procedure we describe is to provide patients with a straightforward method for nose reshaping. This treatment may be carried out in the office under local anesthetic in less than 15 minutes, and as a result, it is comparable to Botox or fillers in the patient's mind [29].

It is extremely well established in the literature [30, 31] that suture procedures are an intrinsic aspect of rhinoplasty and are described as such. To bind the nasal tip to the caudal septum, Joseph [31] utilized sutures. Over time, several additional suture procedures have been presented [32–38]. On the other hand, each of these methods has been proposed as a component of conventional rhinoplasty, and none of them has been presented as a minimally invasive treatment that can be performed on its own to correct nasal issues. On the other hand, our method can be provided as a straightforward, office-based operation that can be carried out under local anesthesia in minutes with almost no downtime. This applies to some patients. Because this operation does not jeopardize the essential anatomical features of the nose, there is no possibility of skin abnormalities associated with LLC excision or difficulties with the internal valves associated with ULC surgery [39, 40].

It is possible to install a single caudal septal suspension suture; however, in certain instances, this may be done at the expense of a retracted columella. When a dorsal suspension is performed for the tip first, it is much simpler to determine the degree of rotation. After that, a septo-columellar suture can be inserted following the degree of rotation without the possibility of the columellar retraction occurring. However, in patients who have an inadequate nasal projection, the use of columellar-septal sutures, which involve dissecting between the medial crura and then suturing them to the septum at a higher position in a tongue-in-groove manner, is effective in achieving an additional one to two millimeters of projection. This technique may also be beneficial for stability in the long-term outcome. If the septum is too lengthy, removing a little section from the anterocaudal portion is possible to lessen the opposing force produced by the septal cartilage's push [39]. It is beneficial to reversely dissect between the upper and lower cartilages to create a space for cartilaginous overlapping [29]. This further reduces the antagonistic effect of the existing structures, particularly the upper cartilages.

The suspension knot can be utilized as a filler in the glabellar region of patients with profound nasofrontal connections to conceal the dorsal prominence during the procedure. The dorsal dissection is an essential component of this technique. It is carried out to achieve fibrosis of the subcutaneous tissue, which is necessary to establish a long-lasting fixation. The quick formation of scar tissue in the skin interface is a biological glue that helps keep the new tip position in place over time [37, 38]. We have found that establishing a solid subcutaneous fibrosis takes at least 3 to 4 weeks. This is based on our own experience. If the suspension is detached before this period, it can be reversed, which the patients may consider an advantage of this surgery. Continuing this study, measuring the nasal length and the nasolabial angle pre- and postoperatively at different intervals could be advantageous. This would allow us to have data that will enable us to precisely estimate the amount of overcorrection required [29].

31.7 Transcutaneous Suture Lifts: Neck

In addition to being the first anatomical region to show signs of aging, the neck also plays a role in the individual's overall identity. Awareness of the neck's aging process is reasonably necessary when it comes to neck rejuvenation. Multiple strategies for neck rejuvenation have been published in the field of research [41]. Skoog [42] described the anatomy of the superficial musculoaponeurotic system (SMAS) in 1974. He also discussed this system's role in the neck's aging. In recent years, there has been an increase in the number of patients interested in minimally invasive surgery, characterized by a low risk of complications and a short recovery period. The use of thread for neck rejuvenation and the concept of the suture suspension neck lift have grown ubiquitous as a convenient and successful technique. However, difficulties have also been observed, such as recurrence, poor correction, and palpability of the sutures. All of these complications have been described.

It was also mentioned by Stuzin et al. [43] that the threaded suture could rip the SMAS layer if the sutures had been introduced when the thread was under tension [43]. Compared to earlier approaches, the elastic lift is more effective, has a longer lifespan, and is conveniently located. The elastic thread is made from a non-absorbable suture material covered with polyester. Because the surface of the polyester is braided rather than barbed, the connective tissue surrounding the suture grows into the braided suture's interstices like that of a ligament [44].

In the past, thread-lifting was accomplished by suspending the ptotic soft tissue with barbed sutures. However, in elastic lifting, the soft tissue is repositioned due to the stretchy nature of the silicone. All patients who underwent mid-face lifting with elastic threads expressed contentment with the outcomes of their procedures, and no significant issues arose throughout the follow-up. Moreover, postoperative improvements were observed in objective outcomes measured using a skin laxity grade score [45].

The concept of neck lifting with a micro-shuttle involves the creation of a percutaneous hammock, which is made up of solid and non-absorbable sutures placed over non-undermined platysma. This hammock is then anchored to fixed loops around the ears via a micro-shuttle needle with two ends. This allows the problem of different depths on the neck to be solved simultaneously. Skin resection is typically not undertaken because the suspension bridge can adjust for the gravitational strain. Instead, skin redraping is accomplished by the intrinsic retraction capability of the skin that has been undermined [46].

References

1. Tong LX, Rieder EA. Thread-lifts: a double-edged suture? A comprehensive review of the literature. Dermatologic Surg. 2019 Jul;45(7):931–40. https://doi.org/10.1097/DSS.0000000000001921.
2. Rachel J, Jamora J. Skin Rejuvenation Regimens. Arch Facial Plast Surg. 2003;5(2):145–9.
3. Kaplan JL. Skin-only facelift. In: Long JN, editor. Medscape. Updated: Feb 27, 2023. https://emedicine.medscape.com/article/1294390-overview#a9. Accessed online at 11 June 2023.
4. Manchot C. Die Hautarterien des Menschlichen Korpes. Leipzig: Vogel; 1889.
5. Whetzel TP, Mathes SJ. Arterial anatomy of the face: an analysis of vascular territories and perforating cutaneous vessels. Plast Reconstr Surg. 1992;89(4):591–603. discussion 604-5
6. Hamra ST. Composite rhytidectomy. Plas Reconstr Surg. 1992;90:1–13.
7. Mani M. Total composite flap facelift and the deep-plane transition zone: a critical consideration in SMAS-release midface lifting. Aesthet Surg J. 2016 May;36(5):533–45.
8. El-Kafrawl HY. Fixed-tension sutures for face and neck lifting. Egypt J. Plast. Reconstr. Surg. 2022;46(1):1–7.
9. Rachel J, Lack E, Larson B. Incidence of complications and early recurrence in 29 patients after facial rejuvenation with barbed suture lifting. Dermatologic Surg. 2010;36(3):348–54.
10. Garvey PB, Ricciardelli EJ, Gampper T. Outcomes in threadlift for facial rejuvenation. Ann Plast Surg. 2009;62(5):482–5.
11. Matarasso A, Pfeifer T. The use of modified sutures in plastic surgery. Plast Reconstr Surg. 2008;122(2):652–8.
12. Villa MT, White LE, Alam M. Barbed sutures: a review of the literature. PRS. 2008;121(3):102–8.
13. Tavares JP, Oliveira CACP, Torres RP, Bahmad F Jr. Facial thread lifting with suture suspension. Braz J Otorhinolaryngol. 2017;83(6):712–9. https://doi.org/10.1016/j.bjorl.2017.03.015. Epub 2017 May 9. PMID: 28549872; PMCID: PMC9449186
14. Paul MD. Complications of barbed sutures. Aesthet Plast Surg. 2008;32:149.
15. Kaminer MS, Bogart M, Choi C, Wee SA. Long-term efficacy of anchored barbed sutures in the face and neck. Dermatologic Surg. 2008;34:1041–7.
16. Villa MT, White LE, Alam M, Yoo SS, Walton RL. Barbed sutures: a review of the literature. Plast Reconstr Surg. 2008;121:102–8.
17. Berry MG, Davies D. Platysma-SMAS plication facelift. J Plast Reconstr Aesthet Surg. 2010;63:793–800.
18. Verpaele A, Tonnard P. Lower third of the face: indications and limitations of the minimal access cranial suspension lift. Clin Plast Surg. 2008;35:645–59.
19. Wu WTL. Barbed sutures in facial rejuvenation. Aesthet Surg J. 2004;24:582–7.
20. Graziosi AC, Beer SMC. Browlifting with thread: the technique without undermining using minimum incisions. Aesthet Plast Surg. 1998;22:120–5.
21. Kalil AF, Fournier PF. Curl lift versus other suture suspension lifts. Cosmet Dermatol. 2006;19:133–7.
22. Ruff GL. Absorbable barbed sutures. Aesthet Surg J. 2006;26:620–8.
23. Ruff G. Technique and uses for absorbable barbed sutures. Aesthet Surg J. 2006;26:620–8.
24. Sulamanidze MA, Paikidze TG, Sulamanidze GM, Neigel JM. Facial lifting with "APTOS" threads: featherlift. Otolaryngol Clin N Am. 2005;38:1109–17.
25. Sulamanidze MA, Fournier PF, Paikidze TG, Sulamanidze GM. Removal of facial soft tissue ptosis with special threads. Dermatologic Surg. 2002;28:367–71.

26. Paul MD. Barbed sutures for aesthetic facial plastic surgery: indications and techniques. Clin Plast Surg. 2008;35:451–61.
27. DeLorenzi CL. Barbed sutures: rationale and technique. Aesthet Surg J. 2006;26:223–9.
28. Badin AZ, Forte MRC, Silva OL. Scarless mid and lower face lift. Aesthet Surg J. 2005;25:340–7.
29. Tiryaki KT. Shuttle lifting of the nose: a minimally invasive approach for nose reshaping. Aesthet Surg J. 2010 Mar;30(2):176–83.
30. Tebbetts JB. Nasal tip sutures: part I. The evolution and nasal tip sutures: part II. The interplays (discussion). Plast Reconstr Surg. 2003;112:1146–9.
31. Joseph J. Nasenplastik und sonstige gesichtplastik. Leipzig: Curt Kabitzsch; 1931.
32. Gruber RP, Friedman GD. Suture algorithm for the broad and bulbous nasal tip. Plast Reconstr Surg. 2002;110:1752–64.
33. Guyuron B, Behmand R. Nasal tip sutures: part II. The interplays. Plast Reconstr Surg. 2003;112:1130–45.
34. Daniel RK. Rhinoplasty: a simplified, three-stitch, opentipsuture technique: part I. Primary rhinoplasty. Plast Reconstr Surg. 1999;103:1491–502.
35. Gruber RP. Suture technique in rhinoplasty by use of the endonasal (closed) approach. Aesthetic Surg J. 1998;18:99–103.
36. Stal S. Nasal tip rotation. In: Gunter JP, Rohrich RJ, Adams WP, editors. Dallas Rhinoplasty: nasal surgery by the masters. St. Louis: Quality Medical Publishing; 2002. p. 402–9.
37. Tebbetts JB. Primary Rhinoplasty: a new approach to the logical and the techniques. St. Louis: Mosby; 1998.
38. Gruber RP. Suture techniques. In: Gunter JP, Rohrich RJ, Adams WP, editors. Dallas Rhinoplasty: nasal surgery by the masters. St Louis: Quality Medical Publishing; 2002. p. 254–70.
39. Guyuron B. Discussion: securing nasal tip rotation through suspension suture technique. Plast Reconstr Surg. 2006;117:1756.
40. Guyuron B. Dynamic interplays during rhinoplasty. Clin Plast Surg. 1996;23:223–31.
41. Kang MS, Kim SH, Nam SM, Park ES. Evaluation of elastic lift for neck rejuvenation. Arch Aesthetic Plast Surg. 2016;22(2):68–73.
42. Skoog TG. Plastic surgery: the aging face. In: Skoog TG, editor. Plastic surgery: new methods and refinements. Philadelphia: W.B. Saunders; 1974. p. 300–30.
43. Stuzin JM, Baker TJ, Baker TM. Refinements in face lifting: enhanced facial contour using vicryl mesh incorporated into SMAS fixation. Plast Reconstr Surg. 2000;105:290–301.
44. Huggins RJ, Freeman ME, Kerr JB, et al. Histologic and ultrastructural evaluation of sutures used for surgical fixation of the SMAS. Aesth Plast Surg. 2007;31:719–24.
45. Kang MS, Shin JS, Nam SM, et al. Evaluation of elastic lift for facial rejuvenation. Arch Aesthetic Plast Surg. 2016;22:20–7.
46. Tiryaki KT, Aksungur E, Grotting JC. Micro-shuttle lifting of the neck: a percutaneous loop suspension method using a novel double-ended needle. Aesthet Surg J. 2016 Jun;36(6):629–38.

Transcutaneous Suture Lifts: Eyebrows 32

Mehmet İhsan Gulmez, Secil Ucar, and Cemal Cingi

32.1 Introduction

The periorbital region, located in the upper third of the face, is of primary importance in reflecting facial aesthetics and expression. People communicate by looking into each other's eyes in their mutual relationships. This causes the periorbital region to be the most conspicuous area of the face. This region includes the eyebrows and eyelids and varies by race, gender, and age. In particular, the eyebrow is known as the mainline of the face and is used as a reference point for all other angles of the face [1]. It forms the upper frame of the eye and expresses youth and attractiveness with its shape and position. Although many authors have tried to define the ideal eyebrow shape and position, it is only possible to achieve this partially. It is not possible to define an ideal eyebrow suitable for every face.

As people age, the eye loses its aesthetic appearance and attractiveness. Aging eyebrows can cause the appearance of fatigue or anger in the person. In this, the effect of the eyebrows falling from their normal position is great. The main reasons for this change over time are gravity and the pulling effect of the muscles working against the frontalis muscle [2]. The frontalis muscle is the only elevator muscle of the eyebrow. Contraction of this muscle causes the forehead to crease transversely

M. İ. Gulmez
Medical Faculty, Department of Otorhinolaryngology, Hatay Mustafa Kemal University, Hatay, Türkiye

S. Ucar
Private International-Prof Clinic, Istanbul, Türkiye

C. Cingi (✉)
Eskisehir Osmangazi University, Medical Faculty, Department of Otorhinolaryngology, Eskisehir, Türkiye
e-mail: cemal@ogu.edu.tr

C. Cingi et al. (eds.), *Minor Interventions, Major Outcomes on the Face*, Comprehensive ENT, https://doi.org/10.1007/978-3-032-01305-7_32

[3, 4]. The depressor muscles of the eyebrow are the procerus, corrugator supercilii, depressor supercilii, and orbicularis oculi. Among the depressor muscles, the corrugator supercilii is the dominant one. The supratrochlear and supraorbital nerves receive the sensation of the forehead. Its motor innervation is via the temporal branch of the facial nerve.

Prolonged hyperactivity of the muscles of the upper third of the face causes three deformities in general: transverse wrinkles of the forehead, droopy eyebrows, and glabellar wrinkles [5]. With the effect of gravity, eyebrow droop begins to show itself in the 20 s and early 30 s. The drooping of the eyebrows is more pronounced in the lateral segment. Some authors attributed this to the fact that the lateral segment receives less support from deep anatomical structures than the medial segment [6]. Some authors have tried to explain this situation with the thought that the frontalis muscle fibers do not extend enough to the lateral part of the eyebrow [7].

32.2 Aesthetic Appearance of the Eyebrow

The aesthetic appearance of the eyebrow is affected by many factors, such as age, race, culture, gender, and fashion. However, periorbital structures also affect the appearance of the eyebrows. Therefore, the eyebrows' size, shape, and position are also different for different faces. It is impossible to talk about an ideal definition suitable for every face for the eyebrow, whose appearance and aesthetics are affected by many factors. On this subject, art historian Johann Winckelmann (1717–1768) stated that in the Greek definition of ideal beauty, the perfect eyebrow makes an arch just above the brow bone, and both eyebrows grow toward the nose [8]. Although this definition is long overdue and far from meeting current fashion needs, it is valuable in reflecting the evolving nature of eyebrow aesthetics. Westmore provides a more recent definition of the ideal eyebrow. Accordingly [9];

1. The medial eyebrow should begin in the same vertical plane as the lateral extent of the ala and the inner canthus.
2. The medial eyebrow ends laterally at an oblique line drawn from the most lateral point of the ala through the lateral canthus.
3. The medial and lateral ends of the eyebrow lie approximately at the same horizontal level.
4. The apex lies on a vertical line directly above the lateral limbus.

Apart from this, other evaluations of the ideal eyebrow are in the literature. Although Ellenbogen agreed with the Westmore criteria, he stated that the hair follicles in the caudal part of the medial border of the brow should start approximately 1 cm above the supraorbital rim [10]. In addition to Westmore, Cook et al. stated that the apex should be more lateral to the lateral canthus [11]. Whitaker et al. stated that the highest point of the eyebrow should be the intersection point of the middle and lateral 1/3 [12]. McKinney stated that the distance between the mid-pupil and the upper eyebrow should be 2.5 cm, and between the upper eyebrow border and the hairline should be approximately 5 cm [13]. Connell said that the distance between the upper eyelid crease and the lower border of the eyebrow should be 15 mm [14]. Matarasso and Terino stated this distance as 16 mm and defined the distance between the mid-pupil as 2.5 cm, between the eyebrow and the supraorbital rim as 1 cm, and between the eyebrow and hairline as 5–6 cm [15].

Gunter stated that an eyebrow aesthetic evaluation without evaluating the entire periorbital region, especially the eyelids, would be insufficient. After reviewing the literature and evaluating his patients, he tried to formulate an attractive eyebrow. Accordingly [16]:

1. The intercantal axis should be tilted slightly upward from medial to lateral.
2. The upper eyelid should cover the iris approximately 1–2 mm.
3. The medial portion of the upper eyelid margin should be in a more vertical plane than the lateral upper eyelid margin.
4. The upper eyelid crease should parallel the lash line and divide the upper eyelid into an upper two-thirds and a lower one-third, never more than 1:1.
5. The medial extension of the supratarsal upper skin fold should not exceed the inner extent of the medial canthus.
6. The lateral extension of the supratarsal upper skin fold should not extend beyond the lateral orbital rim.
7. Minimal scleral show should be observed between the lower eyelid and the iris.
8. The lower eyelid margin should bow gently from medial to lateral, with the lowest point between the pupil and the lateral limbus.

The eyebrow structures of women and men are different. In men, the eyebrow runs just above the orbital rim, while in women, it runs a few millimeters above the rim. In men, the eyebrow is thicker and makes a slight arc; in women, it makes a more aesthetic arc that reaches the highest level in the lateral 1/3.

32.3 Brow Lift Surgery

Eyebrow lift surgery can be performed with the demand for better eyebrow position, structure, symmetry deterioration, or a more aesthetic appearance. Many eyebrow-lifting techniques have been described to date. An endoscopic brow lift, coronal lift, midforehead lift, pretrichial lift, and direct brow lift are some of them. The transcutaneous suture lifting method, mentioned in this section, stands out with its non-invasiveness and acceptable duration of action. Extremely successful results can be obtained with the correct technique applied with the correct threads in the appropriate indication.

32.4 Types of Sutures

We can examine the sutures used in transcutaneous suture lifting techniques under four headings:

1. Polydioxanone (PDO) threads.
2. Poly-L-Lactic acid (PLLA) threads.
3. Polycaprolactone (PCL) threads.
4. Polypropylene threads

32.4.1 Polydioxanone (PDO) Threads

Polydioxanone is a colorless, polymeric, resorbable substance. PDO sutures, which have been used in surgery for a long time, are synthetic, monofilament in structure, and are used in colored form for convenience. It remains for more than 6 months in the body and acts by stimulating fibroblasts to produce more collagen in the treated area [17]. The most commonly used types of PDO sutures in the periorbital region are mono sutures, screw sutures, and COG sutures (Fig. 32.1). Although the cost of gold PDO sutures is higher than other PDO sutures, they are preferred, especially in contour arrangements around the eyes, with their detoxification effect and skin elasticity-supporting feature. Depending on the purpose, these types of sutures can be used alone or in combinations.

32.4.1.1 Mono Threads

Mono threads are straight, barb-free, thin, and monofilament threads. They are placed in the deep dermis and subcutaneous tissue. They create a foreign body reaction and stimulate the immune system and collagen production [18]. It creates a skin

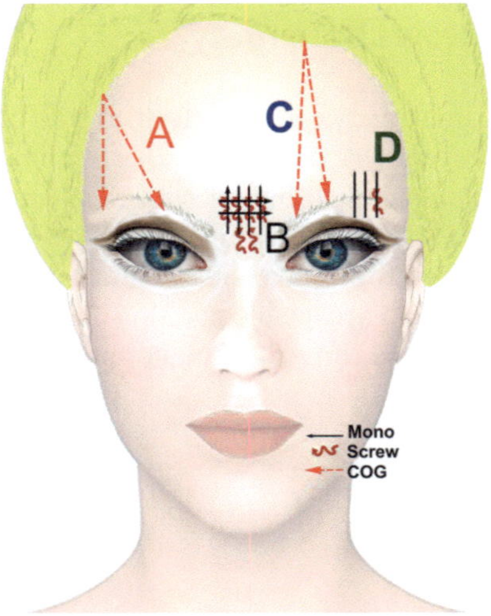

Fig. 32.1 PDO thread applications in eyebrow lifting

tightening, collagen increase, and lifting effect in the applied area [19]. They are also used to remove wrinkles around the eyes and in areas with loss of volume and in eyebrow lifting (Fig. 32.1b, d). The skin-tightening effect is more prominent. It may need to be used with other threads when lifting. They can be used more than once to show the desired effect in the applied area.

32.4.1.2 Screw Threads

Screw threads consist of one or more mono threads wound in a spiral around the insertion needle. The spiral shape causes more volume and lifting effects when placed under the skin [20]. In cases where it is desired to benefit more from these forces, double screw threads, in which two mono threads spiral around the insertion needle, can be used. Screw threads can be used to open deep wrinkles, facelifts, and eyebrow lifts (Fig. 32.1b, d).

32.4.1.3 COG Threads

COG threads are barbed mono threads held under the skin by the hook effect. These spines form a support structure that lifts the overhanging tissue, including the malar region, jawline, and eyebrows [21] (Fig. 32.1a, c).

32.4.2 Poly-L-Lactic Acid (PLLA) Threads

PLLA is a biodegradable and biocompatible thermoplastic aliphatic polyester. It can be easily obtained from natural sources, has no toxic or allergic effects, and has bio-stimulant activity [22]. While the half-life is about 1 month, they are gradually excreted from the body within 9–24 months [23]. It has been used in the European medical community for the treatment of HIV-related facial atrophy for nearly 20 years and was FDA-approved in the USA for this indication in 2004 [24]. It has also been used in aging-related lipoatrophy. It shows its effect not by filling the injected area but by increasing fibroblast proliferation and collagen production.

PLLA threads contain cones of glycolic acid and glycolic polymers in a certain range and number opposite. There is a gap of 2 cm between the opposing cone series. The thread has needles at both ends. These needles are 23 G and 12 cm in size. At the tip of the needle, black lines show the 5 mm border. The line shows the distance to be entered perpendicularly from the skin surface, corresponding to the subcutaneous tissue and the superficial musculoaponeurotic system (SMAS). According to the number of cones, there are three types and lengths of thread with 8, 12, and 16 cones [25, 26]. They are also used in eyebrow lifting, soft tissue lifting, and suspension (Fig. 32.2).

In the application technique, first, the area to be applied is determined, and the appropriate marking is made after the number of cones to be used and the suture length are decided. After sterile conditions are provided, local anesthetic is injected into the needle entry and exit sites. The first needle is placed perpendicular to the skin and advanced to the black mark. Then it is advanced along the vector line, paralleling the skin inside. The thread is pulled until all of the cones of the first

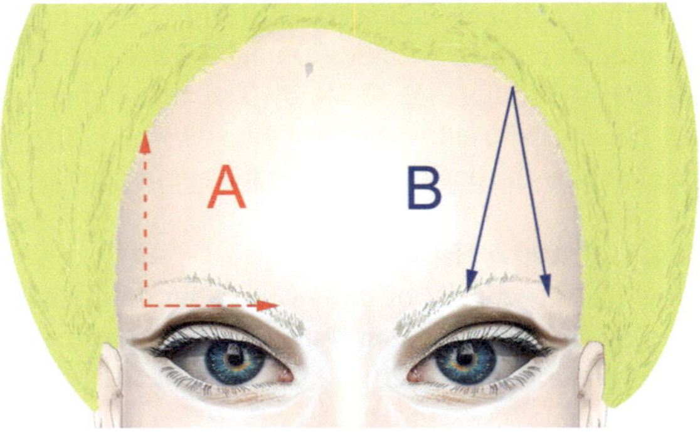

Fig. 32.2 PLLA thread applications in eyebrow lifting

section are inside, and the space between the cones is ensured in the needle entry hole. In this way, the cones are ensured to be seated in the SMAS. Then, it is entered from the same entry point as the other needle and progresses similarly along the other vector line. After all the cones come in and sit in the SMAS, the threads are stretched, and the desired suspension and lifting are done. The process is terminated by deeply cutting the ends of the threads under the skin [25, 26].

32.4.2.1 Brow Lift with L Technique

When performing eyebrow lifting with the L technique, a place between the eyebrow's arc and the eyebrow's lateral end is determined as the entry point first. After properly passing the needle, advance at least 3 cm toward the medial side and exit. After the other needle enters from the same entry point, it moves at least 7 cm toward the superior with a 90-degree angle and exits close to the hairline. The same application is made for the other eyebrow. Both eyebrows' desired application and symmetry are achieved by stretching the threads. The process is terminated by deeply cutting the ends of the threads under the skin [25] (Fig. 32.2a).

32.4.2.2 Brow Lift with V Technique

The entry point is determined at the hairline when performing eyebrow lifting with the V technique. The first needle is entered here and exited right in the middle of the eyebrow arc. The second needle is entered from the same point and exited from the lateral aspect of the eyebrow. The threads are stretched, and the eyebrows are positioned appropriately to ensure the cones are seated. The process is terminated by deeply cutting the ends of the threads under the skin [25] (Fig. 32.2b).

32.4.3 Polycaprolactone (PCL) Threads

Polycaprolactone is a partially crystalline synthetic polyester produced from crude oil and made biodegradable by adding various additives [27, 28]. Its melting point is 60 degrees Celsius. Threads produced from this material have long-lasting effects on the human body, lasting up to 3 years. They are produced in a uniquely serrated or barbed form.

32.4.3.1 Eyebrow Lift with Two Needles

In this technique, two opposite needles from PCL threads are used. The projections of the bilateral superior temporal septum are determined as the entry hole of the needles. Following the local anesthetic injection, the needle is entered through the entry hole and advanced toward the lateral end of the eyebrow arch. Then, proceed along the eyebrow to reach the medial of the eyebrow. From here, the forehead is advanced to the midline, and the needle is exited. Exit from the same point by performing operations on the opposite side symmetrically. The second needle entry points are made approximately 5 mm medial to the first needle entry points. The first needle is advanced through the subcutaneous tissue, while the second is through the deep temporal fascia. The second needle is advanced through the same steps, the forehead midline is exited, and the process is completed [29] (Fig. 32.3).

32.4.3.2 Eyebrow Lift with Double-Needle

The entry point of this technique is where the vertical line passing through the middle of the eyebrow intersects with the hairline. Following the local anesthetic injection, the needle is inserted from the entry point, and the mid-lateral 1/3 intersection of the eyebrow is reached. From here, it moves laterally in the horizontal plane and reaches the lateral eyebrow. Finally, in the vertical plane, it is advanced toward the superior and exits from the lateral of the entry point. The second needle is inserted from the same entry point, and the brow at the mid-medial 1/3 intersection is reached. Proceed symmetrically to the first needle path and exit medial to the entry point. The excess threads are cut after the eyebrow is shaped appropriately [29] (Fig. 32.4a).

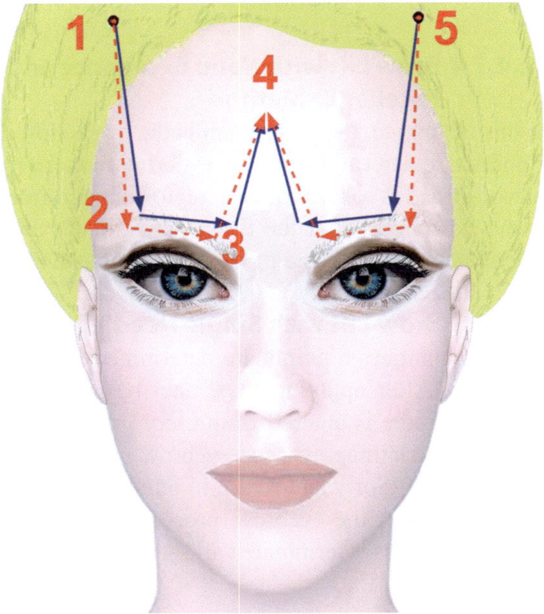

Fig. 32.3 PCL thread applications in eyebrow lifting

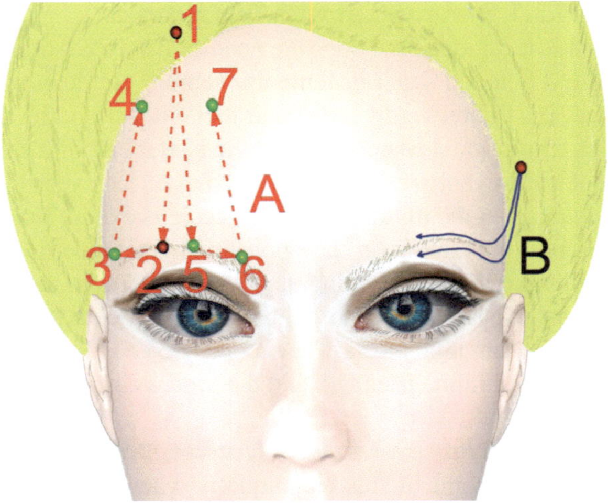

Fig. 32.4 PCL thread applications in eyebrow lifting

32.4.3.3 Eyebrow Lift with Light Lift Thread

In this technique, the projection of the superior temporal septum is determined as the entry point. After the local anesthetic injection, the first thread is entered from the entry point and advanced to the lateral side of the eyebrow. Then, proceed horizontally from the lower border of the eyebrow and exit from the medial side of the eyebrow. The second thread is entered from the same entry point and is advanced approximately 5 mm medial to the first thread to the lateral of the eyebrow. From here, it proceeds horizontally from the upper border of the eyebrow and exits from the medial side of the eyebrow. The process is terminated after the threads are stretched and the eyebrows are shaped appropriately [18, 30] (Fig. 32.4b).

32.4.3.4 Brow Lift with Nano Excellence and Visage Excellence Method

In this technique, the entry point is the projection of the superior temporal septum. 5 points are determined on the eyebrow from lateral to medial as the exit point. A curved thread is passed for each region entered from the entry point and determined as the exit point. After the five placed threads are stretched and the eyebrows are shaped appropriately, the process is terminated [18, 30] (Fig. 32.5).

32.4.3.5 Brow Lift with Single Needle Method

In this technique, 6 points are determined: three on the hairline and three on the eyebrows. After applying local anesthesia to the determined points, the single-threaded needle is entered from entry point number 6 and proceeds to number 7. From here, continue over the eyebrow and go to number 9. From here, proceed to number 8 superiorly and return to number 9 by re-entering 1–2 mm from the side. Continuing over the eyebrow, proceed to number 11 and finally to number 10 to exit. The process is terminated after the appropriate shape is given [29] (Fig. 32.6b).

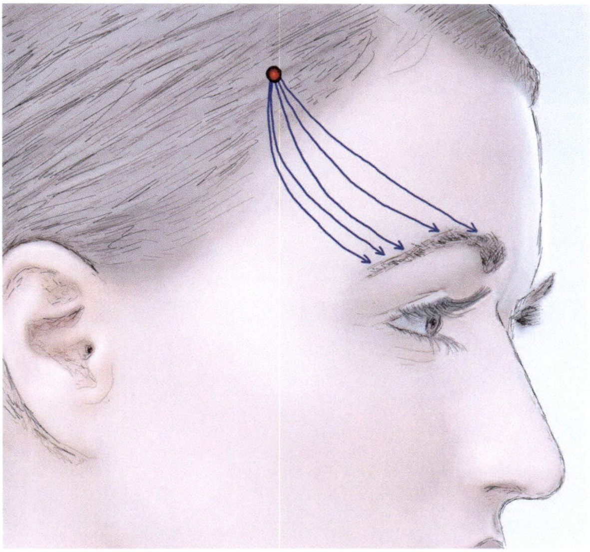

Fig. 32.5 PCL thread applications in eyebrow lifting

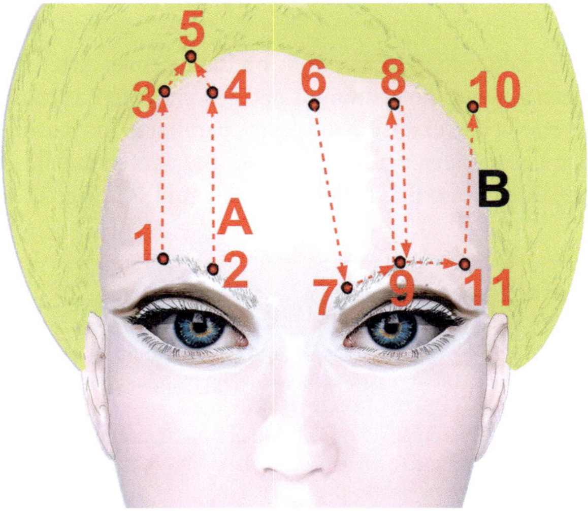

Fig. 32.6 PCL and Polypropylene thread applications in eyebrow lifting

32.4.4 Polypropylene Threads

Polypropylene is a partially crystalline, non-polar, thermoplastic polymer [31]. Threads produced from this material cannot be absorbed in the body. They have unidirectional spines. It enables the thread to advance in one direction and fix the tissue to which it is applied through these spines [32, 33] (Fig. 32.7).

In the eyebrow-lifting technique with polypropylene threads, two points are determined in the lateral and medial thirds of the eyebrow arc, two points on the hairline superiorly in parallel with these points, and the fifth point with a triangular

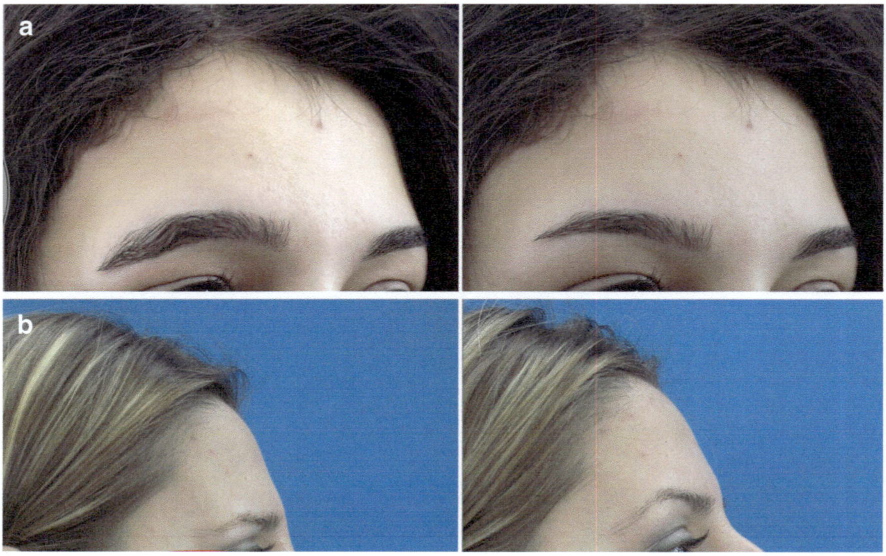

Fig. 32.7 (**a**, **b**) Eyebrow lifting on a patient. (Courtesy of Secil Ucar MD)

apex between the two points on the hairline. After applying local anesthesia to the determined points, straight needles are entered from the determined points on the eyebrow and exit from the points parallel to the hairline on the superior. After giving the desired shape to the eyebrow, the curved needle advances to the top point, and the threads are fixed on the periosteum [34] (Fig. 32.6a).

References

1. Cole EA, Winn BJ, Putterman AM. Measurement of eyebrow position from inferior corneal limbus to brow: a new technique. Ophthalmic Plast Reconstr Surg. 2010;26(6):443–7. https://doi.org/10.1097/IOP.0b013e3181d3dd22.
2. Mesa J, Vasconez LO. Commentary on: transcutaneous brow shaping: a straightforward and precise method to lift and shape the eyebrows. Aesthetic Surg J. 2017;37(8):876–8. https://doi.org/10.1093/asj/sjx134.
3. Benedetto AV, Lahti JG. Measurement of the anatomic position of the corrugator supercilii. Dermatol Surg. 2005;31(8 Pt 1):923–7. https://doi.org/10.1097/00042728-200508000-00006.
4. Hetzler L, Sykes J. The brow and forehead in periocular rejuvenation. Facial Plast Surg Clin North Am. 2010;18(3):375–84. https://doi.org/10.1016/j.fsc.2010.04.002.
5. Yalçınkaya E, Cingi C, Söken H, Ulusoy S, Muluk NB. Aesthetic analysis of the ideal eyebrow shape and position. Eur Arch Oto-rhino-laryngol. 2016;273(2):305–10. https://doi.org/10.1007/s00405-014-3356-0.
6. Knize DM. An anatomically based study of the mechanism of eyebrow ptosis. Plast Reconstr Surg. 1996;97(7):1321–33. https://doi.org/10.1097/00006534-199606000-00001.
7. Lemke BN, Stasior OG. The anatomy of eyebrow ptosis. Arch Ophthalmol. 1982;100(6):981–6. https://doi.org/10.1001/archopht.1982.01030030989019.
8. Romm S. Art, love, and facial beauty. Clin Plast Surg. 1987;14(4):579–83.

9. Westmore MG. Facial cosmetics in conjunction with surgery. Vancouver: Aesthetic PlasticSurgical Society meeting; 1975.
10. Ellenbogen R. Transcoronal eyebrow lift with concomitant upper blepharoplasty. Plast Reconstr Surg. 1983;71(4):490–9. https://doi.org/10.1097/00006534-198304000-00008.
11. Cook TA, Brownrigg PJ, Wang TD, Quatela VC. The versatile midforehead browlift. Arch Otolaryngol Head Neck Surg. 1989;115(2):163–8. https://doi.org/10.1001/archotol.1989.01860260037011.
12. Whitaker LA, Morales LJ, Farkas LG. Aesthetic surgery of the supraorbital ridge and forehead structures. Plast Reconstr Surg. 1986;78(1):23–32. https://doi.org/10.1097/00006534-198607000-00003.
13. McKinney P, Mossie RD, Zukowski ML. Criteria for the forehead lift. Aesth Plast Surg. 1991;15(2):141–7. https://doi.org/10.1007/BF02273847.
14. Connell BF, Lambros VS, Neurohr GH. The forehead lift: techniques to avoid complications and produce optimal results. Aesth Plast Surg. 1989;13(4):217–37. https://doi.org/10.1007/BF01570355.
15. Matarasso A, Terino EO. Forehead-brow rhytidoplasty: reassessing the goals. Plast Reconstr Surg. 1994;93(7):1371–8.
16. Gunter JP, Antrobus SD. Aesthetic analysis of the eyebrows. Plast Reconstr Surg. 1997;99(7):1808–16. https://doi.org/10.1097/00006534-199706000-00002.
17. Wong V, Rafiq N, Kalyan R, Hsenriksen A, Funner A. Hanging by a thread: choosing the right thread for the right patient. J Dermatol Cosmetol. 2017;1(4):86–8.
18. Dursun R, Isık B. Periorbital bölgede ip uygulamaları. In: Baskı 1, Zehra AS, editors. Türkiye Klinikleri. Anklara; 2021. p. 47–54.
19. Hwang U, Lee J, Kang K. Quantitative analysis of polydioxanone thread effects on lid-cheek junction. J Cosmet Med. 2018;2:22–6. https://doi.org/10.25056/JCM.2018.2.1.22.
20. Abraham RF, DeFatta RJ, Williams EF 3rd. Thread-lift for facial rejuvenation: assessment of long-term results. Arch Facial Plast Surg. 2009;11(3):178–83. https://doi.org/10.1001/archfacial.2009.10.
21. Myung Y, Jung C. Mini-midface lift using Polydioxanone cog threads. Plast Reconstr Surg Glob open. 2020;8(6):e2920. https://doi.org/10.1097/GOX.0000000000002920.
22. Garlotta D. A literature review of poly(lactic acid). J Polym Environ. 2001;9(2):63–84. https://doi.org/10.1023/A:1020200822435.
23. Hanke CW, et al. Facial soft-tissue fillers conference: assessing the state of the science. J. Am. Acad. Dermatol. 2011;64(4 Suppl):S66–85, S85.e1-136. https://doi.org/10.1016/j.jaad.2011.02.009.
24. Palm MD, Goldman MP. Patient satisfaction and duration of effect with PLLA: a review of the literature. J Drugs Dermatol. 2009;8(10 Suppl):s15–20.
25. Rezaee Khiabanloo S, Jebreili R, Aalipour E, Saljoughi N, Shahidi A. Outcomes in thread lift for face and neck: a study performed with Silhouette soft and promo happy lift double needle, innovative and classic techniques. J Cosmet Dermatol. 2019;18(1):84–93. https://doi.org/10.1111/jocd.12745.
26. Archer KA, Garcia RE. Silhouette Instalift: benefits to a facial plastic surgery practice. Facial Plast Surg Clin North Am. 2019;27(3):341–53. https://doi.org/10.1016/j.fsc.2019.03.006.
27. Nair NR, Sekhar VC, Nampoothiri KM, Pandey A. 32 – biodegradation of biopolymers. In: Pandey A, Negi S, Soccol B, editors. Current developments in biotechnology and bioengineering. Elsevier; 2017. p. 739–55.
28. Tokiwa Y, Calabia BP, Ugwu CU, Aiba S. Biodegradability of plastics. Int J Mol Sci. 2009;10(9):3722–42. https://doi.org/10.3390/ijms10093722.
29. Yongtrakul P, Sirithanabadeekul P, Siriphan P. Thread lift: classification, technique, and how to approach to the patient. Int J Med Heal Sci. 2016;10:558–66.
30. Sulamanidze M, Sulamanidze G. Facial lifting with Aptos methods. J Cutan Aesthet Surg. 2008;1(1):7–11. https://doi.org/10.4103/0974-2077.41149.
31. Gavrila DE, Victor S, Caramitu A, Mitrea S. Advanced polypropylene and composites with polypropylene with applications in modern medicine. 2020.

32. Monheit GD. Suspension for the aging face. Dermatol Clin. 2005;23(3):561–73., viii. https://doi.org/10.1016/j.det.2005.05.003.
33. Presti P, Yalamanchili H, Honrado CP. Rejuvenation of the aging upper third of the face. Facial Plast Surg. 2006;22(2):91–6. https://doi.org/10.1055/s-2006-947714.
34. Ghalambor A, Pipelzadeh MH. A non-aggressive forehead/brow lift with contour threads: a case report and its application in Iran. Pak J Med Sci. 2006;22(3):320–2.

33 Transcutaneous Suture Lifts: Middle Face

Ergun Sevil, Secil Ucar, and Cemal Cingi

33.1 Introduction

Most of the advances in facelift techniques after the 1990s have been aimed at changing the aging changes of the middle face. Hamra demonstrated for the first time that the middle face improved dramatically with the deep plane facelift, which she described in 1990 [1]. In the later period, nasolabial folding and sagging problems of the malar fat pad were the first structures to be focused on, among the changes that are not addressed by the classical superficial musculaponeurotic system facelift techniques and which are a kind of signature for the early period of the aging middle face [2].

A better understanding of the changes that may occur in skin and soft tissues with aging has enabled the development of new surgical techniques to cope with facial aging. It has also increased physicians' self-confidence in this regard.

Surgical lifting with skin excision, which offers a radical and permanent solution, has been a standard surgical method for decades [3, 4]. The recent understanding of the vectors that must be applied for excellent tissue elevation has helped to position especially the ptotic soft tissues more vertically [5].

In facelift procedures performed with surgical intervention, in addition to general anesthesia complications, possible complications such as infection, skin necrosis, hematomas, seromas, and injury to the facial nerve branches may occur. In

E. Sevil
Medical Faculty, Department of Otorhinolaryngology, Alanya University, Alanya, Turkey

S. Ucar
Private International-Prof Clinic, Istanbul, Türkiye

C. Cingi (✉)
Eskisehir Osmangazi University, Medical Faculty, Department of Otorhinolaryngology, Eskisehir, Türkiye
e-mail: cemal@ogu.edu.tr

C. Cingi et al. (eds.), *Minor Interventions, Major Outcomes on the Face*, Comprehensive ENT, https://doi.org/10.1007/978-3-032-01305-7_33

addition, the long healing process and scar appearance are among its other disadvantages. Therefore, patients prefer to get the same result as a less invasive procedure and quickly return to their daily lives and work.

Since the introduction of thread-lift sutures, their application has gradually spread among many cosmetic medical specialists, with the primary indication of lifting sagged tissues using a minimally invasive closed procedure. It is considered easy to apply after receiving adequate and appropriate training, and it is a relatively less invasive procedure than other surgical lift methods.

Transcutaneous facelift techniques are not a new idea [6, 7]. This procedure involves hanging saggy tissues with transcutaneous sutures passed under the skin of the face and neck, avoiding large incisions and significantly reducing the recovery time [6].

33.2 Anatomy and Physiology

Knowing the facial planes is crucial for safe and effective midline facial surgery. These layers are skin, subcutaneous fat, superficial muscular aponeurotic system (SMAS), parotid masseteric fascia, and parotid gland, respectively, from face to deep [8].

The midface is the area between the orbital mid-horizontal line and the edge of the mandible. The lateral border is the anterior border of the masseter muscle. The medial border is the nasofacial groove and the nasolabial line.

The galea, which forms the superior fascia of the scalp, is tightly attached to the scalp by a fibrous fat layer. The galea is a band of tissue between the abdomen of the frontal and occipital muscles and is also connected to the outer occipital protrusion and the nuchal part of the occipital bone. The galea is divided into superficial and deep layers by stretching forward and wrapping the frontalis muscle. It adheres to the pericranium with loose structures in the deep layer and forms a slip plane; this allows the aponeurosis, which carries the skin, to move over a considerable distance [9, 10].

Galea continues laterally as temporoparietal fascia (TPF). This layer is the direct extension of the SMAS above the zygomatic arch. TPF has no connection with the zygomatic arch. Above the zygomatic arch, TPF can be easily dissected from the superficial layer of the deep temporal fascia, and a separate fat layer called a superficial fat pad is encountered between the two fascia. This fat pad disappears below the middle level of the zygomatic arch. Deep temporal fascia is divided into two layers: superficial and deep. While the deep layer is attached to the medial of the zygomatic arch, the superficial layer is connected to the lateral. Between these two layers, there is an intermediate fat pad. The deep temporal fascia's deep layer can be easily dissected from the intermediate fat pad. However, dissection of the superficial layer of the deep temporal fascia from the intermediate fat pad is more difficult due to the fibrous mesh. A deep fat pad is under the deep layer [11, 12].

The superficial temporal fascia covering the lateral forehead and brow is loosely attached to the deep temporal fascia and firmly attached to the skin above it. The only area where this fascia is durable is the area along the edge of the temporal fossa, located on the frontal bone. This adhesion site is approximately 6 mm wide. This combines the deep galea plan on one side and the pericranium on the other, with all layers of the temporal fascia fixed on the frontal bone. At the end of the lower part, condensation is formed by the superficial temporal fascia ligament structure, the orbital ligament connecting the superficial fascia to the superolateral orbital rim. This structure is also tightly linked to the frontozygomatic suture. Since TPF is also associated with the forehead skin, it connects the skin and the eyebrow lateral rim to the orbital rim [13].

The muscles that provide mimic functions are in the middle face. These muscles also contribute to speech. These muscles are the orbicularis oculi muscle, zygomaticus major and minor muscles, levator labii superioris alaeque nasi muscle, levator angular oris muscle, risorius muscle, and buccinator muscle. The anatomy of the frontal branch, which is the branch of the facial nerve, is also essential for the procedures to be applied to the midface. This branch emerges from the parotid gland and cuts the zygomatic arch approximately in the middle 1/3. The Pitanguy line, which starts 0.5 cm below the tragus and extends 1.5 cm above the lateral eyebrow, is the most commonly used landmark in the course of the temporal branch of the facial nerve [14]. However, since the eyebrow is a somewhat imperfect landmark, the line starting from the lower part of the auricle that divides the line connecting the upper border of the tragus and the lateral canthus into two may be a more consistent approach. Moreover, a more accurate approach to precisely defining the position of the frontal branch of the facial nerve has been reported by Sabini et al. [15].

At the anterior border of the parotid gland, the SMAS becomes the mimetic muscles of the face, including the zygomatic, buccinator, risorius, and other muscles. Above the zygomatic arch, the SMAS becomes the temporoparietal fascia, covering the body of the mandible below and continuing as the platysma [16]. Since the facial nerve runs deep within the SMAS, the dissection on the surface of this layer helps prevent complications.

Various anatomical changes have been proposed that affect midface aging. The critical anatomical marker appears to be the malar fat pad [17, 18].

The malar fat pad provides most of the midface volume. This structure is the concentration of subcutaneous fat in the form of a triangle in the cheek area on the maxilla. The malar fat pad is located superficially on the SMAS and just below the lateral part of the infraorbital rim. The convexity in the middle face creates the young midface appearance [19].

Knowing the complex relationships between fat pads and retaining ligaments will help us understand the soft tissue changes in the aging face. A negative vector image occurs in patients with hypoplastic bone and prominent eyeball structures in the midface region. In addition, if it has a deep eyeball and a prominent midface area, it creates a positive vector image. Such situations involve anatomical differences between patients, making evaluating the mid-facial area challenging.

33.3 Aging in the Midface Area

In facial rejuvenation surgery, the middle oval part of the face is the most challenging. In this section, people change to show facial expressions such as happiness, sadness, anger, etc. The symmetry and balance of the face, which are the essential components of an aesthetically pleasing image, gradually change due to various aging factors. Aging changes in the middle face begin in the early stages of life, and these changes increase over time, creating an older appearance in middle age [20].

Aging vectors change the position and appearance of the face and neck. The sagging of the malar fat pad, a prominent nasolabial fold, a reduction in the anteroposterior length of the face with the reshaping of the maxilla, and the formation of a deep labiodental fold are essential findings related to aging in the midface area [21].

In aging, weakening of the ligaments that support the fat pads occurs over time. The weakening of the zygomatic-cutaneous ligament in the midface causes the malar fat pad to sag. A deeper nasolabial fold occurs when this sagging is combined with the weakening of the orbital ligament that supports the lower eyelid fat pad and orbicularis oculi. In addition, the increased laxity of the skin contributes to the formation of the nasolabial fold. The gap formed between the malar fat pad and the malar eminence due to the sagging of the malar fat pad creates a characteristic hollow appearance. In addition, the formation of orbital fat convexity, together with the pseudogenization of the fat in the lower eyelid region and the separation of the suborbicularis ocular fat pad and malar fat pad complex by the edge of the infraorbital bone, causes double convexity deformity. In time, the ptosis of the malar fat pad continues, and the nasolabial fold becomes more pronounced, with excess skin and volume loss leading to maxillary resorption in the midface aging process [21].

33.4 Patient Selection

Patient selection is essential in the midface lift, as for all surgeries. Mild skin laxity, slight fat pad sagging, and superficial rhythms constitute the patient group suitable for lifting operations. Patients with advanced lipoatrophy, excessive skin laxity, or muscle prolapse, as well as those who want fast results, are not ideal for suture lifting. The best results with suture lifting have been reported in patients with low body fat percentage and prominent bony prominences [22]. Choosing the appropriate thread and suture technique for each patient's defect and concern will increase the procedure's success [23].

33.5 Preoperative Evaluation

After understanding the patient's wishes and complaints, taking photos of the patient and analyzing the face and neck is an indispensable part of the examination process. Various factors determining the appearance of the upper two-thirds of the face should be carefully examined in mid-facelift surgery. Multiple factors, such as temporal and midface sagging degrees, prominence in the nasolabial sulcus, orbital rim clarification, and critical preoperative evaluation components, should be scrutinized. After the surgery, these photos are used by both the patient and the surgeon to assess recovery and medical law.

Jaco's midface classification can be used to assess midface anatomy and aging by physical examination and preoperative photography. In this classification, four variables are used: midface sagging, loss of flexibility, and presence or absence of negative vector or hypoplastic malar eminence [24].

A line perpendicular to the Frankfort horizontal line is drawn below the glabella to evaluate the appropriate projection of the malar region. Suppose the most anterior portion of the midface is behind this line. In that case, the patient is considered to have an incomplete midface projection similar to the negative vector described in periorbital surgery. This classification scheme assesses which of the three classes patients fit into based on the severity of their midface aging [24].

33.6 Technique

Depending on the patient's preference, transcutaneous midface lift procedures can be performed under local or intravenous sedation or general anesthesia. Markings are made when the patient is sitting before surgery. The foundation of mid-facelift procedures has always been the repositioning and support of subcutaneous tissues using absorbable or nonabsorbable sutures.

Mark a vertical line from the superior lateral edge of the malar fat pad about 1–2 cm beyond the hairline in the temporal region to serve as the anchor point for the incision. The mid-pupillary line marks the inferior incision, which is located along the nasolabial fold. Between the two incisions, 0.5% lidocaine and 1:200,000 epinephrine were injected. A local anesthetic is also applied to block the infraorbital and supraorbital nerves. Using a 15-blade instrument about 2 cm long and beveled in the direction of the hair follicles, a temporal incision is performed after the epinephrine has taken effect. A delicate blunt dissection might be executed to reach the deep temporal fascia. A little incision is created with an 11-blade tool close to the nasolabial fold.

Following the nasolabial stab incision, a long, blunt passing instrument is inserted and guided through the malar fat pad to the temporal incision in a subcutaneous plane. The passing device must not pierce the superficial skin or the deeper face muscles, so extreme caution is exercised. A needle driver holds the suture needle while threading a 3–0 Vicryl, PDS absorbable, or 4–0 nylon transparent permanent suture through the instrument's eye. The surgical tool is partially withdrawn through the punctured wound. To avoid completely withdrawing the tip, the device has a mark indicating how near the puncture site should be. The passing instrument is re-advanced to engage the malar fat pad tissue carefully. The needle's insertion path takes a somewhat different route within the malar fat pad. After the fixing incision is closed, the passing instrument's tip is removed, and the suture is dragged out, leaving only the two ends. Afterward, you can secure the suture to the deep temporal fascia using the needle. The malar fat pad is raised to the desired level by applying tension to the suture. Next, the deep temporal fascia is used to anchor the suture. After the incision is closed in layers, the removed region is covered with paper tape and left in place for 3 to 4 days (Figs. 33.1, 33.2, 33.3 and 33.4).

33.7 Types of Sutures

Aptos sutures are made from a 2/0 polypropylene line with notches forming sharp, dented edges. Sumanidze et al. reported that a few threads were pulled subcutaneously with a small incision in the temple area [25]. After the lower thread and needle were removed, the lower thread was cut, and the upper thread was sutured to the temporal muscle fascia after moderate pulling. Sulamidze et al. stated that the Aptos methods were most effective in the midface region. Although they reported soft tissue sagging and weakening about 1 year after the procedure in a study of 4580 patients, they recorded positive results without a complete recurrence of deformities even in the fourth year of the operation [25].

Contour threads with unidirectional barbs are fixed to the fascia. Kaminer et al. described using this suture in 2008 [26]. A 3 mm incision is made on the temporal line. The needle placed in the subcutaneous plane from the incision is advanced in a zigzag pattern. Then, the needle removed from the skin is cut. The thread in the proximal part near the incision is then fixed to the deep fascia.

Multi-anchor suspension sutures containing a monofilament absorbable suture with 5–9 evenly spaced knots have also been described [26]. Sutures are made with 2–0 PDS or Maxon, and 5–7 superficial knots are tied. Eremia and Willoughby reported that these sutures' success showed superior results to those of open facelift surgeries [26, 27].

Approximately nine knots spaced approximately ten millimeters apart are incorporated into the silhouette sutures manufactured by Kloster Methods, Inc., in Corona, California, United States of America. These poly-L-lactic acid cones are absorbable and contained within these knots. The thread is approximately 37.3

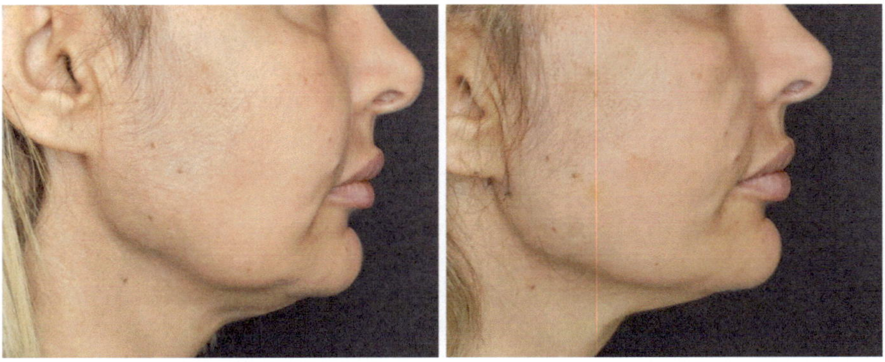

Fig. 33.1 Before and after midface thread lift, Patient 1 side view. (Courtesy of Secil Ucar MD)

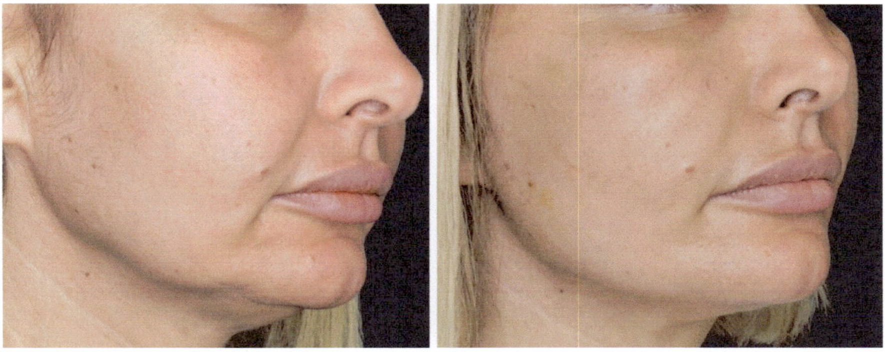

Fig. 33.2 Before and after midface thread lift, Patient 1 three-quarter view. (Courtesy of Secil Ucar MD)

centimeters long, and the sutures are attached to a straight needle measuring 20 centimeters. It is considered that the absorbable cones in Silhouette sutures are the reason why they are believed to last longer than many of the other types of thread lifts. Through the process of a foreign body response, the cones are responsible for initiating an inflammatory response. A significant amount of time is required for the inflammatory process to break down the cones while producing a fibrous capsule that helps maintain the suture's attachment to the connective tissue beneath it [26, 27] (Figs. 33.1, 33.2, 33.3).

Fig. 33.3 Before and after midface thread lift, Patient 2 frontal view. (Courtesy of Secil Ucar MD)

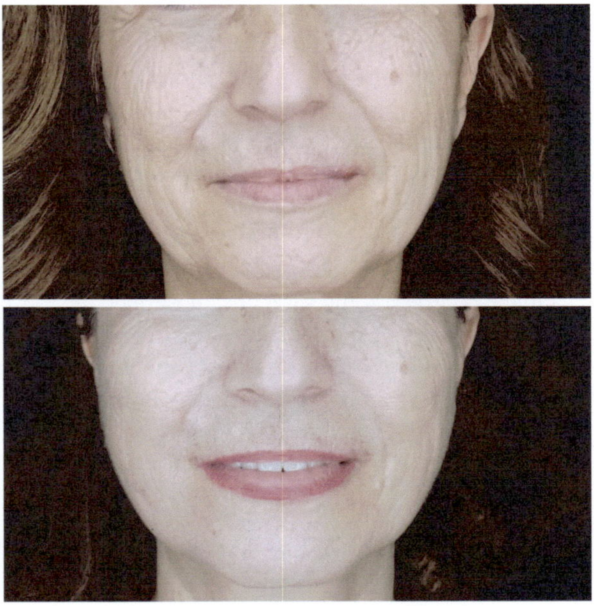

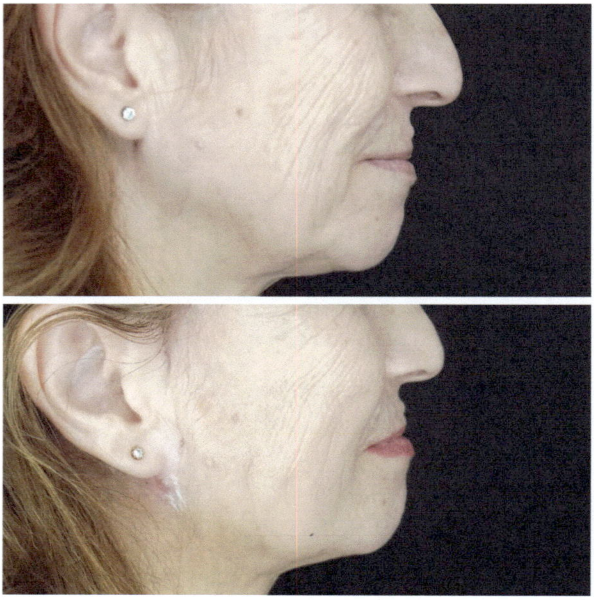

Fig. 33.4 Before and after midface thread lift, Patient 2 side view. (Courtesy of Secil Ucar MD)

33.8 Long-Term Efficiency

The number of studies on the long-term results and satisfaction of patients who underwent facial rejuvenation with transcutaneous sutures needs to be increased [4, 28]. Only some clinical studies are available at the level of evidence 3 [6]. Lycka et al. reported good results from patient interviews and surgical observations in a retrospective analysis of 350 patients. In addition, the authors recommended the transcutaneous suture method in midface lift surgeries instead of traditional surgical procedures due to the low complication rate and high patient satisfaction [29, 33]. Considering the results in terms of duration, it was determined that 117 patients retained 70% of the initial correction over a 12–24-month period [29]. Although the permanent increase was in very few patients, most were satisfied with the results. The fact that sutures increase fibrotic tissue production in soft tissue and support tissue tension may be one of the reasons for successful results [30]. It is known that the collagen matrix of the subcutaneous tissue increases due to fibrosis.

On the contrary, some surgeons questioned the low complication, morbidity, and long-term results of midface lift surgeries with the transcutaneous suture method [22]. Their concerns are that tissue positioning is not maintained long-term, threads are visible, and traction lines are evident or broken when the face is motionless [31].

33.9 Complications

This non-invasive midface lift procedure has some complications and short- and long-term results. Publications on the side effects of a wide variety of alloplastic materials applied to the face have increased, and these complications need to be followed more closely [32, 33]. Although immunological and chemical reactions are not possible against such implants, foreign body reactions or infections may develop [33]. Since the procedure is primarily performed in young patients, surgical sutures may remain under the skin for a long time. It is impossible to obliterate these sutures, so symptoms may worsen over time [33].

The most common complications, such as swelling and bruising, are consistent with most surgical procedures. Skin dimpling or buttoning are also potential adverse events that can occur. Reported complications have been minimal but can include infection, pain, ecchymosis, paresthesia, and inadequate cosmetic results. Commonly, providers have reported suture disruption, suture migration, or suture exposure that may require re-treatment.

References

1. Hamra ST. The deeplane rhytidectomy. Plast Reconstr Surg. 1990;86:53.
2. Quatela VC, Olney DR. Management of the midface. Facial Plast Surg Clin North Am. 2006 Aug;14(3):213–20.
3. Sulamanidze MA, Paikidze TG, Sulamanidze GM, Neigel JM. Facial lifting with "APTOS" threads: featherlift. Otolaryngol Clin N Am. 2005;38:1109–17.
4. Kaminer MS, Bogart M, Choi C, Wee SA. Long-term efficacy of anchored barbed sutures in the face and neck. Dermatologic Surg. 2008;34:1041–7.
5. Paul MD. Barbed sutures for aesthetic facial plastic surgery: indications and techniques. Clin Plast Surg. 2008;35:451–61.
6. Villa MT, White LE, Alam M, Yoo SS, Walton RL. Barbed sutures: a review of the literature. Plast Reconstr Surg. 2008;121:102–8.
7. Salasche SJ, Jarchow R, Feldman BD, Devine-Rust MJ, Adnot J. The suspension suture. J Dermatol Surg Oncol. 1987;13:973–8.
8. Sykes JM, Riedler KL, Cotofana S, Palhazi P. Superficial and deep facial anatomy and its implications for Rhytidectomy. Facial Plast Surg Clin North Am. 2020;28(3):243–51.
9. Quatela VC, Choe KS. Endobrow midface lift. Facial Plast Surg. 2004;20(3):199–206.
10. Knize DM. The importance of the retaining ligamentous attachments of the forehead for selective eyebrow reshaping and forehead rejuvenation. Plast Reconstr Surg. 2007;119(3):1119–20.
11. Babakurban ST, Cakmak O, Kendir S, Elhan A, Quatela VC. Temporal branch of the facial nerve and its relationship to fascial layers. Arch Facial Plast Surg. 2010;12(1):16–23.
12. Vito CQ, Jean PA, Marcelo BA. Endoscopic-assisted facelifting. Facial Plast Surg. 2014;30(4):413–21.
13. Knize DM. Anatomic concepts for brow lift procedures. Plast Reconstr Surg. 2009;124(6):2118–26.
14. Pitanguy I, Ramos AS. The frontal branch of the facial nerve: the importance of its variations in face lifting. Plast Reconstr Surg. 1966;38(4):352–6.
15. Sabini P, Wayne I, Quatela VC. Anatomical guides to precisely localize the frontal branch of the facial nerve. Arch Facial Plast Surg. 2003;5(2):150–2.
16. Mitz V, Peyronie M. The superficial musculo-aponeurotic system (SMAS) in the parotid and cheek area. Plast Reconstr Surg. 1976 Jul;58(1):80–8.

17. Downs B, Wang T. Current concepts in midfacial rejuvenation: facial plastic surgery. Otolaryngol Head Neck Surg. 2008;16:335–8.
18. Casagrande C, Saltz R, Chem R, Pinto R, Collares M. Direct neddle fixation in endoscopic facial rejuvenation. Aesthetic Surg J. 2000;20:361–7.
19. Rohrich RJ, Pessa JE. The fat compartments of the face: anatomy and clinical implications for cosmetic surgery. Plast Reconstr Surg. 2007;119(7):2219–27. discussion 2228–2231
20. Oscar M. Ramirez, the central oval of the face: tridimensional endoscopic rejuvenation. Facial Plast Surg. 2000;16(3):283–98.
21. Emre İE, Çakmak Ö. Ageing face, an overview–aetiology, assessment and management. Otorhinolaryngologist. 2013;6(3):160–6.
22. Flynn J. Suture suspension lifts: a review. Oral Maxillofac Surg Clin North Am. 2005;17:65–76.
23. Sardesai MG, Zakhary K, Ellis DAF. Thread-lifts: the good, thebad, and the ugly. Arch Facial Plast Surg. 2008;10:284–5.
24. Jacono AA, Ransom ER. Anatomic predictors of unsatisfactory outcomes in surgical rejuvenation of the midface. JAMA Facial Plast Surg. 2013;15(2):101–9.
25. Sulamanidze M, Sulamanidze G. APTOS suture lifting methods: 10 years of experience. Clin Plast Surg. 2009;36:281.
26. De BJ, Pizzamiglio R, Theodorou D, Arvas L. Facial rejuvenation and improvement of malar projection using sutures with absorbable cones: surgical technique and case series. Aesth Plast Surg. 2011;35:248.
27. Stein P, Vitavska O, Kind P, Hoppe W, Wieczorek H, Schürer NY. The biological basis for poly-L lactic acid-induced augmentation. J Dermatol Sci. 2015;78:26.
28. Rashid R, Sartori M, White LE, Villa MT, Yoo SS, Alam M. Break-ing strength of 51 barbed polypropylene sutures: rater-blinded, controlled comparison with nonbarbed sutures of various cal-ibers. Arch Dermatol. 2007;2143:869–72.
29. Lycka B, Bazan C, Poletti E, Treen B. The emerging techniqueof the antiptosis subdermal suspension thread. Dermatologic Surg. 2004;30:41–4.
30. Wu WTL. Barbed sutures in facial rejuvenation. Aesthet Surg J. 2004;24:582–7.
31. Paul MD. Complications of barbed sutures. Aesthet Plast Surg. 2008;32:149.
32. DeLorenzi CL. Barbed sutures: rationale and technique. Aesthet Surg J. 2006;26:223–9.
33. Helling ER, Okpaku A, Wang PTH, Levine RA. Complications of facial suspension sutures. Aesthet Surg J. 2007;27:155–61.

The Use of Transcutaneous Sutures to Lift the Nose

34

Sermin Can, Mehmet Akdag, and Cemal Cingi

34.1 Introduction

The shape of the nose tip defines the overall appearance, including its size, shape, angle, and width. Its look is determined by the alar cartilage's position and shape, skin quality, and thickness. Size, strength, curvature, and placement of the tip cartilages and postoperative support of the suspensory ligaments determine the surgical outcome in rhinoplasty. Equally significant are the bridge and hump [1].

In a perfect world, a mid-layer support structure would be visible through the skin after primary rhinoplasty, formed by modifying the tip cartilages through partial excision, transaction, repositioning, suture modification, or augmentation. When a revision is being considered for a rhinoplasty because additional improvement is needed, the most essential part of the surgery is setting the alar cartilage back to how it should be [1].

About 800 BC, in the Hindu book of revelation known as the *Susruta Samhita*, nose reconstruction was covered in the oldest medical literature. However, American surgeon John Roe did not detail a procedure to enhance the nose's aesthetic appeal until 1891. Through direct external incisions, he revealed the underlying osteocartilaginous components to minimize the size of a big nose. To prevent noticeable

S. Can
Department of Otorhinolaryngology, Dicle University Faculty of Medicine, Diyarbakır, Turkey

M. Akdag
Department of Otorhinolaryngology, Dicle University Faculty of Medicine, Diyarbakır, Turkey
e-mail: mehmet.akdag@dicle.edu.tr

C. Cingi (✉)
Eskisehir Osmangazi University, Medical Faculty, Department of Otorhinolaryngology, Eskisehir, Türkiye
e-mail: cemal@ogu.edu.tr

C. Cingi et al. (eds.), *Minor Interventions, Major Outcomes on the Face*, Comprehensive ENT, https://doi.org/10.1007/978-3-032-01305-7_34

scarring of the skin surface, a German surgeon named Jacques Joseph (1896) maneuvered the nose structure through intranasal incisions. This closed method was the norm until the end of the twentieth century [1].

For rhinoplasty to be successful, the nasal skeleton must be in good structural shape before the skin and soft tissues can properly adhere to it. The osteocartilaginous mid-layer of the nose is exposed through trans-cartilaginous, infra-cartilaginous, and inter-cartilaginous incisions in the endonasal (closed) approach. The irregularity can be identified, and its aesthetic alteration is made possible by elevating the underlying skin envelope. The closed procedure is sufficient for many seasoned surgeons to achieve their goals. However, there is less room to maneuver, less visibility, and less exposure when incisions can only be made in the nostrils. Many surgeons are disappointed with the outcomes of closed rhinoplasty due to these limitations. This open approach was revived in the late twentieth century by Anderson, Johnson, Toriumi, Gunter, Rohrich, and Juri, among others. A combination of an external trans-columellar incision and bilateral rimming incision was used. This opened up a lot of space for inspection by lifting the skin of the nose. By bypassing the intraoperative deformation that results from closed delivery procedures, the open technique permits modification of the underlying supporting structure. The underlying abnormality can be more accurately diagnosed, and bone and cartilaginous tissue excision is more precise. Suture alterations and the attachment of cartilage grafts are made more accessible, and the underlying osteocartilaginous structure can be more readily changed [1].

The ability to perform surgical operations that are not possible with a closed method makes open rhinoplasty a more versatile option. Some think the open technique produces a more predictable result because it creates more rigid support and better architectural stability [1].

Most people opt for open rhinoplasty when they want significant alterations to their nose's look or function. However, there are benefits and drawbacks to every approach. The open approach reduces natural nasal support due to its broader exposure and thorough dissection. Because the operation alters every portion of the nose, it must be restored first. While doing an open rhinoplasty to project and shape the nose, it is even more crucial to have strong structural support to avoid postoperative collapse and long-term form loss. Because of this, improved methods of stabilizing the altered intranasal anatomy by cartilage transplant and suture placement during open rhinoplasty have emerged [1].

34.2 Problem

The nose comprises three layers: the outermost layer, which acts as a covering; the middle layer, which is composed of both hard and soft tissues; and the lining, which is thin and vascular and conforms to the contour of the nose. The osteocartilaginous shape predominantly affects the nasal mid-layer, although all the nasal anatomic layers play a role. From an aesthetic standpoint, the shape of the nose's tip dictates the nose's overall appearance, including its angle, length, and position [2]. The alar cartilages shape and support the tip lobule. The aesthetics of the tip are determined by its size, shape, and placement. In a perfect world, the tip cartilages would be altered during primary rhinoplasty via partial excision, transection, repositioning, suture modification, or augmentation to achieve the target outcome [1].

34.3 Relevant Anatomy

Understanding normal and abnormal nasal anatomy is necessary for successful operations. Knowledge of the anatomical relationships between surface contour and its effects on form and function is also required [1].

The nasal architecture consists of the following layers: [1]:

- The nasalis muscle and its corresponding fascia, the outer layer of skin, and the dermis and subcutaneous fat that cover it all: A slack areolar layer separates this outer layer from the supporting layer beneath. The areolar layer offers a safe way to lift the nasal cover and expose the underlying osteocartilaginous structure because it affords a relatively avascular dissection plane.
- The perichondrium and periosteum cover the cartilage and bone in the middle layer, which supports and shapes the skin on the outside. To secure the tip, fibrous ligaments run between the top lateral, alar, and septal cartilages next to each other.

Stratified squamous cells line the inside of the vestibule, and the septal and nasal mucosa line the inside of the nose. Preserving the lining is essential in a standard rhinoplasty procedure. Very little evidence suggests a substantial change to the lining layer.

34.3.1 The Nasal Skin Envelope

In contrast to the thinner, more mobile skin on the dorsum and sidewall, the ala, and tip have thicker, more sebaceous skin. Redraping and contractions over the underlying framework are more familiar with thinner skin. To make the underlying support evident through the overlying skin envelope, a more robust and angular framework is needed for the thick sebaceous skin of the tip, which shrinks less. Rarely is rhinoplasty possible due to highly thick skin [1].

To protect the main blood vessels—arteries, veins, and lymphatics—found in the musculoaponeurotic layer, the nasal skin flap must be raised in the deep areolar plane, somewhat above the bone and cartilage. It is essential to prevent tissue necrosis or excessive scarring in soft tissues [1].

34.3.2 Mid-layer Support

The nasal passages are subdivided into three vaults: the upper bony vault, the middle upper lateral vault, and the lower alar vault [1].

The external valve comprises the inner and outer nostrils, including the caudal border of the alar cartilage, the soft tissue ala, the membranous septum, and the nostril sill. It is located in the lower lateral vault, the tip, and the ala.

The alar cartilages act as a framework to support the nasal tip. Three distinct crus are present in each ala. The intricate cartilage structure is stabilized by a continuous perichondrium that connects the little accessory cartilages that extend from the alar cartilage's most lateral face. The underlying tip cartilages, the thickness of the skin and soft tissues, and the suspensory fibrous attachments to the surrounding septum and upper lateral cartilages dictate the shape and position of the distal nose. These parts work together to keep the lower cartilage vault in place and supported. These ligamentous attachments join the upper lateral cartilages to the cephalic border of the lower lateral cartilages, and they go over the septal angle [1].

Additional ligaments attach the supplementary cartilages to the piriform aperture. Fibrous attachments that link the medial crura to the caudal septum and soft tissue between the medial crura's inferior face and the premaxilla support the crura. Incisions and excisions made during surgery to expose and alter the tip cartilages damage these suspensory ligaments. When the skin is lifted off the underlying cartilage framework, when incisions are made between cartilages, when the alar cartilage is trimmed cephalic, when the septal angle and caudal septum are removed, and when the suspensory ligaments are disrupted, the overall support for the tip is diminished [1].

34.3.3 The Connection Between Nose Shape, Anatomy, and Aesthetics

The nasal tip is an anatomically complex three-dimensional shape. The tip lobule is supported and shaped by the alar cartilage beneath it. As surface anatomy, the skin reflects the size, form, and location of the paired alar cartilages. Each alar cartilage consists of the medial, middle, and lateral crus, and their relative positions determine how the nose looks and moves.

At the medial genu, the medial crus—also known as the columellar breakpoint or the connection of the columella and the lobules—joins the middle crus. The middle crus controls both the columellar/lobular ratio and the cephalad or caudal position [1].

The middle crus connects the medial and lateral crus. Its angle, length, and configuration dictate the infratip lobule's shape, height, and protrusion. Starting at the junction of the columellar and lobular processes, it rotates at an angle known as cephalad angulation. The distance between its interior and exterior is defined by its angle of diversion, which is its lateral angle from the midline. Following its origin, the middle crus continues until it meets the lateral crus, the lateral genu, or domes [1].

The alar cartilage domes dictate the tip's thickness, width, and projection. The superior alar cartilage is bordered by and partially filled with the lateral crura, extending into and filling the tip lobule. Therefore, a tripod is created by two sets of paired crura: one set of medial crura, which are attached to the columella by fibrous tissue and support the lower central leg; the other set of paired crura, which are extended laterally within the tip lobule, forms the two upper spanning legs [1].

If you cut off a leg of the tripod, it will not be able to sustain as much weight. Limb strength and length can be enhanced by grafts or struts for augmentation. A shorter lower leg brings the tip inferior and back. When the top leg is shorter, the tip moves upward and backward toward the shorter leg. The tip will fall back if all three legs are shortened. The tip can be moved forward and to the side by extending the bottom leg.

Skin, compact fat, muscle, and alar cartilage comprise the lower nose, which can become blocked if support is absent. Seventh nerve palsy, causes weakened or overreacted supporting structures, causes vestibular lining stenosis from scarring, or external valve collapse [1].

34.3.4 The Aesthetics

The underlying skeleton is responsible for creating the nasal tip's appearance. Specifically, according to Sheen, a refined tip can be identified by its lateral extensions of the right and left domes, its supratip break, and its columellar break, which are the areas where the tip differentiates from the dorsum [1].

The significance of the tip cartilages to the structure and function of the entire nasal base needs to be more appreciated. In addition to their aesthetic role, the alar cartilages determine the following: the length, width, and position of the columellar cartilages; the form of the nostrils; the location of the alar rim; the alar support and airway potency; and the apparent length of the nose. Restoring or maintaining the medial, middle, and lateral crus anatomical and functional components is essential for a predictable reconstruction.

Surgeons performing rhinoplasty procedures must consider the nasal "gestalt," or proportion, symmetry, and balance of the entire nose. This includes the dorsum, tip, sidewall, and ala. It is essential to have an aesthetic tip [1].

Two lines, which slightly diverge from one another, running from the medial brow ridges to the tip-defining point, define the nasal dorsum as seen from the front. Based on the patient's ethnic origin, the alar bases should be located within a line dropped from the medial canthi. The typical width of the alar flare relative to the alar base is 2 mm. Surgeons must be able to distinguish between alar flare and excessive internal breadth [3]. Symmetry and a little outward flare in the inferior-lateral direction should characterize the alar bases. The alar rim and columella should form a graceful curve from the front, similar to a seagull in flight, with the columella just below the alar rim [1].

In the basal view of the columella and nasal base, you should be able to make out an equilateral triangle. The ideal form for the nose is a teardrop, with the long axis of the nostril extending slightly medially from base to apex [1].

When seen from the side, the perfect dorsal nasofrontal angle would be horizontally between the upper eyelash and the supratarsal fold. The distance between the intersection of the alar rim and the cheek to the tip is used to determine the tip projection. A vertical line drawn next to the most protruding portion of the top lip should be 50–60% ahead of the tip [1].

The ratio of the nasal length to the points that define the tip determines the ideal nasal length. The radix-to-tip distance, which refers to the measurement from the station (the horizontal intersection of the upper and lower lips) to the mentum, should be 0.67 times RT [1].

The four points that define the tip—the tip itself, the break above the tip, the columellar lobular angle, and the other two points—should be able to be used to form two equal triangles. Women ought to have a more noticeable supratip break compared to men. It draws attention to the dorsum and separates it from the tip, adding definition. From the front, the columella and nostril rims should look like gullwing wings because the columella should lie just below the alar rim. At the place where the columella meets the infraction lobule, also known as the columellar breakpoint, the ideal angle is 30–45° [4–7].

The angle of rotation is equal to the tip rotation. Using a perpendicular line to the natural horizontal plane, we draw a straight line through the front and back of the nostrils. In a perfect world, women's rotation angles would be 95–100° while men's would be 90–95° [1].

34.4 Transcutaneous Sutures

Transcutaneous sutures were first used in facial lift surgery by Buncke, who is known as the founder of international microsurgery. Later, Sulamanidze used this suture in facial aesthetic surgery [8, 9]. Various modifications to this suture have recently been developed to increase tip rotation and projection in the nose [8, 9].

Tip surgery is one of the most critical areas of facial aesthetics, and a successful rhinoplasty depends on adequate tip projection and rotation [10]. Some patients with low tip rotation and projection may not need a standard rhinoplasty. Even a slight increase in projection and rotation can provide a satisfactory aesthetic appearance for these patients. This suture technique can reshape the nasal cartilage [11]. However, a suture-only technique is not generally preferred in rhinoplasty. Therefore, patients must be carefully selected.

The fact that both open and closed rhinoplasty surgery are routinely performed under general anesthesia, along with the lengthy operation time, the development of postoperative edema, and the long recovery period, has led surgeons to search for new techniques constantly. Nasal rotation with a transcutaneous suture lift, one of these techniques, is conducted by fixing the nose tip to the nasal bone's periosteum with a nonabsorbable suture [12]. This technique is advantageous for selected patients due to its feasibility with local anesthesia, short recovery time, and low cost.

The nasal tip is anatomically supported by multiple structures over the anterior septum, including Pitanguy's, scroll, and cephalic ligaments that attach to the piriform aperture [13]. Since this minimally invasive technique does not affect the fundamental structures of nasal anatomy, the complication rate seems much lower.

34.5 Patient Selection

Patients with low-type rotation and projection should be selected. The nose skin should not be thick or oily. This technique is viable for patients of all ages [14]. It is not preferred for patients with nasal-obstructing lesions or septal deviation [12].

34.6 Patient Examinations

The structures to be evaluated during a physical examination of the patient include the following [15]:

1. Nasal examination
   (a) Nasal septum
   (b) Internal nasal valve
   (c) Nasal vestibules
2. Nasal bone structure
3. Alar cartilages
4. Nasal type
   (a) Projection
   (b) Rotation
   (c) Symmetry
   (d) Position
5. Nasofrontal angle
6. Nasolabial angle and columella
7. Nasal area
   (a) Width
   (b) Retraction

34.6.1 Surgical Instruments

1. Scalpel number 11
2. 20-gauge IV cannula

3. 4/0 polypropylene suture with a 26-mm needle
4. Kelly–Murphy forceps
5. Fine-tip tenotomy scissors [12, 15]

34.7 Surgical Technique

Patients are advised not to use aspirin, B-blockers, NSAIDs, or herbal medicines before surgery. Usually, a fasting period of 6 h is required before surgery. During surgery, the patient is placed supine. Local anesthesia is administered by an injection of lidocaine (lidocaine HCl 20–0.0125 mg/mL adrenaline; Adeka Drug Co, Istanbul, Turkey) to the nasal dorsum, tip area, columella, and infraorbital region [12]. It takes about 10 min for the local anesthesia to take effect. The skin is sterilized by staining with a povidone-iodine solution. A 20-gauge IV cannula, a 26-mm needle, and a 4/0 polypropylene suture are used during surgery (PROLENE; Ethicon, Somerville, New Jersey, USA). Preoperative marking is carried out with a surgical pen on the frontonasal junction areas of the bilateral lateral nasal wall and in the middle of the columella, approximately to the columella–lobular angle.

Three small incisions are then made at the marked locations with 11 scalpels [16]. During surgery, a 20-gauge IV cannula is introduced through the columellar incision, advanced transcutaneously to the surgeon's right side in the cephalic direction, and removed through the right nasofrontal incision. When the needle tip comes out, the suture is inserted into the needle hole, and then the needle is pulled back until it emerges from the columella incision. One end of the suture should be at the columellar incision and the other at the right nasofrontal incision. The prolene suture is removed from the left nasofrontal incision subperiosteally through the right nasofrontal incision. A 20-gauge IV cannula is passed through the columellar incision and cephalically removed transcutaneously through the left nasofrontal incision. After the suture is placed in the needle hole in the left nasofrontal incision, the needle is withdrawn and removed from the columellar incision [12]. The suture should be passed subperiosteally between both nasofrontal incisions and transcutaneously between the columella and nasofrontal incisions [17]. Then, the depressor septi nasi muscle is cut using tenotomy scissors. The tension of the suture is adjusted according to the desired amount of rotation, and the sutures are tied at the incision in the columella. It should be considered that the amount of rotation will decrease within 2 weeks following surgery, so the rotation should be 30% more than the desired amount [14].

34.8 Postoperative Care

Patients may have mild-to-moderate pain during the postoperative period, and analgesic treatment is ordered for these patients. In the early period, patients can resume their daily activities. Within 2 weeks, the edema is completely resolved. After

2 weeks, a subcision can be made using Kelly–Murphy forceps to open the tiny folds in the nasofrontal areas [14].

34.9 Conclusion

Transcutaneous suture lift is a minimally invasive surgical technique used to increase projection and rotation in type surgery. It is a simple technique that achieves satisfactory results and is advantageous for selected patients as it can be performed under local anesthesia, the recovery time is very short, and the cost and complication rates are low.

References

1. Buchel EW. Tip rhinoplasty. In: Granick MS, editor. Medscape. Updated: Feb 27, 2023 https://emedicine.medscape.com/article/1292616-overview#a10. Accessed online at 15 Apr 2024.
2. Sheen J, Sheen A. Aesthetic Rhinoplasty, vol. 1 and 2. 2nd ed. St. Louis: Mosby; 1987.
3. Rohrich RJ, Malafa MM, Ahmad J, Basci DS. Managing alar flare in Rhinoplasty. Plast Reconstr Surg. 2017 Nov;140(5):910–9.
4. Buckley CE, McArdle A, McInerney NM, O'Broin E. Evaluation of nasal tip definition in closed Rhinoplasty. Plast Reconstr Surg Glob Open. 2016;4(1):e603.
5. Johnson C, Toriumi D. Open structure Rhinoplasty. Philadelphia: Saunders; 1990.
6. Gunter JP, Rohrich RJ. External approach for secondary rhinoplasty. Plast Reconstr Surg. 1987 Aug;80(2):161–74.
7. Juri J. Salvage techniques for secondary rhinoplasty. In: Daniel R, editor. Aesthetic plastic surgery: rhinoplasty. Boston: Little Brown; 1993.
8. Buncke HJ. Surgical methods using one-way suture. Google Patents; 1999.
9. Sulamanidze M, Paikidze T, Sulamanidze G, Neigel JM. Facial lifting with "APTOS" threads: featherlift. Otolaryngol Clin North Am. 2005;38(5):1109–17.
10. Cárdenas JC, Carvajal J, Ruiz AJP. Securing nasal tip rotation through suspension suture technique. Plast Reconstr Surg. 2006;117(6):1750–5.
11. Eroğlu S, Cingi C, Hamilton GS. Suture lift of the nasal tip. Challenges in rhinology. Springer; 2021. p. 277–84.
12. Turhal G, Benzer M, Sahin FF, Midilli R, Karci B, Sahin M, et al. Transcutaneous suture tip plasty: the technique and outcomes. Ann Otol Rhinol Laryngol. 2019;128(9):789–94.
13. Bitik O, Uzun H, Kamburoğlu HO, Dadaci MJ. Nasal tip suspending transfixion suture. Aesthetic Plast Surg. 2014;38(2):309–15.
14. Hernandez-Perez E, Hernandez-Perez JE, Khawaja HA. Transcutaneous lifting of the nose. Dermatology. 2008;21(10):547–54.
15. Cueteaux CG, Shiffman MA. Suture lift of the nasal tip. In: Simplified Facial Rejuvenation. Springer; 2008. p. 321–4.
16. Habesoglu TE, Kulekci SO, Deveci S, Toraman M, Habesoglu MJ. Percutaneous rhinolift procedure for droopy tip. Am J Otolaryngol. 2021;42(4):102988.
17. Serdev NPJMTiR. Transcutaneous and transmucosal Serdev sutures® for nasal tip refinement, Alar Base Narrowing, and Other Corrections 2016:37–56.

35 Transcutaneous Suture Lifts: Lower Face and Mandibular Definition

Ibrahim Hira, Secil Ucar, and Nuray Bayar Muluk

35.1 Introduction

With aging, the superficial part of the skin is first affected, then the skin's and subcutaneous tissues' elasticity decreases, and some changes occur due to volume loss in the tissues, especially the fatty tissue [1]. Age, sun exposure, toxins, and metabolic and hormonal disorders mainly affect this process. The resulting wrinkles, sagging, and volume loss are most noticeable in the face and neck area. As a result of extended life expectancy, increased awareness due to social media, and the desire to be liked, people are resorting to cosmetic procedures more frequently. Cosmetic procedures applied to the face can be classified as surgical (face lift-rhytidectomy) and non-surgical applications. Thread suspension, laser, botulinum toxin, and mesotherapy applications are frequently preferred among non-surgical applications.

Especially in patients with sagging skin in the face and neck area, thread suspension applications, which do not affect the patient's daily activities and work life, are minimally invasive and reliable and are becoming increasingly preferred over surgical methods. It can also be applied together with a surgical facelift [2]. However, it should not be considered as an alternative to surgical facelift. The method chosen for facial rejuvenation also affects the severity of the patient's problems and expectations, the affected areas, the recovery time until returning to daily social activities, and the patient's economic status.

I. Hira
Department of Otorhinolaryngology, Ankara Şereflikoçhisar State Hospital, Ankara, Türkiye

S. Ucar
Private International-Prof Clinic, Istanbul, Türkiye

N. Bayar Muluk (✉)
Faculty of Medicine, Department of Otorhinolaryngology, Kirikkale University, Kırıkkale, Türkiye

C. Cingi et al. (eds.), *Minor Interventions, Major Outcomes on the Face*, Comprehensive ENT, https://doi.org/10.1007/978-3-032-01305-7_35

35.2 Facial Anatomy and Aging

Many intrinsic and extrinsic factors affect the aging process and changes in facial anatomy. Hormonal changes, damage caused by the accumulation of free radicals and cellular waste, mitochondrial aging, shortening of telomeres, and various gene mutations are responsible for intrinsic aging [3–5]. The effect of gravity, sun exposure, intense use of facial muscles, smoking, and other environmental factors lead to the extrinsic aging process [6].

Wrinkles and sagging occur on the face due to decreased skin quality and elasticity, especially with aging. Additionally, volume loss and displacement are observed, especially in fat tissues. While the malar fat pads collapse causes the nasolabial grooves to become prominent, sagging of the labiodental fat pads causes jowl deformity [7]. Over time, mandibular contours are erased, facial volume loss occurs due to fat resorption, fat tissues sag between the ligaments, nasolabial folds become prominent due to sagging of the malar fat pad, the cervico-mental angle become blunt, platysmal bands become prominent and sag, resulting in a "turkey neck" appearance [8]. Another factor that causes these changes is the relaxation of the superficial musculo-aponeurotic system (SMAS), which contains the facial mimic muscles, during the aging process and the decrease in the tonicity of the facial mimic muscles within the SMAS [9, 10]. In addition, as the facial structure changes due to bone resorption with aging, the tree-like ligamentous structures connecting the dermis and periosteum become loose and lose their effect.

The primary purpose of thread suspension applications is to correct these anatomical changes that occur for various reasons by pulling them in the opposite direction of the aging vectors.

35.3 Suture Lift Materials and Mechanism of Efficacy

This technique, first applied by Mitz and Peironye in the 1970s, has become very common among facial rejuvenation techniques today [11]. The threads used in face-lift and rejuvenation techniques are divided into permanent and temporary threads. Following Sulamanidze's APTOS thread applications, which means antiptosis suture, in the treatment of 186 patients with facial ptosis in 1998, Woffles thread applications, Waptos suture applications, Isse indirect barbed thread applications, and Silhouette soft thread applications were developed [12–15]. However, the fact that these threads are not absorbed into the soft tissue of the face and are permanent has been met with dissatisfaction by many patients, and new threads have been developed that are absorbed and disappear in the tissue.

Temporary threads are polyglycolic acid (PGA), polygleocapron (PGCL), polyglactin (PGLA), and poly-L lactic acid (PLLA/PLA), which can be absorbed by the body and eliminated from the body within 6 months to 2 years, mainly benefiting from the biochemical stimulation effect and then the lifting effect. They are threads produced from polydioxanone (PDO) and polycaprolactone (PCL). The most commonly used temporary thread type is PDO suture [16, 17]. PDO threads are fully absorbable, monofilament, synthetic surgical sutures made of PDO sterilized with ethylene oxide. PDO is a usually colorless, crystalline substance with a degradable polymer structure that tissue can break down. PDO thread configurations are mono (basic), twin mono, twisted, twin twisted, duplex, gold, and COG (barbed, serrated) PDO threads [18, 19]. Mono (basic) strings are flat monofilaments, which are the most commonly used and cheaper than other thread types.

PDOs are very widely used threads. Its effect lasts 6–12 months and disappears by turning into water and carbon dioxide. With its biostimulation effect, it is used to eliminate fine wrinkles, tone, tighten, plump, and shape the face and neck area. The type in which mono threads are placed as two braids inside the needle is called twin mono thread. It is used in cases where two threads are placed simultaneously in a single application, ensuring the effect is twice as strong. Twisted threads: They settle under the skin in a spiral shape. These are threads designed to be wrapped around the needle and have high impact and lifting power in the application area. Since they have a high biostimulation effect, they are placed directly into the area to add volume in weak tissue areas, to open wrinkled areas, and to open and correct glabellar lines, nasolabial grooves, and marionette lines. Twin twisted threads are twin helical threads wrapped around the needle, and they are designed to double the impact power with a single application in areas where twisted threads are applied. As for duplex threads prepared as a combination of PDO threads and PGA, while PGA is rapidly absorbed and reduces wrinkles with its acute effect, PDO aims to continue the skin improvement process with its long effect. COG PDO threads are barbed/serrated threads designed in various shapes that are applied to the face with the help of needles or cannulas, which benefit from the lifting and suspension effect. COG applications are more effective in eliminating facial sagging, tightening, and preserving facial symmetry, but their application requires more detailed anatomical knowledge and experience. Most complications related to thread suspension applications develop due to COGs. The barbs are designed to facilitate pulling by being embedded in the subcutaneous SMAS while pulling up on the thread and to prevent slipping by being embedded in the SMAS in the area to be fixed [20, 21].

The threads provide mechanical support, lifting, and fibroblast stimulation to increase collagen production and elastin in the tissue. It also increases the metabolic activity in the tissues, causing an increase in tone and volume. Thus, it provides a reduction in wrinkles and sagging on the face, flattening of hollow areas, and homogenization of tissue color. It stimulates the immune system by creating a foreign body reaction and fibrous bridging within the tissue. It accelerates the wound-healing process with an increase in macrophages. It increases blood and lymph vascular circulation by stimulating angiogenesis. Thus, it facilitates the removal of toxins and edema from the face and increases skin blood circulation. It creates a lipolysis effect by facilitating the excretion of fats with an increase in lymphatic drainage [22–25].

35.4 Indications and Patient Selection

General indications of thread applications in the lower face and neck area; correcting facial asymmetry, eliminating facial sagging, eliminating skin wrinkles, increasing skin tone and turgor, melting excess fat tissue, and reducing nasolabial groove, marionette and jowl line deformities [23, 24].

Serious and uncontrolled psychiatric disorders, unrealistic expectations, drug use, and addiction, serious systemic disease and general condition disorder, local or systemic infection, HIV or other immune system disorders, anticoagulant drug use, pregnancy, allergy, connective tissue diseases, autoimmune tissue. In the presence of conditions such as severe and uncontrolled psychiatric disorders, unrealistic expectations, drug use and addiction, severe systemic disease and general condition disorder, local or systemic infection, HIV or other immune system disorders, anticoagulant drug use, pregnancy, allergy, connective tissue diseases, and autoimmune tissue diseases, thread applications are strictly contraindicated.

35.5 Application

Thread suspension applications (Figs. 35.1a, b, 35.2, 35.3a, b, and 35.4) can be performed under local anesthesia, intravenous sedation, or general anesthesia. The skin is carefully cleaned and covered. Local anesthesia, usually 1% lidocaine and epinephrine, should be injected into the insertion/access area for analgesia and hemostasis. Antibiotic prophylaxis is generally not recommended. However, there are also studies in the literature supporting the use of perioperative single-dose or postoperative antibiotics, and this issue is still controversial [19, 26].

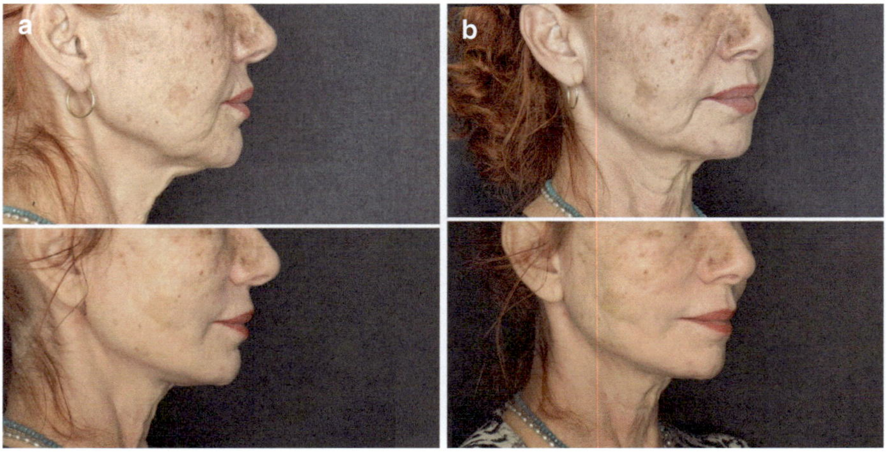

Fig. 35.1 (**a**): Case 1, side view: four double-needle transcutaneous threads were used. (Courtesy of Secil Ucar MD). (**b**): Case 1, three-quarter view: four double-needle transcutaneous threads were used. (Courtesy of Secil Ucar MD)

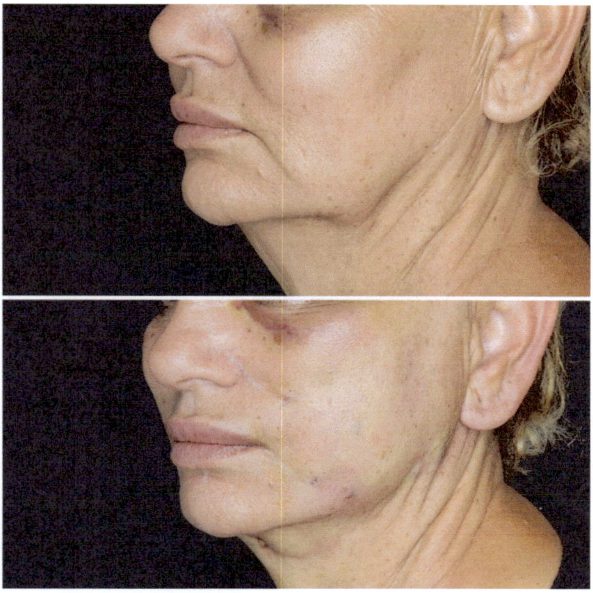

Fig. 35.2 Case 2: four double-needle transcutaneous threads were used. (Courtesy of Secil Ucar MD)

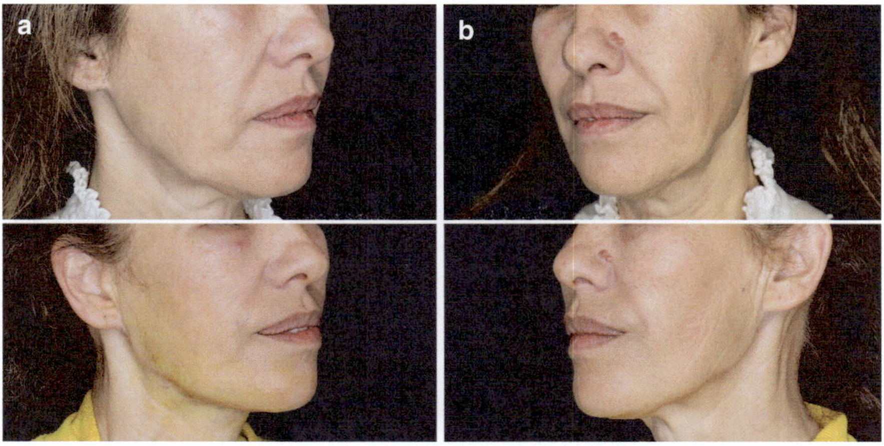

Fig. 35.3 (**a**): Case 3, right side view: four double-needle transcutaneous threads were used. (Courtesy of Secil Ucar MD). (**b**): Case 3, left side view: four double-needle transcutaneous threads were used. (Courtesy of Secil Ucar MD)

An entrance hole is made in the skin, usually with an 18G needle, and the threads are placed under the skin with the help of needles or cannulas. Depending on the type of thread and the desired effect, they are either left in place or pulled together with the tissue to provide a lifting effect. The threads are placed in the SMAS located within the subcutaneous tissue. Vector selection is specific to the patient and is determined by the patient's needs, that is, the desired movement of the tissues and how much mobilization is desired. Vectors are usually placed in a superior-lateral

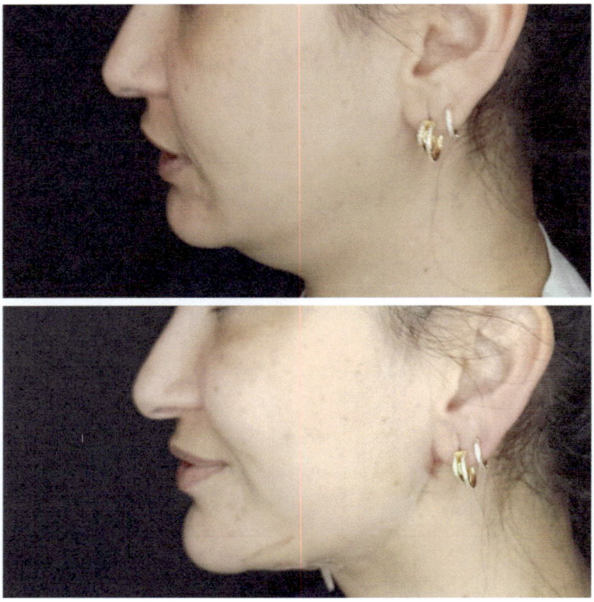

Fig. 35.4 Case 4: four double-needle transcutaneous threads were used. (Courtesy of Secil Ucar MD)

direction. Vertical vectors are recommended for the middle and lower face, and horizontal vectors are recommended for the neck. The length of the threads depends on how much soft tissue is desired and in which direction. Usually, 2–6 stitches are placed on each side for the lower face, mandibular contour, and neck [15]. The threads are placed in the SMAS inside the needle and cannula, and the needle or cannula is inserted into the SMAS.

Cannulas are withdrawn. SMAS is the most suitable area for biostimulation, embedding the threads and/or pulling the tissue up, and correcting the skin. It also allows needles, cannulas, and threads to move easily under the skin and minimizes damage to vessels, nerves, muscles, and fascia under the skin [1, 27].

After the procedure, patients are advised not to lift heavy loads for 3–5 days, not to apply pressure to the procedure area, and not to lean the head forward too much to prevent edema. It is also recommended that excessive movement of the muscles around the mouth, jaw, and neck be avoided for 2–3 weeks [19]. Excessive movement, especially the serrated threads, can be damaged and broken, and since they cannot be integrated into the tissue, their effect may be low and last for a short time.

35.6 Complications

Complications that may be seen in thread suspension applications are pain and bruising in the application area, collapse or painful mass formation at the needle entry points, seroma, hematoma, infection, necrosis, vascular or nerve damage, foreign body reaction, thread breakage, displacement or dislocation, skin along the thread trace retraction and nodule development, dimpled, asymmetry, lipolysis, atrophy, neuropathic pain, fasciculations, involuntary contractions, injury to the parotid gland and Stenson's duct, pseudolymphoma, inclusion cyst and late toxic reactions [19, 28–30].

References

1. Kim BJ, Choi JH, Lee Y. Development of facial rejuvenation procedures: thirty years of clinical experience with face lifts. Arch Plast Surg. 2015;42:521–31.
2. Yu N, Yu P, Liu Z, et al. Elastic thread modified minimal access cranial suspension lift for lower and middle third facial rejuvenation. Medicine (Baltimore). 2020;99(13):e19381. https://doi.org/10.1097/MD.0000000000019381.
3. Gavrilov LA, Gavrilova NS. The reliability theory of aging and longevity. J Theor Biol. 2001;213:527–45.
4. Yokozawa T, Satoh A, Cho EJ. Ginsenoside-Rd attenuates oxidative damage related to aging in senescence-accelerated mice. J Pharm Pharmacol. 2004;56:107–13.
5. Bereiter-Hahn J. Mitochondrial dynamics in aging and disease. Prog Mol Biol Transl Sci. 2014;127:93–131.
6. Gosain AK, Klein MH, Sudhakar PV, et al. A volumetric analysis of soft-tissue changes in the aging midface using high-resolution MRI: implications for facial rejuvenation. Plast Reconstr Surg. 2005;115:1143–52.
7. Mendelson BC, Jacobson SR. Surgical anatomy of the midcheek: facial layers, spaces, and the midcheek segments. Clin Plast Surg. 2008;35:395–404.
8. Kaya KS, Çakmak Ö. Facelift. Curr Pract ORL. 2018;14:84–95.
9. Ghassemi A, Prescher A, Riediger D, et al. Anatomy of the SMAS revisited. Aesth Plast Surg. 2003;27:258–64.
10. Le Louarn C. A new approach to functional anatomy of the lower face: role of the hyoplatysmal ligament, of the platysma and of the depressor labii lateralis. Ann Chir Plast Esthet. 2016;61:101–9.
11. Mitz V, Peironye M. The superficial musculoaponeurotic system in the parotid and cheek area. Plast Reconstr Surg. 1976;58:80–8.
12. Sulamanidze M, Sulamanidze G. APTOS suture lifting methods: 10 years of experience. Clin Plast Surg. 2009;36:281–306.
13. Isse NG, Fodor PB. Elevating the midface with barbed polypropylene sutures. Aesthet Surg J. 2005;25:301–3.
14. Wu WT. Barbed sutures in facial rejuvenation. Aesthet Surg J. 2004;24:582–7.
15. Halepas S, Chen XJ, Ferneini EM. Thread-lift sutures: anatomy, technique, and review of current literature. J Oral Maxillofac Surg. 2020;78:813–20.
16. Modi M. Critical evaluation of suture materials and suturing tecniques in İmplant dentistry. IJCID. 2009;1:31–40.
17. Singhvi MS, Zinjarde SS, Gokhale DV. Polylactic acid: synthesis and biomedical applications. J Appl Microbiol. 2019;127:1612–26.
18. Dennis C, Sethu S, Nayak S, et al. Suture materials current and emerging trends. J Biomed Mater Res Part A. 2016;104:1544–59.
19. Kurmuş GI, Koç E. Polidioksanon İplerle Yüz Germe ve Otolog Yağ Enfeksiyonları. In: Erbağcı Z, editor. Postmenopozal Dönemde Deri, Saç ve Tırnak Bakımı ve Uygun Dermatokozmetik Yaklaşımlar Türkiye Klinikleri 1. Ankara: Baskı; 2018. p. 70–6.
20. Suh DH, Jang HW, Lee SJ, et al. Outcomes of polydioxanone knotless thread lifting for facial rejuvenation. Dermatologic Surg. 2015;41:720–5.
21. Dursun R. Face lifting with threads: types of threads, combinations and complications. Turk Klin J Cosm Dermatol-Special Topics. 2017;10:191–200.

22. Jang HJ, Lee WS, Hwang K, et al. Effect of cog threads under rat skin. Dermatologic Surg. 2005;31:1639–44.
23. Shimizu Y, Terase K. Thread lift with absorbable monofilament threads. J Japan Soc Aesthetic Plast Surg. 2013;35:1–12.
24. Sweden AK. Combination therapy PDO beauty lift threads + LPG. J Clin Exp Dermatol Res. 2014;5:4.
25. Consiglio F, Pizzamiglio R, Parodi PC, et al. Suture-with Resorbable cones: histology and Physico-mechanical features. Aesthet Surg J. 2016;36:122–7.
26. Ferneini EM, Halepas S, Aronin SI. Antibiotic prophylaxis in blepharoplasty: review of the current literature. J Oral Maxillofac Surg. 2017;75:1477.
27. Broughton M, Fyfe GM. The superficial musculoaponeurotic system of the face: a model explored. Anat Res Int. 2013;2013:794682. https://doi.org/10.1155/2013/794682.
28. Winkler E, Goldan O, Regev E, et al. Stensen duct rupture (sialocele) and other complications of the aptos thread technique. Plast Reconstr Surg. 2006;118:1468–71.
29. Karimi K, Reivitis A. Lifting the lower face with an absorbable Polydioxanone (PDO) thread. J Drugs Dermatol. 2017;16:932–4.
30. Tavares JP, Oliveira CACP, Torres RP, et al. Facial thread lifting with suture suspension. Braz J Otorhinolaryngol. 2017;83:712–9.

Transcutaneous Suture Lifts: Neck

36

Sevilay Aynaci, Nuray Bayar Muluk, and Mario Milkov

36.1 Introduction

Loss of neck shape and sagging skin and soft tissues are hallmarks of aging in the lower facial area. Liposuction, open short-scar facelifts (such as MACS-lifting), and percutaneous suspension procedures are the three main categories of minimally invasive treatments for neck rejuvenation [1].

Less invasive procedures for face rejuvenation have been more popular in recent years. After pioneering simple skin excision lifts in the 1970s, surgeons began targeting deeper facial features after learning about the superficial musculoaponeurotic system [2–5]. José Guerrerosantos proposed cervical rhytidoplasty in 1974, which involved elevating and anchoring platysma muscle flaps posterior to the mastoid fascia [6]. In 1980 Illouz pioneered liposuction, a method for non-surgically removing excess fat from the neck. Joel J. Feldman's 1990 article "Corset Platysmaplasty" became the gold standard for neck procedures after seven previous attempts at the area, with the addition of anterior band plication in some instances [3].

The value of volumetric rejuvenation was solidified in the minds of plastic surgeons in the late 1990s [7–9]. This was a fundamental change in perspective, as plastic surgeons began to believe that volume restoration and skin tightening are often required to achieve rejuvenation. Ramirez demonstrated that submental incisions can separate platysma and lip depressors subperiosteally; tugging upwards in the midface can be communicated to the lower face [10]. After making incisions

S. Aynaci
Department of Otorhinolaryngology, Eskisehir City Hospital, Eskisehir, Türkiye

N. Bayar Muluk (✉)
Faculty of Medicine, Department of Otorhinolaryngology, Kirikkale University, Kirikkale, Türkiye

M. Milkov
Faculty of Dental Medicine, Medical University of Varna, Varna, Bulgaria

C. Cingi et al. (eds.), *Minor Interventions, Major Outcomes on the Face*, Comprehensive ENT, https://doi.org/10.1007/978-3-032-01305-7_36

under the skin and behind the ear, Giampapa removed the platysma, undermining soft tissue and permanently fixing interlocking sutures to the mastoid fascia on both sides [11]. The fixation material was an angle loop suture placed close to the mandible's angle. Anatomic suction-assisted lipectomy, platysma imbrication, and controlled tension of interlocking sutures were all necessary. Since volumetric correction seemed more crucial, the following step was to achieve similar outcomes using these methods with even more minor punctures or incisions [1].

36.2 Neck Anatomy

36.2.1 Fascial Layers

The neck has multiple layers of fascia, with superficial and deep fascia being the two primary divisions [12].

The superficial cervical fascia begins at the base of the skull and runs down the body to the axillae and thorax. It encompasses the platysma muscle, external and anterior jugular veins, cutaneous nerves, and superficial lymph nodes. The arrangement is designed to be loose so the neck can move freely [13, 14].

Partitions within the deep cervical fascia include the superficial, middle, and deep layers [15].

- The investing layer, the outermost layer of deep cervical fascia, encircles the sternocleidomastoid and trapezius muscles and is located between the neck muscles and the outermost layer of cervical fascia. It connects to the manubrium, clavicle, and scapula on the underside. The attachment points on the upper side are the mandible, mastoid process, superior nuchal line, and external occipital protuberance [15].
- The pre-tracheal layer, which is the middle layer of deep cervical fascia, extends superiorly from the base of the head to the mediastinum on the underside. A muscular and visceral division characterizes it. The muscular division includes the omohyoid, thyrohyoid, strap, sternohyoid, and sternothyroid muscles. The structures within the visceral division include the pharynx, esophagus, thyroid, parathyroid glands, trachea, and recurrent laryngeal nerve [15].
- The prevertebral layer, which extends from the base of the skull to the mediastinum, is a layer of deep cervical fascia. Together, the alar and prevertebral layers make up this structure. These layers make up the retropharyngeal space, which is located around the cervical vertebrae and deep neck muscles [15].

36.2.2 Strengthening Muscles

A long, thin muscle called the platysma runs from the top of the thorax to the lower lip and cheek. In its regular operation, it draws the center lip downward (through the depressor anguli oris, which contracts the lip commissure inferiorly and is innervated by the facial nerve's marginal mandibular branch). It tightens the neck superficially (through the facial nerve's cervical branch) [16].

The sternal manubrium and the medial clavicle are the sources of the two heads of the sternocleidomastoid muscle. These muscle heads attach to the temporal bone's mastoid process and the superior nuchal line, where they combine. The head turns to face the side that is not contracting, which is how it works. That area is innervated by CN XI [17].

A vast back muscle, the trapezius runs laterally to the scapular spine and inferiorly to the lower thoracic vertebrae, beginning at the external protrusion of the occipital bone. CN XI stabilizes and moves the scapula, which also innervates the trapezius [18].

Among the muscles that extend above the hip socket are the digastric, mylohyoid, and geniohyoid muscles. The hyoid bone and parts of the mandible are attached to these muscles, except the digastric muscle. There are two sides to the digastric muscle; the back side connects to the temporal bone's mastoid process. The hypoglossal nerve (CN XII) is responsible for innervating the geniohyoid. A tributary of the mandibular division of CN V, the mylohyoid nerve supplies the anterior belly of the digastric muscles and the mylohyoid. The back of the stomach is provided with nerve impulses from the facial nerve. As mentioned, their job is to raise the hyoid bone [13].

A group of muscles that are located just below the thyroid and omohyoid bones make up what is called the infrahyoid muscles. The thyrohyoid muscle is the only one not receiving nerve supply from the ansa cervicalis (C1-C3); CN XII innervates it. Starting on the scapula, the omohyoid muscle wraps around the sternocleidomastoid and eventually binds to the hyoid bone. Their names describe the origin and insertion sites of the sternohyoid, sternothyroid, and thyrohyoid muscles [13].

36.3 Aging Process

Both patients and medical professionals frequently overlook the "telltale" signs of aging in the neck in their pursuit of rejuvenation. In many circumstances, it is recommended to combine nonsurgical neck rejuvenation with facial rejuvenation to achieve a more consistent appearance. The neck has a complex network of dermal structures, including the reticular and papillary dermis, fibroseptal network, subcutaneous fat, and underlying fibrous fascia. The layers coordinate their actions to achieve the desired tone and quality [19, 20].

In contrast to the face, which often loses volume and looks older as we get older, the neck can gain fat in the submental compartment and lose definition around the jawline. A saggy or overweight appearance can result from submandibular fat in the preplatysmal compartment [21]. In contrast to overall body fat gain, fat redistribution and neck laxity are unaffected by dietary and exercise changes and frequently worsen following substantial weight loss [22]. Gravitational decline and photodamage, which cause collagen and elastin loss, are both involved in aging, just as they are in the face. Rejuvenation should consider every facet of aging relevant to that individual [19].

36.4 Evaluation

Despite how vague the concept of a young neck may be, precise standards have been established. A young person's neck has a distinct lower jawline, a bulge of the thyroid cartilage, a distinct front edge of the sternocleidomastoid muscle, and a cervical angle ranging from 105 degrees to 120 degrees [23]. The presence of platysmal bands, the extent to which the patient's howling extends into the neck, the degree of preplatysmal and subplatysmal lipolysis, and other similar findings should be considered throughout the evaluation. The platysmal bands' positions, directions, and inter-band distances are documented. The patient should flex the platysma to determine if the bands are dynamic or static [24]. The cervicomental angle and mandibular border can be blunted by platysmal banding, which may result from cervical fascia weakening and contribute to the accelerated aging of the neck (8). Patients who are not good surgical candidates, those who want to postpone or avoid surgery altogether, those whose neck skin laxity is not enough for a surgical facelift, and those who have no intention of ever wanting a facelift are all good candidates for nonsurgical neck tightening. If you lead a hectic lifestyle and do not have time to recover from surgery, nonsurgical skin tightening may be a good option. Furthermore, due to the reduced risk profile, nonsurgical treatment alternatives may be preferred by exceedingly risk-averse patients. They are usually open to undergoing more treatments with less dramatic outcomes in exchange for shorter recovery times. Patients watching their budgets would do well to prioritize nonsurgical treatments over surgical ones. Treatments for nonsurgical skin tightening using local anesthetic are now possible in the comfort of your own office. That means the patient will not have to worry about the dangers and expenses of general anesthesia or the accompanying surgical facility fees [19].

Depending on the patient's anatomy and desired outcomes, it may take a single treatment or a series of treatments, but that's the case with every cosmetic operation. The most dramatic and reliable result is achieved with liposuction, which is used in 81% of cases. However, some patients do not desire surgical intervention due to concerns about ecchymosis, skin laxity, recovery time, vascular or neurologic complications, cost, the possibility of an unnatural result, or medical issues [25, 26].

Surgical, thermal, or chemical stress triggers a cascade of events that most skin-tightening products aim to mimic. In the last stage of wound healing, collagen is realigned, which causes the skin to tighten and collagen to contract [27].

The minimum time required to observe effects is 3–4 months, while the maximum is 6–12 months. Many of the modalities necessitate multiple treatments, with intervals of 4–8 weeks. After 6 months of treatment, it may take another 6–12 months before you notice any changes. Extreme skin laxity, UV damage, or advanced age may restrict the results. These treatments have a range of possible longevity, from 1 to 5 years. The potential outcomes have many moving parts, so it is important to moderate expectations during the initial consultation [19].

36.5 Transcutaneous Suture Lifts—Neck

The under-correction and lack of sustainability of suspension methods have been criticized [1].

The main reason is that most of these suspensions are single-point designs, allowing traction forces to tear tissue at the anchor points. The APTOS Lift and the Happy Lift are examples of barbed suture products. Eight patients with neck-area single-point suspensions showed findings that corroborated this idea. The neck abnormalities returned in every patient after 3 months [1].

When used with an open approach [2] or independently, loop suspensions are an effective and long-lasting process [11, 28]. A loop suspension works by distributing forces that cancel each other out at each point in the loop. The more efficient the tissue-carrying loop is, the less force will be exerted at each point along the loop due to sheer gravity. Another big deal with suspension methods like the APTOS Lift, Happy Lift, and Silhouette is how much money you'll need to buy the products required to do the linked processes. Contrarily, loop suspensions have proven to be both practical and durable. They can be used alone [8, 28] or as a component of an open technique [29, 30]. Creating a carrier loop in the tissue essentially makes tissue resistance fight against itself to balance the shear forces, which is the physical rationale for the long-lasting efficacy of open/closed-loop suspension procedures. At each location in the loop, an opposing force vector acts as a counterbalance. Consequently, the force exerted on opposing suspension-tissue connections is reduced proportionately to the loop's perfection [1].

Compared to other methods, micro-shuttle lifting has several benefits, such as quick treatment (even with local anesthesia), not requiring hospital admission, having a short recovery period, and having inconspicuous punctures. Any prospective product's price tag should be carefully considered as well. This method is inexpensive since the surgeon does not have to spend money on products and can get away with using simple needles and polypropylene sutures. The safety of micro-shuttle lifting should be considered. Postoperative numbness, hematoma, skin slough, or facial nerve damage is unlikely [31, 32]. By avoiding interlocking and instead running the threads that suspend the neck continuously from ear to ear. It provides a seamless bridge for the sliding neck system. The elderly patient population was satisfied with less-than-ideal outcomes since they refused to undergo open surgery under any circumstances [1].

References

1. Tiryaki KT, Aksungur E, Grotting JC. Micro-shuttle lifting of the neck: a percutaneous loop suspension method using a novel double-ended needle. Aesthet Surg J. 2016;36(6):629–38. https://doi.org/10.1093/asj/sjw001. Epub 2016 Feb 23
2. Tiryaki KT. Shuttle lifting of the nose: a minimally invasive approach for nose reshaping. Aesthet Surg J. 2010;30(2):176–83.
3. Feldman JJ. Corset platysmaplasty. Plast Reconstr Surg. 1990;85(3):333–43.
4. Skoog T. Plastic surgery: new methods and refinements. Philadelphia: Saunders; 1974.
5. Mitz V, Peyronie M. The superficial muscul-oaponeurotic system (SMAS) in the parotid and cheek area. Plast Reconstr Surg. 1976;58(1):80–8.
6. Guerrerosantos J. Surgical correction of the fatty fallen neck. Ann Plast Surg. 1979;2(5):389–96.
7. Donofrio LM. Fat distribution: a morphologic study of the aging face. Dermatologic Surg. 2000;26(12):1107–12.
8. Pessa JE. An algorithm of facial aging: verification of Lambros's theory by three-dimensional stereolithography, with reference to the pathogenesis of midfacial aging, scleral show, and lateral suborbital trough deformity. Plast Reconstr Surg. 2000;106(2):479–88. discussion 489–490
9. Pessa JE. The potential role of stereolithography in the study of facial aging. Am J Orthod Dentofacial Orthop. 2001;119(2):117–20.
10. Ramirez OM, Robertson KM. Comprehensive approach to rejuvenation of the neck. Facial Plast Surg. 2001;17(2):129–40.
11. Giampapa V, Bitzos I, Ramirez O, Granick M. Long-term results of suture suspension platysmaplasty for neck rejuvenation: a 13-year follow-up evaluation. Aesth Plast Surg. 2005;29(5):332–40.
12. Roesch ZK, Tadi P. Anatomy, head and neck, neck. In: StatPearls [Internet]. Treasure Island: StatPearls Publishing; 2024. [Updated 2023 Jul 24]. Available from: https://www.ncbi.nlm.nih.gov/books/NBK542313/.
13. Kohan EJ, Wirth GA. Anatomy of the neck. Clin Plast Surg. 2014 Jan;41(1):1–6.
14. Guidera AK, Dawes PJ, Fong A, Stringer MD. Head and neck fascia and compartments: no space for spaces. Head Neck. 2014 Jul;36(7):1058–68.
15. Warshafsky D, Goldenberg D, Kanekar SG. Imaging anatomy of deep neck spaces. Otolaryngol Clin N Am. 2012 Dec;45(6):1203–21.
16. Hwang K, Kim JY, Lim JH. Anatomy of the platysma muscle. J Craniofac Surg. 2017 Mar;28(2):539–42.
17. Bordoni B, Jozsa F, Varacallo M. StatPearls [Internet]. In: Anatomy, head and neck, sternocleidomastoid muscle. Treasure Island: StatPearls Publishing; 2023.
18. Ourieff J, Scheckel B, Agarwal A. StatPearls [Internet]. In: Anatomy, back, trapezius. Treasure Island: StatPearls; 2023.
19. Sturm A, Shokri T, Ducic Y. Nonsurgical rejuvenation of the neck. Clin Plast Surg. 2023 Jul;50(3):497–507. https://doi.org/10.1016/j.cps.2022.12.014.
20. Locketz GD, Bloom JD. Percutaneous radiofrequency technologies for the lower face and neckfacial. Plast Surg Clin North Am. 2019;27(3):305–20.
21. Hatef DA, Koshy JC, Sandoval SE, et al. The submental fat compartment of the neck. Semin Plast Surg. 2009;23(4):288–91.
22. Park JH, Kim JI, Park HJ, et al. Evaluation of safety and efficacy of non-invasive radiofrequency technology for submental rejuvenation. Lasers Med Sci. 2016;31(8):1599–605.
23. Ellenbogen R, Karlin JV. Visual criteria for success in restoring the youthful neck. Plast Reconstr Surg. 1980;66(6):826–37.
24. Rohrich RJ, Savetsky IL, Cohen JM, et al. Effective treatment of platysmal bands with neurotoxin. Plast Reconstr Surg Glob Open. 2020;8(6):e2812.

25. Jianu DM, Filipescu M, Jianu SA, et al. The synergy between lasers and adipose surgery in face and neck rejuvenation: a new approach from personal experience. Laser Ther. 2012;21(3):215–22.
26. Schlessinger J, Weiss SR, Jewell M, et al. Perceptions and practices in submental fat treatment: a survey of physicians and patients. Skinmed. 2013;11(1):27–31.
27. Gentile RD. Renuvion/J-plasma for subdermal skin tightening facial contouring and skin rejuvenation of the face and neck. Facial Plast Surg Clin North Am. 2019;27(3):273–90. https://doi.org/10.1016/j.fsc.2019.03.001. Epub 2019 May 22
28. Tiryaki KT. Shuttle lifting of the face: a percutaneous purse string suture suspension method for facial rejuvenation. Presented at the 19th International Society of Aesthetic Plastic Surgery, February 10–13, 2008, Melbourne.
29. Tonnard P, Verpaele A. The MACS-lift short scar rhytidectomy. Aesthet Surg J. 2007;27(2):188–98.
30. Nahai FN. The submandibular gland in the neck. Aesthet Surg J. 2006;26(4):471.
31. Baker DC. Complications of cervicofacial rhytidectomy. Clin Plast Surg. 1983;10(3):543–62.
32. Matarasso A, Elkwood A, Rankin M, Elkowitz M. National plastic surgery survey: face lift techniques and complications. Plast Reconstr Surg. 2000;106(5):1185–95. discussion 1196

Part VI

Mesotherapy

Mesotherapy: Overview

37

Fatih Savran, Murat Songu, and Andrew A. Winkler

37.1 Introduction

The mesoderm develops into connective tissue, muscular, and circulatory systems from the three embryological germ layers (ecto-, meso-, and endoderm) [1].

Mesotherapy (from the Greek mesos, "middle," and therapeia, "to treat medically") is a nonsurgical cosmetic drug treatment [2].

Skin injections for therapeutic purposes date back to ancient Chinese and Indian medicine. In 1847, Karl Baunscheidt thought that a drug could have an effect even if injected superficially and dermally 2 mm deep. In 1853, a Scottish doctor named Alexander Wood injected dermic morphine to provide relief in many painful conditions. In 1860, Bartolomeo Guala began to practice systematic hypodermic therapy. In 1867, Gaetano Primavera in Naples conducted the first experiment to assess the extent of drug absorption in the urine after hypodermic administration. In 1870, doctors injected distilled water into the dermis during the Franco-Prussian War to relieve arthritic pain. In 1885, William Halsted reported that intradermal inoculation of sterile water induces local anesthesia. In 1894, Pietro Orlandini, a Venetian physician, suggested dermal punctures to treat certain types of localized pain. In 1941, George D. Gammon and Isaac Starr demonstrated that sterile water inoculation has an analgesic effect on or near the skin [3]. Dr. Michel Pistor coined the term "mesotherapy" in an article titled "Revealing an effect of procaine local and pathology in

F. Savran (✉)
Sancaktepe Regional Hospital, Department of Otolaryngology, Istanbul, Turkey

M. Songu
Songu Private Clinic, Izmir, Turkey

A. A. Winkler
University of Colorado School of Medicine, Department of Otolaryngology, Aurora, CO, USA
e-mail: andrew.winkler@cuanschutz.edu

C. Cingi et al. (eds.), *Minor Interventions, Major Outcomes on the Face*, Comprehensive ENT, https://doi.org/10.1007/978-3-032-01305-7_37

man" (A Brief Description of New Properties of Locally Applied Procaine in Human Pathology), which he published in La Presse Medicale in 1958. It began with Pistor intravenously injecting procaine into a partially deaf person to treat an acute asthma attack. With procaine, the standard treatment for an acute asthma attack at the time, Pistor noticed that the patient's hearing improved for a few hours. When Pistor noticed this situation, he started injecting procaine into the superficial dermis in areas close to the ear. Again, surprisingly, some patients showed relief from neck pain. Following this, Pistor coined the term mesotherapy to describe mesoderm therapy [3–5].

The French Academy of Medicine recognized mesotherapy in 1987 and accepted it as a part of traditional medicine [6, 7]. In 2004, analyzing preclinical and clinical trials, Sergio Maggiori proposed the term "local intradermal therapy" (LIT) to emphasize that superficial inoculation enables clinical effects to be achieved with a lower drug dose. LIT has become one of the best-known and most widely practiced microinvasive techniques for treating various local clinical conditions [3].

Mesotherapy is performed in structures derived from the mesoderm beyond the embryonic stage of human development. It is a minimally invasive technique consisting of intra or subcutaneous injection of microscopic amounts of various mixtures of natural plant extracts, homeopathic agents, pharmaceuticals, vitamins, and other bioactive substances through multiple dermal punctures [2, 8]. In mesotherapy, drugs and other substances are injected into the mesoderm (fat and connective tissue layer under the skin). Mesotherapy injections aim to stimulate the injected tissues for various purposes [2, 5].

Mesotherapy, also known as intradermotherapy, does not mean the treatment of any particular condition; it describes only one method of drug delivery [2]. Currently, local intradermal therapy (mesotherapy, LIT) is based on the hypothesis that the drug applied in the superficial layer of the skin allows a more prolonged pharmacological effect at the administration site and beyond. Preclinical studies have shown that intradermal administration of anti-inflammatory, anesthetic, and antibiotic substances allows a reduced dose and a prolonged effect in the tissues below the injection site (skin, muscle, and joint) compared to intramuscular administration. Also, an excellent antibody response is obtained after intradermal injection of an antigen compared to intramuscular administration. This suggests a lower dose inoculated into the dermis may achieve a more significant effect than a deep injection. This technique alters the normal absorption kinetics of the injected drug, significantly slows systemic absorption, and allows distribution in tissues below the inoculation site [3]. Other claimed advantages for mesotherapy include inexpensive equipment, relatively little training requirement for providers, rapid and undiluted delivery of drugs to the target site, much lower dosage requirements for drugs, faster accumulation of benefits, minimal invasiveness, no accompanying pain, and no hospitalization [8]. Before mesotherapy became an acceptable treatment method in cosmetic dermatology, it was primarily accepted in many fields, such as pain management, sports medicine, and rheumatology [2].

37.2 Theories About the Effective Mechanism of Mesotherapy

37.2.1 Pastor's Reflex Theory

Mesotherapy affects the inhibitory mechanisms at the dermal level, affecting the reactions in the "visceral-medullary-cerebral" pathway at the lateral medullary level. This dermal inhibitory stimulus occurs both mechanically (via needles) and through the pharmacological effects of drugs.

37.2.2 Microcirculatory Theory

Mesotherapy agents stimulate local microcirculation in damaged tissue.

37.2.3 Mesodermic Theory

It affects the cells related to the immune system in the dermis.

37.2.4 Third Circulation Theory

With the help of interstitial tissue, mesotherapy agents are thought to reach deeper tissues and provide higher concentrations in target tissues, increasing their therapeutic effects [9].

In mesotherapy, the aim is to deliver the products as a depot up to 4 mm deep with intradermal injections. If necessary, the products used are diluted within the framework of the treatment parameters, and multiple injections are planned to be repeated at regular intervals in the area of the pathology. The frequency of application is determined according to these criteria [4]. Products used in mesotherapy are drugs or cocktails that dissolve in water and do not adversely interact when applied together. In mesotherapy applications, 4, 6, 8, and 13 mm long (27, 30, 32, 34 G) needle tips are preferred. The application can be done manually or using mesotherapy guns. In treating skin lesions, rollers and microneedling instruments are also preferred for standard and homogeneous treatment today [6]. Different injection techniques can be used in mesotherapy:

(i) Epidermal technique.
(ii) Papular technique, in which reagents are injected into the dermo-epidermal junction.
(iii) Intradermal injection (page method), in which the injections are penetrated to a depth of 2–4 mm and given at an angle of 30–60°.

(iv) Point injection into the deep dermis. Generally, the practitioner determines the injected formula or cocktail based on the patient's needs. For this reason, standardized formulas are not available [5].

After applying topical anesthetic creams to the application area, painless injections are applied to the skin area with fine and small needles. Intradermal application is called the Nappage technique. It has recently been used in multi-injection devices, including pneumatic and electronic devices [6]. It is necessary to follow some rules when choosing the substances applied in mesotherapy. It should be hydrosoluble, not an oily solution. Medicines prepared from fatty substances, except propylene glycol, are not used in mesotherapy. It should be at a suitable pH and isotonic. It should be tolerable at the subepidermal level and must be able to interact with receptors in the tissue. It should not be an allergen, and the patients must be questioned as to whether they have ever had an allergic reaction to the substance used. It must be physically and chemically suitable. Ideally, effects and side effects should be defined, and there should be synergistic, not antagonistic, effects between multiple medications [10, 11]. Many substances are used in mesotherapy.

37.3 Indications and Medications Used

Primarily accepted in pain management, sports medicine, and rheumatology, mesotherapy is advocated in treating various conditions such as chronic pain, vascular disease, psoriasis, and rheumatoid arthritis [12, 13]. Its analgesic effect has been used to treat conditions such as cancer, neuralgia, arthritis, and other musculoskeletal conditions, as well as vascular stasis-derived diseases and medical conditions. Mesotherapy is widely accepted in cosmetic medicine to eliminate cellulite, reduce fat, promote weight loss, treat aging skin, reduce sagging skin, reduce acne scars and stretch marks, and rejuvenate the hands and neck [1, 2, 14, 15]. However, there is insufficient information on formulations, techniques, doses, and toxicology, and the scientific literature describing the use of certain substances is limited. These formulations, methods, and dosages may vary depending on the experience of the practicing physician.

Phytological and pharmacological agents control inflammation in rheumatoid arthritis, while connective tissue activators such as silica, biotin, and proteolytic enzymes are used for ligament tears and tendon degeneration. In acute sports injuries, 1–3 sessions are usually applied. At least 15 sessions may be required for chronic conditions such as cellulite and fine wrinkles. In such cases, injections are also recommended once a year or even every 6 months.

In mesotherapy, vasodilators, anti-inflammatory drugs, muscle relaxants, proteolytic enzymes, vitamins, minerals, plant extracts, vaccines, antibiotics, hormones, hormone blockers, and anesthetics are injected. Phosphatidylcholine and deoxycholate have also been used in subcutaneous injections. Most mesotherapy formulas contain a vasodilator. The reason for this is unclear, but recent studies have shown that the vasodilator results in faster clearance or reuptake of injected phosphatidylcholine and deoxycholate. Therefore, a vasodilator may be helpful for patients where systemic uptake of the injected drug is desired [5].

The most common painful conditions in which mesotherapy is utilized are discopathy; pathologies that cause neck, back, and lower back pain, such as arthrosis; joint injuries of the shoulder and knee; soft tissue pathologies, such as bursitis, tendinitis, and synovitis; rheumatoid diseases such as rheumatoid arthritis and ankylosing spondylitis; and carpal tunnel syndrome nerve entrapment pathologies such as sciatica. It is used by mixing local anesthetic, myorelaxant, and non-steroidal anti-inflammatory substances in acute locomotor system pathologies. In chronic conditions, circulation regulators such as pentoxifylline derivatives are added to this mixture [4].

Mesotherapy applied to the face area is popular among nonsurgical skin rejuvenation methods. Mesotherapy injections made using vitamins, minerals, some homeopathic agents, and natural proteins are called "mesoglow" when used for skin rejuvenation and "mesolift" when applied to gain tone. The most common and most straightforward mesotherapy formulation for facial skin rejuvenation involves the injection of a multivitamin solution into the dermis over multiple sessions. It has been reported that mesotherapy applied on the face reduces wrinkles, increases elasticity, and improves pigmentation, but it has yet to be proven. Subdermally applied vitamin injections are claimed to regenerate cells, activate fibroblasts, and stimulate collagen and elastin production [2, 6, 16]. In antiaging studies, applications are made for skin rejuvenation, renewal, and repair. To prevent the formation of wrinkles, patients in their mid-20s are recommended mesotherapy anti-aging treatments, and treatments for the face, neck, arms, and hands are recommended several times a year [2]. All injections of vitamins, minerals, peptides, amino acids, hyaluronic acid (HA), and mesotherapy products supporting collagen synthesis should be applied to the face, neck, and décolleté to a depth of 2–2.5 mm. The injected amounts per injection are limited to a maximum of 0.02–0.05 ml, and the distance between the two injection points should be 1–2 cm in the epidermis. The amount of product to be used in a single session is between 2.5 and 5 ml, depending on the application area and skin condition [4]. Mesotherapy mixed with botulinum toxin has become famous for body shaping and point weight loss [2].

Ten sessions are recommended once a week for skin rejuvenation. 17 β Estradiol 1 ml, procaine 2 ml, vitamin C 3 ml, mesocaine 2 ml, glycosaminoglycans (GAG) 0.5–1 ml, hyaluronic acid 2 ml, and trissilinol 0.5% 2 ml are drugs used for skin rejuvenation.

Procaine is a local anesthetic and vasodilator that is soluble in water. Procaine is an ester of PABA and deanol and is the primary drug of mesotherapy. It aids in increasing the absorption of other medications. It is available in 1% and 2% forms. Vitamin C (L-ascorbic acid) is a widely used supplement that is felt to strengthen the immune system. Ascorbic acid is an antioxidant that protects tissues from damage by free radicals. It supports connective tissue and is used in collagen production. Vitamin C is required for the hydroxylation process during the synthesis of collagen proteins. In this way, it is theorized that more muscular collagen tissue is formed. It also inhibits melanin synthesis.

Glycosaminoglycans (GAG) contain chondroitin-4-sulfate, chondroitin-6-sulfate, dermatan sulfate, and heparan sulfate. GAGs support collagen fibrils by binding to proteins in the extracellular matrix. GAG injection stimulates collagen production and development and stabilizes collagen fibrils. GAGs are used in mesotherapy to treat striae, skin wrinkles, and alopecia. Local edema, erythema, and ecchymosis may occasionally occur at the injection site.

Hyaluronic acid (HA) is a natural substance necessary for all living organisms. It is found in high concentrations in the connective tissue and liquid around the eyes. Hyaluronic acid is in the form of a gel in the skin tissue. It fills the space between collagen and elastic fibrils; their role in the skin tissue is to transport vital substances to the cells during blood circulation, moisturize the skin, and protect the tissues by acting as a cushion against mechanical and chemical damage. As a result of environmental factors (such as sunlight and air pollution) and aging, hyaluronic acid in the tissue is broken down and damaged over time. In recent years, synthetic forms of HA have been used in cosmetic dermatology to treat wrinkles. It is applied along the wrinkles on aged and damaged skin using the point or tunneling technique. In addition to hyaluronic acid used as a direct filler, combined hyaluronic acid preparations can be used for mesolift purposes. Products containing hyaluronic acid can be injected Nappage, point, or intradermally [10].

For wrinkle treatment, dimethyl amino ethanol (DMAE) 25 mg/ml 1 ml, Timomodulina 1 ml, Alpha lipoic acid 1 ml, GAG 0.5 ml, procaine 2% 1 ml, 17β Estradiol 2 ml, and Procaine 2% 1 ml can be used.

It is used around the eyes, mentum, forehead, nasolabial, malar, chin edges, mentum, and forehead. DMAE is a naturally sourced substance obtained from salmon. It is felt to strengthen and stabilize the membranes of skin cells. Dramatically tightens facial, eyelid, and neck muscles for a youthful appearance. Alpha lipoic acid is a substance found in various foods and can also be synthesized in the body. Alpha lipoic acid and its reduced form, dihydrolipoic acid, show antioxidant properties. It achieves this antioxidant effect by catching free radicals, chelating with metals, increasing the reusability of other antioxidants, and repairing oxidative damage. It can reduce its toxic effects by forming chelates with heavy metals. It helps to maintain blood glucose balance by affecting the signaling pathways of insulin. Due to its impact on oxidative stress and glucose balance, it can prevent the formation and progression of diabetic complications and neurodegenerative diseases [10, 17].

For skin tension, DMAE 25 mg/ml, Timomodulina 1 ml, Alpha lipoic acid 50 mg/ml 2 ml, GAG 1 ml, sodium pyruvate 2 ml, procaine 1 ml, vitamin C 2 ml, sodium bicarbonate 8% 1 ml, procaine 1 ml, or 17β estradiol can be used. Estradiol injection is thought to play a role in skin tightening in premenopausal and menopausal women. Pyruvate is a derivative of lactic acid. It stimulates collagen synthesis from fibroblasts and has a lipolytic effect. The main indication of pyruvate is antiaging [6, 10].

Mesotherapy methods are an important treatment option for androgenic hair loss in women, the early onset of androgenic hair loss in men, postpartum hair loss in women, and regional hair loss such as scalp, beard, and eyebrows. Cocktails prepared from procaine, lidocaine, biotin, pantheon, trental, fonzylene, multivitamins, vitamin A, oligo-elements, antiandrogens, and finasteride products are frequently preferred today. Treatment can be performed with 2.5–3 ml of product in each session, once a week for the first month, once every 15 days for the second month, and once a month after that. 30-gauge 4 mm needles can be used. Treatment should continue for 6 months. The recommended mixture includes the following:

1. D-Panthenol 2 ml, Biotin 2 ml, Buflomedil 2 ml, Lidocaine 2 ml
2. Mesocaine 2 ml, Finasteride 2 ml, Trissilinol 2 ml, Biotin 2 ml [4, 6]

While lipolytic drugs and drugs that increase microcirculation are used in the upper region of the belly and waist circumference, medicines that cause edema and fibrosis are used in the hip and thigh regions. While some have proposed vascular and inflammatory theories to explain the appearance of cellulite, the best evidence supports gender-based structural differences in the organization of female subcutaneous fat that produces the pits and cavities characteristic of cellulite. Injection depth can vary up to 13 mm depending on the depth of lubrication and cellulite. Approximately 0.2–0.4 ml of product is applied to each point at 5–8 cm intervals. Especially in treating cellulite, proteolytic products, collagenase, and hyaluronidase, which dissolve fibrous bands, should be used cautiously as they can cause allergic reactions. Adipolitic active substances that remove free fatty acids and triglycerides from adipocytes: yohimbine alpha, tratricol, aminophylline, euphyllin, alcaxantina (alcacopha and aminophylline), phosphatidylcholine, deoxycholate, L carnitin, caffeine, and coenzyme A. Circulatory regulators: benzopyrones (coumarin), buflomedil, melilot-rutine, ginkgo biloba, pentoxyphyllin, procain, and lidocaine. These substances can be used as a mixture [1, 4].

In stages 1 and 2 cellulite: rutina + mellilotus 2 ml + procaine 2 ml, buflomedil 2 ml + trissilinol 2 ml + alcachofra-artichoke 2 ml, pentoxifylline 2 ml + ginko biloba 2 ml + benzopyrone 2 ml.

In stages 3 and 4 cellulite: rutina + mellilotus 2 ml + trissilinol 2 ml + buflomedil 1 ml + loimbina 0.5% 0.5–1 ml, pentoxifylline 2 ml + ginko biloba 2 ml + artichoke 2 ml +, tratricole 350 mcg 2 ml + procaine 2 ml + aminophylline 2 ml can be used.

The importance of compliance with diet and exercise increases even more in stage 3 and advanced cellulite. The results of the application begin to be seen from the sixth month. Esberiven (Rutin-melilot extract, Sweet Clover extract) contains 50 mg of rutoside and 200 mg of melilot extract. 200 mg of extract contains 1 mg of coumarin. Coumarin improves lymphatic circulation and blood circulation by increasing peristaltic contractions. Rutoside is a bioflavonoid known as "Vitamin P." It reduces capillary fragility, has an anti-edema effect, and shows a lymphokinetic effect. Rutoside provides vasoconstriction and increases capillary resistance. Fonzilan (Buflomedil, Lofton) is a vasodilator and opens the precapillary sphincters. It is beneficial for smokers. Pentoxifylline inhibits phosphodiesterase, providing lipolysis. It facilitates the passage of erythrocytes through capillaries. It allows erythrocytes to change shape. Methylxanthines such as aminophylline and caffeine exert lipolytic effects by inhibiting the phosphodiesterase enzyme [6, 10] (Figs. 37.1, 37.2, and 37.3).

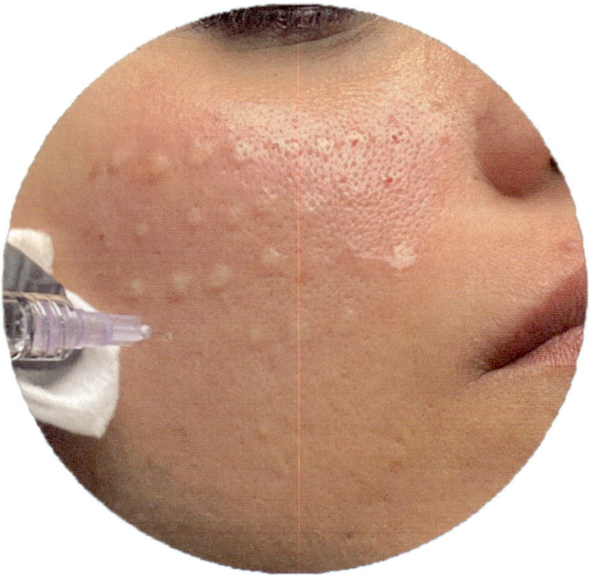

Fig. 37.1 Mid-face mesotherapy (Xela Rederm). (Courtesy of Murat Songu MD)

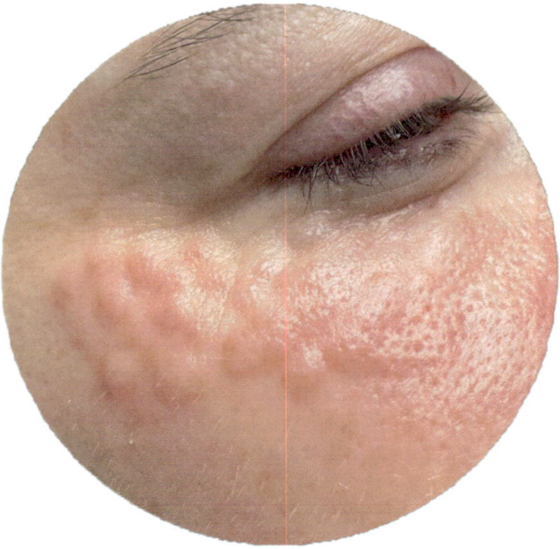

Fig. 37.2 Under eye treatment (Papular technique). (Courtesy of Murat Songu MD)

37.4 Contraindications

It is not recommended to apply mesotherapy to pregnant women, breastfeeding mothers, uncontrolled hyperthyroidism, bleeding diathesis disorders, poor general condition, advanced heart and cancer patients. Active skin disease or infection in the application area also is a contraindication. In addition, regional slimming

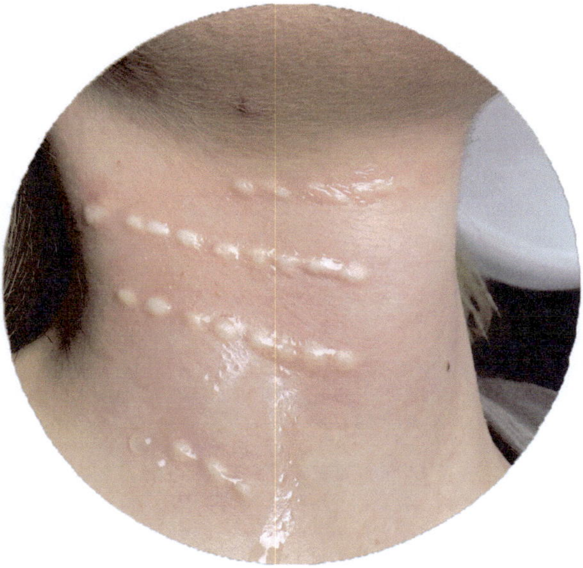

Fig. 37.3 Neck treatment (Papular technique). (Courtesy of Murat Songu MD)

applications are not recommended for kidney and liver disorders and lymphatic and circulatory disorders [7].

37.5 Side Effects

Traditional mesotherapy techniques and medications have been associated with atypical mycobacterial infections, urticaria, and lichenoid drug eruptions. Worsening of psoriasis is increasingly related to non-tuberculosis atypical mycobacterial infections, manifesting as late-onset skin and soft tissue infections, but mainly if mesotherapy is performed with poor aseptic measures by nonprofessional practitioners or if nonquality-controlled substances and drugs are injected. Pain is typically minimal during and after superficial injections. The injected areas may bleed temporarily and show signs of inflammation that resolve within a few days. After the application, bruising and swelling at the injection site are the most common side effects [2, 5, 7]. Complications such as post-inflammatory hyperpigmentation, ecchymosis, prolonged swelling and tenderness (lasting for several months), ulceration, and hematoma formation, although rare, may occur [5, 12]. Other side effects in publications include subcutaneous nodule formation, localized urticaria pigmentosa, and a lichenoid eruption [18, 19]. There are life-threatening risks, such as embolism, but they have not been reported in the medical literature.

37.6 Conclusion

Mesotherapy has become a frequently applied treatment today due to low-dose products and few side effects. Pain therapy is now used in many areas of the body. Mesotherapy for skin rejuvenation, alopecia, and lipolysis are all being explored. Although it is widely used today, it is still a treatment method with many unknowns, including the efficacy of different mesotherapy products and the most effective treatment protocols.

References

1. Rotunda AM, Avram MM, Avram AS. Cellulite: is there a role for injectables? J Cosmet Laser Ther. 2005;7(3–4):147–54.
2. Atiyeh BS, Ibrahim AE, Dibo SA. Cosmetic mesotherapy: between scientific evidence, science fiction, and lucrative business. Aesth Plast Surg. 2008;32(6):842–9.
3. Mammucari M, Maggiori E, Russo D, Giorgio C, Ronconi G, Ferrara PE, Canzona F, Antonaci L, Violo B, Vellucci R, Mediati DR, Migliore A, Massafra U, Bifarini B, Gori F, di Carlo M, Brauneis S, Paolucci T, Rocchi P, Cuguttu A, Di Marzo R, Bomprezzi A, Santini S, Giardini M, Catizzone AR, Troili F, Dorato D, Gallo A, Guglielmo C, Natoli S. Mesotherapy: from historical notes to scientific evidence and future prospects. ScientificWorldJournal. 2020;2020:3542848. https://doi.org/10.1155/2020/3542848. PMID: 32577099; PMCID: PMC7305548.
4. Braccini F, Dohan Ehrenfest DM. Intérêt des thérapies combinées en médecine esthétique pour le traitement du vieillissement du visage: toxine botulique, fillers et mésothérapie [Advantages of combined therapies in cosmetic medicine for the treatment of face aging: botulinum toxin, fillers and mesotherapy]. Rev Laryngol Otol Rhinol (Bord). 2010;131(2):89–95. French. PMID: 21284223.
5. Matarasso A, Pfeifer TM. Mesotherapy and injection lipolysis. Clin Plast Surg. 2009;36(2):181–92.
6. Siquier-Dameto G, Boadas-Vaello P, Verdú E. Intradermal treatment with a hyaluronic acid complex supplemented with amino acids and antioxidant vitamins improves cutaneous hydration and viscoelasticity in healthy subjects. Antioxidants (Basel). 2024;13(7):770. https://doi.org/10.3390/antiox13070770. PMID: 39061838; PMCID: PMC11274003.
7. Metin N, Karapınar T, Turan Ç. Lip mesotherapy with dexpanthenol in the treatment of isotretinoin-induced cheilitis. J Cosmet Dermatol. 2022;21(10):4684–90. https://doi.org/10.1111/jocd.14993. Epub 2022 May 10. PMID: 35426210.
8. Sivagnanam G. Mesotherapy-the french connection. J Pharmacol Pharmacother. 2010;1(1):4–8.
9. Gökdemir G. Mesotherapy and platelet-rich plasma for the treatment of hair loss. Turkderm. 2014;48(S1):74–9.
10. Liao X, Cheng F, Jiang Y. Efficacy and safety of mesotherapy with tranexamic acid versus vitamin C in the treatment of melasma: a meta-analysis and systemic review. J Cosmet Dermatol. 2024;23(9):2785–92. https://doi.org/10.1111/jocd.16353. Epub 2024 May 1. PMID: 38693699.
11. Vedamurthy M. Mesotherapy. Indian J Dermatol Venereol Leprol. 2007;73(1):60–2. https://doi.org/10.4103/0378-6323.30661. PMID: 17314456.
12. Matarasso A, Pfeifer TM. Mesotherapy for body contouring. Plast Reconstr Surg. 2005;115(5):1420–4.
13. Kalil A. Approach and contribution COS DERM. Cosmet Dermatol. 2006;19(12):753–8.
14. Polat M, Üstün H. A case of mesotherapy-induced panniculitis. Cutan Ocul Toxicol. 2016;35(2):163–4.

15. Doerr TD. Lipoplasty of the face and neck. Curr Opin Otolaryngol Head Neck Surg. 2007;15(4):228–32.
16. Scarano A, Qorri E, Sbarbati A, Gehrke SA, Frisone A, Amuso D, Tari SR. The efficacy of hyaluronic acid fragments with amino acid in combating facial skin aging: an ultrasound and histological study. J Ultrasound. 2024;27(3):689–97. https://doi.org/10.1007/s40477-024-00925-5. Epub 2024 Jun 24. PMID: 38913131; PMCID: PMC11333785.
17. Nagaja SA, John RS, Swetha G, Kumar SP, Krishnan M. Injectable platelet-rich fibrin and hyaluronic acid mesotherapy for management of actinic elastosis of lower eyelids: a case series. Cureus. 2024;16(9):e68429. https://doi.org/10.7759/cureus.68429. PMID: 39360098; PMCID: PMC11445689.
18. El Hawa M, Shahla WA, Fares C, Saade D. Non-facial skin rejuvenation of the neck, chest, and hands. Part one: using injections. J Cosmet Dermatol. 2025;24:e16624. https://doi.org/10.1111/jocd.16624. PMID: 39548357.
19. Bessis D, Guilhou JJ, Guillot B. Localized urticaria pigmentosa triggered by mesotherapy. Dermatology. 2004;209(4):343–4.

Mesotherapy: Available Products and Their Applications

38

Caner Kesimli, Cemal Cingi, and Andrew A. Winkler

38.1 Introduction

Mesotherapy consists of multiple intradermal or subcutaneous injections of a mixture of compounds (plant extracts, homeopathic agents, medicines, vitamins, and other bioactive substances) in minute dosages are administered utilizing tiny gauge needles. This technique is used to treat medical disorders, primarily those that are localized, as well as cosmetic conditions. The name "meso" may be translated to "middle" and "mean." This refers to the injection method, which is placed into the middle layer of skin or "intradermotherapy" and the "mean dose" of the medication that is administered, a dose that falls somewhere in the middle of alternative medicine and homeopathy [1, 2].

Mesotherapy is not a treatment for any specific ailment; it is merely a means of medication delivery [3]. It does not refer to any particular therapeutic approach. Mesotherapy is administered into structures *derived* from mesoderm. Mesoderm ceases to exist beyond the embryonic stage of human development [1].

C. Kesimli
Istinye University, Medical Faculty, Department of Otorhinolaryngology, Istanbul, Turkey

C. Cingi (✉)
Eskisehir Osmangazi University, Medical Faculty, Department of Otorhinolaryngology, Eskisehir, Türkiye
e-mail: cemal@ogu.edu.tr

A. A. Winkler
University of Colorado School of Medicine, Department of Otolaryngology, Aurora, CO, USA
e-mail: andrew.winkler@cuanschutz.edu

C. Cingi et al. (eds.), *Minor Interventions, Major Outcomes on the Face*, Comprehensive ENT, https://doi.org/10.1007/978-3-032-01305-7_38

38.2 Mesotherapy

The aging process is a complicated and multifaceted phenomenon that impacts every organ in the body, including the skin [4, 5]. In clinical terms, aging skin becomes thin, dry, and pale, as well as having visible wrinkles and decreased suppleness [6, 7]. The accumulation of elastotic material in the papillary and mid-dermis, a process known as solar elastosis, and quantitative changes in collagen, which are represented by a decrease in biosynthesis and volume [7], are two of the histological alterations related to aged skin.

Mesotherapy is a technique that has been employed in recently to rejuvenate and tone the skin [8, 9]. It was initially reported in France by Michel Pistor [10]. To stimulate the biosynthetic ability of fibroblasts and facilitate interaction between cells, this technique involves the non-invasive transdermal injection of vitamins, enzymes, hormones, hyaluronic acid, and natural plant extracts into the skin. This technique aims to increase collagen and elastin production [11, 12]. The following are some of the injection methods that can be utilized in mesotherapy:

(i) The intra-epidermal technique
(ii) The papular technique, in which reagents are injected into the dermo-epidermal junction
(iii) The nappage method, in which injections penetrate to a depth of 2–4 mm and are delivered at an angle of 30–60°
(iv) Point-by-point injection into the deep dermis [13–15]

Mesotherapists frequently use medications approved by the FDA for functions not examined by the FDA [16]. The FDA does not assert that such off-label use by physicians violates its regulations, and even the courts have ruled that off-label usage does not intrinsically constitute carelessness or medical malpractice unless it is contraindicated or used experimentally for a given condition [17]. In contrast, another school of thought contends that combining medications and other components in mesotherapy formulations produces a new drug that the FDA has yet to approve for application. As a result, in this application, mesotherapy combinations are not an "off-label" use, but rather have not been evaluated by the FDA [18]. In conclusion, the practice of mesotherapy not only continues to exist but also continues to expand (Figs. 38.1, 38.2, and 38.3).

38.2.1 Lip Mesotherapy

Among the mucocutaneous adverse effects of isotretinoin (ISO), the most common are dry lips and cheilitis, which account for 90–100% of all cases [19]. The objective evaluation of the severity of ISO-related cheilitis is accomplished by the utilization of the Isotretinoin Cheilitis Grading Scale (ICGS), which was created by Orneals et al. [20]. Cheilitis and lip dryness associated with ISO are dose-dependent, predictable, and a manageable condition [19]. Currently, the treatment for

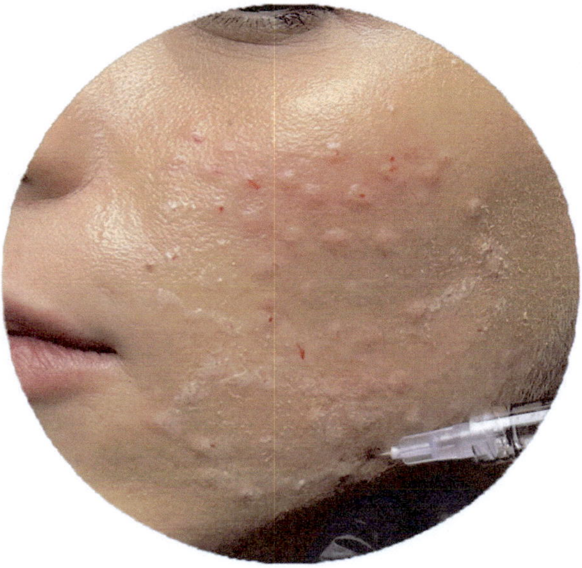

Fig. 38.1 Mid and lower face mesotherapy (Xela Rederm). (Courtesy of Murat Songu MD)

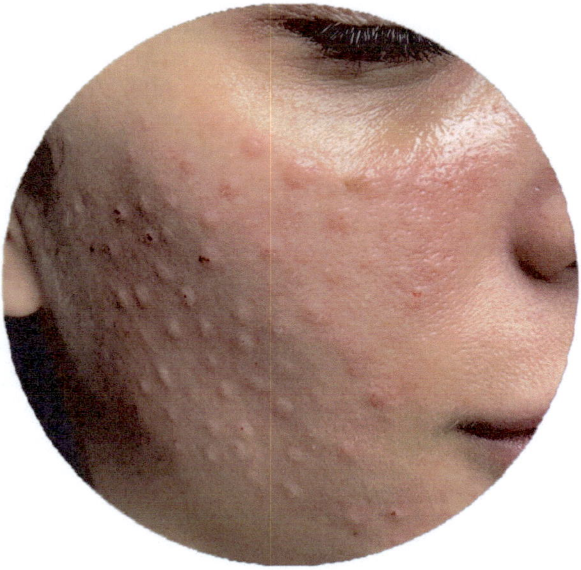

Fig. 38.2 Mid and lower face mesotherapy (Jalupro). (Courtesy of Murat Songu MD)

ISO-related cheilitis [19] involves the application of hydrating and emollient items to ease the symptoms of the condition. Dexpanthenol, often known as DXP, is an alcohol derivative of pantothenic acid. It is a component of the B complex vitamins and a necessary factor of a healthy epithelium [21, 22]. Within the skin and mucous membranes, DXP undergoes enzymatic degradation to form pantothenic acid.

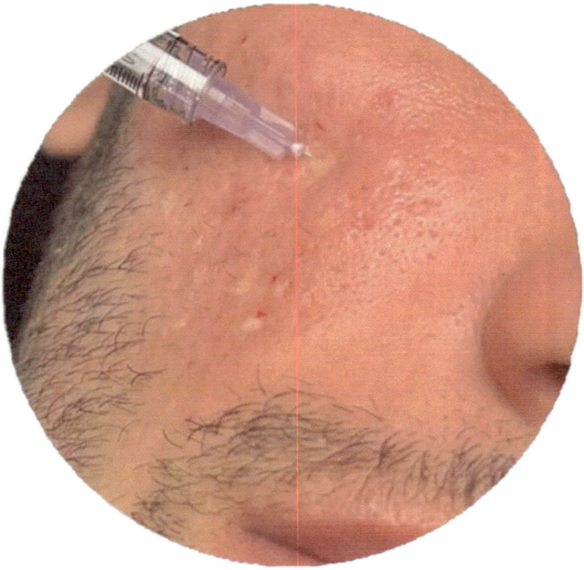

Fig. 38.3 Mid and lower face mesotherapy on a male patient (Cytocare). (Courtesy of Murat Songu MD)

Additionally, it is involved in creating glutathione, ATP, and coenzyme A, all of which have a protective effect against the harm caused to mucosa [22–24]. Additionally, DXP, which possesses antioxidant and anti-inflammatory properties, can be used locally and administered systemically [21]. Additionally, enhanced fibroblast proliferation and quicker re-epithelialization in wound healing are two dermatological effects attributed to the topical application of dexpanthenol [21, 25].

38.2.2 Lipolysis

Mesotherapy is the buzzword in the world of cosmetics, specifically in the "melting fat" fad that is aimed at treating cellulite and producing weight loss. Mesotherapy is used to produce "injection lipolysis." Presently, mesotherapy is gaining allure mainly for non-surgical cosmetic applications, like removal of disfiguring fat (cellulite) [26] in thighs, buttocks, hips, legs, arms, and facial areas [27], including eye pads [28]; skin rejuvenation, to minimize wrinkles and tighten loose skin, body contouring [29], striae [28], vitiligo, hyperpigmentation, acne [30], and alopecia.

The drugs found to be effective in the elimination of unwanted fat deposits and skin rejuvenation include phosphatidylcholine (PC), L-carnitine, aminophylline, hyaluronidase, collagenase, glycolic acid, retinoic acid, multivitamins (A, D, E, K), trace elements [minute quantities of zinc, copper, selenium, chromium, and manganese], an acetylcholine analog dimethylaminoethanol (DMAE), lidocaine, and others [31].

The following is a list of the proposed mechanisms for the numerous chemicals in eliminating undesirable fat. PC exhibits lipolytic action through its influence on the permeability of the adipocyte membrane, which in turn leads to fat mobilization. To enhance the fat-dissolution capabilities of PC using the disintegration of adipocytes, some individuals incorporate minute amounts of sodium deoxycholate [27] into the formulation, a bile salt detergent used by the body to dissolve fat. It is believed that thyroid preparations, aminophylline, and isoproterenol can promote the release of insulin, which in turn assists in the breakdown of fat cells [17].

When cellulite is present, the bands of fibrous tissue generated between fat lobules are broken down by the enzymes hyaluronidase and collagenase. Exfoliating the skin (peels) is what glycolic acid does. Anti-aging of the skin is aided by vitamin E, an antioxidant; vitamin K affects clotting mechanisms and, as a result, regulates the microcirculation of the skin; DMAE causes myofibril contraction and smoothens the lax skin; and trace elements are essential for regulating turnover and repair of skin cells [31]. Vitamin A is responsible for regulating the turnover of skin cells and keratinization. Vitamin C enhances collagen synthesis and reduces hyperpigmentation by inhibiting melanin production.

38.2.3 Biorejuvenation

In a preliminary trial conducted on a limited population of individuals ($n = 20$), mesotherapy with numerous microinjections of hyaluronic acid was reported helpful for skin photoaging. Ultrasound validated this, but not all patients responded similarly [32].

38.2.4 Alopecia

An intermittent vaginal injection of recombinant human follicle-stimulating hormone (rhFSH) every 3 days has been successfully employed in women who are undergoing in vitro fertilization (IVF) treatment, primarily to reduce the frequency of hospital visits [33]. This is an example of how the concept of mesotherapy has been expanded to explore new indications and treatment endpoints.

Pharmaceuticals are among the various substances, plant extracts, vitamins, and other components utilized in mesotherapy treatments. Mesotherapy does not have a uniform formulation, and its components can vary depending on the indication. Both anecdotal reports and the physician's experience are the basis for the components and combination of the injected material. There has been no evidence to support the hypothesis that the components have a particular mode of action. The textbook [34, 35] is the best resource to consult if one is looking for comprehensive information regarding indications, drugs, doses, and procedures.

38.3 Treatment Characteristics and Injection Techniques

Treatment sessions for non-cross-linked hyaluronic acid (HA) ranged from one to six at weekly to bimonthly, whereas sessions for cross-linked HA ranged from one to three at 4–36 weeks. A follow-up was conducted between the ages of 4 and 62 weeks. 23–32 gauge needles with lengths ranging from 4 to 13 mm were utilized in most experiments. Mesogun, nanomicroneedles with nanochip, skin roller, and microneedling were some methods used in the research to deliver HA. The injections were carried out through a total volume of 0.5–8 cc and were administered through 10–1000 injection points (0.01–0.3 cc/point). The injections' depth and distance ranged from 0.2 to 6 mm and from 0.2 mm to 2 cm, respectively. The serial micropuncture technique was the most commonly utilized injection technique. Others used the nappage (pilotage) methodology, depot, and micro-linear methods [34]. One study found that the depot technique (mid-to-deep dermis injection) was significantly more effective than the pilotage technique (superficial dermal injection) in improving biophysical measurements such as anisotropy, hydration, and skin roughness.

The authors found that patients were more satisfied with the depot technique than with the pilotage technique (superficial dermal injection) [35]. In addition, Kim et al. reported that Restylane Vital caused a substantial improvement in skin texture and increased dermal thickness when applied using the dermal approach. On the other hand, subcutaneous injections revealed only improved hydration [36]. Satardinova et al. reported no significant difference in efficacy between the serial micropuncture and the biosynthetic point (BAP) used in the Profhilo HA injection technique [37]. The BAP technique involves five subdermal bolus injections on each side of the face.

38.4 Mesotherapy Formulations

Mesotherapy formulations typically contain vitamins, amino acids, antioxidants, and coenzymes. These substances can have antioxidant effects, promote collagenases, enhance cell regeneration, generate the necessary energy for DNA synthesis and cell reconstruction, and modulate biochemical homeostasis. The only exception to this is non-cross-linked HA. Mesotherapy chemicals were utilized in 14 trials for facial rejuvenation, and the outcomes were inconsistent [34]. The effectiveness of non-cross-linked HA on fine lines was investigated in both static and dynamic rhytids.

Furthermore, improvement in skin texture, roughness, firmness, brightness, homogeneity, facial pore size, hydration, and viscoelastic features was demonstrated by assessment using wrinkle grading scales, global esthetic improvement scales (GAIS), patient evaluation, and a three-dimensional camera [34, 38–40]. Changes were observed in the skin. The reduction of facial pores and improvement in skin hydration were found to have a favorable effect on the appearance of the skin. Several biophysical tests and colorimetry demonstrated an improvement in the hydration of the skin, both superficial and deep, as well as in erythema, the pH of the skin, and the production of sebum [38–42]. Histological and ultrasonic examinations revealed an increase in the thickness of the epidermis and the dermis, fibroblast activity, neoangiogenesis, an elevated level of epidermal growth factor, and the deposition of collagen. Additionally, there was a decrease in interleukin (IL)-1, IL-6, and matrix metalloproteinase-1 [34].

In addition to its antioxidant and moisturizing benefits, adding mannitol to mesotherapy products based on HA can further enhance HA's long-term effectiveness by scavenging reactive oxygen species (ROS) and delaying the breakdown of HA. Moreover, it can reduce swelling and inflammatory reactions that occur after injection. The effectiveness of non-cross-linked HA coupled with mannitol was investigated in two separate experiments. During the 3-month follow-up, they reported that the patients were moderately to highly satisfied [35, 43]. Furthermore, a considerable improvement in biophysical parameters of skin (anisotropy, skin hydration, elasticity, and roughness) and dermal thickness was demonstrated using a cutometer, Visio probe, and echography, and this improvement lasted for 2–3 months [35, 43].

References

1. Sivagnanam G. Mesotherapy – the french connection. J Pharmacol Pharmacother. 2010;1(1):4–8.
2. Le Coz J. History of mesotherapy. 2005. Available from: http://www.mesotherapyworldwide.com/images/pdf/AJM_Vol_3_200511_40.pdf. Accessed on 21 Nov 2009.
3. Rotunda A, Kolodney MS. Mesotherapy and phosphatidylcholine injections: historical clarification and review. Dermatologic Surg. 2006;32:465–80.
4. Yaar M, Gilchrest BA. Photoaging: mechanism, prevention and therapy. Br J Dermatol. 2007;157:874–87.
5. Farage MA, Miller KW, Berardesca E, et al. Clinical implications of aging skin: cutaneous disorders in the elderly. Am J Clin Dermatol. 2009;10:73–86.
6. Makrantonaki E, Zouboulis CC. Molecular mechanisms of skin aging: state of the art. Ann N Y Acad Sci. 2007;1119:40–50.
7. El-Domyati M, El-Ammawi TS, Medhat W, et al. Electro-optical synergy technique: a new and effective non-ablative approach to skin aging. J Clin Aesthet Dermatol. 2010;3:22–30.
8. Atiyeh BS, Ibrahim AE, Dibo SA. Cosmetic mesotherapy: between scientific evidence, science fiction, and lucrative business. Aesth Plast Surg. 2008;32:842–9.
9. Toledo LS. Emerging techniques in aesthetic plastic surgery. Clin Plast Surg. 2009;36:177–80.
10. Pistor M. What is mesotherapy? Chir Dent Fr. 1976;46:59–60.
11. Amin SP, Phelps RG, Goldberg DJ. Mesotherapy for facial skin rejuvenation: a clinical, histologic, and electron microscopic evaluation. Dermatologic Surg. 2006;32:1467–72.
12. Lacarrubba F, Tedeschi A, Nardone B, et al. Mesotherapy for skin rejuvenation: assessment of the subepidermal low-echogenic band by ultrasound evaluation with cross-sectional B-mode scanning. Dermatol Ther. 2008;21(Suppl):1–5.
13. Vedamurthy M. Mesotherapy. Indian J Dermatol Venereol Leprol. 2007;73:60–2.
14. Iorizzo M, De Padova MP, Tosti A. Biorejuvenation: theory and practice. Clin Dermatol. 2008;26:177–81.

15. El-Domyati M, El-Ammawi TS, Moawad O, El-Fakahany H, Medhat W, Mahoney MG, Uitto J. Efficacy of mesotherapy in facial rejuvenation: a histological and immunohistochemical evaluation. Int J Dermatol. 2012;51(8):913–9.
16. FDA Statement on Lipo-Dissolve. 2008. Available from: http://www.cbs46.com/print/15186454/detail.html. Accessed on 21 Nov 2009.
17. Weaver KA, Figura J. Mesotherapy and the off-label use of approved drugs. Available from: http://www.mesotherapyworldwide.com/images/pdf/AJM_Vol_4_2006_58.pdf. Accessed on 21 Nov 2009.
18. ASPS guiding principles for mesotherapy/injection lipolysis. 2008. Available from: http://www.plasticsurgery.org/Documents/Medical_Profesionals/Health_Policy/ASPS-Guiding-Principles-for-Mesotherapy-Injection-Lipolysis-7-08.pdf. Accessed on 22 Nov 2009.
19. Bagatin E, Costa CS. The use of isotretinoin for acne–an update on optimal dosing, surveillance, and adverse effects. Expert Rev Clin Pharmacol. 2020;13(8):885–97.
20. Ornelas J, Rosamilia L, Larsen L, et al. Objective assessment of isotretinoin-associated cheilitis: isotretinoin cheilitis grading acale. J Dermatol Treat. 2016;27(2):153–5.
21. Ebner F, Heller A, Rippke F, Tausch I. Topical use of dexpanthenol in skin disorders. Am J Clin Dermatol. 2002;3(6):427–33.
22. Wojtczak L, Slyshenkov VS. Protection by pantothenic acid against apoptosis and cell damage by oxygen free radicals-the role of glutathione. BioFactors. 2003;17(1–4):61–73.
23. Turgut O, Ay AA, Turgut H, Ay A, Kafkas S, Dost T. Effects of melatonin and dexpanthenol on antioxidant parameters when combined with estrogen treatment in ovariectomized rats. Age. 2013;35(6):2229–35.
24. Slyshenkov VS, Dymkowska D, Wojtczak L. Pantothenic acid and pantothenol increase biosynthesis of glutathione by boosting cell energetics. FEBS Lett. 2004;569(1–3):169–72.
25. Metin N, Karapınar T, Turan Ç. Lip mesotherapy with dexpanthenol in the treatment of isotretinoin-induced cheilitis. J Cosmet Dermatol. 2022;21(10):4684–90.
26. Leibaschoff G. Mesotherapy and cellulite. Am J Mesother. 2006;4:53.
27. Rotunda AM, Suzuki H, Moy RL, Kolodney MS. Detergent effects of sodium deoxycholate are a major feature of an injectable phosphatidylcholine formulation used for localized fat dissolution. Dermatologic Surg. 2004;30:1001–8.
28. Rittes PG. Stretch marks – striae. Am J Mesother. 2005;3:11–36. Available from http://www.mesotherapyworldwide.com/images/pdf/AJM_Vol_3_200511_36.pdf. Accessed on 21 Nov 2009.
29. Matarasso A, Pfeifer TM. Plastic Surgery Educational Foundation DATA Committee. Mesotherapy for body contouring. Plast Reconstr Surg. 2005;115:1420–4.
30. Bryant R. Controversial mesotherapy: could it be the next Botox? Dermatol Times. 2004;25:1. Available from http://www.modernmedicine.com/modernmedicine/article/articleDetailjs-pid=137281. Accessed on 21 Nov 2009.
31. Exract from mesotherapyedmonton.com. Available from: http://mesotherapy0.tripod.com/id4.html. Accessed on 21 Nov 2009.
32. Lacarrubba F, Tedeschi A, Nardone B, Micali G. Mesotherapy for skin rejuvenation: assessment of the subepidermal low-echogenic band by ultrasound evaluation with cross-sectional B-mode scanning. Dermatol Ther. 2008;21:S1–5.
33. Hsu CC, Hsu CT. Conception using vaginal administration of gonadotrophins in IVF: a case report. Reprod Biomed Online. 2006;12:170–3.
34. Iranmanesh B, Khalili M, Mohammadi S, Amiri R, Aflatoonian M. Employing hyaluronic acid-based mesotherapy for facial rejuvenation. J Cosmet Dermatol. 2022;21(12):6605–18.
35. Taieb M, Gay C, Sebban S, Secnazi P. Hyaluronic acid plus mannitol treatment for improved skin hydration and elasticity. J Cosmet Dermatol. 2012;11(2):87–92.
36. Kim J. Effects of injection depth and volume of stabilized hyaluronic acid in human dermis on skin texture, hydration, and thickness. Arch Aesthet Plast Surg. 2014;20(2):97–103.
37. Satardinova E. Hybrid cooperative complexes of high and low molecular weight hyaluronans for facial skin rejuvenation in the oriental mongoloid face: a case series. Aesthet Med. 2019;5:14–9.

38. Trong HN, Phuong TV, Van TN, et al. The efficacy and safety of hyaluronic acid microinjection for skin rejuvenation in Vietnam. Maced J Med Sci. 2019;7(2):234–6.
39. Cesare B, Roberto C, Giuseppe N, Luca G, Carlo DA. Face rejuvenation: a new combinated protocol for biorevitalization. Acta Biomed. 2018;89(3):400.
40. El-Domyati M, El-Ammawi TS, Moawad O, et al. Efficacy of mesotherapy in facial rejuvenation: a histological and immunohistochemical evaluation. Int J Dermatol. 2012;51(8):913–9.
41. Qian W, Zhang YK, Hou Y, et al. Effect analysis of intradermal hyaluronic acid injection to treat enlarged facial pores. J Cosmet Dermatol. 2018;17(4):596–9.
42. Grand-Vincent A, Boisnic S, Salomon C, Prinderre P, Piccerelle P. Clinical assessment of a mesotherapy formulation for skin rejuvenation in healthy volunteers. J Cosmet Dermatol Sci Appl. 2017;7(4):291–305.
43. Baspeyras M, Rouvrais C, Liégard L, et al. Clinical and biometrological efficacy of a hyaluronic acid-based mesotherapy product: a randomised controlled study. Arch Dermatol Res. 2013;305(8):673–68.

Part VII

Facial Skin Rejuvenation and Scar Treatments

Acne Scars

39

Nagihan Bilal, Nuray Bayar Muluk, and J. Regan Thomas

39.1 Introduction

Acne is a persistent inflammatory skin disorder. It will continue to be a problem for roughly 30% of these individuals into adulthood. While lesions are most frequently discovered on the face, they can also be detected on the back and the chest [1].

When a person reaches puberty, a series of genetic and hormonal events begin to take place, which ultimately leads to the development of acne. Oil production in the sebaceous glands of the face, back, and chest increases as the hormone levels associated with developing secondary sexual characteristics rise. Those genetically predisposed to the condition have a process known as follicular hyperkeratosis, characterized by a thickening of the lining of the wall of the duct of the oil gland. Eventually, this thickening will cause the duct to become blocked, resulting in the buildup of oil beneath the skin in the form of comedones, more generally known as blackheads. There is a proliferation of bacteria within these comedones known as *Corynebacterium acnes*. These bacteria create free fatty acids, which irritate the skin. When this process is allowed to continue, it can result in pustular and cystic lesions, both of which have the potential to rupture and leave scars [1].

N. Bilal
Izmir Bakircay University Cigli Research and Education Hospital,
Department of Otorhinolaryngology, Izmir, Turkey

N. Bayar Muluk (✉)
Faculty of Medicine, Department of Otorhinolaryngology, Kırıkkale University,
Kırıkkale, Türkiye

J. R. Thomas
University of New Mexico School of Medicine, Albuquerque, NM, USA

C. Cingi et al. (eds.), *Minor Interventions, Major Outcomes on the Face*,
Comprehensive ENT, https://doi.org/10.1007/978-3-032-01305-7_39

39.2 Pathophysiology

Several different factors contribute to the development of acne vulgaris. Genetics plays a significant role [2, 3]. The following four elements, which interact with one another, are responsible for the development of acne [2, 4]:

Several factors contribute to acne, including the release of inflammatory mediators into the skin, follicular hyperkeratinization, which leads to the subsequent clogging of the follicle, follicular colonization by *Cutibacterium acnes* (formerly known as *Propionibacterium acnes*), and excessive sebum production.

Before hyperkeratinization, inflammatory responses have been demonstrated to take place, according to research investigations. Cytokines produced by CD4+ T cells and macrophages activate local endothelial cells, which then up-regulate inflammatory mediators in the vessels surrounding the pilosebaceous follicle [5]. These mediators include vascular cell adhesion molecule-1 (VCAM-1), intercellular adhesion molecule-1 (ICAM-1), and human leukocyte antigen (HLA)–DR.

In follicular hyperkeratinization, there is an increase in the proliferation of keratinocytes and a decrease in desquamation, which results in the formation of microcomedones loaded with keratin and sebum [6].

The anaerobic organism known as *C. acnes*, formerly *P. acnes*, is found in acne lesions. Inflammation is triggered by the presence of *C. acnes*, formerly *P. acnes*, by several methods. Through the production of proinflammatory mediators that can diffuse through the follicular wall, *C. acnes*, formerly known as *P. acnes*, can promote inflammation. Activation of the toll-like receptor two on monocytes and neutrophils has been demonstrated by studies involving *C. acnes*, which was formerly known as *P. acnes* [7]. Proinflammatory cytokines, such as interleukins 12 and 8, as well as tumor necrosis factor, are produced as a result of activation of the toll-like receptor 2, which in turn leads to the creation of these chemicals. The fact that some people acquire inflammatory acne vulgaris while others do not may also be explained by the fact that they have a hypersensitivity to *C. acnes*, which was initially known as *P. acnes* [8]. A further important element in the development of acne vulgaris is the presence of abundant sebum. A variety of hormones and mediators are responsible for controlling the synthesis and excretion of sebum. Regarding sebum production and release, androgen hormones are essential [9]. There is a correlation between the amount of comedone acne that is present in prepubescent girls and the amount of the adrenal androgen dehydroepiandrosterone sulfate (DHEAS) that is circulating in the bloodstream [2, 3, 10, 11].

Many other mediators and receptors, including growth hormone, insulin-like growth factor, and peroxisome proliferator-activated receptors, are also responsible for regulating the sebaceous gland and may play a role in the development of acne [12, 13]. Moreover, the sebaceous gland operates as a neuroendocrine-inflammatory organ, and it is stimulated by hormones that release corticotrophins in reaction to stress and regular functions [14].

39.3 Etiology

Genetic predisposition is the primary factor that contributes to the development of acne. Additionally, other aggravating variables have been identified.

Acne can be exacerbated by the use of hair pomades and cosmetic products [15].

Steroids, lithium, certain antiepileptics, and iodides are examples of medications that have the potential to encourage the development of acne [6, 16].

The development of acne vulgaris may be triggered by several endocrine problems, including polycystic ovarian syndrome, congenital adrenal hyperplasia, and other conditions associated with excess androgens. An exacerbation may even be brought on by pregnancy [16, 17].

Several causes that might aggravate the condition include mechanical occlusion caused by headbands, shoulder pads, backpacks, or underwire bras [8, 18].

The presence of much sunshine can either help acne or make it worse. In any event, exposure to ultraviolet light will age the skin [2].

39.4 Treatment

39.4.1 Atrophic Scars

39.4.1.1 Chemical Peels

Chemical peeling refers to applying chemicals to the skin to destroy the damaged layers on the surface and speed up the skin's repair [19, 20].

In addition to treating scars and skin infections, chemical peeling is also used to reverse the symptoms of aging on the skin. Acne scars are particularly susceptible to the effects of chemical peeling. The most common clinical indications for facial chemical peeling are dyschromias, wrinkles, and acne scars [21, 22].

Glycolic Acid

In addition to being soluble in alcohol, glycolic acid is an alpha hydroxy acid generated from sugars found in fruit and milk. Glycolic acid exerts its effects by reducing the thickness of the stratum corneum, fostering epidermolysis, and distributing melanin from the basal layer. It does this by boosting the release of IL-6, which promotes the expression of the genes for dermal hyaluronic acid and collagen [23]. The operation is well tolerated, and patient compliance is excellent; however, glycolic acid peels should not be performed on patients who have contact dermatitis, are pregnant, or have a hypersensitivity to glycolates. On the other hand, the side effects, which may include irritation or transient hyperpigmentation, are not significantly noteworthy [24]. Several studies demonstrated that the amount of skin damage caused by glycolic acid peels grows in a manner that depends on both the dose and the amount of time—compared to solutions containing free acid, the acid contained at the higher concentration (70%) caused more damage to the tissue than the acid contained at the lower concentration (50%). There is a correlation between a decrease in pH and an increase in the transmembrane permeability coefficient, which provides a plausible explanation for the efficacy of glycolic acid in treating skin conditions [25]. Five consecutive 70% glycolic acid sessions every 2 weeks [19] have yielded the most favorable outcomes for acne scars.

Jessner's Solution

A combination of salicylic acid, resorcinol, and lactic acid in 95% ethanol is an excellent superficial peeling agent. Dr. Max Jessner developed this combination. Regarding its chemical and structural properties, resorcinol is like phenol. Additionally, it improves the penetration of other agents by disrupting the weak hydrogen bonds in keratin [26]. Lactic acid is an alpha hydroxy acid responsible for corneocyte detachment and the stratum corneum's subsequent desquamation [27].

For the same reason that other superficial peeling agents are readily tolerated, Jessner's peels are also. In addition to delayed or aberrant wound healing, active inflammation, dermatitis, or infection of the area that has to be treated are also considered general contraindications. Isotretinoin therapy should be administered within 6 months following peeling. Because allergic contact dermatitis and systemic allergic reactions to resorcinol are uncommon, these conditions must be considered absolute contraindications [19, 28, 29].

Pyruvic Acid

Pyruvic acid is a powerful peeling agent that also comes as an alpha-keto acid [30]. Additionally, it can induce the development of new collagen and the formation of elastic fibers [31]. In addition, it possesses keratolytic, antibacterial, and sebostatic properties. For the treatment of mild acne scars, it has been suggested that either 40% or 70% pyruvic acid be utilized [32, 33]. During therapy, you may have desquamation, crusting in areas of weaker skin, acute stinging, and a burning feeling. These are all potential adverse effects. Pyruvic acid produces vapors that stink and irritate the upper respiratory mucosa [19]. Because of this, it is essential to ensure appropriate ventilation during the application process.

Salicylic Acid

Regarding the treatment of acne scars, salicylic acid is considered to be among the most effective peeling agents [34]. In addition to being a beta hydroxy acid agent, it can also remove intercellular lipids covalently connected to the cornified envelope surrounding cornified epithelioid cells. Throughout numerous sessions, three to five times, every 3–4 weeks, the most effective concentration for acne scars is 30% [35–37]. When you peel with salicylic acid, you will experience only minor and temporary adverse effects. Among these are erythema and dryness of the skin. This treatment treats dark skin because persistent postinflammatory hyperpigmentation or scarring is uncommon [38]. Some symptoms associated with salicylism or salicylic acid toxicity include rapid breathing, tinnitus, hearing loss, dizziness, abdominal cramps, and symptoms related to the central nervous system. This was seen when salicylic acid at a concentration of 20% was applied to 50% of the body's surface [36]. More than 1000 patients have been peeled by Grimes using the current

20% and 30% ethanol formulations that are on the market, and he has not identified any instances of salicylism [19, 39].

Trichloroacetic Acid

A German dermatologist, P.G. Unna, was the first to describe trichloroacetic acid (TCA) as a peeling agent. This description was made in the year 1882. When TCA is applied to the skin, it induces protein denaturation, also known as kerato-coagulation, which results in a white frost that can be easily noticed [40]. It is combined with 100 mL of distilled water to get the necessary concentration for chemical peeling. Several parameters determine the extent of tissue penetration and harm caused by a TCA solution. These factors include the amount of TCA employed, the anatomic site, and the skin preparation. To successfully perform a peel, choosing suitable TCA-concentrated solutions is essential. When the concentration of TCA is between 10% and 20%, it produces a very light superficial peel that does not penetrate below the stratum granulosum. The 25% and 35% concentrations make a light superficial peel with diffusion encompassing the entire epidermis thickness. The concentration between 40% and 50% can cause injury to the papillary dermis. Finally, when the concentration exceeds 50%, it causes injury that extends to the reticular dermis. Unfortunately, using TCA concentrations higher than 35% TCA can result in adverse effects that are difficult to foresee, such as scarring. Therefore, 35% TCA is the only way to achieve the desired medium-depth chemical peel. Using TCA at concentrations that are more than 35% is something that should be avoided. The treatment of isolated icepick scars or, in certain instances, isolated lesions may be the treatment of choice (TCA CROSS) [41]. When carried out correctly, peeling with TCA has the potential to be one of the most satisfying methods in the treatment of acne scars; nevertheless, it is not recommended for dark skin due to the high risk of hyperpigmentation [19, 42].

39.4.2 Hypertrophic Scars

Silicone Gel

Silicone-based products are among the most frequent and successful options for the prevention of hypertrophic acne scars as well as the treatment of these scars. The silicone gel was integrated into treating hypertrophic acne scars from the beginning to overcome the challenges of managing silicone sheets. Furthermore, silicone gel has several benefits, including being clear, drying quickly, not irritating the skin, and not causing maceration. Moreover, it may treat severe scars and uneven skin parts. The mechanism of action has yet to be completely understood; however, numerous ideas [43] have been proposed. These hypotheses include the following: (1) the rise in hydration, (2) the increase in temperature, (3) the protection of the scar, (4) the increased tension of oxygen levels, and (5) the effect on the immune system. At the moment, there is only one observational open-label study that has been carried out on 57 specific patients. In this particular trial, the gel was applied to the scars twice a day for 8 weeks, and they showed an average improvement in thickness that was judged to be between 40% and 50% when compared to the baseline [19].

When treating hypertrophic scars that have already formed, the gel should be administered in modest amounts, twice daily, for at least 8 weeks to produce a suitable aesthetic result. While it is advised that the exact dosage be taken for at least 12–16 weeks for prevention, the treatment should be initiated as soon as possible after the danger of a patient acquiring hypertrophic acne scars has been established [19].

It is possible to administer treatment with silicone gel to patients of any age, including women in childbearing months. In addition, the silicone gel can be utilized throughout the year, particularly during the seasons [19].

Intralesional Steroid Therapy

Steroid injections administered intralesionally are among the most frequently used therapies for hypertrophic scars and keloids. You can use it on its own or as a component of various therapeutic procedures. In addition to alleviating symptoms such as itching and discomfort, corticosteroids can reduce scars' volume, thickness, and texture when appropriately used [44]. In addition to their anti-inflammatory qualities, it has been hypothesized that steroids exert vasoconstrictor and antimitotic activity. The mechanisms of action have yet to be explained. The reduction of oxygen and nutrients to the scar, along with the inhibition of the proliferation of keratinocytes and fibroblasts [44] and the stimulation of digestion of collagen deposition through the block of a collagenase inhibitor, the alpha-2-microglobulin [45], are the two distinct mechanisms that are thought to be responsible for the arrest of pathological collagen production by steroids. The needle on the syringe has to be held in an upright position throughout the injection [46]. It is usually ideal for the injections to be preceded by the administration of anesthetic creams or to be coupled with injections of lidocaine [19, 45]. This is because the injections will be more effective.

Cryotherapy

Cryotherapy with liquid nitrogen can greatly improve the clinical appearance of hypertrophic scars and keloids and also determine the total regression of these scars [19].

The low temperatures obtained during cryotherapy sessions produce a slowdown of blood flow, which in turn causes the formation of an intraluminal thrombus resistant to anoxia and tissue necrosis [47]. The success of this treatment is heavily influenced by several critical criteria, including the scar's age and size. Cryotherapy is most effective for treating scars that are younger and smaller in size [48].

Pulsed Dye Laser

In the 1980s, Apfelberg et al. [49] and Castro et al. [50] were the first to propose using lasers to treat hypertrophic scars and keloids. Since then, more lasers with a variety of wavelengths have been launched. Unfortunately, laser therapy for hypertrophic scars has only had a limited amount of success in the past, as a significant number of patients have experienced only a slight improvement [51–53].

Surgery

W-plasty is the most effective method for the repair of prominent facial scars [54]. The scar is disrupted due to this therapeutic technique, which makes the lesion less noticeable. Autologous skin transplants, full-thickness or composite fat-skin grafts, are an additional beneficial alternative for wound closure with little stress. This is especially true in the context of cosmetic surgery. According to research, the retro- and preauricular sites and the neck are the most desirable donor sites for skin grafts that are utilized to treat face abnormalities [55].

References

1. Teenage acne scarring can be prevented and treated. https://www.medscape.com/viewarticle/412155. Accessed online at 11 June 2023.
2. Rao J. Acne vulgaris. In: James WD, editor. Medscape. Updated; 2020. https://emedicine.medscape.com/article/1069804-overview#a9. Accessed online at 11 June 2023.
3. Goulden V, McGeown CH, Cunliffe WJ. The familial risk of adult acne: a comparison between first-degree relatives of affected and unaffected individuals. Br J Dermatol. 1999;141(2):297–300.
4. Thiboutot D, Gollnick H, Bettoli V, Dréno B, Kang S, Leyden JJ, et al. New insights into the management of acne: an update from the Global Alliance to Improve Outcomes in Acne group. J Am Acad Dermatol. 2009;60(5 Suppl):S1–50.
5. Jeremy AH, Holland DB, Roberts SG, Thomson KF, Cunliffe WJ. Inflammatory events are involved in acne lesion initiation. J Invest Dermatol. 2003;121(1):20–7.
6. Norris JF, Cunliffe WJ. A histological and immunocytochemical study of early acne lesions. Br J Dermatol. 1988;118(5):651–9.
7. Kim J, Ochoa MT, Krutzik SR, et al. Activation of toll-like receptor 2 in acne triggers inflammatory cytokine responses. J Immunol. 2002;169(3):1535–41.
8. Webster GF. Inflammatory acne represents hypersensitivity to Propionibacterium acnes. Dermatology. 1998;196(1):80–1.
9. Pochi PE, Strauss JS. Sebaceous gland activity in black skin. Dermatol Clin. 1988;6(3):349–51.
10. Lucky AW, Biro FM, Simbartl LA, Morrison JA, Sorg NW. Predictors of severity of acne vulgaris in young adolescent girls: results of a five-year longitudinal study. J Pediatr. 1997;130(1):30–9.
11. Baek JH, Ahn SM, Choi KM, Jung MK, Shin MK, Koh JS. Analysis of comedone, sebum and porphyrin on the face and body for comedogenicity assay. Skin Res Technol. 2016;22(2):164–9.
12. Trivedi NR, Cong Z, Nelson AM, Albert AJ, Rosamilia LL, Sivarajah S, et al. Peroxisome proliferator-activated receptors increase human sebum production. J Invest Dermatol. 2006;126(9):2002–9.
13. Smith TM, Cong Z, Gilliland KL, Clawson GA, Thiboutot DM. Insulin-like growth factor-1 induces lipid production in human SEB-1 sebocytes via sterol response element-binding protein-1. J Invest Dermatol. 2006;126(6):1226–32.
14. Zouboulis CC, Böhm M. Neuroendocrine regulation of sebocytes – a pathogenetic link between stress and acne. Exp Dermatol. 2004;13(Suppl 4):31–5.
15. Davis EC, Callender VD. A review of acne in ethnic skin: pathogenesis, clinical manifestations, and management strategies. J Clin Aesthet Dermatol. 2010;3(4):24–38.
16. Momin SB, Peterson A, Del Rosso JQ. A status report on drug-associated acne and acneiform eruptions. J Drugs Dermatol. 2010;9(6):627–36.
17. Mango D, Ricci S, Manna P, Miggiano GA, Serra GB. Clinical and hormonal effects of ethinylestradiol combined with gestodene and desogestrel in young women with acne vulgaris. Contraception. 1996;53(3):163–70.

18. Basler RS. Acne mechanica in athletes. Cutis. 1992;50(2):125–8.
19. Fabbrocini G, Annunziata MC, D'Arco V, De Vita V, Lodi G, Mauriello MC, Pastore F, Monfrecola G. Acne scars: pathogenesis, classification and treatment. Dermatol Res Pract. 2010;2010:893080. https://doi.org/10.1155/2010/893080.
20. Ghersetich I, Brazzini B, Lotti T. Chemical peeling. In: Lotti TM, Katsambas AD, editors. European handbook of dermatological treatments. 2nd ed. Berlin: Springer; 2003.
21. Ghersetich I, Teofoll P, Gantcheva M, Ribuffo M, Puddu P. Chemical peeling: how, when, why? J Eur Acad Dermatol Venereol. 1997;8(1):1–11.
22. Landau M. Chemical peels. Clin Dermatol. 2008;26(2):200–8.
23. Bernstein EF, Lee J, Brown DB, Yu R, Van Scott E. Glycolic acid treatment increases type I collagen mRNA and hyaluronic acid content of human skin. Dermatologic Surg. 2001;27(5):429–33.
24. Javaheri SM, Handa S, Kaur I, Kumar B. Safety and efficacy of glycolic acid facial peel in Indian women with melasma. Int J Dermatol. 2001;40(5):354–7.
25. Becker FF, Langford FPJ, Rubin MG, Speelman P. A histological comparison of 50% and 70% glycolic acid peels using solutions with various pHs. Dermatologic Surg. 1996;22(5):463–5.
26. Rook A, Wilkinson DS, Ebling FJG. Textbook of dermatology. Oxford: Blackwell Scientific; 1972.
27. Van Scott EJ, Yu RJ. Hyperkeratinization, corneocyte cohesion and alpha hydroxy acids. J Am Acad Dermatol. 1984;11(5):867–79.
28. Lynch BS, Delzell ES, Bechtel DH. Toxicology review and risk assessment of resorcinol: thyroid effects. Regul Toxicol Pharmacol. 2002;36(2):198–210.
29. Barbaud A, Modiano P, Cocciale M, Reichert S, Schmutz J-L. The topical application of resorcinol can provoke a systemic allergic reaction. Br J Dermatol. 1996;135(6):1014–5.
30. Griffin TD, Van Scott EJ, Maddin S. The use of pyruvic acid as a chemical peeling agent. J Dermatol Surg Oncol. 1989;15:1316.
31. Monheit GD. Medium-depth combination peels. Dermatol Ther. 2000;13(2):183–91.
32. Van Scott EJ, Yu RJ. Alpha hydroxy acids: therapeutic potentials. Can J Dermatol. 1989;1(5):108–12.
33. Berardesca E, Cameli N, Primavera G, Carrera M. Clinical and instrumental evaluation of skin improvement after treatment with a new 50% pyruvic acid peel. Dermatologic Surg. 2006;32(4):526–31.
34. Unna PG. Therapeutiques generales des maladies de la peau. 1882.
35. Lazo ND, Meine JG, Downing DT. Lipids are covalently attached to rigid corneocyte protein envelopes existing predominantly as β-sheets: a solid-state nuclear magnetic resonance study. J Invest Dermatol. 1995;105(2):296–300.
36. Swinehart JM. Salicylic acid ointment peeling of the hands and forearms: effective nonsurgical removal of pigmented lesions and actinic damage. J Dermatol Surg Oncol. 1992;18(6):495–8.
37. Imayama S, Ueda S, Isoda M. Histologic changes in the skin of hairless mice following peeling with salicylic acid. Arch Dermatol. 2000;136(11):1390–5.
38. Grimes PE. The safety and efficacy of salicylic acid chemical peels in darker racial-ethnic groups. Dermatologic Surg. 1999;25(1):18–22.
39. Fabbrocini G, De Padova MP, Tosti A. Chemical peels: what's new and what isn't new but still works well. Facial Plast Surg. 2009;25(5):329–36.
40. Dinner MI, Artz JS. The art of the trichloroacetic acid chemical peel. Clin Plast Surg. 1998;25(1):53–62.
41. Slavin JW. Trichloroacetic acid peels. Aesthet Surg J. 2004;24(5):469–70.
42. Al-Waiz MM, Al-Sharqi AI. Medium-depth chemical peels in the treatment of acne scars in dark-skinned individuals. Dermatologic Surg. 2002;28(5):383–7.
43. Berman B, Perez OA, Konda S, et al. A review of the biologic effects, clinical efficacy, and safety of silicone elastomer sheeting for hypertrophic and keloid scar treatment and management. Dermatologic Surg. 2007;33(11):1291–302.
44. Mustoe TA, Cooter RD, Gold MH, et al. International clinical recommendations on scar management. Plast Reconstr Surg. 2002;110(2):560–71.

45. Kelly AP. Medical and surgical therapies for keloids. Dermatol Ther. 2004;17(2):212–8.
46. English RS, Shenefelt PD. Keloids and hypertrophic scars. Dermatologic Surg. 1999;25(8):631–8.
47. Boutli-Kasapidou F, Tsakiri A, Anagnostou E, Mourellou O. Hypertrophic and keloidal scars: an approach to polytherapy. Int J Dermatol. 2005;44(4):324–7.
48. Rusciani L, Rossi G, Bono R. Use of cryotherapy in the treatment of keloids. J Dermatol Surg Oncol. 1993;19(6):529–34.
49. Apfelberg DB, Maser MR, Lash H. Preliminary results of argon and carbon dioxide laser treatment of keloid scars. Lasers Surg Med. 1984;4(3):283–90.
50. Castro DJ, Abergel RP, Meeker C. Effects of the Nd:YAG laser on DNA synthesis and collagen production in human skin fibroblast cultures. Ann Plast Surg. 1983;11(3):214–22.
51. Norris JEC. The effect of carbon dioxide laser surgery on the recurrence of keloids. Plast Reconstr Surg. 1991;87(1):44–53.
52. Lawrence WT. In search of the optimal treatment of keloids: report of a series and a review of the literature. Ann Plast Surg. 1991;27(2):164–78.
53. Sherman R, Rosenfeld H. Experience with the Nd:YAG laser in the treatment of keloid scars. Ann Plast Surg. 1988;21(3):231–5.
54. Wolfram D, Tzankov A, Pülzl P, Piza-Katzer H. Hypertrophic scars and keloids—a review of their pathophysiology, risk factors, and therapeutic management. Dermatologic Surg. 2009;35(2):171–81.
55. Riedel F, Hormann K. Plastic surgery of skin defects in the face. Principles and prospective. HNO. 2005;53(12):1020–36.

Post-Traumatic Scars

40

Enes Gungor, Nuray Bayar Muluk, and J. Regan Thomas

40.1 Introduction

Persons of any age or ethnicity can develop scarring as a result of trauma. Scars caused by atrophic scarring are lower and thinner than the surrounding skin. Even though they are thicker and raised above the skin, hypertrophic scars remain within the initial injury's boundaries. Scars that are keloid are raised and extend beyond the borders of the initial damage. Traumatic scars can negatively impact the physical, psychological, and social well-being of patients. Scar tightening, also known as contractures, frequently occurs over joints and can restrict normal movement and the capacity to participate in activities of daily living that are considered normal. How people perceive themselves and how others perceive them can be impacted by disfigurement, which may even result in those individuals experiencing emotions of depression or worry. There is a high probability that traumatic scars will result in discomfort, itching, and other unpleasant feelings [1].

E. Gungor
Department of Otorhinolaryngology, Etimesgut Sait Erturk State Hospital, Ankara, Turkey

N. Bayar Muluk (✉)
Faculty of Medicine, Department of Otorhinolaryngology, Kırıkkale University, Kırıkkale, Türkiye

J. R. Thomas
University of New Mexico School of Medicine, Albuquerque, NM, USA

C. Cingi et al. (eds.), *Minor Interventions, Major Outcomes on the Face*, Comprehensive ENT, https://doi.org/10.1007/978-3-032-01305-7_40

40.2 Definition

Keloids and hypertrophic scars have been known as atypical responses to trauma for ages. Keloids are an abnormal scarring condition. However, the finding of a histopathologic distinction between these two entities is relatively new [2], despite the fact that morphologic differences between them have been recognized for many years.

One definition of a keloid is an atypical scar extending beyond the boundaries of the spot where the skin damage occurred. Keloids are characterized by the clinical appearance of a raised amorphous growth, as shown in the first two photos below. Keloids are commonly linked with pruritus and pain inside the affected area. Using scanning electron microscopy, one may observe several unique characteristics: the presence of collagen fibers randomly organized inside a dense connective tissue matrix. The collagen bundles that make up normal scars are oriented in a manner parallel to the skin's surface, as shown in the third image below [3].

Certain body parts, such as the sternum, the deltoid region of the upper arm, and the upper back, are more likely to develop keloid development than other parts of the body. Because these regions are likewise prone to elevated levels of muscle and skin stress, it is possible that their link with keloids can be explained [4]. Although amelanotic areas, such as the palms of the hands or the soles of the feet, have significant levels of skin tension and motion, keloids are not connected with these areas of the skin. Earlobes, the mandibular border, and the posterior neck are the areas of the head and neck most frequently affected by the development of keloid tumors. Because the earring post is positioned posteriorly, the earlobe is often damaged on the posteromedial surface most of the time. There is a low incidence of involvement in the middle one-third of the face [2].

There is a lack of complete understanding of the particular etiologic variables responsible for the formation of keloids, except trauma. Even though keloids are typically associated with elements that are detrimental to the healing process of wounds, such as infection, excessive tension, foreign substances, and repetitive trauma, they can also develop in clean and uncomplicated wounds [2].

The term "hypertrophic scar" refers to a scar that has become wider or more unattractive because it does not extend beyond the confines of the incision where it was initially formed. In contrast to keloids, the hypertrophic scar eventually reaches a particular size and either becomes stable or returns to its original size. Comparable to keloids, hypertrophic scars are linked to elements that are detrimental to the healing process of wounds [2].

In contrast to keloid formation, hypertrophic scarring does not exhibit any tendency toward racial or familial majority. A scanning electron microscope examination reveals collagen bundles that have been flattened and are oriented in a parallel fashion. Like keloids, these scars have a more significant proportion of type III collagen than typical wounds. This is another similarity between the two. Hypertrophic scars are more prone to appear in the same anatomical regions as keloids (e.g., the mandibular border), most likely due to the increased tension in these areas [2].

40.3 Pathophysiology

With the exception of tissue trauma, the precise etiologic variables connected with the formation of keloids are difficult to ascertain. Nevertheless, keloids have been observed in situations without associated trauma. Keloids and hypertrophic scars are both related to adverse wound healing characteristics, such as infection and increased wound tension [2].

There needs to be a clearer comprehension of the pathophysiology of keloids. According to the theory, fibroblasts and myofibroblasts are the cells accountable for the accumulation of a dense extracellular matrix composed of glycosaminoglycans and collagen, respectively. Several investigations have found that the fibroblasts found within keloids produce a higher amount of fibronectin than previously thought [2].

An allergic immunoglobulin E (IgE)–mediated reaction is one of the many hypotheses proposed to explain the mechanism of keloid development. This response is thought to result in a lower percentage of mature cross-linked collagen and a higher fraction of soluble collagen. A second idea suggests that the initiation of keloid formation can be attributed to either an insufficient amount of melanocyte-stimulating hormone (MSH) or an excessive amount of MSH. The fact that specific stages of life, such as pregnancy and puberty, are connected with an increase in MSH and subsequent keloid formation lends credence to this notion. A third explanation considers the likelihood that keloid formation could be caused by microvascular blockage and the following hypoxia that happens as a result. There have been more recent studies that have reported an increased expression of interleukin-6 (IL-6) in the pathophysiology of keloids, as well as the role of insulin-like growth factor-1 (IGF-1) and the IGF-1 receptor axis in the invasive activity of keloids [2].

It is quite likely that genetic factors play a role in the creation of keloids. This is because keloids are more widespread in specific families and populations. In fibroblasts derived from keloids, it has been discovered that DeltaNp63 is overexpressed and p53 is underexpressed [5].

40.4 Classification of Traumatic Scars

To make clinical management more manageable, physicians frequently categorize traumatic scars into four distinct categories: hypertrophic scar, atrophic scar, flat (superficial) scar, and keloid scar. This classification is based on the histological and morphological characteristics of the scars [6, 7]. Based on the growth phase, they are also classified as mature scars, immature scars, linear scars, and widespread scars [8]. In addition, they are classified as linear scars and widespread scars. The color, erythema, texture, thickness, and flexibility of scars are some of the qualities essential for classification. In the consensus report for laser treatment of traumatic scars published in 2014 by Dr. Anderson et al. [9], traumatic scars were classified taking considerations of scar dyschromia (i.e., erythematous, hyper-pigmented, or hypo-pigmented), scar type (i.e., hypertrophic, flat, or atrophic), body location of the scar (i.e., face, neck, or limbs), and patient characteristics (i.e., skin type and comorbid conditions). This classification was developed to assist clinicians in selecting appropriate lasers and variables for treatment. It emphasized that the laser selection should focus on dyschromia and the relative scar thickness or atrophy, as these characteristics are the most prominent appearance features of traumatic scars [6, 9].

40.5 Treatment

Because there is no known cure for traumatic scarring, it is essential to have excellent early wound care and injury prevention strategies to reduce the amount of scarring that occurs. Several treatments, including physical therapy, pressure, and others, can assist in reducing the growth of contractures following an injury. Medical professionals, such as dermatologists, plastic surgeons, physical and occupational therapists, and psychiatrists, may be included in treating scars. Other professionals may also assist in the process of scar camouflage. Treatments commonly used include irradiation, cryotherapy with liquid nitrogen, silicone gel sheeting, injectable chemotherapeutic drugs (such as fluorouracil), and topical and injectable corticosteroids. The use of tissue fillers is one method for treating atrophic scars. In treating red scars, lasers that target blood vessels are frequently utilized. Additionally, more recent ablative (destructive) and nonablative fractional lasers have significantly advanced treatment for specific individuals who have traumatic scars, but it is typically necessary to undergo numerous treatments simultaneously. Surgical intervention may be required in severe scars and contractures [1].

40.5.1 Management of Hypertrophic Scars and Keloids

Hypertrophic Scars

When hypertrophic scars are positioned in an anatomical region conducive to treatment, they can typically be treated with simple excision, provided wound closure can take place without undue tension. Sometimes, steroid injections are necessary, but this is contingent upon the specific wound and the patient [2].

Keloids

A simple excision treatment for keloids has a recurrence rate that ranges from 50% to 80%. It has been suggested that both complete excision and near-total excision (leaving behind a tiny remnant of keloid on the periphery sections of the incision) are viable options [2].

Mechanical pressure through compression devices is recommended for treatment that does not include surgery. The application of pressure has the potential to break up collagen bundles and soften the keloid mass; however, to achieve a meaningful effect, the therapy must be administered for extended periods (more than

23 hours per day for 6 months). Unfortunately, when it comes to the head and neck, there are a lot of areas that cannot be affected by applying pressure [2].

Nitrogen mustard, tetroquinone, antihistamines, retinoic acids, zinc, vitamin A, vitamin E, and verapamil are some treatments that have been tried and tested, and the results have been mixed [2].

Interferon (IFN) therapy is utilized because it can inhibit the production of collagen in dermal fibroblasts [2].

Cold-knife excision, followed by postoperative injection of intralesional steroid, is one of the most frequently utilized combination therapies for keloids. In most cases, the injection into the lesion only occurs 2–3 weeks after the operation, then is repeated 3–4 weeks later [2].

Treatment of Traumatic Scars Using Laser and IPL

The interaction between lasers and infrared light (IPL) and tissue is based on the passage of light through the tissue and the subsequent absorption of photons, which will then be converted into heat, pressure (photoacoustic effect), as well as photochemical and photobiological reactions. The notion of selective photothermolysis of laser and light was initially presented by Dr. Rox Anderson and colleagues [10] from Harvard Medical School in 1983. Laser and light selectively impact the irradiated capillaries, pigment, or scar tissue when the right wavelength, exposure time, and energy are utilized. Laser and light are mainly absorbed by hemoglobin, melanin, water, or collagen in the skin. Since then, numerous laser and light devices have been invented, and dermatologists and plastic surgeons are currently utilizing them to treat scars, vascular diseases, pigmented diseases, and hair removal. As a result of the observation of the histological characteristics of scars, which include abnormal microvascular growth and abnormal collagen fiber arrangement, a wide range of laser and light modalities have been developed and implemented to prevent and treat traumatic scars. These modalities are primarily based on the principles of selective photothermolysis and fractional photothermolysis [6].

Targeted Laser or Light Devices for the Vascular System

For the treatment of traumatic scars, the laser and light modalities that are utilized the most frequently are the pulsed dye laser (PDL), ablative and nonablative fractional lasers, and intense pulsed light (IPL). It is possible to achieve the goal of closing the local capillaries and reducing the blood supply for the creation of scar tissue by using photodynamic therapy (PDL) (585 nm or 595 nm), potassium titanyl phosphate laser (532 nm), and intense pulsed light (IPL) (400–1200 nm; 500–600 nm). These treatment methods specifically target hemoglobin in red blood cells within vessels. To efficiently remove scar vasculature, it is necessary to have a pulse duration that is less than the time it takes for hemoglobin to relax thermally. It was also found that PDL was able to reduce the production of connective tissue growth factor (CTGF) in keloid patients [11] as well as in keloid fibroblasts that were cultured in vitro [12]. The tissue growth factor/small mothers against decapentaplegic (TGF/SMADs) pathway, which is highly expressed in keloid and hypertrophic scars [6], was shown to be the pathway that led to the discovery of CTGF as a powerfully profibrotic growth factor.

Fractional Lasers

Using a novel approach to skin treatment known as fractional photothermolysis, the fractional laser can generate microscopic thermal injury zones precisely controlled in terms of their width (less than 500 µm), depth, and density. These zones are encircled by a reservoir of epidermal and dermal tissue that has been spared, thereby enabling lightning-fast repair of laser-induced thermal injury [13, 14]. This technology makes treating patients with high energy possible while reducing the likelihood of scarring and hypopigmentation [15]. Ablative fractional lasers, such as the carbon dioxide laser with a wavelength of 10,600 nm and the erbium: yttrium-aluminum-garnet (Er: YAG) laser with a wavelength of 2940 nm, employ water as the target chromophore and generate columns of vaporized tissue that are surrounded by coagulated tissue and eschar. Forty-eight hours after the ablation, the vaporized columns are filled with epidermal cells that are entirely continuous, and the levels of heat shock proteins (Hsp-72 and Hsp-42) remain elevated for months [16, 17]. In histology, mature burn scars treated with fractional carbon dioxide laser showed a reversion toward a fetal collagen profile, with increased type III collagen and decreased type I collagen [18]. This was observed in patients who had undergone the treatment.

Additionally, the collagen architecture of treated scars was more similar to that of normal skin [18]. The process of collagen modeling induced by fractional carbon dioxide laser therapy may be due to the production of molecular changes. These changes include an increase in the expression of TGF-β3 and matrix metalloproteinase-1 and a decrease in the expression of basic fibroblast growth factor [6, 19].

Radiofrequency Therapy for Scars Caused by Trauma

The micro-plasma radiofrequency technique was developed as a technology that performs minimum ablation. To induce mild ablation of the epidermis and the formation of microchannels of the dermis on scar tissue, it makes use of radiofrequency energy to stimulate the nitrogen in the air, which results in the formation of a grid of high-energy foci known as plasma sparks. These sparks release heat as they return to their steady state, which occurs when they return to their steady state.

In recent years, micro-plasma radiofrequency has obtained good results for the treatment of traumatic scars as well as acne scars [20, 21]. This has been accomplished in conjunction with fractional technology. The fractional micro-plasma radiofrequency technology (FMRT) has emerged as a technology comparable to the ablative fractional laser. Both ablation and thermal coagulation characterize this technology, and it can cause the neogenesis of collagen and the remodeling of the epidermis and dermis. According to histological investigations, fractional mirror radiation therapy (FMRT) generates shallow and broad microchannels, like craters.

In contrast, fractional carbon dioxide lasers generate narrow, deep microchannels resembling cones [22]. However, hyperpigmentation has been considered to be a significant adverse effect associated with laser treatment in patients with Fitzpatrick skin type III or IV [6]. Micro-plasma radiofrequency is also effective and safe for post-burn hyperpigmentation, which indicates its application for treating traumatic scars in patients with Fitzpatrick skin type III or IV.

References

1. Jagdeo J, Shumaker PR. Traumatic scarring. JAMA Dermatol. 2017;153(3):364.
2. Kokoska MS. Hypertrophic scarring and keloids. In: Meyers AD, editor. Medscape. Updated; 2022. https://emedicine.medscape.com/article/876214-overview#a4. Accessed online at 12 June 2023.
3. McGinty S, Siddiqui WJ. Keloid. StatPearls; 2022.
4. Ogawa R, Okai K, Tokumura F, Mori K, Ohmori Y, Huang C, et al. The relationship between skin stretching/contraction and pathologic scarring: the important role of mechanical forces in keloid generation. Wound Repair Regen. 2012;20(2):149–57.
5. De Felice B, Ciarmiello LF, Mondola P, Damiano S, Seru R, Argenziano C, et al. Differential p63 and p53 expression in human keloid fibroblasts and hypertrophic scar fibroblasts. DNA Cell Biol. 2007;26(8):541–7.
6. Fu X, Dong J, Wang S, Yan M, Yao M. Advances in the treatment of traumatic scars with laser, intense pulsed light, radiofrequency, and ultrasound. Burns Trauma. 2019;7:1.
7. Tripathi PB, Nelson JS, Wong BJ. Posttraumatic laser treatment of soft tissue injury. Facial Plast Surg Clin North Am. 2017;25(4):617–28.
8. Gold MH, McGuire M, Mustoe TA, Pusic A, Sachdev M, Waibel J, et al. International Advisory Panel on Scar M: updated international clinical recommendations on scar management: part 2–algorithms for scar prevention and treatment. Dermatol Surg. 2014;40(8):825–31.
9. Anderson RR, Donelan MB, Hivnor C, Greeson E, Ross EV, Shumaker PR, et al. Laser treatment of traumatic scars with an emphasis on ablative fractional laser resurfacing: consensus report. JAMA Dermatol. 2014;150(2):187–93.
10. Anderson RR, Parrish JA. Selective photothermolysis: precise microsurgery by selective absorption of pulsed radiation. Science. 1983;220(4596):524–7.
11. Yang Q, Ma Y, Zhu R, Huang G, Guan M, Avram MM, et al. The effect of flashlamp pulsed dye laser on the expression of connective tissue growth factor in keloids. Lasers Surg Med. 2012;44(5):377–83.
12. Zhu R, Yue B, Yang Q, Ma Y, Huang G, Guan M, et al. The effect of 595 nm pulsed dye laser on connective tissue growth factor (CTGF) expression in cultured keloid fibroblasts. Lasers Surg Med. 2015;47(2):203–9.
13. Manstein D, Herron GS, Sink RK, Tanner H, Anderson RR. Fractional photothermolysis: a new concept for cutaneous remodeling using microscopic patterns of thermal injury. Lasers Surg Med. 2004;34(5):426–38.
14. Jih MH, Kimyai-Asadi A. Fractional photothermolysis: a review and update. Semin Cutan Med Surg. 2008;27(1):63–71.
15. Uebelhoer NS, Ross EV, Shumaker PR. Ablative fractional resurfacing for the treatment of traumatic scars and contractures. Semin Cutan Med Surg. 2012;31(2):110–20.
16. Hantash BM, Bedi VP, Kapadia B, Rahman Z, Jiang K, Tanner H, et al. In vivo histological evaluation of a novel ablative fractional resurfacing device. Lasers Surg Med. 2007;39(2):96–107.
17. Laubach HJ, Tannous Z, Anderson RR, Manstein D. Skin responses to fractional photothermolysis. Lasers Surg Med. 2006;38(2):142–9.
18. Ozog DM, Liu A, Chaffins ML, Ormsby AH, Fincher EF, Chipps LK, et al. Evaluation of clinical results, histological architecture, and collagen expression following treatment of mature burn scars with a fractional carbon dioxide laser. JAMA Dermatol. 2013;149(1):50–7.

19. Qu L, Liu A, Zhou L, He C, Grossman PH, Moy RL, et al. Clinical and molecular effects on mature burn scars after treatment with a fractional CO(2) laser. Lasers Surg Med. 2012;44(7):517–24.
20. Halachmi S, Orenstein A, Meneghel T, Lapidoth M. A novel fractional micro-plasma radio-frequency technology for the treatment of facial scars and rhytids: a pilot study. J Cosmet Laser Ther. 2010;12(5):208–12.
21. Wang S, Mi J, Li Q, Jin R, Dong J. Fractional microplasma radiofrequency technology for non-hypertrophic post-burn scars in Asians: a prospective study of 95 patients. Lasers Surg Med. 2017;49(6):563–9.
22. Shin MK, Choi JH, Ahn SB, Lee MH. Histologic comparison of microscopic treatment zones induced by fractional lasers and radiofrequency. J Cosmet Laser Ther. 2014;16(6):317–23.

Chemical Peeling 41

Ayşe Karaoğullarından, Nuray Bayar Muluk,
Heather Yeakel, and Jarrod Keeler

41.1 Introduction

Chemical "peeling" is when a chemical substance applied to the skin causes controlled destruction of the epidermis, whether or not it is part of the dermis, leading to skin renewal and reshaping [1]. Chemical peeling is a noninvasive procedure in some skin diseases and cosmetic areas. It causes damage to the skin with different chemicals, allowing the skin to reshape and look younger [2]. The first findings of this method were seen in Ancient Egyptian papyrus, and it was understood that the skin was tried to be repaired in various ways. Cleopatra taking milk baths and French women smoothing their skin with old wine show how ancient chemical peeling methods date back to ancient times. Occasionally, sour milk, stale wine, and animal fats have been used for skin regeneration [3, 4]. In recent years, alpha hydroxy acids (AHAs), which are very effective in keratinization disorders, have increased and have begun to be used frequently in many skin diseases and dermo-cosmetic areas. Chemical peeling aims to damage the skin layers to the desired depth and treat various lesions by taking advantage of wound healing during

A. Karaoğullarından
Adana City Hospital, Department of Otorhinolaryngology, Adana, Turkey

N. Bayar Muluk (✉)
Faculty of Medicine, Department of Otorhinolaryngology, Kırıkkale University, Kırıkkale, Türkiye

H. Yeakel
Department of Otolaryngology-Head and Neck Surgery, St. Luke's University Health Network, Bethlehem, PA, USA
e-mail: heather.yeakel@sluhn.org

J. Keeler
Otolaryngology & Facial Plastic and Reconstructive Surgery, Specialty Physician Associates, St. Luke's Medical Center, Bethlehem, PA, USA

C. Cingi et al. (eds.), *Minor Interventions, Major Outcomes on the Face*, Comprehensive ENT, https://doi.org/10.1007/978-3-032-01305-7_41

regeneration. Chemical peeling: It is used to treat a variety of skin lesions such as photodamage, pigment disorders, scars, and acne vulgaris.

41.2 Anatomy

Knowing the layers that make up the skin is essential to understanding the types of chemical peels and their mechanisms of action [3]. The skin has three layers: epidermis, dermis, and hypodermis (subcutaneous tissue).

- *Epidermis:* From surface to profound. It consists of four avascular layers: stratum corneum, stratum granulosum, stratum spinosum, and stratum basale. The fifth layer, the stratum lucidum, lies below the stratum corneum and is found on the palms of the hands and soles of the feet. Keratinocytes, located in layers other than the stratum basale, produce the protein called keratin, which is found in hair and nails.
  - *The stratum corneum* is a protective layer of squamous cells rich in keratin.
  - *Stratum spinosum* is a layer whose cells are connected by desmosomes. Between them are Langerhans cells and macrophages.
  - *Stratum basale* connects the epidermis to the dermis. There are melanocytes, which produce melanin pigment, and Merkel cells, which are responsible for the sensory stimulation of touch.
- *Dermis:* Contains hair follicles, sebaceous glands, nerves, and blood vessels.
  - *Papillary layer:* It consists of finger-like projections connecting the dermis and epidermis, intertwined with the stratum basale.
  - *Reticular layer:* It consists of elastin and collagen fibers that give the skin elasticity and tensile strength.
- *Hypodermis (subcutaneous tissue):* It is the deepest layer of the skin. It consists of loose connective tissue and fatty tissue.

41.3 Types of Chemical Peeling

Chemical peeling affects the more superficial epidermis and deepens into the lower layers of the skin, the papillary and reticular dermis [4]. This depth may vary depending on the content of the applied substance, concentration, and application method [5]. Chemical peeling applications are classified as very superficial, superficial, medium, and deep peeling according to the depth of the effect area, the damage caused, and the degree of effectiveness (Table 41.1) [6].

- *Very superficial peeling:* It is the damage of the stratum corneum with 10–20% trichloroacetic acid (TCA), low-potency glycolic acid, salicylic acid (SA), and retinoic acid. These are very mild peelings of the stratum corneum and are often called home peelings.

Table 41.1 Classification of chemical peeling

	Peeling agent	Depth of penetration	İndications	Complications
Very superficial	30–50% glycolic acid, AHA, Jessner's solution, 20–30% resorcinol	Stratum corneum	Acne, mild photoaging	Erythema
Superficial peel	50–70% glycolic acid, Jessner's solution, 40–50% resorcinol, BHA (salicylic acid), TCA (10–30%)	Stratum corneum to papillary dermis	Acne, pigmentary disorders (melasma), photoaging	Erythema, hyperpigmentation, acneiform rash
Medium depth peel	70% glycolic acid, 35–70% TCA, combination (CO_2 + 35% TCA; Jessner's solution + 35% TCA; 70% glycolic acid + 35% TCA)	Papillary dermis to upper reticular dermis	Photoaging, actinic keratosis, fine rhytids, superficial atrophic scars	Erythema, hyperpigmentation, herpes reactivation, solar lentigo
Depth peel	Baker–Gordon, phenol 88%	Mid-reticular dermis	Pigmentary disorders, severe photoaging, scars	İnfections depigmentation, scar, erythema, herpes reactivation, cardiac arrhythmias, pain

Adapted from Ref. [6]
AHA α-hydroxy acid, *BHA* β-hydroxy acid, *TCA* trichloroacetic acid

- *Superficial peeling:* 10–35% TCA, 10–25% Jessner's solution, alpha hydroxy acid (AHA), salicylic acid (SA), and tretinoin solution can be used in the superficial peeling process. Peeling off the top layer of the epidermis, the stratum corneum, creates a more vital epidermis. The renewal of keratinocytes in the basal layers of the epidermis is stimulated, and collagen production in the dermis increases.

Indications for superficial peeling include photoaging (roughness, yellow spots, fine lines, keratosis, and solar lentils), pigment disorders (melasma, post-inflammatory), and acne [5, 7]. Glycolic acid, an α-hydroxy acid, is the most widely used superficial peel [8]. A new development, β-lipohydroxy acids, are unique salicylate derivatives in that they have antibacterial, antifungal, and anti-inflammatory properties in addition to their exfoliative abilities. Given this anti-inflammatory effect, β-lipohydroxy acid peels are preferably used in patients predisposed to develop post-inflammatory hyperpigmentation (PIH). Chemical peeling with glycolic acid is a well-tolerated and safe treatment method for active acne vulgaris. Salicylic acid peeling for active acne vulgaris is more suitable for treating patients with darker skin and shows earlier healing than glycolic acid [9].

Other examples of superficial peels include Jessner's solution (resorcinol, lactic acid, and salicylic acid in ethanol), 10–15% TCA, and tretinoin [8].

- *Medium-depth peeling:* It affects the entire epidermis and papillary dermis and may penetrate the upper reticular dermis. In this case, skin renewal occurs from follicle epithelial cells that form new epidermis layers and stimulate collagen and elastin synthesis. It is effective in pigment changes, treatment of mild to moderate wrinkles, photoaging, and actinic keratosis.
- *Deep peeling:* Removes the epidermis, penetrates the middle reticular dermis, and causes protein coagulation. It causes necrosis and inflammation in the epidermis, papillary, and reticular dermis. Epidermal regeneration develops from follicular epithelial cells, and elastin and collagen synthesis continue for years after peeling [10, 11]. 35–50% TCA, Jessner's solution, 35% TCA combination, 70% glycolic acid, and 35% TCA combination, or 88% phenol can be used. Clinical indications for deep chemical peeling include severe photoaging, pigment disorders, and scars [5]. Croton oil and phenols mixed in various combinations are the active ingredients of deep peeling. Male skin is unsuitable for deep peeling treatment due to its thickness [8]. Treatment with phenols is excruciating and requires general anesthesia or deep sedation. Additionally, the risk of heart failure associated with its use limits its clinical benefit. Cardiac monitoring is required, and therefore, laser resurfacing is often preferred [5].

41.4 Chemical Peeling Agents

The actual peeling agent is the first and most important equipment for performing chemical peels. There are various chemical agents used for this purpose. pH, where 50% of the chemical is in free acid form, is the pKa of the chemical agent. A lower pK is associated with stronger peeling when choosing the chemical agent. Although there is a wide variety of products used for chemical peeling, the most commonly used compounds in the clinic are [12]:

41.4.1 Hydroxy Acids—Fruit Acids (AHAs)

Fruit acids: glycolic acid (obtained from sugar cane, GA), malic acid (obtained from apples), tartaric acid (obtained from grapes), mandelic acid, lactic acid (obtained from milk), and citric acid (obtained from fruits). The biological activities of GA depend on the type of acid, its concentration, pH, carrier and formulation, the general structure of the skin area, and the duration of contact with the skin. Low concentrations cause 5–10% corneolysis. Concentrations as high as 50–70% cause epidermolysis. GA is an exfoliative agent that causes epidermolysis with peeling of the skin by preventing corneocyte adhesion and keratinocyte accumulation in the stratum granulosum [13, 14]. It causes dermal remodeling by stimulating fibroblasts [15]. The risk of complications is low, even in people with dark skin [16]. Some studies have shown hydroxy acids have an anticarcinogenic effect [17]. It is used for superficial and medium-depth peeling in acne treatment. It has bactericidal effects on propionibacterium acnes [18]. It is neutralized with an alkaline solution such as sodium bicarbonate or normal saline.

LA is another α-hydroxy acid (derived from sour milk or blueberries) used in adjuvant therapy for acne, alone or in combination with other exfoliating agents. LA reduces corneocyte adhesion and removes dead skin cells. It has been shown to reduce melanin synthesis by directly inhibiting the tyrosinase enzyme, thus revealing skin-whitening effects [19]. LA is a safe peeling with few side effects.

Mandelic acid is an aromatic α-hydroxy acid commonly used to treat mild to moderate acne. Similar to other α-hydroxy acids, mandelic acid induces exfoliation of the epidermis by reducing corneocyte adhesion. It is a large molecule with antibacterial properties [20]. Therefore, mandelic acid is better tolerated on the skin and is often used as an alternative to GA peeling [16]. Mandelic acid peeling is formulated as a combined peeling with SA (20% SA, 10% mandelic acid) [19].

41.4.2 B-Hydroxy Acid (BHA)

Salicylic acid is a 2-hydroxybenzoic acid (from the willow tree) used mainly in superficial peeling due to its strong keratolytic and comedolytic properties [21]. It promotes the peeling of the upper lipophilic layers of the stratum corneum. It can penetrate comedones due to its lipophilic properties. These chemical properties make it successful in acne patients [22]. Additionally, its anti-inflammatory properties have been stated [21]. 5–30% SA is used for superficial peeling in acne. At these concentrations, this peel is safe and self-limiting; therefore, neutralizing agents are not required.

41.4.3 Jessner Solution (Resorcinol + Lactic + Salicylic + Ethanol)

Jessner solution combines resorcinol, salicylic acid, and lactic acid in 95% ethanol. The development of allergic contact dermatitis to resorcinol may limit the use of this product. It has been shown that its combination with TCA increases its effectiveness in treating melasma and acne scars and reduces post-inflammatory erythema [23]. Corneolysis enhances the effect of other keratolytic agents.

41.4.4 Resorcin

Pyruvic acid: It is an α-keto acid that converts to lactic acid. It quickly penetrates the dermis and causes epidermolysis in a short time. It is antimicrobial and induces collagen-elastin synthesis.

41.4.5 Trichloroacetic (TCA)

TCA is obtained from acetic acid by chlorination of three hydrogen ions. The most important feature of this agent is that it induces re-epithelialization, dermal remodeling, and cosmetic improvement through the coagulation of dermal and epidermal proteins [24]. TCA acts on epidermal cells by inducing growth factors and cytokines [25]. Specifically, platelet-derived growth factor increases in the cytoplasm of keratinocytes immediately after contact with TCA but returns to normal levels within 24 h. This release of growth factors before necrosis enables TCA to cause re-epithelialization and dermal regeneration. TCA can be used in superficial, mid-depth, and deep peeling, depending on the concentration applied. It is considered a gold standard agent for chemical peel applications. Generally, higher concentrations penetrate faster and denature greater amounts of protein, creating deeper peeling and associated with higher complications. 10–35% concentrations are used in superficial peeling and eliminate superficial pigmentation changes and superficial wrinkles. 35–50% concentrations provide moderate peeling, improve deeper wrinkles, pigmentations, and scars, and increase skin firmness. It is the most effective agent used in the treatment of acne scars. However, it should not be used in dark-skinned individuals as it may cause hyperpigmentation [6]. The "Chemical Reconstruction of Skin Scars" technique, in which TCA is applied only on the lesion in acne scars, is a recently described and effective method. High concentration (50–100%) TCA: especially in atrophic scars, it is applied to the base of the scar structure for a few seconds until whitening appears. These applications are performed at 4-week intervals, and effective results can be obtained [26]. It is applied in two to three sessions at 2- to 4-week intervals [1, 6]. It is also used in melasma, photoaging, under-eye circles, actinic keratosis, xanthelasma, seborrheic keratosis, and acanthosis nigricans.

41.4.6 Phenol

It provides deep chemical peeling and high penetration into the reticular dermis [27]. This agent is usually used as a 3-way Baker-Gordon solution (3 ml 88% phenol, eight drops septisol, and three drops Croton oil with 2 ml distilled water). Croton oil is responsible for deep penetration. It causes coagulation necrosis of dermal and epidermal proteins. It activates dermal fibroblasts and stimulates new collagen synthesis. Chemical peeling applied with phenol is very painful and causes cardiac arrhythmias and kidney-liver toxicity. Therefore, it is appropriate to perform it under operating room conditions.

41.5 Chemical Peeling

Each agent for chemical peeling has a different mechanism of action (Table 41.2). Epidermolysis provides smoother skin, especially in the stratum corneum. Peels that reach the stratum basale, where melanocytes are located, improve irregular pigmentation. Peelings that reach the papillary and reticular dermis increase the skin's elasticity by affecting elastin and collagen. All these compounds have a desquamation-increasing effect on the skin; thus, the cell cycle is accelerated. They peel the surface of the stratum corneum layer, making the skin smoother.

When peeling agents are combined, the risk of complications is reduced, and clinical results are better [6]. Various companies have developed superficial chemical peeling products by combining TCA and BHA. Again, various forms of Jessner's solution are available for sale. Combining TCA with Jessner's solution results in lower TCA concentrations, providing deeper penetration and minimizing complications such as scarring [28].

These agents reduce sebum secretion in acne, have a comedolytic effect, and cause keratolysis. They also show anti-inflammatory and antibacterial effects [6]. As the number of superficial peelings applied to treat mild and moderate acne increases, the response to treatment increases. While improvement is generally observed in inflammatory and non-inflammatory lesions, the effect is minimal in nodulocystic lesions [29]. In a study by Dréno et al., SA was used and found effective in both inflammatory and non-inflammatory lesions [29]. In addition, the 30% SA peeling application did not cause the development of pain, erythema, bleeding, crust, or post-inflammatory hyperpigmentation (PIH) in treating acne. It has been reported that it provides an effective treatment [30]. They also stated that peeling with SA suits dark-skinned patients with hyperpigmentation due to its whitening effect. It is more effective than GA in comedones and papules [9].

Chemical peels, lasers, and other light treatments can treat PIH (post-inflammatory hyperpigmentation). Still, these methods should be cautiously applied, as they may cause pigmentation [31]. The combination of SA peeling and retinoid showed a better effect in treating PIH than using treatment methods alone, was well tolerated, and had a lower recurrence rate. The important thing is to raise patients' awareness that PIH lesions will pass over time.

Table 41.2 Mechanism of action of the distinct peeling agents

Agent	Mechanism of action
A-hydroxy acids	Low concentrations (5–10%) produce corneolysis High concentrations (50–70%) induce epidermolysis
Jessner solution (resorcinol + lactic + salicylic + ethanol)	Corneolysis, increasing the effect of other keratolytic agents
Trichloroacetic acid	Coagulative necrosis of dermal and epidermal proteins, keratolytic effect (desguamation)
Phenol	Coagulation of dermal and epidermal proteins

Adapted from Ref. [13]

41.5.1 Chemical Peeling Preparation and Application

Before applying TCA, the skin is cleaned with alcohol or acetone and degreased to ensure homogeneous penetration of the agent. Topical anesthesia is not recommended, as it may cause vasoconstriction and affect the concentration of the agent. TCA is applied with cotton swabs and gauze until the desired effect occurs. Evaporated water and moisturizing cream can then relieve the burning sensation. The peeling is covered using retinol cream.

The application method of other peeling agents is similar. Glycolic acid peels are applied in successive layers with gauze or a brush until the patient begins to experience intense stinging, redness, and whitish areas. Peeling is initially applied for a maximum of 3 min. Consecutive sessions may take longer, depending on the patient's tolerance. A grayish color indicates excessive penetration and should be avoided. Glycolic acid peels are neutralized with bicarbonate and continue until the patient reports itching in all areas.

The characteristic of salicylic acid peelings is that the patient reports a very intense but temporary burning sensation at the beginning of the procedure. Two or four layers are applied. To accelerate the crystallization process, ventilation of the patient should be avoided. Salicylic acid peels are usually removed with water to relieve pain.

Several placebo-controlled studies have shown that prior preparation with topical retinoids when using TCA peels accelerates regeneration [26, 32]. Combination with retinoids facilitates healing by reducing the risk of complications and accelerating epidermal regeneration [32]. This is to compress the stratum corneum layer, increase epidermal thickness, increase glycosaminoglycan concentration, increase vascularity, and reduce melanin synthesis. It is sufficient to use retinoic acid or retinol for 2–4 weeks before chemical peeling [33].

Combined peels minimize side effects and accelerate regeneration by using lower concentrations with a synergistic effect between different ingredients. Combinations of TCA with other cosmetic products have been investigated, and their synergistic effects have been demonstrated [27]. TCA has been used in skin rejuvenation methods and other techniques such as botulinum toxin injection and carbon dioxide laser. It has also been combined with other exfoliating agents such as phenol, Jessner's solution, and tretinoin.

41.5.2 Application

1. Appropriate patient selection is made.
2. The patient is informed about the procedure and has a consent form signed. Photographic documentation is prepared for comparison.
3. For the treatment to be successful, preliminary preparations must be made.

    (a) The patient's hair is removed with a bonnet.
    (b) The patient's face is cleaned with cleansing agents (alcohol, ether, or acetone).

   (c) Vaseline or protective creams can prevent damage to the lips, nose, and eye corners.
   (d) Eyes and ears are covered with cotton.

4. The chemical peeling agent is applied to the desired areas with the help of an applicator or a brush.
5. The first application time is aimed to be 2–3 min.
6. While applying the chemical peeling agent, the patient is asked to rate the burning sensation he/she feels on a scale from 1 to 10.
7. If the patient gives 8–10 points for this burning sensation, the procedure is not continued.
8. There should be at least 5 min between repeated applications.
9. After the peeling process, the acid is neutralized by applying a neutralizer or water to the treatment area.
10. After the procedure, moisturizer is applied to the face. The patient is told not to go out in the sun and to use moisturizer until the skin returns to normal [5]. The moisturizing time of the skin may vary depending on whether the procedure is superficial or medium deep.
11. "Peeling" application sessions are individually arranged according to the patient's skin type and the skin's tolerance to the chemical agent.
12. Care should be taken to ensure that there are at least 2 weeks between two sessions for superficial peeling and at least 6 months for medium-depth peeling.

Patient selection is very important in chemical peeling applications. First, a detailed anamnesis should be taken from the patient before the session. Which peeling agent will be used for which patient and the neutralization process varies for each patient? In addition, the indications, contraindications, and complications of the peeling process should be well known.

41.5.3 Indications for Chemical Peeling

1. Photoaging
2. Actinic keratosis
3. Pigmentary dyschromias
4. Senile lentigo
5. Acne
6. Acne scars
7. Seborrheic keratosis

41.5.4 Contraindications of Chemical Peeling

1. Bad doctor-patient relationship
2. Psychological problems
3. Unrealistic expectations

4. Poor general health and nutritional status
5. Use of oral contraceptives and drugs that may cause photosensitivity (e.g., tetracycline)
6. Having received isotretinoin treatment in the last 3–6 months for superficial peeling and in the last 6–12 months for medium-deep peeling
7. Active infection and open wounds
8. Active herpes virus infection

41.5.4.1 Relative Contraindications

1. Medium or deep peeling must have been done within 3–12 months.
2. Recent facial surgery.
3. Abnormal scar formation such as keloid formation and delayed wound healing.
4. Radiotherapy history.
5. Fitzpatrick skin type IV, V, VI (Classification of skin color according to its reactions to sun exposure) [34].
6. Aspirin allergy for salicylic acid peeling.
7. Use of anticoagulants.
8. Intensive smoking.
9. Pregnancy/breastfeeding.
10. Risk of exposure to intense sunlight.
11. Previous surgical interventions (must wait at least 6 months).

41.6 Side Effects and Complications

Chemical peeling is a very simple procedure that is widely used today. However, there may be some undesirable changes in the skin after the procedure. However, not all of these changes can be considered as complications. Therefore, these changes are examined in two groups: expected side effects and complications.

41.6.1 Expected Side Effects

Changes that can be seen in many patients after the procedure and resolve spontaneously are temporary erythema, milia, and acne-like rash.

41.6.2 Complications

41.6.2.1 Immediate Complications

Including skin edema, burning, itching sensation, and blistering. Among the complications that require urgent treatment, the most serious is anaphylactic shock. In addition, eye damage may occur if the chemical agent splashes into the eye. When phenol is used as a chemical agent, liver and kidney function tests should be checked, and attention should be paid to cardiac arrhythmia [35]. Ringing in the ears, shortness of breath, and nausea may occur due to salicylic acid [36].

Table 41.3 General post-peeling complications

Immediate	Persistent erythema, edema
Late	Hyperpigmentation Hypopigmentation Depigmentation Demarcation lines Vesicles, blisters, scabs Milium Acneiform rash Infections (herpes reactivation, bacterial
Medium and deep	Atrophic scars Cardiac arrhythmias (phenol) Laryngeal edema Exacerbation of a dermatosis Infectious toxic shock syndrome

Adapted from Refs. [9, 36, 37]

41.6.2.2 Late Complications

1. Peeling line on the neck following tear drops
2. Infections due to viral and bacterial causes (staphylococcal, streptococcal, pseudomonas, herpes simplex)
3. Acneiform eruptions
4. Ecchymosis in the infraorbital region
5. Post-inflammatory hyperpigmentation (Fitzpatrick skin type 4-5-6) [37]
6. Erythema lasting longer than 3 weeks should be closely monitored for scar tissue formation
7. Deep chemical burn
8. Atrophic or hypertrophic scar formation
9. Systemic (cardiac, renal, hepatic, hematological)

In conclusion, chemical peeling is a safe and effective method that treats several cosmetic skin problems. It can be easily applied in hospitals, outpatient clinics and examination environments. To improve the cosmetic result and avoid possible complications, it is necessary to know the correct indications, tell the patient realistic expectations, and have a broad knowledge of the agent's application technique. As important as the application of chemical peeling is, post-application care and close follow-up of the patient are also very important (Table 41.3) [9, 36, 37].

References

1. Chen X, Wang S, Yang M, Li L. Chemical peels for acne vulgaris: a systematic review of randomised controlled trials. BMJ Open. 2018;8(4):e019607. https://doi.org/10.1136/bmjopen-2017-019607.
2. Perić S, Bubanj M, Bubanj S, Jančić S. Side effects assessment in glicolyc acid peelings in patients with acne type I. Bosn J Basic Med Sci. 2011;11(1):52–7. https://doi.org/10.17305/bjbms.2011.2624.

3. Meaike JD, Agrawal N, Chang D, Lee EI, Nigro MG. Noninvasive facial rejuvenation. Part 3: physician-directed-lasers, chemical peels, and other noninvasive modalities. Semin Plast Surg. 2016;30(3):143–50. https://doi.org/10.1055/s-0036-1584818.
4. McLafferty E, Hendry C, Alistair F. The integumentary system: anatomy, physiology and function of skin. Nurs Stand (Royal College of Nursing (Great Britain): 1987). 2012;27(3):35–42. https://doi.org/10.7748/ns2012.10.27.7.35.c9358.
5. Kontochristopoulos G, Platsidaki E. Chemical peels in active acne and acne scars. Clin Dermatol. 2017;35(2):179–82. https://doi.org/10.1016/j.clindermatol.2016.10.011.
6. O'Connor AA, Lowe PM, Shumack S, Lim AC. Chemical peels: a review of current practice. Australas J Dermatol. 2018;59(3):171–81. https://doi.org/10.1111/ajd.12715.
7. Roberts WE, Miller N. Optimized patient outcomes with the novel modality of corrective chemical peel and neurotoxin on same-day treatment. J Drugs Dermatol. 2024;23(1):1349–54.
8. Berson DS, Cohen JL, Rendon MI, Roberts WE, Starker I, Wang B. Clinical role and application of superficial chemical peels in today's practice. J Drugs Dermatol: JDD. 2009;8(9):803–11.
9. Al-Talib H, Al-Khateeb A, Hameed A, Murugaiah C. Efficacy and safety of superficial chemical peeling in treatment of active acne vulgaris. An Bras Dermatol. 2017;92(2):212–6. https://doi.org/10.1590/abd1806-4841.20175273.
10. Truchuelo M, Cerdá P, Fernández LF. Chemical peeling: a useful tool in the office. Peeling químico, una herramienta útil en la consulta. Actas dermo-sifiliograficas. 2017;108(4):315–22. https://doi.org/10.1016/j.ad.2016.09.014.
11. Mangat DS, Tansavatdi K, Garlich P. Current chemical peels and other resurfacing techniques. Facial Plast Surg: FPS. 2011;27(1):35–49. https://doi.org/10.1055/s-0030-1270422.
12. Rendon MI, Berson DS, Cohen JL, Roberts WE, Starker I, Wang B. Evidence and considerations in the application of chemical peels in skin disorders and aesthetic resurfacing. J Clin Aesthet Dermatol. 2010;3(7):32–43.
13. Clark E, Scerri L. Superficial and medium-depth chemical peels. Clin Dermatol. 2008;26(2):209–18. https://doi.org/10.1016/j.clindermatol.2007.09.015.
14. Salam A, Dadzie OE, Galadari H. Chemical peeling in ethnic skin: an update. Br J Dermatol. 2013;169(Suppl 3):82–90. https://doi.org/10.1111/bjd.12535.
15. Sharad J. Glycolic acid peel therapy – a current review. Clin Cosmet Investig Dermatol. 2013;6:281–8. https://doi.org/10.2147/CCID.S34029.
16. Sarkar R, Bansal S, Garg VK. Chemical peels for melasma in dark-skinned patients. J Cutan Aesthet Surg. 2012;5(4):247–53. https://doi.org/10.4103/0974-2077.104912.
17. Dainichi T, Ueda S, Isoda M, Koga T, Kinukawa N, Nose Y, Ishii K, Amano S, Horii I, Furue M. Chemical peeling with salicylic acid in polyethylene glycol vehicle suppresses skin tumour development in hairless mice. Br J Dermatol. 2003;148(5):906–12. https://doi.org/10.1046/j.1365-2133.2003.05282.x.
18. Takenaka Y, Hayashi N, Takeda M, Ashikaga S, Kawashima M. Glycolic acid chemical peeling improves inflammatory acne eruptions through its inhibitory and bactericidal effects on Propionibacterium acnes. J Dermatol. 2012;39(4):350–4. https://doi.org/10.1111/j.1346-8138.2011.01321.x.
19. Usuki A, Ohashi A, Sato H, Ochiai Y, Ichihashi M, Funasaka Y. The inhibitory effect of glycolic acid and lactic acid on melanin synthesis in melanoma cells. Exp Dermatol. 2003;12(Suppl 2):43–50. https://doi.org/10.1034/j.1600-0625.12.s2.7.x.
20. Garg VK, Sinha S, Sarkar R. Glycolic acid peels versus salicylic-mandelic acid peels in active acne vulgaris and post-acne scarring and hyperpigmentation: a comparative study. Dermatol Surg. 2009;35(1):59–65. https://doi.org/10.1111/j.1524-4725.2008.34383.x.
21. Arif T. Salicylic acid as a peeling agent: a comprehensive review. Clin Cosmet Investig Dermatol. 2015;8:455–61. https://doi.org/10.2147/CCID.S84765.
22. Handog EB, Datuin MS, Singzon IA. Chemical peels for acne and acne scars in asians: evidence based review. J Cutan Aesthet Surg. 2012;5(4):239–46. https://doi.org/10.4103/0974-2077.104911.
23. Safoury OS, Zaki NM, El Nabarawy EA, Farag EA. A study comparing chemical peeling using modified Jessner's solution and 15% trichloroacetic acid versus 15% trichloro-

acetic acid in the treatment of melasma. Indian J Dermatol. 2009;54(1):41–5. https://doi.org/10.4103/0019-5154.48985.
24. Lee JB, Chung WG, Kwahck H, Lee KH. Focal treatment of acne scars with trichloroacetic acid: chemical reconstruction of skin scars method. Dermatol Surg. 2002;28(11):1017–21. https://doi.org/10.1046/j.1524-4725.2002.02095.x.
25. Yonei N, Kanazawa N, Ohtani T, Furukawa F, Yamamoto Y. Induction of PDGF-B in TCA-treated epidermal keratinocytes. Arch Dermatol Res. 2007;299(9):433–40. https://doi.org/10.1007/s00403-007-0781-6.
26. Hevia O, Nemeth AJ, Taylor JR. Tretinoin accelerates healing after trichloroacetic acid chemical peel. Arch Dermatol. 1991;127(5):678–82.
27. Landau M. Combination of chemical peelings with botulinum toxin injections and dermal fillers. J Cosmet Dermatol. 2006;5(2):121–6. https://doi.org/10.1111/j.1473-2165.2006.00237.x.
28. Dayan E, Rohrich RJ. Jessner's solution with trichloroacetic acid chemical peel: optimizing outcomes and safety. Plast Reconstr Surg Glob Open. 2019;7(5):e2250. https://doi.org/10.1097/GOX.0000000000002250.
29. Dréno B, Fischer TC, Perosino E, Poli F, Viera MS, Rendon MI, Berson DS, Cohen JL, Roberts WE, Starker I, Wang B. Expert opinion: efficacy of superficial chemical peels in active acne management–what can we learn from the literature today? Evidence-based recommendations. J Eur Acad Dermatol Venereol: JEADV. 2011;25(6):695–704. https://doi.org/10.1111/j.1468-3083.2010.03852.x.
30. Dainichi T, Ueda S, Imayama S, Furue M. Excellent clinical results with a new preparation for chemical peeling in acne: 30% salicylic acid in polyethylene glycol vehicle. Dermatol Surg. 2008;34(7):891–9. https://doi.org/10.1111/j.1524-4725.2008.34174.x.
31. Thiboutot DM, Dréno B, Abanmi A, Alexis AF, Araviiskaia E, Barona Cabal MI, Bettoli V, Casintahan F, Chow S, da Costa A, El Ouazzani T, Goh CL, Gollnick H, Gomez M, Hayashi N, Herane MI, Honeyman J, Kang S, Kemeny L, Kubba R, et al. Practical management of acne for clinicians: an international consensus from the Global Alliance to Improve Outcomes in Acne. J Am Acad Dermatol. 2018;78(2 Suppl 1):S1–S23.e1. https://doi.org/10.1016/j.jaad.2017.09.078.
32. Kim IH, Kim HK, Kye YC. Effects of tretinoin pretreatment on TCA chemical peel in Guinea pig skin. J Korean Med Sci. 1996;11(4):335–41. https://doi.org/10.3346/jkms.1996.11.4.335.
33. Vagotis FL, Brundage SR. Histologic study of dermabrasion and chemical peel in an animal model after pretreatment with Retin-A. Aesth Plast Surg. 1995;19(3):243–6. https://doi.org/10.1007/BF00451097.
34. Starkman SJ, Mangat DS. Chemical peels: deep, medium, and light. Facial Plast Surg: FPS. 2019;35(3):239–47. https://doi.org/10.1055/s-0039-1688944.
35. Costa I, Damasceno PS, Costa MC, Gomes K. Review in peeling complications. J Cosmet Dermatol. 2017;16(3):319–26. https://doi.org/10.1111/jocd.12329.
36. Monheit GD. Medium-depth chemical peels. Dermatol Clin. 2001;19(3):413–25, vii. https://doi.org/10.1016/s0733-8635(05)70282-5.
37. Roberts WE. Chemical peeling in ethnic/dark skin. Dermatol Ther. 2004;17(2):196–205. https://doi.org/10.1111/j.1396-0296.2004.04020.x.

Laser Peeling

42

Osman Erdoğan, Ali Seyed Resuli, and Desiderio Passali

42.1 Introduction

The face is the part of the body that other people first notice. Human interaction begins with evaluating body language and facial expressions before verbal communication. Therefore, facial skin conditions are essential for understanding their general body health, age, self-care, and attractiveness. While the appearance of the skin with wrinkles, spots, drooping appearance, and non-homogeneous reflection of light is associated with aging, on the contrary, smooth, taut skin reflects the light homogeneously refers to youth.

Throughout history, people have used many methods to renew the skin surface to look younger and more beautiful. Skin peeling, the general name of these methods, is the artificial exfoliation of the outermost layer of the epidermis, sometimes extending deeper, with physical and chemical means [1]. The Assyrians, Egyptians, Babylonians, and Indians used pumice to exfoliate the facial skin physically [1, 2]. Salicylic acid, acetone, resorcinol, solution of formaldehyde, phenol, beta-naphthol, glacial acetic acid, mercurial salts, sulfur, and solid CO_2 are chemicals used for skin peeling [1].

Aging slows skin cell turnover, reduces its ability to retain moisture, and decreases collagen, elastin, and fat cell production [3]. Skin photoaging, a common aesthetic problem, is characterized by dyschromia, rhytids, telangiectasia, textural changes, keratosis, elastosis, erythema, and skin thinning. Ablative skin resurfacing

O. Erdoğan (✉)
VM Medical Park Ankara Hospital, Department of Otorhinolaryngology, Ankara, Turkey

A. S. Resuli
İstanbul Yeni Yüzyıl University, Faculty of Medicine, Department of Otorhinolaryngology, Istanbul, Turkey

D. Passali
IFOS Former President, ORL Head and Neck Surgery, University of Siena, Siena, Italy

C. Cingi et al. (eds.), *Minor Interventions, Major Outcomes on the Face*, Comprehensive ENT, https://doi.org/10.1007/978-3-032-01305-7_42

is the primary treatment for reversing the signs of photoaging [4]. Thanks to the advances in laser technology in recent years, lasers have been used intensively in the treatment of skin lesions, skin resurfacing, and rejuvenation. This chapter will focus on ablative laser systems used in skin rejuvenation and treatment of superficial lesions.

42.2 History of Laser Technology

Laser originated as an acronym for "light amplification by stimulated emission of radiation." With the understanding of the concept of stimulated emission put forward by Albert Einstein in 1917, which forms the basis of the laser theory, the first laser emerged as a ruby crystal emitting red light by Maiman in 1959. Goldman started to use it in the medical treatment for various skin diseases in 1963 [5–7]. Although the CO_2 laser was discovered by Patel in 1963, after the articulated arm was developed by Polanyi in 1968, its use in medical applications has become widespread, especially in resurfacing for rhytid and acne scarring [8–10]. Many vascular lesions have been successfully treated with the argon laser since the 1970s [11]. Following the widespread use of CO_2 and argon laser for cutaneous lesions, complications such as hypertrophic scar (most commonly), pigment changes, atrophic scar, infection, pain, bleeding, prolonged healing, benign reactive proliferation, and local anesthesia have been reported [10, 12].

The theory of selective photothermolysis, which aims to focus the energy directed by laser application on the target tissue and reduce its effect on the surrounding tissues, was put forward by Anderson and Parish in 1983 [13]. They developed a simple model and tried to predict what wavelength, pulse duration, and exposure dose would induce selective thermal and mechanical damage to these structures. Which target will be affected, the microscopic scale of this selective effect, and the required exposure doses are related to this theory.

It is important to explain two basic principles in understanding selective photothermolysis. First, if a photon of a selected wavelength is absorbed explicitly by a pigmented target, a selective heat increase occurs in that target tissue. This increase in heat is proportional to the photon absorbed, which is calculated by multiplying the radiation's intensity with the tissue's absorption coefficient. Second, as the target tissue is exposed to the laser, it heats up, spreading this heat equally to the surrounding tissues. The selective effect causes denaturation, vaporization, carbonization, or destruction of the target tissue with sufficient laser exposure while causing minimal damage to the surrounding tissue. For this, the thermal relaxation time, determined according to the dimension and thermal properties of the tissue and defined as the time required for the tissue to decrease to half of the peak temperature reached as a result of laser exposure, must be known. Laser exposure with a pulse duration shorter than the thermal relaxation time allows the target to cool, causing minimal thermal injury to the surrounding tissues and creating a selective effect on the target tissue [14].

After the theory of selective photothermolysis was introduced, pulsed lasers replaced continuous wave CO_2 and argon lasers, which caused non-selective damage to the target tissue because of prolonged laser exposure. According to pulse duration, these laser systems are classified as long-pulsed (microsecond to millisecond), including pulsed dye laser; very short-pulsed (nanosecond to picosecond), including quality-switched ruby, alexandrite, and neodymium: yttrium-aluminum-garnet; superpulsed CO_2 lasers [15].

Picosecond lasers became widespread after the theory of selective photothermolysis and are especially preferred in tattoo treatment. A computer simulation study conducted by Ho et al. in 2002 reported that the photoacoustic effect is the primary mechanism in the fragmentation of tattoo particles. Fragmenting the tattoo particles quickly (10–100 picoseconds) without increasing the melting point minimizes the heat damage to the surrounding tissues. The steam-carbon reaction makes these fragmented particles almost transparent [16].

A new concept called fractional photothermolysis in skin treatment was introduced in 2004 by Manstein et al. According to this concept, micro-thermal wounds called microscopic treatment zones (MTZ) are formed according to a specific geometric pattern, regardless of the chromophore in the tissue. Each non-contiguous MTZ produces necrotic debris surrounded by living tissue under the intact stratum corneum. Fractional photothermolysis provided significant reduction of side effects in photoaged skin treatment, limited epidermal and dermal necrosis sharply in MTZ, epidermal healing in these MTZ wounds taking less than 1 day, and reduction of erythema and oozing seen in ablative techniques [17].

Significant historical developments in lasers for skin lesions include more precise exposure of the target tissue with the laser beam, minimizing surrounding tissue exposure to the laser beam and accelerating the healing due to lesion-specific treatment. Thanks to the developing technology, more adjustable laser systems enable more specific lesion treatment. In this context, physicians should have more detailed information about laser systems before starting the treatment to provide more effective treatment.

42.3 Ablative Laser Techniques

42.3.1 Carbon Dioxide Laser

Continuous wave CO_2 laser systems with a wavelength of 10,600 nm absorbed by the water in the tissue have been used for skin resurfacing since the 1980s. These systems caused complications due to the wide pulse range, extensive thermal damage around the target tissue, and microvascular coagulation in the dermis. These complications included pigment changes, demarcation lines, prolonged erythema, and scarring [18, 19]. After understanding the selective photothermolysis theory from the 1990s, pulsed CO_2 laser systems with short pulse intervals and providing cooling of the chromophore began to be used [19]. Ultrapulse CO_2 laser for skin ablation requires three times less energy than continuous wave CO_2 laser.

Theoretically, if the same size lesion and amount of energy are used with the ultrapulse CO_2 laser, more volume and deeper ablation can be performed compared to the continuous wave CO_2 laser. At the same time, less surrounding tissue damage occurs [20]. The duration and severity of postoperative erythema correlate with laser energy and several passes [21]. Compared to the Er: YAG laser, although wound healing takes longer, tissue tightening and fibroplasia are more pronounced. Thus, longer-lasting results can be obtained with the CO_2 laser compared to the Er: YAG laser system [22]. In addition, it causes better bleeding control compared to Er: YAG systems, while it causes more thermal damage, charring, and scar formation [23].

Four parameters determine the effect of fractional CO_2 laser on tissue: (1) Power refers to the energy delivered to the tissue with each shot. It can vary between 5 and 100 mJ/microbeam and affects the amount of ablation. (2) Pitch is the ratio of the entire area to the treated area. As this parameter decreases, the treated area increases, and the healing time and discomfort increase. (3) Dwell time defines the pulse duration, and as it increases, thermal damage increases. (4) The microbeam diameter differs between devices and determines the penetration depth. The practitioner should approach the lesion by considering these four parameters. For example, a small microbeam diameter is used for deep ablation, and a large diameter is used for superficial ablation. Pitch parameters should be increased for faster recovery and more comfortable operation [23].

The histological basis of the efficacy of the fractional CO_2 laser on scars, rhytids, pore size reduction, pigment changes, and photodamage is neocollagenesis and fibrosis developing 3 months after the treatment [24]. It provides contraction that shortens the dermal collagen up to one-third of its length by changing its triple helical structure after heating [25]. Stimulated cell proliferation, balanced collagen organization, and prevented excessive fibrosis were obtained with the modulatory effects of increasing fibroblast growth factor (FGF) secretion and suppressing transforming growth factor beta (TGF-β) secretion [26]. Hence, synergistic benefit can be achieved in collagen synthesis with platelet-rich plasma (PRP), which contains growth factors such as platelet-derived growth factor (PDGF), TGF-β, vascular endothelial growth factor (VEGF), fibroblast growth factor (FGF), epidermal growth factor (EGF), and keratinocyte growth factor (KGF), applied together with fractional CO_2 [27, 28]. Activating different cytokine pathways by changing the amount of applied laser energy provides lesion-specific laser energy values [29]. Follicular stem cells in the pilosebaceous unit play an initiating role in the healing of the epidermal layer after fractional CO_2 laser. This explains why hairy skin areas heal faster and have fewer complications [4]. After a fractional CO_2 laser, granulation tissue appears for up to 3 days, and reepithelialization can occur in 1 week with a fractional CO_2 laser [23, 30].

Although the CO_2 laser is very effective in skin smoothing, rhytid reduction, removing lentigines, and tightening the skin, the fractional CO_2 laser is preferred due to the shortened healing process [31]. CO_2 laser treatment provides excellent cosmetic improvement on the perioral, periorbital, and glabellar rhytids. Superficial wrinkles are eliminated, and deep wrinkles are significantly improved. It also provides tightening in previously loose and folded skin [32]. With fractional CO_2, not only is improvement achieved in rhytids, but also improvement continues until at least 6 months after treatment and is permanent even after 2 years [33, 34]. In the fractional CO_2 laser treatment of wrinkles and rhytids caused by photodamage, recovery is observed in the late period due to the activation of the collagen remodeling process and an increase in collagen 1 and 3 density [35–38]. In a split-face study, an approximate 23% reduction in wrinkle depth was observed 3 months after the treatment with the fractional CO_2 laser. According to the Fitzpatrick wrinkle score, 64% improvement was noted on the treated side [39]. Improving wrinkles also increases the quality of life regarding the skin condition [40].

A hypertrophic scar is a benign proliferation formed by fibrosis and an increase in type 1 and 3 collagen in the dermis layer. TGF-β plays a vital role in the formation of hypertrophic scarring and other fibrotic conditions. Matrix metalloproteinase (MMP) type 3, a collagenase, reduces collagen. In treating hypertrophic scar with fractional CO_2 laser, clinical improvement occurs with an increase in MMP 1 and a decrease in TGF, FGF, and type 1 and 3 collagen [41]. While improvement is observed in hypertrophic scars with fractional CO_2 laser treatment applied 6 months after the injury, this effect is also seen in the treatment of early-stage (1 month after injury) hypertrophic scars [42, 43]. Histologically, after the laser treatment of keloid and hypertrophic scars, collagen decreases in the first month and returns to normal in the third month. This is explained as the reduction of collagen in the tissue because of the removal of disorganized obsolete collagen by fractional photothermolysis and then the normalization of its quantity and quality with the synthesis of new collagen [44]. While collagen bundles are arranged in random directions in keloid scars, the density of collagen bundles decreases after fractional CO_2 laser treatment, and collagen bundles show more parallel arrangement [45].

In treating acneiform scars after severe acne episodes, there is no late-period hypopigmentation and permanent scarring with fractional CO_2 laser [46–48]. Early effects such as erythema, serosanguinous, oozing, petechiae, and edema are not permanent [36, 46, 47, 49]. Patients with Fitzpatrick skin type 4–6 have an increased risk of hyperpigmentation. Therefore, to avoid the adverse effects of hyperpigmentation, deep fractional CO_2 laser should be preferred instead of superficial fractional CO_2 laser, which causes more epithelial damage, especially in patients with skin type 4 [48, 50]. There is approximately 70% improvement in scar depth after treatment, which is attributed to the deeper dermal penetration of the fractional CO_2 laser compared to the continuous CO_2 laser [46]. In an ex vivo study, this effect is supported by tissue ablation and thermal effect reaching a depth of 1 mm [51]. Scar type and laser energy affect acneiform scar treatment. A high-energy laser is more effective than a low-energy laser in scar healing. Rolling scars respond better than icepick scars, while boxcar scars show a higher risk of adverse reactions [52]. The addition of intradermal PRP increases the acne scar correction power of the fractional CO_2 laser [27, 53–55].

42.3.2 Erbium: YAG Laser

Er: YAG laser with a wavelength of 2940 nm in the mid-infrared visible light spectrum was developed as an alternative to the CO_2 laser in the 1990s and has 10–15 times the water absorption compared to the CO_2 laser with a wavelength of 10,600 nm. Therefore, the ablation threshold value on the skin is 1.6 J/cm^2, while it is 5 J/cm^2 in the CO_2 laser. Er: YAG laser requires less energy for ablation, resulting in less surrounding tissue damage [56]. With the CO_2 laser, the first pulse exposes the dermis, and the residual heat causes charring in the dermis, which makes it difficult for the next pulse to penetrate. However, controlled ablation depth can be achieved with the Er: YAG laser [57]. Er: YAG laser causes less hypertrophic scarring than CO_2 laser because it is more specific to water, has less penetration depth, causes less surrounding tissue damage, and prevents damage to deep pilosebaceous structures that allow normal epithelialization [58].

Knowing the advantages and disadvantages of both methods facilitates the selection of the appropriate method. While the benefits of the CO_2 laser include more tissue contraction, excellent bleeding control, and good long-term results thanks to the continuation of collagen remodeling, the disadvantages include the prolonged postoperative period, hypopigmentation, and scar development potential. The advantages of the Er: YAG laser are shorter postoperative recovery, fewer complications, and being more controlled and titratable by adjusting the number of passes and the amount of energy, while the disadvantages include minimal tissue contraction, intraoperative bleeding, more laser passages that increase the operation time, and limited collagen remodeling, which is essential for the requirement and scar revision [59, 60]. Collagen contraction is 1–4% immediately after the procedure and 0–14% in the long term [59]. Er: YAG laser increases the concentration of type 1, 3, and 4 collagen and triggers neo-collagen formation [61].

Low-energy Er: YAG lasers effectively treat mild to moderate lesions in acneiform scars. CO_2 and Er: YAG hybrid laser systems, low and high-energy dual-mode Er: YAG laser systems, and variable-energy Er: YAG laser systems can be used in moderate and severe acne scars as they provide deep tissue penetration, better bleeding control, and better collagen contraction [62].

While low-energy Er: YAG laser is preferred in the superficial treatment of mild to moderate photoaging and rhytids, high-energy Er: YAG laser gives similar results to CO_2 laser without thermal injury in deep rhytids [63–65]. Biomechanical evaluation of high-energy Er: YAG laser reveals increased skin thickness and decreased laxity, similar to superficial burns [66, 67]. Although there is a histological similarity between Er: YAG laser and superficial burns in terms of damage to deep dermal vessels, Er: YAG laser does not cause damage to the surrounding tissue, while in superficial burns, all cell types in the reticular dermis are impaired [68]. Superficial and deep wrinkles can be successfully treated with the Er: YAG laser, but bleeding problems often occur in deep laser applications. Therefore, the Er: YAG/CO_2 combination and the variable Er: YAG or CO_2 laser are recommended for deep wrinkles [69].

42.3.3 Erbium: YSSG Laser

Er: YSSG laser has a wavelength of 2790 nm and has more water absorption than the conventional CO_2 laser and less water absorption than the Er: YAG laser. In addition to rapid vaporization, it provides deeper penetration than the Er: YAG laser, which allows for more balanced absorption and coagulation. Compared to Er: YAG and CO_2 laser, sufficient collateral thermal damage occurs to ensure hemostasis without causing thermal damage as in CO_2 laser [4, 23]. It improves the treatment of rhytids, periorbital wrinkles, and dyspigmentation [70, 71].

42.3.4 Combined CO_2/Er: YAG Laser Systems

Synergistic and minimal adverse effects are aimed in laser treatment with the combination of 10,600 nm CO_2 laser and 2940 nm Er: YAG laser. An animal study reported that this combination provided earlier neovascularization and vessel budding compared to CO_2 laser and early termination of the inflammatory response, resulting in a transparent skin area. Early termination of the inflammatory process accelerates reepithelialization and minimizes erythema [72].

With CO_2/Er: YAG combined treatment on human skin, well-controlled and minimal adverse effects and no scar formation were observed. According to the mechanism described by Trelles et al., a partial epidermal window is opened with the Er: YAG laser in the first shot, and the partial epidermis and dermis layers are irradiated with the second non-ablative CO_2 laser shot. With the third Er: YAG shot, the partial epidermis layer is ablated, the dermis is exposed, and a coagulation and denaturation pattern is created in the dermis by irradiating the exposed dermis layer with the non-ablative CO_2 laser with 50% overlap with this shot. Thus, step-by-step shots provide minimal and deep residual thermal damage and reduce adverse effects [73].

The balanced progression of the inflammatory process completes wound healing. Excessive inflammation causes increased angiogenesis and prolonged clinical erythema. In addition, nonviable tissue at the wound site prolongs inflammation. Goldman et al. used the Er: YAG laser to remove residual tissue after the CO_2 laser because of its minimal thermal effect. Thus, although there was no difference in wrinkle improvement with a single treatment, inflammation and vascularization are decreased [74]. In a study by Utley et al., after 1 week of laser treatment, less collagen damage and thermal necrosis were observed in CO_2 laser treatments, followed by Er: YAG and Er: YAG alone, compared to Er: YAG treatments, followed by CO_2 and CO_2 alone. The similarity of thermal necrosis and collagen damage in CO_2 laser treatments followed by Er: YAG and Er: YAG alone was attributed to the partial removal of necrosis tissue after CO_2 laser by Er: YAG [75]. In the study conducted by Greene et al., after 4–6 months of treatment, they achieved the most extended recovery period with the CO_2 laser alone, the shortest with the Er: YAG laser alone, and an intermediate recovery period with the CO_2/Er: YAG combination [76].

Histologically, the amount of collagen doubles approximately 3 months after the treatment with the combination of Er: YAG and CO_2 laser. Although the increase in the amount of collagen is similar to that achieved with the CO_2 laser alone, minimal thermal damage is achieved compared to the CO_2 laser alone [77]. Long-term neo collagen density and thickness were reported to be highest in the CO_2 laser alone, least in the Er: YAG laser alone, and intermediate in the CO_2 and Er: YAG combination [76].

The patients found the CO_2/Er: YAG laser combination more satisfactory in normalizing skin texture and color than the Er: YAG laser alone. Clinically, the degree of improvement in skin texture and wrinkles was higher in combination therapy [78].

42.4 Patient Selection

Patient selection plays a vital role in the success of laser treatment. While non-motion-related rhytids in the periorbital and perioral areas respond better to laser therapy, movement-related rhytids in the glabella and forehead areas are less responsive [79]. Fitzpatrick type 1–3 is the most suitable skin type for most laser treatments [80]. In a pilot study, fractional CO_2 laser was safe in Fitzpatrick type 4–5 skin types [81]. While Er: YAG laser is preferred in patients with superficial dyspigmentation and darker skin, the CO_2 laser is more suitable for diffuse lentigines and more severe dyspigmentation [4].

Laser therapy should be avoided in pregnant and breast-feeding patients. Due to the hormonally increased risk of hyperpigmentation, patients receiving estrogen therapy should be warned before treatment. In pediatric patients, low-energy fractional CO_2 laser causes less pain and can effectively treat hypertrophic scars [82]. In prolonged topical or systemic steroid use, immunological deficiencies, and collagen vascular diseases, skin healing may be delayed, and even atrophic scarring may develop after laser treatment [4]. Patients should be questioned in terms of postinflammatory hyperpigmentation history, hypertrophic scar and keloid susceptibility, and retinoid use. There are debates about stopping the use of retinoids 6–12 months before laser treatment or not discontinuing the use of them [83]. Laser ablation should be avoided in patients with Koebnerizing skin diseases (such as vitiligo, lichen planus, and psoriasis) and epilepsy [32, 84].

42.5 Adverse Effects and Complications

42.5.1 Erythema

Erythema is one of the most common adverse effects of laser therapy. Unless erythema is prolonged, it should be considered the usual effect of laser therapy. Especially in CO_2 laser treatment, erythema is common because more thermal damage is created in the dermis. There may be an increase in erythema within 1–3 days after laser treatment. Erythema may resolve in 1 day if low power is used, whereas erythema may last longer than 1 week at high power settings and dwell times. Persistent erythema is defined as erythema lasting longer than 6 months. Intense erythema should be treated with potent topical steroids, which may herald scar formation. In addition, topical ascorbic acid can reduce erythema due to its anti-inflammatory effect. Vitamin C can be used after epithelialization, as there will be more erythema due to its irritant effect [23, 85].

42.5.2 Postinflammatory Hyperpigmentation

Transient postinflammatory hyperpigmentation is the most common side effect. It is seen in 33% of all patients and almost all with Fitzpatrick type 4–6 skin type [85]. It is more common in darker skin tones. It is seen in 5% of the periorbital area and 17–83% of other facial areas after CO_2 resurfacing. Hyperpigmentation can be seen within 3–6 weeks after treatment. Applying hydroquinone compounds, light glycolic acid peels, and glycolic, azelaic, or retinoid acid creams after treatment accelerates the improvement of hyperpigmentation [79]. Its incidence was significantly reduced using fractional laser therapy instead of full-field laser therapy [86]. Short-term application of topical corticosteroids after ablative laser therapy reduces the risk of postinflammatory hyperpigmentation [87]. Avoiding sunlight for several weeks before and after treatment and starting sunscreen with an anti-inflammatory agent after laser treatment is essential in reducing the risk of postinflammatory hyperpigmentation [86, 88]. It has also been reported that fusidic acid is superior to erythromycin cream in reducing the risk of PIH [89].

42.5.3 Hypopigmentation

Hypopigmentation is a delayed side effect that occurs more than 6 months after treatment and is difficult to treat [79]. It occurs due to the interruption of melanogenesis due to irreversible damage to melanocytes. True hypopigmentation is rare and is associated with previous dermabrasion and phenol peeling treatments or aggressive laser therapy [85].

42.5.4 Infection

The risk of viral, bacterial, and fungal infections is high in the first week until epithelialization is complete [85]. Despite antiviral prophylaxis, herpes infection is seen in 2–7% of cases after laser treatment [79]. The risk of bacterial infection after laser treatment is 0.1% [90]. The most common bacterial agents are S. aureus and Pseudomonas, and the most common fungal agents are Candida species. Signs of infection are acute-onset pain, burning, or itching. Other signs include erythema, crusting, exudation, and pustular lesions [91].

Contrary to the commonly used antiviral prophylaxis, the benefit of using antibacterial drugs after laser treatment has not been proven. Instead, antibacterial therapy should be used if infection is suspected because there is a risk of systemic disease and scarring. Oral tetracycline-based antibiotics can be used for moderate to severe acne flares [79]. The frequency of fungal infection is 0–1.2%. Since cutaneous candidiasis can be confused with acne and milia, its diagnosis is difficult. Therefore, patients should be questioned in terms of diseases that predispose to candidiasis, such as diabetes, angular cheilitis, immunosuppression, or vaginal candidiasis. Topical or systemic fluconazole can be used in its treatment [85, 86].

42.5.5 Scar

Scar formation can be seen between 2 and 4 weeks after laser treatment. While it can be seen in 2–4% of all laser treatments, it has been reported to decrease to 0% after fractional CO_2 laser [49, 86]. Scar formation occurs due to improper adjustment of laser parameters or overlapping laser pulses [79]. Areas such as the infraorbital region, mandible, or anterior neck should be treated cautiously as they have less pilosebaceous unit and less vascularity and are more prone to scar formation. Post-treatment wound infection and contact dermatitis may cause scarring [85, 92].

42.5.6 Acne Flare

Increased sebum production due to aberrant follicular re-epithelialization and thermal damage to the pilosebaceous unit may trigger acne formation [91]. There is a predisposition to acne exacerbation in the first week in patients with a history of acne and after 6 weeks in patients without a history of acne. Topical erythromycin, clindamycin, tretinoin, glycolic acid, or azelaic acid can be used in its treatment [85].

References

1. Eller JJ, Wolff S. Skin peeling and scarification: in treating pitted scars, pigmentations and specific facial blemishes. J Am Med Assoc. 1941;116:934–8.
2. Brody HJ, Monheit GD, Resnik SS, Alt TH. A history of chemical peeling. Dermatol Surg. 2000;26:405–9.
3. Bertossi D, Giampaoli G, Lucchese A, et al. The skin rejuvenation-associated treatment: fraxel laser, microbotox, and low G prime hyaluronic acid: preliminary results. Laser Med Sci. 2019;34:1449–55.
4. Agrawal N, Smith G, Heffelfinger R. Ablative skin resurfacing. Facial Plast Surg. 2014;30:55–61.
5. Einstein A. Zur quantentheorie der strahlung. Phys Z. 1917;18:121–8.
6. Maiman T. Stimulated optical radiation in ruby. Nature. 1960;187:493–4.
7. Goldman L, Blaney DJ, Kindel DJ, et al. Pathology of the effect of the laser beam on the skin. Nature. 1963;197:912–4.
8. Patel CKN. Selective excitation through vibrational energy transfer and optical maser action in N2-CO_2. Phys Rev Lett. 1964;13:617–9.
9. Stellar S, Polanyi TG. Lasers in neurosurgery: a historical overview. J Clin Laser Med Sur. 1992;10:399–411.

10. Bernstein LJ, Kauvar AN, Grossman MC, Geronemus RG. The short- and long-term side effects of carbon dioxide laser resurfacing. Dermatol Surg. 1997;23:519–25.
11. Apfelberg DB, Maser MR, Lash H, Rivers J. The argon laser for cutaneous lesions. JAMA. 1981;245:2073–5.
12. Olbricht SM, Stern RS, Tang SV, et al. Complications of cutaneous laser surgery: a survey. Arch Dermatol. 1987;123:345–9.
13. Anderson RR, Parrish JA. Selective photothermolysis: precise microsurgery by selective absorption of pulsed radiation. Science. 1983;220:524–7.
14. Parrish JA, Anderson RR, Harrist T, et al. Selective thermal effects with pulsed irradiation from lasers: from organ to organelle. J Invest Dermatol. 1983;80:75–80.
15. Tanzi EL, Lupton JR, Alster TS. Lasers in dermatology: four decades of progress. J Am Acad Dermatol. 2003;49:1–34.
16. Ho DD, London R, Zimmerman GB, Young DA. Laser-tattoo removal—a study of the mechanism and the optimal treatment strategy via computer simulations. Laser Surg Med. 2002;30:389–97.
17. Manstein D, Herron GS, Sink RK, et al. Fractional photothermolysis: a new concept for cutaneous remodeling using microscopic patterns of thermal injury. Laser Surg Med. 2004;34:426–38.
18. Scheuer JF, Costa CR, Dauwe PB, et al. Laser resurfacing at the time of rhytidectomy. Plast Reconstr Surg. 2015;136:27–38.
19. Sandel HD, Perkins SW. CO_2 laser resurfacing: still a good treatment. Aesthet Surg J. 2008;28:456–62.
20. Clementoni MT, Pedrelli V, Zaccaria G, et al. New developments for fractional co 2 resurfacing for skin rejuvenation and scar reduction. Facial Plast Surg Clin North Am. 2020;28:17–28.
21. Trelles MA, Mordon S, Svaasand LO, et al. The origin and role of erythema after carbon dioxide laser resurfacing. Dermatol Surg. 1998;24:25–9.
22. Trelles MA, Shohat M, Urdiales F. Safe and effective one-session fractional skin resurfacing using a carbon dioxide laser device in super-pulse mode: a clinical and histologic study. Aesthet Plast Surg. 2011;35:31–42.
23. Alexiades-Armenakas MR, Dover JS, Arndt KA. Fractional laser skin resurfacing. J Drugs Dermatol. 2012;11:1274–87.
24. Hessler J, Trujillo O. Combining laser resurfacing and facial rejuvenation surgery. Facial Plast Surg. 2021;37:233–9.
25. Walia S, Alster TS. Prolonged clinical and histologic effects from co_2 laser resurfacing of atrophic acne scars. Dermatol Surg. 1999;25:926–30.
26. Nowak KC, McCormack M, Koch RJ. The effect of superpulsed carbon dioxide laser energy on keloid and normal dermal fibroblast secretion of growth factors: a serum-free study. Plast Reconstr Surg. 2000;105:2039–48.
27. Aal AMA, Ibrahim IM, Sami NA, Kareem IMA. Evaluation of autologous platelet-rich plasma plus ablative carbon dioxide fractional laser in the treatment of acne scars. J Cosmet Laser Ther. 2017;20:106–13.
28. Abdel-Maguid EM, Awad SM, Hassan YS, et al. Efficacy of stem cell-conditioned medium vs. platelet-rich plasma as an adjuvant to ablative fractional CO_2 laser resurfacing for atrophic post-acne scars: a split-face clinical trial. J Dermatol Treat. 2019;32:1–24.
29. Prignano F, Campolmi P, Bonan P, et al. Fractional CO_2 laser: a novel therapeutic device upon photobiomodulation of tissue remodeling and cytokine pathway of tissue repair. Dermatol Ther. 2009;22:8–15.
30. Wright EJ, Struck SK. Facelift combined with simultaneous fractional laser resurfacing: outcomes and complications. J Plast Reconstr Aesthet Surg. 2015;68:1332–7.
31. Glaser DA, Semchyshyn NL, Carniol PJ. Carbon dioxide laser resurfacing, fractionated resurfacing and YSGG resurfacing. In: Carniol PJ, Sadick NS, editors. Clinical procedures in laser skin rejuvenation. CRC Press; 2007. p. 27.
32. Brightman LA, Brauer JA, Anolik R, et al. Ablative and fractional ablative lasers. Dermatol Clin. 2009;27:479–89.

33. Carniol PJ, Hamilton MM, Carniol ET. Current status of fractional laser resurfacing. JAMA Facial Plast Surg. 2015;17:360–6.
34. Clementoni MT, Galimberti M, Tourlaki A, et al. Random fractional ultrapulsed CO_2 resurfacing of photodamaged facial skin: long-term evaluation. Laser Med Sci. 2013;28:643–50.
35. Rahman Z, MacFalls H, Jiang K, et al. Fractional deep dermal ablation induces tissue tightening. Laser Surg Med. 2009;41:78–86.
36. Walgrave SE, Ortiz AE, MacFalls HT, et al. Evaluation of a novel fractional resurfacing device for treatment of acne scarring. Laser Surg Med. 2009;41:122–7.
37. Katz B. Efficacy of a new fractional CO_2 laser in the treatment of photodamage and acne scarring. Dermatol Ther. 2010;23:403–6.
38. de Filippi Sartori J, Osaki TH, Osaki MH, et al. "Split-face" evaluation of collagen changes induced by periorbital fractional CO_2 laser resurfacing. Aesthet Surg J. 2021;42:239–48.
39. Karsai S, Czarnecka A, Jünger M, Raulin C. Ablative fractional lasers (CO_2 and Er:YAG): a randomized controlled double-blind split-face trial of the treatment of peri-orbital rhytides. Laser Surg Med. 2010;42:160–7.
40. Kohl E, Meierhöfer J, Koller M, et al. Fractional carbon dioxide laser resurfacing of rhytides and photoaged skin – a prospective clinical study on patient expectation and satisfaction. Laser Surg Med. 2015;47:111–9.
41. Qu L, Liu A, Zhou L, et al. Clinical and molecular effects on mature burn scars after treatment with a fractional CO_2 laser. Laser Surg Med. 2012;44:517–24.
42. Hultman CS, Edkins RE, Wu C, et al. Prospective, before-after cohort study to assess the efficacy of laser therapy on hypertrophic burn scars. Ann Plas Surg. 2013;70:521–6.
43. Tan J, Zhou J, Huang L, et al. Hypertrophic scar improvement by early intervention with ablative fractional carbon dioxide laser treatment. Laser Surg Med. 2021;53:450–7.
44. Azzam OA, Bassiouny DA, El-Hawary MS, et al. Treatment of hypertrophic scars and keloids by fractional carbon dioxide laser: a clinical, histological, and immunohistochemical study. Laser Med Sci. 2016;31:9–18.
45. El-Zawahry BM, Sobhi RM, Bassiouny DA, Tabak SA. Ablative CO_2 fractional resurfacing in treatment of thermal burn scars: an open-label controlled clinical and histopathological study. J Cosmet Dermatol. 2015;14:324–31.
46. Chapas AM, Brightman L, Sukal S, et al. Successful treatment of acneiform scarring with CO_2 ablative fractional resurfacing. Laser Surg Med. 2008;40:381–6.
47. Samuthrsindh K, Helbig D, Paasch U, et al. Prospective, uncontrolled examination of ablative fractional photothermolysis on Asian and Caucasian skin. Med Laser Appl. 2011;26:3–9.
48. Shamsaldeen O, Peterson JD, Goldman MP. The adverse events of deep fractional CO_2: a retrospective study of 490 treatments in 374 patients. Laser Surg Med. 2011;43:453–6.
49. Hunzeker CM, Weiss ET, Geronemus RG. Fractionated CO_2 laser resurfacing: our experience with more than 2000 treatments. Aesthet Surg J. 2009;29:317–22.
50. Sriprachya-Anunt S, Fitzpatrick RE, Goldman MP, Smith SR. Infections complicating pulsed carbon dioxide laser resurfacing for photoaged facial skin. Dermatol Surg. 1997;23:527–35.
51. Hantash BM, Bedi VP, Chan KF, Zachary CB. Ex vivo histological characterization of a novel ablative fractional resurfacing device. Laser Surg Med. 2007;39:87–95.
52. Li B, Ren K, Yin X, et al. Efficacy and adverse reactions of fractional CO_2 laser for atrophic acne scars and related clinical factors: a retrospective study on 121 patients. J Cosmet Dermatol. 2022;21:1989–97. https://doi.org/10.1111/jocd.14868.
53. Lee JW, Kim BJ, Kim MN, Mun SK. The efficacy of autologous platelet rich plasma combined with ablative carbon dioxide fractional resurfacing for acne scars: a simultaneous split-face trial. Dermatol Surg. 2011;37:931–8.
54. Gawdat HI, Hegazy RA, Fawzy MM, Fathy M. Autologous platelet rich plasma: topical versus intradermal after fractional ablative carbon dioxide laser treatment of atrophic acne scars. Dermatol Surg. 2014;40:152–61.
55. Wu N, Sun H, Sun Q, et al. A meta-analysis of fractional CO_2 laser combined with PRP in the treatment of acne scar. Laser Med Sci. 2021;36:1–12.

56. Perez MI, Bank DE, Silvers D. Skin resurfacing of the face with the Erbium:YAG laser. Dermatol Surg. 1998;24:653–9.
57. Sanniec K, Afrooz PN, Burns AJ. Long-term assessment of perioral rhytide correction with erbium. Plast Reconstr Surg. 2019;143:64–74.
58. Goldberg DJ, Meine JG. Treatment of photoaged neck skin with the pulsed Erbium:YAG laser. Dermatol Surg. 1998;24:619–21.
59. Alster TS. Cutaneous resurfacing with CO_2 and Erbium: YAG lasers: preoperative, intraoperative, and postoperative considerations. Plast Reconstr Surg. 1999;103:619–32.
60. Brauer JA, Patel U, Hale EK. Laser skin resurfacing, chemical peels, and other cutaneous treatments of the brow and upper lid. Clin Plast Surg. 2013;40:91–9.
61. El-Domyati M, Abd-El-Raheem T, Abdel-Wahab H, et al. Fractional versus ablative erbium:yttrium-aluminum-garnet laser resurfacing for facial rejuvenation: an objective evaluation. J Am Acad Dermatol. 2013;68:103–12.
62. Keyal U, Huang X, Bhatta A. Laser treatment for post acne scars – a review. Nepal J Med Sci. 2013;2:165–70.
63. Khatri KA, Machado A, Magro C, Davenport S. Laser peel: facial rejuvenation with a superficial erbium:YAG laser treatment. J Cutan Laser Ther. 2009;2:119–23.
64. Pozner JN, Goldberg DJ. Superficial erbium:YAG laser resurfacing of photodamaged skin. J Cosmet Laser Ther. 2009;8:89–91.
65. Jasin ME. Achieving superior resurfacing results with the erbium:YAG laser. Arch Facial Plast Surg. 2002;4:262–6.
66. Medved F, Wurm A, Held M. Facial microcirculatory and biomechanical skin properties after single high energy (Er):YAG laser application. Laser Surg Med. 2017;49:891–8.
67. Hersant B, SidAhmed-Mezi M, Chossat A, Meningaud JP. Multifractional microablative laser combined with spatially modulated ablative (SMA) technology for facial skin rejuvenation. Laser Surg Med. 2017;49:78–83.
68. Castro DJ, Abergel RP, Johnston KJ, et al. Wound healing: biological effects of Nd:YAG laser on collagen metabolism in pig skin in comparison to thermal burn. Ann Plas Surg. 1983;11:131–40.
69. Weinstein C. Erbium laser resurfacing: current concepts. Plast Reconstr Surg. 1999;103:602–16.
70. Ross EV, Swann M, Soon S, et al. Full-face treatments with the 2790-nm erbium:YSGG laser system. J Drugs Dermatol. 2009;8:248–52.
71. Lee JW, Kim BJ, Kim MN, Lee CK. Treatment of periorbital wrinkles using a 2,790-nm yttrium scandium gallium garnet laser. Dermatol Surg. 2010;36:1382–9.
72. Trelles MA, García-Solana L, Calderhead RG. Skin resurfacing improved with a new dual wavelength Er:YAG/CO_2 laser system: a comparative study. J Clin Laser Med Surg. 1999;17:99–104.
73. Trelles MA, Allones I, Luna R. One-pass resurfacing with a combined-mode erbium: YAG/ CO_2 laser system: a study in 102 patients. Br J Dermatol. 2002;146:473–80.
74. Goldman MP, Manuskiatti W. Combined laser resurfacing with the 950-microsec pulsed CO2 + Er:YAG lasers. Dermatologic Surg. 1999;25:160–3.
75. Utley DS, Koch RJ, Egbert BM. Histologic analysis of the thermal effect on epidermal and dermal structures following treatment with the superpulsed CO_2 laser and the Erbium:YAG laser: an in vivo study. Laser Surg Med. 1999;24:93–102.
76. Greene D, Egbert BM, Utley DS, Koch RJ. In vivo model of histologic changes after treatment with the superpulsed CO_2 laser, Erbium:YAG laser, and blended lasers: a 4- to 6-month prospective histologic and clinical study. Laser Surg Med. 2000;27:362–72.
77. Goldman MP, Marchell N, Fitzpatrick RE. Laser skin resurfacing of the face with a combined CO_2/Er:YAG laser. Dermatologic Surg. 2000;26:102–4.
78. Goldman MP, Marchell NL. Laser resurfacing of the neck with the combined CO_2/Er:YAG laser. Dermatologic Surg. 1999;25:923–5.
79. Alster TS, Doshi S. Laser skin resurfacing. In: Burgess CM, editor. Cosmetic dermatology. Heidelberg: Springer; 2005.

80. Allemann IB, Kaufman J. Fractional photothermolysis—an update. Laser Med Sci. 2010;25:137–44.
81. Tan KL, Kurniawati C, Gold MH. Low risk of postinflammatory hyperpigmentation in skin types 4 and 5 after treatment with fractional CO_2 laser device. J Drugs Dermatol. 2008;7:774–7.
82. Won T, Ma Q, Chen Z, et al. The efficacy and safety of low-energy carbon dioxide fractional laser use in the treatment of early-stage pediatric hypertrophic scars: a prospective, randomized, split-scar study. Laser Surg Med. 2022;54:230–6.
83. Tannous Z. Fractional resurfacing. Clin Dermatol. 2007;25:480–6.
84. Buzina DS, Lipozenčić J, Mokos ZB, et al. Ablative laser resurfacing: is it still the gold standard for facial rejuvenation? Acta Dermatovenerol Croat. 2010;18:190–4.
85. Alster TS, Lupton JR. Treatment of complications of laser skin resurfacing. Arch Facial Plast Surg. 2000;2:279–84.
86. Hamilton MM, Kao R. Recognizing and managing complications in laser resurfacing, chemical peels, and dermabrasion. Facial Plast Surg Clin North Am. 2020;28:493–501.
87. Cheyasak N, Manuskiatti W, Maneeprasopchoke P, Wanitphakdeedecha R. Topical corticosteroids minimise the risk of postinflammatory hyperpigmentation after ablative fractional co_2 laser resurfacing in Asians. Acta Dermatol Venereol. 2015;95:201–5.
88. Wanitphakdeedecha R, Phuardchantuk R, Manuskiatti W. The use of sunscreen starting on the first day after ablative fractional skin resurfacing. J Eur Acad Dermatol. 2014;28:1522–8.
89. Wei M, Li L, Zhang XF, et al. Fusidic acid cream comparatively minimizes signs of inflammation and postinflammatory hyperpigmentation after ablative fractional CO_2 laser resurfacing in Chinese patients: a randomized controlled trial. J Cosmet Dermatol. 2021;20:1692–9.
90. Metelitsa AI, Alster TS. Fractionated laser skin resurfacing treatment complications: a review. Dermatologic Surg. 2010;36:299–306.
91. Chwalek J, Goldberg DJ. Ablative skin resurfacing. Curr Probl Dermatol. 2011;42:40–7.
92. Aslam A, Alster TS. Evolution of laser skin resurfacing. Dermatologic Surg. 2014;40:1163–72.

Hypertrophic Scar, Keloid, and Their Treatment

43

Neslihan Sari, Nuray Bayar Muluk, and J. Regan Thomas

43.1 Introduction

Keloidal scars (KS) and hypertrophic scars (HTS) cause cosmetic issues, physical impairment, and psychological and social challenges [1, 2]. Both KS and HTS result from abnormal fibrous wound healing in response to trauma, surgery, inflammation, and burns, stemming from a lack of regulation in wound healing mechanisms. They occur in 30–90% of patients. Both types are raised, firm scars formed from excessive production of fibrinogen and collagen during the healing process. Symptoms like pruritus, pain, and pressure are associated with KS and HTS, but the primary concern is aesthetic disfigurement [3]. While they both display the same inflammatory fibroproliferative process, differences exist between HTS and KS. HTS remains confined to the injury site and may regress over time, whereas KS extends beyond the initial injury borders and does not typically regress. On histological examination, HTS typically exhibits hypertrophic collagen in a wavy pattern, while KS lacks a distinct collagen pattern, featuring thick and uniformly stained collagen fibers known as keloidal or hyalinized collagen [4] (Fig. 43.1).

N. Sari (✉)
Department of Otorhinolaryngology, Mardin Training and Research Hospital, Mardin, Turkey

N. Bayar Muluk
Faculty of Medicine, Department of Otorhinolaryngology, Kırıkkale University, Kırıkkale, Türkiye

J. R. Thomas
University of New Mexico School of Medicine, Albuquerque, NM, USA

C. Cingi et al. (eds.), *Minor Interventions, Major Outcomes on the Face*, Comprehensive ENT, https://doi.org/10.1007/978-3-032-01305-7_43

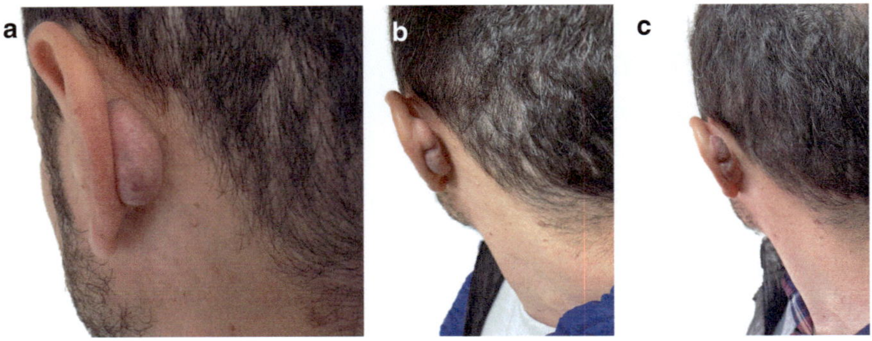

Fig. 43.1 (**a**) The keloid was seen on the posterior surface of the auricle of a 31-year-old male after conchal cartilage harvesting for rhinoplasty. That patient had a previous surgical excision of a skin lesion, but the keloid recurred. (**b**) The patient used silicon-containing cream and two-dose cryotherapy one month apart. (**c**) The early period after the cryotherapy session

43.2 Incidence

Genetic, systemic, local, and lifestyle factors contribute to the formation, intensity, and duration of HTS/KS. HTS and KS peak during the second and third decades, presenting with equal gender distribution [5]. This phenomenon is thought to be due to increased turnover in younger populations, elevated collagen production, and a more active immune system [6, 7]. Genetic factors are more significant in KS formation. The incidence in darker-pigmented populations ranges from 4.5% to 16%. The highest prevalence occurs in the African population, followed by Asian and Hispanic populations, and less frequently in Caucasians. A positive family history is strongly associated with KS formation, although no specific gene has been identified. Rare genetic syndromes, including Rubinstein-Taybi and Goeminne syndromes [8], can increase the risk of developing KS [8]. Systemic factors include hormonal influences, hypertension, and high levels of circulating inflammatory cytokines [9, 10]. An increased incidence of KS formation is observed during puberty and pregnancy, with a reduction in size during menopause [8]. Juvenile-onset KS shows female predominance [11]. Additionally, a higher incidence of hyperimmunoglobulin E and allergic symptoms has been noted in KS-affected patients compared to those with HTS, suggesting a role for mast cells in etiopathogenesis. An association with blood type A has also been observed. Local factors involve mechanical stress on wounds or scars [10]. Although genetic predisposition is not as prominent in HTS, it is more common among individuals with darker complexions. HTS tends to occur in areas of skin that are subject to stretching due to increased tension [6]. Reports indicate that the incidence of developing HTS is between 40% and 70% following a surgical procedure and between 33% and 91% after burns [7] (Fig. 43.2).

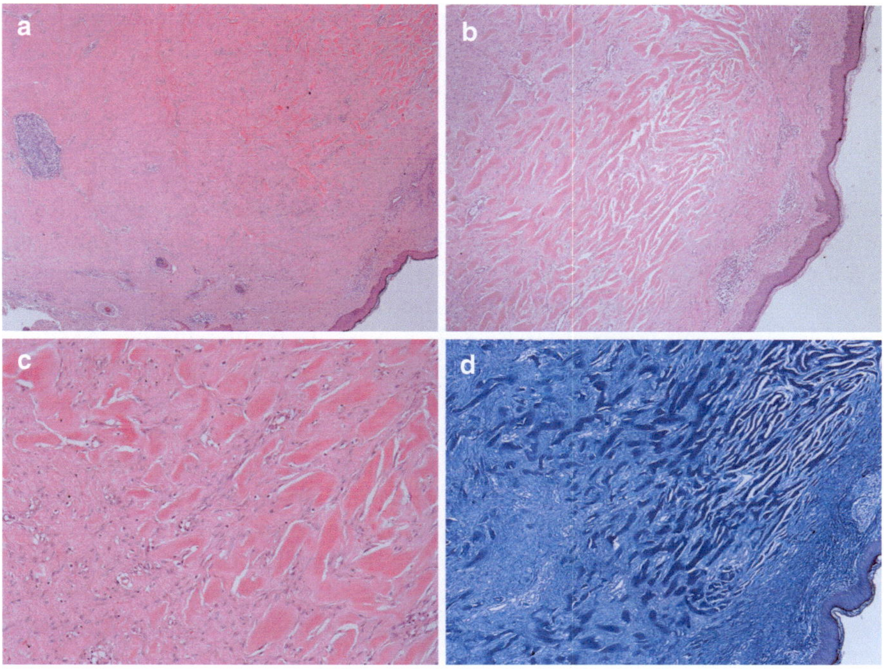

Fig. 43.2 (**a**) Hematoxylin and eosin staining of keloid tissue in the patient seen above demonstrates the abundant collagen deposition within the dermis and the presence of the keloid-associated lymphoid tissues containing micro-vessels and inflammatory cells (H&E, 10X). (**b**) At higher magnification; keloidal collagen is clearly seen (H&E, 20X). (**c**) Keloidal collagen are seen at 40hpf on hematoxylin and eosin (H&E, 40X). (**d**) On Masson's trichrome, collagen bundles are well demarcated and disorganized, involving two-thirds of the dermis with a normal appearance of papillary dermis and epidermis

43.3 Clinical Characteristics

HTS do not grow outside the area of the original wound, whereas KS grow laterally beyond the border of the wound. In clinical practice, many lesions exhibit intermediate growth and appearance characteristics that make it difficult to determine whether they are KS or HTS [4]. Generally, HTS occurs with injury within 4–8 weeks and has rapid growth for up to 6 months, then regresses, eventually leading to a flat scar with no symptoms. HTS scar formation is rare after the excision of the original lesion. KS tends to recur following excision. KS appears as firm, mildly tender, bosselated tumors with a shiny surface and sometimes telangiectasia with focal areas of ulceration. The borders of the tumor are well demarcated but irregular in outline. HTS has a similar appearance but is usually linear if following a surgical scar or papular or nodular, following inflammatory and ulcerating lesions. Both lesions are commonly pruritic, but KS may even cause significant pain and hyperesthesia. HTS has no predilection sites (but commonly occurs in extensor surfaces), whereas predominant anatomic sites, anterior chest, shoulders, earlobes, upper arms, and cheeks, have a higher predilection for KS formation [5, 12, 13].

43.4 Pathophysiology

Wound healing occurs in three phases: inflammation, proliferation, and remodeling. After a wound occurs, platelet degranulation, activation, and clotting cascades form a fibrin plug. Platelet degranulation releases various growth factors that act as chemotactic agents, recruiting neutrophils, macrophages, epithelial cells, mast cells, and fibroblasts. This first phase lasts 48–72 h. Next, the proliferative phase endures for up to 3–6 weeks. Recruited fibroblasts synthesize reparative tissue. This granulation tissue consists of procollagen, elastin, proteoglycans, and hyaluronic acid, forming a repair framework that facilitates vascular ingrowth. Modified fibroblasts, which contain actin filaments, initiate wound contraction. Once the wound is closed, the immature scar transitions into the final maturation phase, which lasts several months. The abundant extracellular matrix is degraded, and immature type 3 collagen transforms into mature type 1 collagen. In HTS and KS, there is a disruption of the fundamental process of wound healing, caused by a dysfunction in the underlying regulatory mechanism that leads to persistent inflammation, excessive collagen synthesis, or deficient matrix degradation and remodeling, resulting in an imbalance between anabolic and catabolic phases, although KS is more sustained and aggressive [5].

43.5 Histopathology of HTS and KS

In HTS and KS, the epidermis and papillary dermis have normal structures. HTS has dermal nodules with more collagen fibers running in different directions. But KS contains thick and uniformly stained collagen fibers called keloidal or hyalinized collagen. Keloidal collagen distinguishes HTS and KS. The absolute keloidal collagen threshold is not known to accurately distinguish two lesions. Another feature of KS is that it shows strong inflammation in the dermis at the place where the lesion meets healthy skin [4].

43.6 Prevention

Avoiding all unnecessary wounds and surgical manipulations in any patient, regardless of whether they are prone to KS/HTS, is the ideal approach to preventing pathological scarring. Achieving rapid epithelialization within 10–14 days is essential to minimize excessive scarring. Wounds under tension due to movement, body location, or tissue loss carry a higher risk of scarring. In the case of a cutaneous injury, promptly closing wounds with minimal or no tension is crucial. Debridement of contaminated wounds, adequate hemostasis, gentle handling of tissues, and limiting foreign bodies, such as debris and braided polyfilamentous sutures like polyglactin or silk, are necessary. Adequate tissue nutrition should be ensured through diet [13, 14]. Mid-chest incisions should be avoided, and incisions should follow the natural lines of the skin. In head and neck surgery, the aesthetic subunits of the face must be considered when selecting incision sites. In facial procedures, subcutaneous sutures should be applied only when necessary. Wound healing and the aesthetic outcome of scar formation can be improved through massage or the application of a greasy ointment.

Pressure therapy, silicone gel sheeting, and flavonoid (quercetin and kaempferol) containing scar creams are used for prophylaxis. Imiquimod 5% cream, a topical immunoresponse modifier, is used in the treatment of genital warts, basal cell carcinoma, and actinic keratoses. It increases collagen breakdown and alters the expression of apoptosis-associated genes. It positively affects KS in the postoperative period [5].

43.7 Treatment

Most therapeutic approaches may be used for both HTS and KS. However, distinguishing between HTS and KS is important before initiating any treatment [5]. The Japan Scar Workshop (JSW) scar scale (JSS) is a diagnostic algorithm for KS, HTS, and mature scars. Mature scars have a score of 5 or less, while scores between 6 and 15 indicate HTS, and scores of 16 or more indicate KS. KS should be treated in specialized medical facilities with combination therapies due to a high likelihood of resistance to treatment [4].

43.7.1 Surgery

For complicated wounds and delayed closure in HS, simple excision is utilized. For Z and W, plasty results in wide scars, excision, and narrowing of the scar, altering the scar's direction. Z-plasty aims to extend the reduced wound distance and align the central axis of the scar parallel to skin creases. Z-plasty is preferred for hypertrophic scars crossing joints or wrinkle creases at a right angle. For facial scars, W-plasty is favored because every scar can be oriented along skin creases when it is shifted. In facial surgery, full-thickness skin grafts or composite fat-skin grafts serve as alternatives to achieve wound closure with minimal tension. The preferred donor sites for facial grafts are the retroauricular and preauricular areas, as well as the neck and upper lip [3].

Excision is not recommended as monotherapy for keloids due to the high recurrence rate, which ranges from 45% to 100%. Therefore, intramarginal surgical excision of a keloid is advised to avoid stimulating collagen synthesis. Surgical therapy should be accompanied by adjuvant treatments such as pressure, corticosteroids, and radiotherapy [15].

43.7.2 Pressure

Pressure therapy has been used for decades to treat KS and HTS. Several hypotheses exist regarding its mechanism of action. By decreasing oxygen levels in the tissues, it reduces perfusion and collagen synthesis. Additionally, pressure is thought to increase apoptosis, decrease scar hydration, stabilize mast cells, and reduce angiogenesis [16]. In rehabilitation centers, manual or mechanical massage therapy is employed to treat scars and burns [13].

43.7.3 Topical Silicone Gel

It serves as a first-line therapy for minor KS and HTS [17]. The proposed mechanism of action enhances hydration and creates an occlusive environment that regulates fibroblasts and decreases collagen synthesis [18, 19]. Silicone is applied as a cream, spray, gel cushion, or sheeting [20]. Two weeks after primary wound closure, a duration of 12–24 h is recommended for 2–3 months [15].

43.7.4 Laser Therapy

The most commonly used lasers in scar management are the pulsed-dye laser (PDL) and fractional lasers. Combining treatments with intralesional medications and laser therapy is utilized for HS and KS. KS is more resistant to standard therapies; therefore, other modalities should be considered [21]. However, the most promising option is PDL. It may require 2–6 treatments to achieve improved scar resolution. Its mechanism of action involves causing local ischemia by destroying blood vessels, promoting neo-collagenesis, dissociating disulfide bonds in collagen for realignment, and reducing fibroblast proliferation. Side effects can include hyper or hypopigmentation and postoperative purpura [5].

43.7.5 Corticosteroids

Several corticosteroids are employed in scar management, including triamcinolone acetonide (TAC), hydrocortisone acetate, dexamethasone, and methylprednisolone, with TAC being the most widely used. Corticosteroid injections reduce fibroblast proliferation, collagen, and glycosaminoglycan synthesis while suppressing pro-inflammatory mediators. TAC can be used alone or in conjunction with other treatment modalities. Response rates to corticosteroid injections vary, showing regression rates of 50–100% after one year. The recurrence rate stands between 33 and 50% after 5 years. Potential side effects include telangiectasia, atrophy, steroid acne, pigmentary changes, necrosis, ulceration, systemic side effects, and pain at the injection site [22].

43.7.6 Botulinum Toxin

Botulinum toxin is a neurotoxin that temporarily induces flaccid paralysis of striated muscle for 2–6 months. Botox affects fibroblast activity and reduces tension around the scar through muscular chemo-immobilization [23].

43.7.7 Radiation

Superficial X-rays, electron beam therapy, and low- or high-dose-rate brachytherapy have been utilized for scar reduction with favorable results. The mechanism of action involves inhibiting neovascular buds and proliferating fibroblasts, which leads to reduced collagen synthesis. However, it must be administered with caution due to the risk of carcinogenesis, particularly in the breast and thyroid areas [5].

43.7.8 Cryotherapy

Cryotherapy causes vascular damage, resulting in tissue necrosis. It is used either as monotherapy or in conjunction with other treatment methods such as intralesional steroid injection. Various delivery methods for cryotherapy include spray, contact probes, and intralesional needle probes. Its side effects include hypopigmentation, blistering, pain, delayed healing, and infection. For larger lesions, multiple sessions are required. Intralesional cryotherapy for the treatment of KS shows favorable results in terms of volume reduction and alleviating complaints of pain and pruritus. However, complete scar eradication has not been established, and recurrences have been observed. The average decrease in scar volume ranged from 51% to 63% [24, 25].

43.7.9 5-Fluorouracil (5-FU)

5-FU, a pyrimidine analog, inhibits fibroblast proliferation, angiogenesis, and collagen synthesis. Intralesional 5-FU can be used alone or in combination with other forms of keloid treatments. Side effects include skin erythema, pain, and ulceration [26].

43.7.10 Tranilast

It has been identified as an anti-allergic agent used in allergic diseases. Additionally, it is used as an oral medication in the treatment of HTS/KS [4, 27].

43.7.11 Emerging Treatments

Stem cell therapy accelerates wound repair by enhancing migration, angiogenesis, and recapitalization through paracrine signaling. Mesenchymal stem cells secrete growth and differentiation factors that regulate the inflammatory and immune responses involved in wound healing. Fat grafting also improves scar appearance and supports tissue regeneration in burns with KS. Adipose stem cells can differentiate into various tissues, aiding in soft-tissue maturation and remodeling [15].

Verapamil is a calcium channel blocker that promotes the degradation of scar tissue by inducing pro-collagenase secretion. It has been employed in combination with intralesional steroid injections, cryotherapy, and PDL [28].

Interferons are cytokines; one of their functions is to reduce fibrosis, enhance healing, and lead to lower recurrence rates when used in combination therapies for KS.

Bleomycin, a chemotherapy agent, reduces collagen expression and increases apoptosis. It is administered via intralesional injection, dermojet injection, or tattooing to treat HTS and KS.

ACE inhibitors are commonly used to treat hypertension and inhibit the generation and action of Ang II in tissues. The local renin-angiotensin system has been shown to modulate collagen production and wound healing, playing a role in fibrotic diseases [15].

Imiquimod 5% cream, onion extract, and immunotherapy are used in the prevention and treatment of HTS and KS [3, 29].

References

1. Leventhal D, Furr M, Reiter D. Treatment of keloids and hypertrophic scars: a meta-analysis and review of the literature. Arch Facial Plast Surg. 2006;8:362–8.
2. Yuan FL, Sun ZL, Feng Y, et al. Epithelial-mesenchymal transition in the formation of hypertrophic scars and keloids. J Cell Physiol. 2019;234:21662–9.
3. Wolfram D, Tazankov A, Pülzl P, et al. Hypertrophic scars and keloids – a review of their pathophysiology, risk factors, and therapeutic management. Dermatol Surg. 2009;35:171–81.
4. Ogawa R, Akita S, Akaishi S, et al. Diagnosis and treatment of keloids and hypertrophic scars-Japan scar workshop consensus document 2018. Burns Trauma. 2019;27:1–39.
5. Gauglitz GG, Korting HC, Pavicic T, et al. Hypertrophic scarring and keloids: pathomechanisms and current and emerging treatment strategies. Mol Med. 2011;17:113–25.
6. Butzelaar L, Ulrich MM, Mink van der Molen AB, et al. Currently known risk factors for hypertrophic skin scarring: a review. J Plast Reconstr Aesthet Surg. 2016;69:163–9.
7. Mahdavian Delavary B, van der Veer WM, Ferreira JA, et al. Formation of hypertrophic scars: evolution and susceptibility. J Plast Surg Hand Surg. 2012;46:95–101.
8. Robles DT, Berg D. Abnormal wound healing: keloids. Clin Dermatol. 2007;25:26–32.
9. Ogawa R. Keloid and hypertrophic scars are the result of chronic inflammation in the reticular dermis. Int J Mol Sci. 2017;18:606.
10. Ogawa R, Dohi T, Tosa M. The latest strategy for keloid and hypertrophic scar prevention and treatment: the Nippon Medical School (NMS) Protocol. J Nippon Med Sch. 2021;88:2–9.
11. Noishiki C, Hayasaka Y, Ogawa R. Sex differences in keloidogenesis: an analysis of 1659 keloid patients in Japan. Dermatol Ther. 2019;9:747–54.

12. Glass DA 2nd. Current understanding of the genetic causes of keloid formation. J Investig Dermatol Symp Proc. 2017;18:S50–3.
13. Al A, Gauglitz G, Barret JP. Up-to-date approach to manage keloids and hypertrophic scars: a useful guide. Burns. 2014;40:1255–66.
14. Slemp AE, Kirschner RE. Keloids and scars: a review of keloids and scars, their pathogenesis, risk factors, and management. Curr Opin Pediatr. 2006;18:396–402.
15. Ojeh N, Bharatha A, Gaur U, et al. Keloids: current and emerging therapies. Scars Burn Heal. 2020;10:1–18.
16. Macintyre L, Baird M. Pressure garments for use in the treatment of hypertrophic scars – a review of the problems associated with their use. Burns. 2006;32:10–5.
17. Gold MH, McGuire M, Mustoe TA, et al. International Advisory Panel on Scar Management. Updated international clinical recommendations on scar management: Part 2 – Algorithms for scar prevention and treatment. Dermatol Surg. 2014;40:825–31.
18. Reish RG, Eriksson E. Scar treatments: preclinical and clinical studies. J Am Coll Surg. 2008;206:719–30.
19. Puri N, Talwar A. The efficacy of silicone gel for the treatment of hypertrophic scars and keloids. J Cutan Aesthet Surg. 2009;2:104–6.
20. Ud-Din S, Bayat A. New insights on keloids, hypertrophic scars, and striae. Dermatol Clin. 2014;32:193–209.
21. Khetarpal S, Kaw U, Dover JS, et al. Laser advances in the treatment of burn and traumatic scars. Semin Cutan Med Surg. 2017;36:185–91.
22. Morelli Coppola M, Salzillo R, Segreto F, et al. Triamcinolone acetonide intralesional injection for the treatment of keloid scars: patient selection and perspectives. Clin Cosmet Investig Dermatol. 2018;11:387–96.
23. Sohrabi C, Goutos I. The use of botulinum toxin in keloid scar management: a literature review. Scars Burn Heal. 2020;6:1–13.
24. Guix B, Henriquez I, Andrés A, et al. Treatment of keloids by high-dose-rate brachytherapy: a seven-year study. Int J Radiat Oncol Biol Phys. 2001;50:167–72.
25. van Leeuwen MC, Bulstra AE, Ket JC, et al. Intralesional cryotherapy for the treatment of keloid scars: evaluating effectiveness. Plast Reconstr Surg Glob Open. 2015;3:e437.
26. Khalid FA, Mehrose MY, Saleem M, et al. Comparison of efficacy and safety of intralesional triamcinolone and combination of triamcinolone with 5-fluorouracil in the treatment of keloids and hypertrophic scars: Randomised control trial. Burns. 2019;1:69–75.
27. Darakhshan S, Pour AB. Tranilast: a review of its therapeutic applications. Pharmacol Res. 2015;91:15–28.
28. Boggio RF, Boggio LF, Galvão BL, et al. Topical verapamil as a scar modulator. Aesthetic Plast Surg. 2014;38:968–75.
29. Zurada JM, Kriegel D, Davis IC. Topical treatments for hypertrophic scars. J Am Acad Dermatol. 2006;55:1024–31.

Part VIII

Oral Beauty and Dental Aesthetics

Beauty of the Face: Features of Male Teeth

44

Zeynep Çukurova Yılmaz and Nurcan Aksaka

44.1 Introduction

Cosmetic dentistry has always been part of daily dental practice. Therefore, changing the smile's appearance is one of the most common reasons presented to the dentist as part of the comprehensive treatment plan of an individual because aesthetics has built confidence and success in the present era. Male dental appearance has some different aesthetics from female dental aesthetics. In our society, the role of men is typically emphasized through their physical activities, while women are more related to attractiveness. Male facial and dental characteristics differ when compared to females to achieve the role of their life. For this rationale, the male teeth proportion and smile lines vary slightly from the female teeth proportions. Women are stereotypically shown to fit society's smile condition precisely, while men are notably shown more permissibly. Presently, society has shown a shift in the predominance of male-dominant traits. Several factors are responsible for the change in the appearance of the male smile, ultimately vitalizing confidence and making the individual successful. This chapter will assist the dentist in considering the effect of a male smile under the light of contemporary dental aesthetics to reflect on whether it is currently accepted or is just dictated by the dental concept of what appears to be a triumphant male smile. The objectives of this study were to analyze various factors affecting male teeth aesthetics. The futuristic view, recognition, and application of such factors may have positive consequences on male smile attitudes and thus present more acceptable male smile criteria in the future [1, 2].

Z. Çukurova Yılmaz (✉)
Dentoper Dental Clinic, Fethiye, Turkey

N. Aksaka
Faculty of Dentistry, Periodontology Department, Istanbul Medipol University, Istanbul, Turkey

C. Cingi et al. (eds.), *Minor Interventions, Major Outcomes on the Face*, Comprehensive ENT, https://doi.org/10.1007/978-3-032-01305-7_44

44.2 Background and Significance

In the past, men's preferred aesthetics were very different. In contrast, overweight individuals were preferred in history and medieval times, and more robust and sleeker individuals between 20 and 30 were preferred male figures in the classic period. Nowadays, especially since the nineteenth century and with the beginning of alterations in the social order, sports clubs are gaining importance as an area of struggle. They have started caring for their physical appearance, and the harmoniously drawn bodies are much preferred. A beautiful smile is one of our primary goals for maintaining a beautiful and cared-for appearance. Attractive smiles, facial aesthetics, and white and aesthetically designed teeth are fashionable with the concept of eternity. Everyone, regardless of age or sex, desires a beautiful smile [3].

In many cultures, the latest standards of smile aesthetics are individuals' straight, chalk-like white, and large-toothed smiles. However, some cultures include pregnancy, fertility, rebirth, and faith because of the gap between the teeth, especially the triangular gap between the central incisors, which afterward forms the teeth of the baby, the wisdom teeth, and an aesthetic feature that should not be removed. It may be perceived as showing attitude, seriousness, and influence. At the same time, in another culture where social adaptation is essential, it may be called showy and cause people to laugh with good intentions. A nice smile is expressed in every culture to show how these evaluations differ. Still, there are many examples where the influences of oral and dental health parameters on people are evaluated differently in different cultures. With the information obtained from the studies conducted, practices belonging to tooth-white cultures and especially men in different world geographies are described [3, 4].

44.3 Anatomy of Male Teeth

Concerning males, there is intrinsic beauty if we can respect and understand male anatomical features. Male dentition is more extensive, so structured dental aesthetic rules cannot be applied. However, structure without refinement is primitive. This is true of males' teeth: they have the right enamel thickness, especially at the incisal edge, which matches the inner layer structure. The cortex/structure thickens over time, contributing to the bluish-gray opacity of males' teeth with dentin exposed. The enamel layer has to compensate for this dentin thickness variation. If the dentin layer is thick, as is typical in men, the enamel must present a rounded mamelon outline with the central tip closer to the incisal edge and a very convex lingual slope.

Male dentition usually has a heterodont parabola proportion. The lateral incisal edge is shorter and more cervical, and progressively, the length increases toward the canines. Considering the dental morphological differences between males and females, male teeth size is more significant than female teeth, considering both length and width. This greater size, combined with other anatomical characteristics, influences the dental proportions, the space between teeth/smile, and the form/shape of the dental arches, influencing smile aesthetics. The enamel is the most mineralized structure in our bodies, with a mineral concentration of approximately 96% by weight. Anybody and dental factors and physiological processes affecting the enamel can indirectly influence the shade. Inflammation and ischemia of the pulp tissue usually result in a darkly stained tooth caused by the hemodynamic by-products diffusing into the dentinal tubules [2, 4].

44.4 Differences from Female Teeth

After any dental aesthetic treatment, the final result should reflect the facets of the patient's personality. The teeth belonging to a man should not reflect the characteristics of female teeth; our sex and character shape the teeth. Therefore, it is helpful to identify at first the differences between male and female teeth. From children's teeth to natural teeth, there is a significant difference in the teeth' length, width, and form. This difference is conditioned first by the biotype and the sexual characteristics of each patient. For females, the narrow teeth are relatively common, as the stance remains large compared to the body of the tooth. Also, the tooth's crown corresponding to the cervical line is increased, with the mesiodistal size barely accentuated. Though the male sex initially had large-dimension teeth, the degree of wear is higher than in females; their initial size dramatically diminishes, forcing men to consider the aesthetic treatment of their teeth to improve appearance. The alignment of teeth is essential for dental composition. Suppose there is an errant one or a missing tooth. In that case, it is noteworthy that through prosthetic rehabilitation, the dentist or technician can alter the geometry, alignment, and dimensions of the final teeth—modifications that will lead to an enhancement in the final appearance of the dental units, linking these with the main characteristics of the patient and producing a desired smile, as seen from the patient's perspective [2, 3].

44.5 Factors Influencing Male Teeth Aesthetics

Biological, genetic, environmental, cultural, and lifestyle factors influence a male smile. People tend to classify men as dominant or not. They usually perceive a face as dominant when it belongs to a socially dominant person, such as a man. Huge body diversity is shaped primarily by our genotype and altered by aging and environmental factors. Smokers are rated relatively highly on attractiveness and sociability, with no differences in healthiness. This perception results from cultural exposure that has taught us to have specific aesthetic preferences influenced by lifestyle trends and market interests. Knowledge of the factors affecting facial and dental appearance is necessary to choose improvement methods and develop a treatment system or protocol to plan aesthetically satisfactory results. Despite many similarities, men and women display differences in their smiles. Such invariability relies on a multifactorial phenomenon that is both biologically and culturally determined. The missing treatment proposals for male patients influence the need for this narrative review. Smiling in private, work, and social environments can improve men's mental health. All the differences mentioned earlier can be used to identify critical needs for treatment strategies [2, 4].

44.6 Genetics and Ethnicity

Among the multitude of factors that define beauty and appearance, genetics is one of the most important. Twin studies conducted in the early twenty-first century resulted in calculated heritability values of 51% for dental dimensions. Tooth size, shape, and alignment are also highly genetically dominated traits. Malocclusion, crowding, and the need for orthodontic treatment have multifactorial etiological explanations, with heredity starting from 40%. Therefore, the overall dental health and the size and shape of teeth are influenced by genetic predisposition. The dentist can establish if the patient has a pleasant smile by combining proportions and ratios or dimensions with position. Key factors that can guide our decisions in treatment planning are, for example, the indirect Vintage Ideal Proportions Approach for the front teeth or the rule of golden percentage for the upper center teeth, both defined mathematically.

A difference in various dental shapes was discovered in population genetics. A study comparing faunal samples from different regions established that combined tooth shape frequencies significantly differed among the populations. The male facial aesthetic is also considerably affected by genetic and environmental factors. A slight focus group felt North America's male aesthetic had attributes quite suitable for Far Eastern and Oriental ethnic groups. Multiple variations of tooth size and shape were also noticed among different ethnicities, where a significant occlusal discrepancy might appear even if they do not fit into the standard international dental layout. The combined influence of genetic and environmental factors creates significant differences in dental appearance. That is why every treatment goal should be accomplished according to the needs and requests of each patient, whose main aesthetic is their cultural background. A culturally sensitive practice acknowledges the importance of the sociocultural influences that impact the enhancement of the presenting facial aesthetic [2, 4].

44.7 Techniques and Procedures for Enhancing Male Teeth Aesthetics

Male aesthetic preferences differ from female aesthetic preferences, and men represent a significant part of the population seeking techniques and procedures to enhance their smiles. The main reason men do not bring this theme to a dental consultation could be the need for more conversation between them and the professionals, hindering the advancement of dental aesthetics in these patients. This section presents conventional and brand-new techniques to enhance male dental aesthetics. Male patients are primarily interested in invasive treatments, which may require a psychological approach to advocate for conservative treatments. Addressing them and discussing treatment options for dental aesthetic enhancements is essential. New technologies are available, from digital smile design to 3D printed models. They offer many solutions; however, patients must see the model in reality—in their mouth—to decide which treatment line to choose [2, 4].

There are several ways to enhance the dental appearance of male patients. Bonding is one of the most commonly used minimally invasive techniques; however, there is no need for an exaggerated look for males. On the contrary, an excessively masculine appearance may be perceived negatively. Aesthetics should be within the limits, and the patient must understand what look he wants. It should be documented and diagnosed whether an orthodontic or prosthetic treatment, multiple or single-tooth restoration, implant, or crown lengthening will be feasible with the line of treatment that the patient chooses. Exact procedures for diastema closure, veneers, and implants were proposed. It is also essential that bonding and the veneers obtained by males have a shape and texture perpendicular to the surface. Beveled incisal edges can be proposed for some male patients. In the following pages, orthodontics and surgery are also discussed [2, 4].

Sexual dysmorphism refers to the difference in size, form, and appearance of the teeth between males and females when tooth alignments are evaluated. Although it is impossible to prove it, the literature suggests that gender may affect the shape and form of the teeth [5]. Cultural differences must also be considered when determining the appearance of teeth according to gender. When it comes to the teeth' forms, structures, and colors, it is frequently observed that people exhibit features belonging to both sexes in their teeth appearance.

It is possible to determine sex from many parts of the body, such as the skull and bones. Sex determination becomes a vital process as it plays a leading role in the identification of a person and poses a significant problem for forensic cases where body integrity has been compromised. Therefore, determining gender from teeth can also be essential in solving forensic cases [6].

44.8 Incisal Edges and Incisal Embrasures

Morphology, crown, and root lengths of the teeth differ for male and female sexes. The position and appearance of the incisal edges of the incisors are of great importance for smile aesthetics. The age and gender of the patient affect the length of the incisal edge. The average crown length for maxillary teeth is between 10.4 and 11.2 mm. Considering the width and height of the maxillary anterior teeth, it has been shown that the average crown lengths are higher in men than in women [7]. Although it changes with aging, the average incisal appearance in men is 1.91 mm [8].

The gaps between the cutting edges of the teeth are called incisal embrasures. Aging and gender may alter the shape of these embrasures. In men, the incisal embrasures appear square and blunter. Additionally, a shallower embrasure indicates advanced age and masculinity.

In Western culture, masculinity is characterized by vigor and sharp lines. According to Frush and Fisher, "the typical male appearance is cubic, hard, built and energetic" [9]. Therefore, jagged teeth with sharper edges and square and angular incisors may be perceived as masculine. However, this view varies according to the individual. Therefore, it is essential to plan treatment by considering the individual's aesthetic perception, character traits, and wishes. Observing darker shaded teeth in men compared to women in the same age group may also be possible [10].

44.9 Golden Portion and Tooth Ratio

Various tooth width ratios have been assessed throughout the years; the most well-known is the golden proportion. The golden proportion was first utilized for teeth by Lombardi [1]. Levin then applied this proportion to dental aesthetics, suggesting that the width of the maxillary lateral incisor should be 0.618 of the maxillary central incisor and that the lateral incisor should be 0.618 of the width of the canine in a frontal view [5]. A meta-analysis offered six pieces of research that evaluated male and female participants' tooth width ratios. In the six trials, 395 males and 446 women were assessed. The tooth width ratio of the lateral incisor to the central incisor was not different between men and women ($P = .22$). A significant difference ($P < .001$) was seen in the tooth width ratio between the canine and lateral incisors, suggesting that male individuals had a higher ratio of canines to lateral incisors than female participants. In summary, men had a higher canine-to-lateral incisor tooth width ratio than women [11].

When observing an ideal smile, several factors must be considered, including the symmetrical composition of teeth, color, and forms. It has been suggested that, among other things, a patient's emotions, sex, gender, age, gingival arrangement, and facial form could all affect the form of their teeth [12]. Beforehand, it is known that the pre-established four conventional tooth forms (oval, triangular, rectangular, and square) do appear in the population; however, it corresponds to a low percentage of people, so with the new research, the perception changes. In a study among four hundred and sixty students (285 female; 175 male), it was found that the population under study had the highest percentages of hybrid tooth shapes, including TO (20.87% total; 21.4% female and 20% male), SOS (20.65% total; 21.4% female and 19.43% male), and OR (19.57% total; 17.89% female and 22.29% male). In contrast, the oval was the most common form among the pure basic forms (6.52% total; 7.37% female and 5.15% male). The result was the suggestion of five novel hybrid tooth shapes, which are as follows: SOF (square-oval with flat lateral incisors), OR (oval-rectangular), TR (triangular-rectangular), and SOS (square-oval with scalloped lateral incisors) [7].

From a clinical perspective, there is no association between gender and tooth forms; instead, when it comes to aesthetic procedures, trials must be conducted and patient ideas must be taken into account, taking into consideration not just one particular tooth form but their entire range (Figs. 44.1 and 44.2).

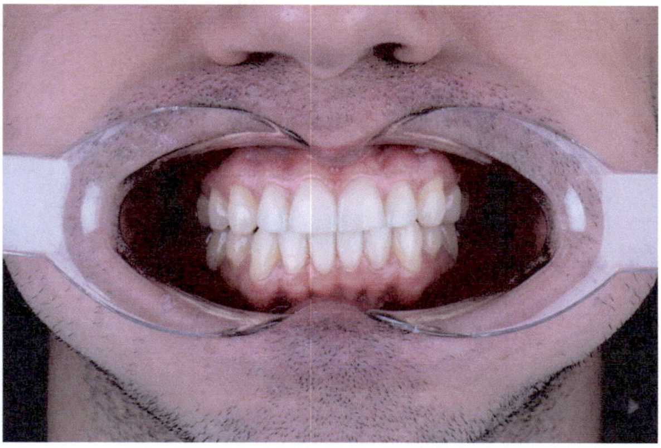

Fig. 44.1 Aesthetic male teeth, frontal view

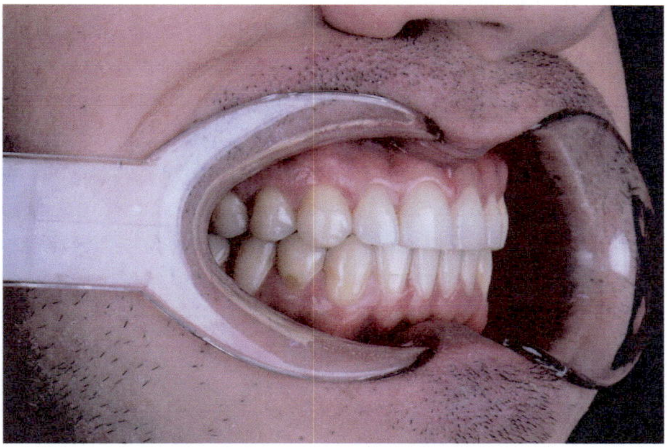

Fig. 44.2 Aesthetic male teeth, side view

44.10 Conclusion

Some distinguishing features of male smiles are more noticeable than others. Initially, a man's smile is more beautiful with straight teeth. Teeth in good alignment are highly prized because they provide the impression of vitality and strength. The shade of one's teeth is also significant; having pearly whites is an asset. Having white teeth makes people think their teeth are healthy, which is a plus in and of itself.

It is commonly believed that men should have slightly more extensive and prominent teeth to project an image of confidence and strength. This does not mean they must be enormous, but they should be proportional to a man's face to bring out his best features.

Proper tooth alignment and positioning are the foundation of a perfect male grin. When issues arise, patients can get their teeth straightened using state-of-the-art orthodontic treatments, including braces and clear aligners, which are customized to fit each patient's specific dental structure.

An attractive grin features symmetry and balance. Teeth that are misaligned relative to one another can throw off the appearance of facial harmony, which is why orthodontics is used. This necessitates considering the teeth' dimensions, form, and placement, particularly the front incisors, which are the most noticeable when grinning. Because even little misalignments can throw off the smile's balance, achieving symmetry in orthodontic treatment frequently necessitates meticulous planning and accuracy. The ultimate aim is a balanced and proportionate smile that enhances the face as a whole.

A gorgeous smile is set against the backdrop of gums. The primary goal of orthodontic treatment is maintaining normal gum health and visible gum. A gummy smile, where the gums protrude too much, or receding gums, which make the teeth look overly long, are both aesthetic issues that can diminish the attractiveness of a smile. The gold standard is a perfectly proportioned gum line that subtly frames each tooth and adds to rather than takes away from a smile. This requires a thorough evaluation of the gums' condition and, if necessary, procedures to fix abnormalities at the gum line.

When getting that perfect smile, tooth shape and color are major factors. Orthodontics, in collaboration with other dental specialists, typically addresses these factors. Teeth whitening can create a brighter smile, while chips or unusually shaped teeth can be corrected with reshaping procedures. Teeth in good alignment and with consistent color and shape help create a beautiful smile.

Regarding orthodontic treatment, bite function is just as crucial as appearance. The perfect smile makes biting, chewing, and speaking easier. Orthodontists ensure a good bite by paying great attention to the relationship between the front and back teeth. In addition to protecting the health of the teeth and gums, a properly aligned bite can lessen the likelihood of problems, including jaw pain, TMJ disorders, and uneven tooth wear.

References

1. Pham TAV, Nguyen PA. Morphological features of smile attractiveness and related factors influence perception and gingival aesthetic parameters. Int Dent J. 2022;72(1):67–75. https://doi.org/10.1016/j.identj.2021.02.001.
2. Cracel-Nogueira F, Pinho T. Assessment of the perception of smile esthetics by laypersons, dental students and dental practitioners. Int Orthod. 2013;11(4):432–44. English, French. https://doi.org/10.1016/j.ortho.2013.09.007.
3. Althagafi N. Esthetic smile perception among dental students at different educational levels. Clin Cosmet Investig Dent. 2021;13:163–72. https://doi.org/10.2147/CCIDE.S304216.
4. Alhammadi MS, Halboub E, Al-Mashraqi AA, Al-Homoud M, Wafi S, Zakari A, Mashali W. Perception of facial, dental, and smile esthetics by dental students. J Esthet Restor Dent. 2018;30(5):415–26. https://doi.org/10.1111/jerd.12405.
5. Lombardi ME, Levin EI. Dental esthetics and the golden proportion. J Prosthet Dent. 1978;40:244–52.
6. Banerjee A, Kamath VV, Satelur K, Rajkumar K, Sundaram L. Sexual dimorphism in tooth morphometrics: an evaluation of the parameters. J Forensic Dent Sci. 2016;8(1):22–7.
7. Sterrett JD, Oliver T, Robinson F, Fortson W, Knaak B, Russell CM. Width/length ratios of normal clinical crowns of the maxillary anterior dentition in man. J Clin Periodontol. 1999;26:153–7.
8. Roy S. The eight components of a balanced smile. J Clin Orthodont JCO. 2005;39:155–67.

9. Frush JP, Fisher RD. Introduction to dentogenic restorations. J Pros Dent. 1955;5:586–95.
10. Esan TA, Olusile AO, Akeredolu PA. Factors influencing tooth shade selection for completely edentulous patients. J Contemp Dent Pract. 2006;7:80–7.
11. Londono J, Ghasemi S, Lawand G, Dashti M. Evaluation of the golden proportion in the natural dentition: a systematic review and meta-analysis. J Pros Dent. 2023;129(5):696–702.
12. Mahn E, Walls S, Jorquera G, Valdés AM, Val A, Sampaio CS. Prevalence of tooth forms and their gender correlation. J Esthet Restor Dent. 2018;30(1):45–50. https://doi.org/10.1111/jerd.12341.

45 Aesthetic Considerations In Orthodontic Treatment of Adults

Ece Bozok

45.1 Introduction

Using fixed orthodontic equipment as a treatment method has increasingly become the standard in orthodontic practice worldwide. According to the findings of epidemiological research [1, 2], around thirty percent of the average population has either a moderate or a significant requirement for orthodontic treatment. Despite this, since the development of the acid-etch process and its application for the bonding of orthodontic brackets, one of the key concerns has been to restore the enamel surface to a state that is as close to its initial state as feasible while minimizing the amount of enamel loss that occurs after treatment. Alterations to enamel can occur due to bonding, debonding, and clean-up methods. These alterations include enamel loss brought on by etching, decalcification, and scratches on the enamel [3]. The unfavorable effects on the color and aesthetics of enamel related to the alterations stated above should also be considered, in addition to the structural faults discussed previously [4].

45.2 The Aesthetic Paradigm

45.2.1 The Golden Proportion/Divine Proportion

Fibonacci numbers—The series of increasing numbers looks like it was generated by adding the two most recent numbers. For example, 0–55, 1, 2, 3, 5, 8, 13, 21, 34, 55, etc. The sum of all additions is exactly 1.618 times that of all previous additions, and this ratio will be maintained indefinitely. Also, the increment from one number

E. Bozok (✉)
Faculty of Dentistry, Department of Orthodontics, Istanbul Medipol University, Istanbul, Turkey

C. Cingi et al. (eds.), *Minor Interventions, Major Outcomes on the Face*, Comprehensive ENT, https://doi.org/10.1007/978-3-032-01305-7_45

to the next in this series is 0.618. The foundation of the Golden Section [5–7] is this 1.618 ratio of the Fibonacci numbers.

45.2.2 The Golden Section

The term "repeated ratio" describes dividing a surface into related but distinct pieces. Originally known as the Phi/Divine Proportion, the "Golden Proportion" is human history's most important recurring ratio. Its value is 1.618:1 [5–7].

45.2.3 Genetic Implications of the Logarithmic Spiral and the Golden Section

Even the most basic prehistoric creatures, like snails, have a logarithmic spiral. Practical uses of the divine ratio in healthcare. The mandible is aesthetically attractive because of the golden ratio between the corpus axis (XiPm) and the condylar axis (Xi-Co). When measured from the apex of the condyle, the corpus axis was in perfect proportion to the condylar axis in all normal mandible composites [8].

45.2.3.1 Macroesthetics

The initial step is to spot any irregularities, including a crooked or uneven jawline, an excess or shortage of mandibles, or an uneven face, from various views of the face. (from a macro aesthetic standpoint) [9, 10].

45.3 Facial Proportion

45.3.1 Vertical Division

The facial thirds provide the most useful framework for analyzing the vertical proportions of the face from the side and front angles. Optimal facial divisions include three equal halves [5]:

- Tragus to glabella in the upper body
- From the opharic to subnasion
- At the base, subnasion to the gonion. Two uneven halves make up the bottom third of the face:

  (a) A quarter of the subnasion to the gonion is the same as the subnasion to the lip commissures.
  (b) The commissures of the lips to the gonion are equal to two-thirds of the subnasion to the gonion.

- Raising the lower 1/3 of the jaw:
  - (a) An overabundance of teeth on top of the jaw,
  - (b) Class III malocclusion,
- Short stature in the bottom half:
  - (a) an underdeveloped jawbone in the upper jaw, or
  - (b) Mandibular retrusion.

45.3.2 Horizontal Division

A perfectly proportional form has an equal central, medial, and lateral half. When a person's eyes are equally spaced and wide, that's when their medial and central fifths are determined. Center your nose within the fifth and make sure its width is equal to or slightly broader than the fifth's [9]. This will make your nose seem its finest.

45.3.3 Balance and Symmetry

The midline of the face is the defining feature of facial symmetry. The midline separates the face into the right and left sides by passing through its center and a portion of the lip (also known as Cupid's bow). Inherently harmonious and lovely faces have more symmetric and identical sides, bringing them closer to bilateral duplication or mirror images (horizontal symmetry) [5].

45.4 Miniesthetics

45.4.1 Smile Type: Vertical Tooth and Lip Relationship

At least 75% of the maxillary crown should be visible when smiling for social acceptance, and no more than 4 mm of gingiva or incisor crown lip coverage is allowed [11]. Slightly overlapping your upper lip with the gum line of your top central incisor will give you a picture-perfect smile [12]. Using the amount of gingival and incisor show, Tjan et al. [13] classified smiles as low, moderate, or high. A normal grin should reveal between seventy-five and one hundred percent of the maxillary crown. With a low smile, your field of vision drops below 75%. An elevated smile, or "gummy smile," reveals the full length of the crown and a continuous strip of gingiva [14]. If you have a low smile type and would want your upper teeth to be longer, you have a few options: arch wires, anterior vertical elastics, Class II elastics (which can move the occlusal plane forward), or orthognathic surgery [11]. As an option to prolong the lifespan of a prosthetic crown, orthodontic treatment or porcelain laminate veneers may be recommended [14]. Many dental problems can lead to an overjet, an overbite, a huge gap between the lower and upper jaws while the patient is at rest, an overabundance of vertical space in the front of the mouth, or an enlarged muscle that elevates the top lip, all of which can result in a high grin type. Orthognathic surgeons have several alternatives for correcting a high smile type, including segregated arch mechanics for maxillary incisor intrusion and intrusion with temporary anchorage devices [11]. Since orthodontic treatment might exacerbate the issue due to too retracted maxillary incisors or an anterior tilting of the occlusal plane, orthognathic surgery should be considered for cases of vertical maxillary excess without significant repose exposure of maxillary teeth [15]. In normal or low-angle cases, a molar extrusion is an option; however, when there is sufficient incisor display, a deep bite, and a deep Spee curve, the suggested technique is the active intrusion of the mandibular incisors [14]. Flaring incisors make them look worse when resting or smiling but better when standing up straight [16].

45.4.2 Transverse Dimension of Smile

The buccal corridor is created when a patient smiles by the space where the buccal surfaces of the back teeth meet the corners of their lips [17]. Buccal canals are said to provide the impression of a more natural look. The arch's transverse breadth should coincide with the face's width for aesthetic reasons. The best way to predict how the dental arches will look and feel after treatment is to look at the shape of the mandibular arch and the width of the intercanine gap between the mandibles. A narrow, collapsed arch shape is associated with poor transverse dimension features, so orthodontic treatment is favorable from an aesthetic standpoint [16]. It may be required to expand the maxillary arch if it appears narrowed, regardless of whether it is caused by cross-biting. For people with the right form and width of the maxillary arch, applying buccal crown torque to canines and premolars angled toward the palate can make a smile look fuller [14]. On the other hand, people with buccally flared posteriors shouldn't get expansion [11]. Relapse [14] results from intentionally overexpanding the buccal corridor, which flattens the grin arc, gives teeth a denture-like appearance, and puts the bite out of kilter. Researchers have correlated less appealing smiles and wider buccal corridors [18]. Both groups obtained identical findings when assessing buccal corridors [19].

45.5 Microesthetics

45.5.1 Tooth Proportions

Smiles that adhere to the golden ratio are those in which the canine's apparent width is 62% of the lateral incisor's width, the first premolar's apparent width is 62% of the canine's apparent width, and the lateral incisor's apparent width is 62% of the central incisor's width. This ratio is useful when determining the size of a lateral after treatment for abnormally small lateral incisors or when reducing canines to replace them due to congenitally absent laterals [11]. It is important to properly preserve microesthetics during extraction therapy because smiles after extractions depart more from the golden proportion ratios than smiles without extractions [20].

45.5.2 Height–Width Relationships

Eighty percent of a tooth's height should be its breadth [11]. A range of 0.75 to 0.85 has been proposed by Sterrett et al. [21] as the optimal. The breadth and length of the central incisor might range from 8.1 to 8.6 mm and 9.5 to 10.2 mm, respectively [22]. When the height is too high, the teeth look tapered, and when it's too low, they look square. In cases of disproportionate length, the treatment technique is affected by factors such as the sulcular depth of the incisors, lip level, relative crown length, and amount of incisal wear [23]. Periodontal crown lengthening is done in situations with vertical gingival encroachment, facial laminates are utilized for deformed crowns, and bonding or laminates are used to restore the missing portion of the crown in cases of reduced crown height [11].

45.5.3 Connectors and Embrasures

The region between teeth is called the connector area, and the triangles that lie incisal to that area are called embrasures [24]. As the central incisors give way to the premolars, the contact points migrate gingivally, widening the incisal embrasure. The connector length between two maxillary incisors should be half of the crown length, ideal for the 50-40-30 ratio of the maxillary anterior teeth, and so on [25]. The interdental papilla fills the gingival embrasure, and the embrasures are typically bigger than the connectors. Short interdental papillae cause unsightly black triangles to grow above the connectors to open gingival embrasures. Due to orthodontic therapy, adults with periodontal disease or very crowded or rotated maxillary incisors may develop black triangles. The recommended method involves orthodontic root paralleling and interproximal stripping to reshape the teeth, followed by space closure [11]. Dental reshaping may be necessary to prevent black triangles. Thus, patients at risk should be informed of this [26].

45.5.4 Gingival Height, Shape, and Contour

Aesthetic dental appearance cannot be achieved without proportionate gingival height. The canine gingival and central incisor margins are typically parallel, with the lateral incisor margin 1.5 mm below. This should be remembered when the canines take the position of the laterals [11]. The canines and elliptical-shaped maxillary central incisors have gingival zeniths positioned distal to the tooth's long axis. Gingival symmetry is key, so make sure the long axis of the tooth and the gingival zenith coincide with the shape of your maxillary and mandibular incisors [27]. Periodontal procedures such as gingivectomy or crown lengthening remove excess gingiva to create a more desirable gumline contour, whereas tissue grafts, guided tissue regeneration, and nonsurgical orthodontic extrusion are common methods for treating gingival recession [22].

45.5.5 Tooth Shade and Color

An aesthetically beautiful smile results from a gradual shading pattern that begins at the midline and moves posteriorly. The lightest and brightest are the maxillary central incisors; subsequently, the teeth become less so. Maxillary laterals are a shade darker than the central incisors, but otherwise, they have a comparable tint. The canines have the highest chroma (color saturation) and are the darkest teeth in the mouth. However, the color of the first two premolars is more similar to that of the laterals, making them lighter than the canines [22]. As a result of facial enamel wearing away and secondary dentin production, teeth grow darker and less shiny as we age [11].

45.5.5.1 Enamel Color Variables

Research has demonstrated that enamel bonding and debonding processes impact enamel color factors [3, 28]. Procedures for removing resin after debonding [28] and the ability of resin tags to penetrate enamel structures to depths of up to 50 mm can cause enamel color changes [3]. Debonding and cleaning treatments cannot reverse resin impregnation into the enamel structure [29], and discoloration of the enamel can happen due to the direct absorption of food colorants or products caused by orthodontic appliance deterioration [30]. The fact that these resin residues remain in the enamel tags that cover the middle third of the buccal surface for an extended period makes the color stability of these materials crucial for the color of the teeth. Also, the enamel surface could become rougher and change color due to post-debonding treatments that remove adhesive residues using rotary abrasive tools or handheld equipment [1, 31, 32].

References

1. Chen Q, Zheng X, Chen W, Ni Z, Zhou Y. Influence of orthodontic treatment with fixed appliances on enamel color: a systematic review. BMC Oral Health. 2015;15(31) https://www.medscape.com/viewarticle/842445_2. Accessed online at 8 July 2024
2. Borzabadi-Farahani A. An insight into four orthodontic treatment need indices. Prog Orthod. 2011;12:132–42.
3. Sandison RM. Tooth surface appearance after debonding. Br J Orthod. 1981;8:199–201.
4. Hosein I, Sherriff M, Ireland AJ. Enamel loss during bonding, debonding, and cleanup with use of a self-etching primer. Am J Orthod Dentofacial Orthop. 2004;12:717–24.
5. Bamal R, Kumar A, Pareek PK, Jaswal A. Esthetics in orthodontics: a review. Int J Dent Med Sci Res. 2021;3(6):664–71.

6. Raj V. Esthetic paradigms in the interdisciplinary management of maxillary anterior dentition – a review. J Esthet Restor Dent. 2013;25(5):295–304.
7. Ricketts RM. The biologic significance of the divine proportion and Fibonacci series. AJODO. 1982;81(5):351–70.
8. Ricketts RM. The golden divider. J Clin Orthod. 1981;15(11):752–9.
9. Meshramkar R, Mathur P, Navya NB, Gupta M, Lekha K. A study to evaluate the role of macro-, micro-, and miniesthetics in an attractive smile. Int J Prosthodont Restorat Dent. 2019;9(4) https://www.ijoprd.com/abstractArticleContentBrowse/IJOPRD/19693/JPJ/fullText. Accessed online at 8 July 2024
10. Proffit WR. Contemporary orthodontics. St. Louis: Mosby Elsevier; 2007.
11. Proffit WR, Fields HW, Sarver DM. Contemporary orthodontics. 5th ed. St. Louis: Elsevier, Mosby; 2012.
12. Hulsey CM. An esthetic evaluation of lip-teeth relationships present in the smile. Am J Orthod. 1970;57(2):132–44.
13. Tjan AH, Miller GD, The JG. Some esthetic factors in a smile. J Prosthet Dent. 1984;51(1):24–8.
14. Zachrisson BU. Esthetics in tooth display and smile design. In: Nanda R, editor. Biomechanics and esthetic strategies in clinical orthodontics. St. Louis: Elsevier Saunders; 2005. p. 110–30.
15. Ackerman JL, Proffit WR. Soft tissue limitations in orthodontics: treatment planning guidelines. Angle Orthod. 1997;67(5):327–36.
16. Sarver DM, Ackerman MB. Dynamic smile visualization and quantification: Part 2. Smile analysis and treatment strategies. Am J Orthod Dentofacial Orthop. 2003;124(2):116–27.
17. Frush JP, Fisher RD. The dynesthetic interpretation of the dentogenic concept. J Prosthet Dent. 1958;8(4):558–81.
18. Janson G, Branco NC, Fernandes TM, Sathler R, Garib D, Lauris JR. Influence of orthodontic treatment, midline position, buccal corridor and smile arc on smile attractiveness. Angle Orthod. 2011;81(1):153–61.
19. Sarver DM, Ackerman JL. Orthodontics about face: the re-emergence of the esthetic paradigm. Am J Orthod Dentofacial Orthop. 2000;117(5):575–6.
20. Tauheed S, Shaikh A, Fida M. Microaesthetics of the smile: extraction vs. non-extraction. J Coll Physicians Surg Pak. 2012;22(4):230–4.
21. Sterrett JD, Oliver T, Robinson F, Fortson W, Knaak B, Russell CM. Width/length ratios of normal clinical crowns of the maxillary anterior dentition in man. J Clin Periodontol. 1999;26(3):153–7.
22. Sharma PK, Sharma P. Dental smile esthetics: the assessment and creation of the ideal smile. Semin Orthod. 2012;18(3):193–201.
23. Kovich V. Esthetics and anterior tooth position: an orthodontic perspective. Part I: Crown length. J Esthet Dent. 1993;5(1):19–23.
24. Sarver DM. Principles of cosmetic dentistry in orthodontics: Part 1. Shape and proportionality of anterior teeth. Am J Orthod Dentofacial Orthop. 2004;126(6):749–53.
25. Morley J, Eubank J. Macroesthetic elements of smile design. J Am Dent Assoc. 2001;132(1):39–45.
26. Singh S, Singla L, Anand T. Esthetic considerations in orthodontics: an overview. Dent J Adv Stud. 2021:1–5.
27. Gurel G. The science and art of porcelain laminate veneers. London: Quintessence Publishing (IL); 2003.
28. Fleming GJ. Advances in dental materials. Prim Dent J. 2014;3:54–61.
29. Øgaard B, Rølla G, Arends J. Orthodontic appliances and enamel demineralization. Part 1. Lesion development. Am J Orthod Dentofacial Orthop. 1998;94:68–73.
30. Maijer R, Smith DC. Corrosion of orthodontic bracket bases. Am J Orthod. 1982;81:43–8.
31. de Araujo EB, Zis V, Dutra CA. Enamel color change by microabrasion and resin-based composite. Am J Dent. 2000;13:6–7.
32. van Waes H, Matter T, Krejci I. Three-dimensional measurement of enamel loss caused by bonding and debonding of orthodontic brackets. Am J Orthod Dentofacial Orthop. 1997;112:666–9.

The "Pink Aesthetic Concept" in Facial Beauty

46

Nurcan Aksaka and Zeynep Çukurova Yılmaz

46.1 Introduction

Although personal perception of beauty varies according to ethnicity, periods, socio-cultural situation, and many other environmental factors, the perception of facial aesthetics is mainly consistent with the general population. The harmony of the general outlines of the face with the teeth and gums that appear during speech and smile should be in a way that meets aesthetic expectations to complete facial aesthetics. Therefore, dentists have developed various diagnostic and treatment methods to achieve this face–mouth harmony. The treatment should be decided after carefully evaluating the patient's characteristics, character, and aesthetic expectations. In addition, the possible results and limitations of the treatment should be explained to the patient in detail.

Proper dental anatomy, tooth alignment, and occlusion are insufficient to ensure facial aesthetics. The gingiva surrounding these teeth is also expected to meet specific criteria during function or the smile. The perfect harmony between "pink aesthetics" (gingival aesthetics) and "white aesthetics" (dental aesthetics) is the key to an ideal smile.

N. Aksaka
Faculty of Dentistry, Periodontology Department, Istanbul Medipol University, Istanbul, Turkey

Z. Çukurova Yılmaz (✉)
Dentoper Dental Clinic, Fethiye, Turkey

C. Cingi et al. (eds.), *Minor Interventions, Major Outcomes on the Face*, Comprehensive ENT, https://doi.org/10.1007/978-3-032-01305-7_46

46.2 Health of Gingiva

Dentofacial aesthetics plays a significant role in an individual's social attractiveness; patients with a regular and aligned relationship between their incisors are generally regarded as more charming, popular, and intelligent and have a higher chance of landing a job than those with an inconsistent relationship between these teeth [1].

The smile analysis always comes first in the aesthetic evaluation process before periodontal or prosthodontic therapy. The interactions between the teeth, the lip structure, and the gingival scaffold are the fundamental components of a smile. A smile that harmoniously combines the "pink" (periodontal) and "white" (teeth) aesthetics is the ideal one. When treating excessive gingival exposure in "gummy" smiles or tooth exposure in gingival recession, advancements in periodontology have improved aesthetic results. The area of the oral mucosa that covers the jaw's alveolar processes and encircles the tooth necks is called the gingiva.

46.3 Gingival Morphology

46.3.1 Color

The vascular blood supply, pigment-containing cells' presence, and keratinization's thickness and level are typically reflected in the coral pink or pale pink of the marginal and attached gingivae [2]. Understanding pink aesthetics is crucial because it will enable medical professionals to adjust the gingival region of dental prostheses to the soft tissues.

A distinct mucogingival line separates the connected gingiva from the nearby alveolar mucosa, which is pink and stippled in contrast to the alveolar mucosa's red, smooth, and glossy appearance. Gingival color varies slightly according to individual pigmentation. There is a broad range of colors that are determined by the amount of melanogenesis, the degree of epithelial cornification, the depth of epithelialization, and the gingival vascularity configuration [3].

Gingival color changes can be caused by inflammation or disease, and they frequently appear in the form of a reddish, purple, or even bluish tint. Gingival color is a significant sign of overall gingival health and should be appropriately examined and monitored to diagnose and treat various oral health disorders.

46.3.2 Gingival Biotype

The term "gingival biotype" refers to the thickness of the gingiva in the faciopalatal/labiolingual dimension. "Thick-flat" and "thin-scalloped" gingiva biotypes were identified. A thick tissue biotype was defined as a gingival thickness greater than 2 mm, and a thin tissue biotype as a gingival thickness less than 1.5 mm [4].

A large zone of keratinized tissue and solid bone architecture characterizes a thick gingival biotype. This biotype is also more tolerant of trauma. However, a scalloped gingival contour and a narrow strip of keratinized tissue point to a weak bone architecture highly susceptible to injury or inflammation.

The initial thickness of the gingiva can influence the potential success of restorative procedures like implants. It is postulated that individuals with thin gingival biotypes are more susceptible to developing periodontal or gingival disease. The thick, flat tissue biotype is essential to an implant's aesthetic appeal. Therefore, the adequate thickness of the attached gingiva is crucial because a thin and sensitive gingival edge may cause recession following trauma, surgery, or inflammatory injuries. In contrast, thick gingival tissue is more accessible to manipulate, maintains vascularity, and aids in wound healing both before and after surgery [5].

46.3.3 Interdental Papilla

The interdental papilla is an essential component of the gingiva's anatomy. Several factors can cause it to decrease height, ultimately forming an open embrasure region known as a "black triangle." Patients often complain about black triangles because they can be very unpleasant. Clinicians must comprehensively understand the available therapy choices to manage this clinical condition effectively (Fig. 46.1).

The portion of the gingiva that occupies the area between the contact points of adjacent teeth is called the interdental papilla. It is supported laterally by the tooth margins and the underneath alveolar bone [6]. At the anterior teeth, the interdental papilla has a pyramidal shape. Two papillae in posterior regions are connected by a concave saddle region known as a "col." The col may exhibit para or nonkeratinization [7]. The loss in interdental papilla can be caused by several things, such as bone resorption in the alveolar ridge due to periodontal disease, where the distance from the point of contact should be at least as excellent as 5 mm in regular teeth [8].

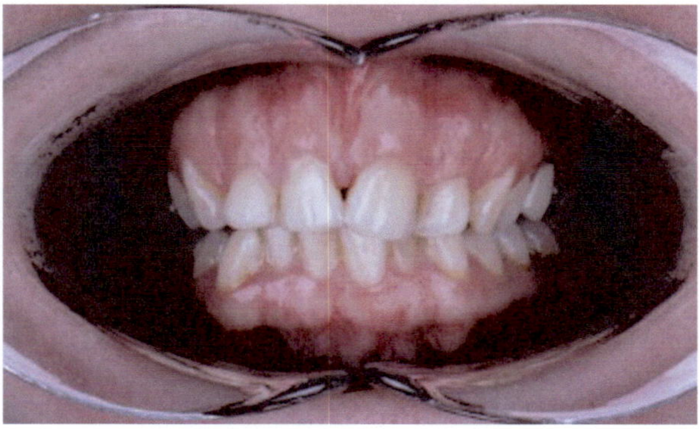

Fig. 46.1 The black triangle refers to an open embrasure between teeth (between 11 and 21 numbered teeth)

46.3.4 Gingival Zenith Point

The lips designate the aesthetic zone and constitute the smile's framing. The quantity of the gingival show is determined by its position when smiling. During treatment planning, gingival contours must be considered to forecast the final aesthetic outcome and achieve the best outcomes in gingival contour rehabilitation (crown lengthening, implant, restorative, and orthodontic therapy). The gingival line, which connects the tangents of the gingival zeniths of the canine and central incisor, is an essential aspect of gingival morphology. The gingival zenith is the most apical feature of the free gingival margin [9]. It was stated that this significant landmark has a particular spatial orientation in the mesiodistal and apical-coronal directions. The zenith of the central incisor should be at the distal third, the lateral incisor in the middle, and the cuspid can range from the anterior third through to the distal third. The zenith's location will contribute to the tooth's desired axial inclination by altering the long axis' line angle position (Fig. 46.2) [10].

Generally, dentists and orthodontists agree that smiles with gingival zenith modifications more significant than 1 mm are more aesthetically pleasing. Asymmetric gingival zeniths are less appealing than symmetrical gingival zeniths.

46.3.5 Gingival Contour

The form and thickness of the gingiva's margins from the tooth's crown are referred to as the gingival contour. Sharp interdental papillae and equally tapering gingival margins at the tooth's cervical edge are characteristics of the ideal gingival contour. These days, gingival form and contour recontouring is a relatively straightforward process.

An implant differs significantly from a tooth at the crystal bone and mucosa level. Unlike natural incisor teeth with a triangular cross section, implants have a smaller diameter and a circumferential form. To replicate the proper dental emerging profile, careful and suitable treatment of a temporary restoration may aid in developing the peri-implant soft tissue's shape [11]. Su et al. recently identified the critical and subcritical contours as distinct regions within the trans gingival zone

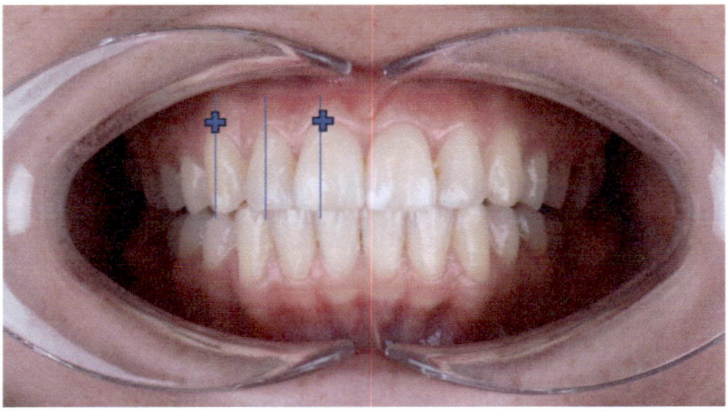

Fig. 46.2 The gingival line, which is the line connecting the tangents of the gingival zeniths of the canine and central incisor

based on the peri-implant gingival tissues' reaction to abutment/crown contour alterations [12]. The subcritical contour refers to the deeper area and affects the peri-implant soft tissue support, affecting the gingival color. The critical contour is the most superficial area and will affect the gingival level and zenith location. Optimizing the peri-implant soft tissue architecture requires alterations to the vital and subcritical shapes of the restorative emergence profile.

46.4 Important Anatomic Landmarks

46.4.1 Incisal Edge Position

An essential consideration in the planning of anterior teeth aesthetic rehabilitation is the examination of the incisal embrasure. A pleasing grin is defined by the pattern of form created by the incisal embrasures and the spaces between the maxillary anterior teeth against the darker background of the mouth. The pattern of the intervals between the embrasures starts distally, between the central incisors, and continues in that direction. The size and volume of incisal embrasures grow as they move away from the midline (Fig. 46.3).

The treatment strategy for aesthetic rehabilitations should consider the contact between the central incisors, symmetry, position of the incisal edges, width, contact points, and embrasures. Following the individual assessment, confirming how the central incisors relate to the other teeth and the face is essential. The ideal relationship between the maxillary central incisors and the midline of the face should be linear, straight, and transverse to the horizontal plane. Contact between the maxillary central incisors should always be parallel to the facial midline, even when it is impossible to align the facial midline with the dental midline.

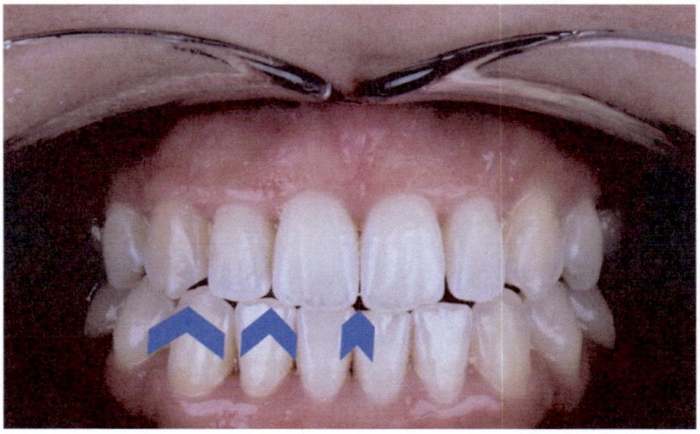

Fig. 46.3 The incisal embrasure between the central and lateral incisors should be more significant than the incisal embrasure between the central incisors. The same aspect as the incisal embrasure between the canine and lateral incisor should be more significant than the incisal embrasure between the lateral and central incisors

46.4.2 Optimal Smile

A beautiful smile is an essential part of facial aesthetics. Expressing our emotions freely and without fear increases our self-confidence and improves our ability to communicate with other people. This expression also positively affects the other party's opinion about our beauty and character.

When smiling, the levator muscles contract first, lifting the upper lip to the nasolabial fold. Then, the levator labii superior muscles of the upper lip, the zygomaticus major muscles, and the superior fibers of the buccinator lift the lip and fold upward, allowing the smile. In an optimal smile, the incisal edges of the maxillary anterior teeth should be parallel to the lower lip. Symmetrical positioning of the corners of the mouth, upper lip curvature in harmony with the gingival margins, minimal buccal corridor appearance, and appropriate dental components are other elements required for an aesthetic smile [13].

Although a 1–2 mm gingival appearance during a smile is aesthetically acceptable, the "gummy smile," in which more than 2–3 mm of gingiva is visible, makes many patients aesthetically unpleasant. The most common cause of this condition has been reported as hyperactivity of the upper lip muscles. In addition, skeletal disorders, short anterior crown lengths, and passive eruption are among the etiologic factors [14].

Tjan et al. classified the smile line as low, average, and high. A low smile line is when less than 75% of the clinical crown length is visible, and an average smile line is when 75–100% of the clinical crown length, interproximal papilla, and 1–2 mm of gingiva are visible and is considered ideal. A gummy smile refers to a high smile line [15].

According to the Mercado-Rosso classification, a type 1 gummy smile, characterized by a thin lip and barcode-shaped wrinkles that usually disappear during the smile, is associated with inadequate maxillary support. In a type 2 gummy smile, the upper lip is thicker, has fewer perioral wrinkles, and is raised more in the canine and lateral region. This is due to an imbalance between the levator muscles' strength and the soft tissues' resistance. The type 3 form is the most severe and has a vast smile, including molars, due to the excessive strength of the zygomatic muscles [16].

If the gummy smile must be treated to meet aesthetic expectations, the most appropriate method should be selected after a detailed clinical and radiographic examination. Gingivectomy, lip repositioning, botulinum toxin A injections (Botox), or orthognathic surgery are used for gummy smile treatment [17, 18].

46.5 Treatment of "Black Triangles" in Facial Aesthetics

Many factors, such as periodontal diseases and their surgical or non-surgical treatments, iatrogenic factors, orthodontic treatments, anatomical factors, and traumatic tooth brushing, can cause interdental papillary loss [19]. The loss of this soft tissue, an essential part of the gingiva, forms "black triangles" that negatively affect facial aesthetics and cause many patient complaints. Therefore, reconstruction of the interdental papilla is one of the essential goals of periodontal treatment. Papillary rebuilding is one of the most challenging and least predictable procedures in periodontology due to the poor blood supply to the area, and there is yet to be a consensus among clinicians on the superiority of the available methods [20]. It is up to the clinician's experience to choose and perform the most appropriate non-surgical or surgical procedure for the patient.

If a papillary loss has occurred due to traumatic oral hygiene, it is essential to detect it early. Discontinuing the traumatic use of the wrong toothbrush or interdental brush and providing the patient with appropriate brushes and the correct oral hygiene method can allow for papillary re-epithelialization and complete filling of the papilla. It may be possible to reshape the interdental papilla with restorative or orthodontic treatment without surgical intervention [7].

Suppose there is papillary loss due to abnormal tooth shape. In that case, the contours of the teeth can be reshaped, and the contact points of the teeth can be moved more apically, thus eliminating the black triangular appearance. With orthodontic treatment, diastemas between the teeth can be closed, and a contact point can be created between neighboring teeth. This may provide some degree of displacement of the papilla in the coronal direction. Again, if divergent roots cause a black triangle appearance, the papilla can be filled between the teeth with root movement [21].

Different surgical techniques focus on papilla reconstruction, such as pedicle soft tissue grafts flaps, semilunar coronally repositioned flaps, envelop type flaps, guided tissue regeneration (GTR) therapy, and dermal matrix autogenous skeletal and connective tissue grafts. Subepithelial connective tissue graft has been recognized as the gold standard among surgical techniques [22]. These procedures, however, still demand significant surgical knowledge and involve risks of clinical consequences. They also have a high morbidity rate and are unpredictable [23]. In addition, injections of fillers such as HA into the papillary region after local anesthesia are among the non-invasive methods [24, 25].

46.6 Treatment of Gingival Recessions

The gingival margin displacement apical to the tooth's cementoenamel junction is called gingival recession. This condition, frequently encountered in clinical practice, causes tooth sensitivity, root caries, and aesthetic problems in patients [26].

Recession can affect a single tooth or a group of teeth. Before treating gingival recessions, etiologic factors should be identified, and a detailed clinical evaluation should be performed. The amount of keratinized gingiva, the size and location of the recession, the biotype of the gingival tissue, and local factors such as faulty fillings, tooth positions, and traumatic factors should be identified, and all conditions that may impair healing should be eliminated [27]. Periodontal diseases should be treated, and harmful habits such as excessive tooth brushing should be changed to new methods suitable for the patient.

Surgical or non-surgical approaches can be performed to treat gingival recessions. Prosthetic, restorative, or orthodontic approaches may be helpful depending on the recession's severity. The surgical intervention to address aesthetic concerns is to cover the root surface and create a new marginal border compatible with the adjacent teeth' gingiva. The coronally advanced flap technique is commonly performed in gingival recession treatment with connective tissue obtained from the palatal region [28]. Laterally positioned flaps, double papilla flaps, guided tissue regeneration, free gingival graft, tunnel technique, or modified coronally positioned flaps are other methods that can be used for root closure [29, 30].

The choice of technique depends on the severity of the recession, its location, the number of teeth affected, the amount of keratinized gingiva apical or lateral to the recession, the gingival biotype, and the clinical skill and experience of the physician [31]. Even if the treatment outcome is not predictable in all cases, choosing the appropriate treatment method after determining all etiologic factors will positively affect the final result.

46.7 Aesthetic Crown Lengthening

Short clinical crown lengths due to caries, tooth wear, fractures, passive eruption, trauma, etc., can negatively affect facial aesthetics. A crown lengthening procedure is necessary to achieve aesthetic harmony in such cases.

Periodontal health, oral hygiene, crown root ratio, furcation access, endodontic status of the tooth, and the amount of keratinized tissue should be evaluated before the crown lengthening procedure. In the presence of gingival overgrowth, gingivectomy with a scalpel or laser may be sufficient to achieve aesthetic harmony. When a flap operation is indicated, it is essential to remove enough bone to preserve the suprarenal tissue attachment (attachment epithelium and suprarenal connective tissue), which is approximately 2 mm [32]. If the suprarenal attachment is not preserved, periodontal health may be compromised, and complications such as gingival recession, pocket formation, and bone resorption may occur.

Prosthetic restorations must be made six months after bone surgical operations [33]. Otherwise, the position of the gingival margin may alter between 2 and 4 mm after the final prosthetic restoration. The gingival recession that may occur after permanent restoration will again negatively affect aesthetics.

46.8 Bone and Soft Tissue Augmentations

For an implant-supported restoration to support the aesthetic appearance, there must be sufficient supportive bone and soft tissue in the related area. The implants must be positioned parallel at right angles into the bone. In cases of bone loss, bone grafts can be used alone or supported by an absorbable or non-absorbable barrier membrane to fill the complex tissue deficiency. Autogenous grafts, xenografts, allografts, synthetic grafts, or a combination of these materials can create bone in the lateral and vertical direction at the implant site [34]. Peri-implant soft tissue thickness is also essential for maintaining aesthetics in the future. In some cases, soft tissue deficiency can be performed in the same session as bone augmentation, but in most cases, a second surgery is required for soft tissue augmentation.

46.9 Conclusion

As a result of increasing individual awareness, society's aesthetic expectations have increased considerably. To meet these expectations, clinicians must adopt new technology, research new materials and treatment techniques, listen carefully to patients' wishes, and work multidisciplinary.

References

1. Pithon MM, Nascimento CC, Barbosa GC, Coqueiro RS. Do dental esthetics have any influence on finding a job. Am J Orthod Dentofacial Orthop. 2014;146(4):423–9.
2. Newman MG, Takei H, Klokkevold PR, Carranza FA. Newman and Carranza's clinical periodontology. Elsevier Health Sciences; 2018. p. 29.
3. Dummett CO, Gupta OP. The DOPI assessment in gingival pigmentation. J Dent Res. 1966;45:122.
4. Rathee M, Rao PL, Bhoria M. Prevalence of gingival biotypes among young dentate North Indian population: a biometric approach. Int J Clin Pediatr Dent. 2016;9(2):104–8.
5. Sharma P, Bawa SKS, Chauhan P, Malhotra D. Gingival biotype: a key to successful aesthetics–its role and functions–observation-based research. Eur J Dent Oral Health. 2024;5(2):9–12.
6. Cohen B. Pathology of the interdental tissues. Dental Practit. 1959;9:167–73.
7. Patel M, Guni A, Nibali L, et al. Interdental papilla reconstruction: a systematic review. Clin Oral Invest. 2024;28:101. https://doi.org/10.1007/s00784-023-05409-0.
8. Tarnow DP, Magner AW, Fletcher P. The effect of the distance from the contact point to the crest of bone on the presence or absence of the interproximal dental papilla. J Periodontol. 1992;63(12):995–6.
9. Pawar B, Mishra P, Banga P, Marawar PP. Gingival zenith and its role in redefining esthetics: a clinical study. J Indian Soc Periodontol. 2011;15(2):135–8. https://doi.org/10.4103/0972-124X.84382.
10. Waliszewski M. Restoring dental appearance: a literature review. J Prosthodent. 2005;93:386–94.
11. Gallucci GO, Belser UC, Bernard JP, Magne P. Modeling and characterization of the CEJ for optimization of esthetic implant design. Int J Periodont Restorat Dent. 2004;24:19–29.
12. Su H, Gonzalez-Martin O, Weisgold A, Lee E. Considerations of implant abutment and crown contour: critical contour and subcritical contour. Int J Periodont Restorat Dent. 2010;30:335–43.
13. Alaqeely R, AlRowis R, AlSeddiq A, AlShehri F, Aldosari M. Influence of gingival display on smile attractiveness assessed by Saudi Arabian laypersons and dental professionals. Sci Rep. 2023;13(1):18718.
14. Sabri R. The eight components of a balanced smile. J Clin Orthod. 2005;34(3):155–67.
15. Tjan AH, Miller GD, The JG. Some esthetic factors in a smile. J Prosthet Dent. 1984;51:24–8. https://doi.org/10.1016/S0022-3913(84)80097-9.
16. Mercado-García J, Rosso P, Gonzalvez-García M, Colina J, Fernández JM. Gummy smile: mercado-rosso classification system and dynamic restructuring with hyaluronic acid. Aesthetic Plast Surg. 2021;45(5):2338–49.

17. Hunt O, et al. The influence of maxillary gingival exposure e on dental attractiveness ratings. Eur J Orthod. 2002;24(2):199–204.
18. Polo M. Botulinum toxin type A in the treatment of excessive gingival display. Am J Orthod Dentofacial Orthop. 2005;127(2):214–8.
19. Singh VP, Uppoor AS, Nayak DG, Shah D. Black triangle dilemma and its management in esthetic dentistry. Dent Res J (Isfahan). 2013;10(3):296–301.
20. Kandaswamy S, Goonewardene M, Tennant MC. Changes in interdental papillae height following alignment of the anterior teeth. Aust Orthod J. 2007;23(1):16–23.
21. Carnio J, Carnio AT. Papilla reconstruction: interdisciplinary consideration for clinical success. J Esthet Restor Dent. 2018;30(6):484–91.
22. Carranza N, Zogbi C. Reconstruction of interdental papilla with an underlying subepithelial connective tissue graft: technical considerations and a case reports. Int J Periodont Restorat Dent. 2011;31(11):e45–50.
23. Anitua E, Troya M, Orive G. Plasma rich in growth factors promote gingival tissue regeneration by stimulating fibroblast proliferation and migration and by blocking transforming growth factor-beta1-induced myodifferentiation. J Periodontol. 2012;83(8):1028–37.
24. da Silva Thaiz Z, Rogério M, Rafael SF, Aline d O, Indira CDS, Letícia d SP, et al. Hyaluronic acid for repairing interdental papilla in esthetic area: case report. Rev Clin Periodoncia Implantol Rehabil Oral [Internet]. 2019;12(3):157–8.
25. Alhabashneh R, Alomari S, Khaleel B, Qinawi H, Alzaubi M. Interdental papilla reconstruction using injectable hyaluronic acid: a 6 month prospective longitudinal clinical study. J Esthet Restor Dent. 2021;33(3):531–7.
26. Daprile G, Gatto MR, Checchi L. The evolution of buccal gingival recessions in a student population: a 5-year follow-up. J Periodontol. 2007;78:611–4.
27. Imber JC, Kasaj A. Treatment of gingival recession: when and how? Int Dent J. 2021;71(3):178–87.
28. de Sanctis M, Zucchelli G. Coronally advanced flap: a modified surgical approach for isolated recession-type defects: three-year results. J Clin Periodontol. 2007;34:262–8.
29. Hofmanner P, Alessandri R, Laugisch O, et al. Predictability of surgical techniques used for coverage of multiple adjacent gingival recessions – a systematic review. Quintessence Int. 2012;43:545–54.
30. Aroca S, Molnar B, Windisch P, et al. Treatment of multiple adjacent Miller class I and II gingival recessions with a Modified Coronally Advanced Tunnel (MCAT) technique and a collagen matrix or palatal connective tissue graft: a randomized, controlled clinical trial. J Clin Periodontol. 2013;40:713–20.
31. Stefanini M, Marzadori M, Aroca S, et al. Decision making in root-coverage procedures for the esthetic outcome. Periodontol. 2000;2018(77):54–64.
32. Jepsen S, Caton JG, Albandar JM, et al. Periodontal manifestations of systemic diseases and developmental and acquired conditions: consensus report of workgroup 3 of the 2017 World Workshop on the Classification of Periodontal and Peri-Implant Diseases and Conditions. J Periodontol. 2018;89(suppl 1):S237–48.
33. Brägger U, Lauchenauer D, Lang NP. Surgical lengthening of the clinical crown. J Clin Periodontol. 1992;19(1):58–63.
34. Fagan MC, Owens H, Smaha J, Kao RT. Simultaneous hard and soft tissue augmentation for implants in the esthetic zone: report of 37 consecutive cases. J Periodontol. 2008;79:1782–8.

Orthodontic Management of Smile Aesthetics

47

Kemal Devrim İşçi

47.1 Introduction

Aesthetic perception becomes an increasingly important criterion in orthodontic treatment. That is why an aesthetic smile has emerged as an indispensable concept and gives direction to treatment. Social, psychological, and physical factors determine a smile. Even if the physical factor of a smile is highly standard, the subjective aspect of this smile is the most critical parameter. It is thought that negative teeth appearance may cause disturbances in patients' daily lives even though there is no handicapping or pain related to dental and facial appearance. Corrections of alignment, spacing, and aesthetic factors in a malocclusion mainly remedy the smile. There are three pathways in general orthodontic treatment strategies for correcting or creating an aesthetic smile. The first option is the alignment of crowded teeth or the reconstruction of arches with spacing. The second is eliminating gingival and/or buccal vestibular avulsions. Soft tissue rearrangements or restorations are achieved thirdly.

Orthodontics has traditionally been considered as the area involved in the correction of facial disfigurements as well as the tendency and necessity caused by malocclusion. In addition to functional and biological analyses, treatment planning for correcting dentofacial deformity has benefited from aesthetic evaluations for many years. However, the photographic and cinematographic industries have enhanced the popularity of the aesthetic perceptions and valuations of the population. The patient's primary concern is their facial and dental/oral appearance change. The loss of teeth and their structural and functional change naturally reflected their occlusions and took place in artistic works. Thus, the smile can be considered a product of both the individual and the society and indicates a symbol of happiness and

K. D. İşçi (✉)
Faculty of Dentistry, Department of Orthodontics, İstanbul Galata University, Istanbul, Turkey

C. Cingi et al. (eds.), *Minor Interventions, Major Outcomes on the Face*, Comprehensive ENT, https://doi.org/10.1007/978-3-032-01305-7_47

well-being. The discussion for the reconstruction of a smile consists of at least three stages: the peri-treatment phase smile, the immediate smile, and the long-term reconstructed smile after treatment. Suffice it to say that the orthodontic treatment planning is directly related to the patient's smile.

Teeth framed by upper and lower lips, gum and tissue sculpting, and the sum of spaces and gaps are just a few aspects that contribute to a beautiful smile. Observable features of a well-proportioned smile include the amount of gum tissue exposed when smiling, the shape of the smile arch, the proportion of the teeth, any changes in dental axial inclination or midline misalignment, the distance between the buccal surface and the gums, the height and shape of the gingiva, the presence of diastema, and the color of the teeth. Each component may be considered independently, but they must all work together to form a whole that produces the desired visual outcome. People nowadays have different expectations when they seek dental treatment and are more conscious and critical about their smiles. Therefore, it is essential to understand what the public considers appropriate smiling features when deciding on a specific dental treatment.

A flawless grin results from numerous factors, each critical to varying degrees. Dental professionals must be well-versed in defining the sweet spot where their aesthetic smile knowledge meets the individual's perception. A dentist's competencies are the skills and knowledge they need to do their job well. A person's smile is an essential component of their social interactions and a description of their facial beauty and delicateness [1]. The primary objective of this research was to detail the many aesthetic factors and techniques that go into creating a picture-perfect grin.

When you smile, it is like a curve that straightens everything out. A smile is a crucial facial expression for conveying friendship, agreement, and gratitude, among the most important facial expressions. In the last ten years, smile design and analysis have become essential tools for orthodontic diagnosis and treatment planning [2, 3]. Patients often seek treatment due to a desire for aesthetics [4]. A beautiful, balanced smile is one of the most important goals of modern orthodontic treatment. This goal is achieved through the subspecialty of micro aesthetics, which focuses on the details of individual teeth; gingival aesthetics on the gums; macro aesthetics on the placement of individual teeth in groups; and facial aesthetics [3]. The development of standards for evaluating facial forms and the direction of orthodontic treatment is a direct outcome of the many studies conducted on facial features [5]. Results from the occlusal relationship were the mainstay of orthodontic treatment for quite some time. These days, occlusion and soft tissues must work in tandem for orthodontic treatment to be considered modern. A professional can learn about the hierarchy of aesthetic choice by observing the impact of smile attractiveness components. So, it is crucial to understand how orthodontic treatment affects the aesthetics of a smile. Researchers have recently focused more on the midline position, axial midline angulation, buccal corridor, and smile arc, contributing to a beautiful smile [6].

Our ability to extrapolate increases after we grasp the grin's significance within the face's context. When it comes to how attractive a person seems, it has a bearing on their physical appearance and mental traits. Perception and evaluation of an individual are greatly affected by the presence or absence of harmful changes to their skin. A person's sexuality, IQ, emotional stability, dominance, and behavioral intentions while interacting with others can all be negatively impacted by changes. These traits become readily apparent when dental treatment improves the smile's aesthetics. You have probably seen how cosmetic treatments boost patients' confidence and well-being [7, 8].

47.2 The Ideal Smile

The gesture of a genuine grin is intricate. When people express themselves through it, it often goes a long way [9]. Perceived health and success are also linked to the perfect grin. Good oral hygiene is shown when there are no signs of inflammation, calculus deposits, discolored teeth, broken restorations, or ugly gums. According to Ruelkellerman's research, people are more likely to be loyal, honest, and conscientious when their teeth are in a healthy alignment [1].

47.3 Classification of Smile

Many authors have classified grins into distinct types. For example, Ackerman et al. [2] identified two kinds of smiles.

The voluntary social smile, or posed smile, is characterized by the following: the lips part slightly due to mild contraction of the muscles that lift them, and the teeth and, occasionally, the gingival scaffold are shown.

The involuntary grin, also known as the enjoyment smile, unposed smile, or Duchenne smile, occurs when the muscles responsible for pressing down on the gums and cheeks contract to their maximum capacity. This allows the lips to expand fully and the front teeth to be exposed as much as possible. This smile is induced by laughing or intense pleasure.

Stage II, Forced Smile, was the classification given by Peck and Peck [10].

47.4 Smile Assessment

Photographs and video recordings are the main clinical tools for smile evaluations. Clinical examinations are standard in dentistry, but recording patients' information is equally important. Consequently, images have traditionally served as the benchmark [7].

However, in contrast to filming one's smile, the reliability of images has lately come under scrutiny. This is because smiling is a complex and dynamic activity involving multiple facial muscles interacting to create varied dentolabial architectural positions [7].

There are three distinct patterns of smiling that Rubin [11] identifies. When people greet each other in social situations or strange places like the elevator, they often display the commissure smile [11], usually called the Mona Lisa smile. The commissures are drawn upward in this smile, revealing or concealing the teeth. Cuspid smiles, often called social smiles, are the second form of a smile. Its usage in self-portraits shared on social media has spread over the world. This type of smile displays anterosuperior teeth, naturally or not, by consistently drawing the top lip upward. Many patients find that it helps them hide undesirable smile changes, including a gingival smile, which allows for a more accurate examination. A complicated grin [11] is the third type of smile pattern, defined by a broad upper lip movement and a movable lower lip. This method of accurately portraying patients' smile designs is also known as spontaneous smile, which is typically involuntary. Camara [9] argues that complex smiles should form the basis of aesthetic planning since social smiles might not reflect reality since they reflect learned voluntary movements [7].

It is evident that effectively recording a patient's smile in real-time using static images is challenging. Getting the patient to smile also makes taking good pictures harder since everyone has their own sense of humor [9] (Fig. 47.1).

47.5 Necessary Features of a Better Smile

First, the smile arc; second, the ratio and symmetry of the maxillary central incisors; third, the ratio of the anterior to the posterior teeth; fourth, the presence of an anterosuperior space; fifth, the gingival design; sixth, the levels of gingival exposure; seventh, the buccal corridor; eighth, the midline and tooth angulation; ninth, the details—tooth color and anatomical shape; and tenth, the lip volume [7].

The "dominance of central incisors" is defined by the central incisors, which are the most prominent teeth in the upper jaw, and the alignment of the teeth on the back of the mouth, from canine to canine or first premolar to first premolar, is specifically considered. Simply put, the central incisors are the show-stopping stars of a grin. So, "dominance of central incisors" [7] is closely related to commandments 1–4.

47.5.1 Smile Arc: Vertical Placement of Maxillary Incisors

The maxillary central incisors are essential for a smile, which is where aesthetic planning should start [1, 10, 12]. When you smile, the first commandment says your upper teeth should be in the best possible vertical position. When planning an aesthetic procedure, that is the initial stage [7].

47.5.2 Maxillary Central Incisor Ratio and Symmetry

The ratio and symmetry of the maxillary central incisors are altered after the vertical location of the incisors has been established. Therefore, it is imperative to attain the ideal width-height (W/H) ratio and symmetry of central incisors, as stated in the

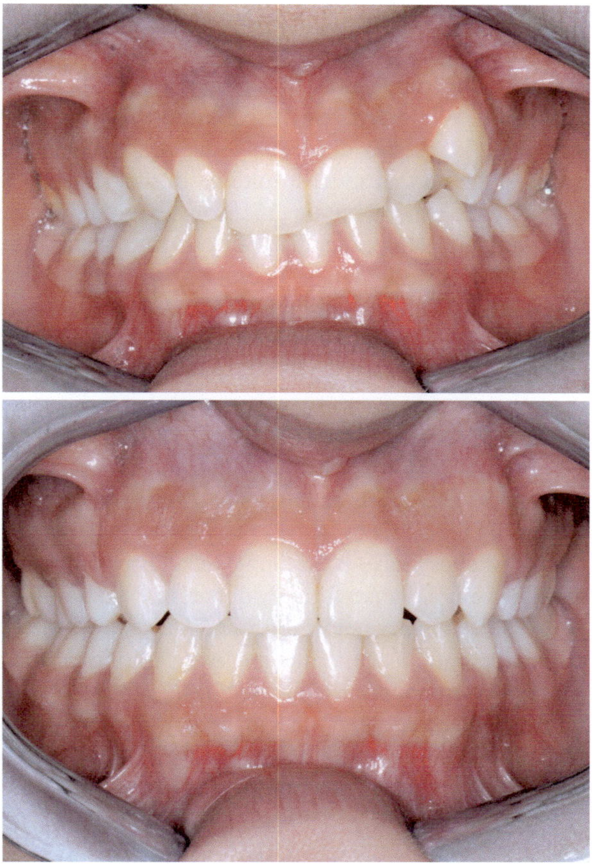

Fig. 47.1 Orthodontic management of teeth. Up: Before treatment. Down: After treatment

second commandment. To find the W/H ratio, the physician needs to take note of the clinical crown width and height of the maxillary central incisors. Consequently, he must consider the more aesthetically pleasing 75 to 85% ratios [13]. Central incisors with proportions closer to 75% will have a more extended pattern that women generally like, while incisors with proportions closer to 85% will have a broader pattern that men typically approve of [7].

47.5.3 Anterior-Superior Tooth Proportion

The next step after achieving the perfect vertical location of maxillary incisors, W/H ratio, and maximum symmetry between central incisors is adjusting the percentage between anterosuperior teeth. The golden ratio, first published by Levin in 1978 [14], is the basis for this characteristic, which is extensively considered in dentistry. In frontal view, teeth have a width-to-projection ratio [7].

47.5.4 Anterosuperior Spaces' Existence

The aesthetic zone's diastema perception has been the subject of much scholarly discussion. While doing so, it sparks a great deal of debate. The question that needs answering is whether diastemas in the aesthetic zone are attractive or not. The evidence suggests that modest midline diastemas (less than 2.0 mm) may be undetected by the general public [15]. Some well-known artists may have diastemas and find them appealing; this discovery might explain. This conclusion [15] should be questioned as well, though, because it is overly optimistic about the effect of midline diastemas on grin aesthetics. Are diastemas between 1.0 and 2.0 mm invisible to the naked eye? [7].

47.5.5 Design of the Gingiva

Aesthetic dentistry also has to consider the architecture of the gingiva. When describing the perfect gingival shape when smiling, the words "pink aesthetics" and "red aesthetics" have been employed. "The canine gingival margin must coincide with the central incisors gingival margin, whereas the lateral incisors gingival margin must be slightly below this line," states one dental textbook as a necessary condition for optimal aesthetic gingiva. Smiling to the fullest is assured with this parameter. If dentists use the previously indicated criteria, they may place the incisal edge of the central incisors at the same level as or slightly higher than the canines in cases where their lengths are equal [16]. Consequently, unsightly grins, such as plane or inverted arcs, may be created [7].

47.5.6 Gingival Exposure

Measuring the number of exposed teeth and gums in the aesthetic zone is crucial to have a beautiful smile. Gingival exposure is defined as the degree to which the grin line is high, medium, or low, as stated by Tjan et al. [17].

According to the literature, gingival tissue exposure when smiling is not bad [15, 18, 19]. Consistent with other research [15, 18], we discovered in a prior study [19] that 3.0 mm is the upper limit for gingival tissue exposure. As a result, a gingival exposure of at most 3.0 mm is appropriate, but values over this mark are unsightly. Considering the various types of smiles—high, medium, and low—and these results, the 6th commandment implies that the most aesthetic option is a high grin with gingival exposure of no more than 3.0 mm, followed by a medium smile and a low smile.

47.5.7 Buccal Corridor

When you smile, the buccal corridor is the area on both sides of your mouth that separates the vestibular surface of your exposed posterior teeth from the lip commissure [20, 21]. Typically, a narrow maxillary dental arch is seen after a sizable buccal corridor, an intermediate corridor after dental arches of intermediate transverse dimensions, and a narrow or nonexistent corridor is associated with severe transverse dental arches. Whether buccal corridor oversmiling is more aesthetically pleasing is a topic on which the literature is divided. Some research shows that various buccal corridors have little effect on smile aesthetics, while other research finds the reverse to be true. At the Federal University of Bahia, we did some further research and came to the same conclusion: intermediate buccal corridors are more aesthetically pleasing than wide or narrow ones. More expansive buccal passages are considered more unsightly, in line with this tendency [22, 23].

47.5.8 Midline and Tooth Angulation

Midline deviation, like the buccal corridor, is a contentious aspect of grin aesthetics. But ordinary people do not even notice it. According to research, average people cannot detect midline variations of more than three or four millimeters [15, 18]. That is why it is acceptable to hold some well-known artists and models up as examples of beauty standards even though they have a significant midline deviation [7].

47.5.9 Anatomical form and Tooth Color

It is common practice to carry out the procedures that make up this commandment during the orthodontic finishing phase. Dental whitening, contact lens adjustment, and incisal edge reshaping in the aesthetic zone are the three operations essentially outlined in the 9th commandment that can help with aesthetic refinement [7].

47.5.10 Lip Fullness

Finally, the structure surrounding and framing a smile—the lips—is the subject of the last commandment. The modern beauty standard includes a large, attractive smile, fuller lips, and more visible upper teeth when smiling, at rest, and speaking [7].

47.6 Measurement of Smile Characteristics

As an unintended side effect of orthodontic treatment, the grin arc can be flattened using one of three methods: [2]

Suppose the incisor-lip position at rest is not considered or monitored. In that case, the smile arc may be flattened after the maxillary incisors are overinsured to fix an overbite or a gingival grin. In addition to flattening the smile arc, the patient may experience the aging effects mentioned earlier [24] and a low lip line when smiling and at rest, caused by the careless use of archwires with accentuated curves. The grin arc can be flattened, and the patient's lip line can become low when smiling and at rest due to the careless usage of archwires with accentuated curves, which can age the patient in the same way as stated above [25].

47.6.1 Bracket Alignment

Do not utilize the same bracket heights for a reverse smile arc, a flat smile, or a parallel smile. Bracket placements should be patient-specific, considering the angle between the incisal margins and the curvature of the lower lip [26], to attain the most aesthetically pleasing grin arc. For example, a reverse smile arc [25] calls for higher-than-usual bracket placement on the central incisors of the maxilla and progressively lower bracket placement on the lateral incisors and canines.

Orthognathic surgery, intermaxillary elastics, and extraoral forces can all influence the cant of the occlusal plane. For example, a nonconsonant grin arc can be produced when the incisal margins shift away from the lower lip due to an upward cant in the maxillary occlusal plane. In contrast, an unsightly grin arc will result from the lower lip covering the upper incisal margins due to an excessively clockwise tilt of the occlusal plane. Attrition from central incisor shortening, thumb sucking, and other behaviors; excessive posterior vertical growth (often shown in brachyfacial patterns); and the muscles of the lower lip are further factors that might impact the grin arc [27]. When the curvature of the incisal margins does not correspond with the border of the lower lip when smiling, it affects both the lip line and the smile arc, which is caused by the inclination of the maxillary incisors. An everted lower lip is seen with excessively proclined incisors, while the lower lip partially covers uprighted or reclined incisors [25].

47.7 Clinical Guidelines For Improving Smile Aesthetics

47.7.1 Vertical Dimension

If you want your teeth to look their best when smiling and talking, follow these tips: Look at the patient's teeth from the front for an accurate cosmetic assessment. To get an "eye-to-eye" view [2, 27] while the patient is seated in the dental chair, tilt their head to one side of the headrest.

Pictures of the lips at rest should be taken before and after treatment to document the spontaneous gingival exhibition of the maxillary incisors. A brief film showing the patient smiling and excitedly speaking can also help capture this spontaneous event.

When you smile, the curvature of the upper teeth's incisors should align with the lower lip's inside. Standard practice dictates that the maxillary central incisors be half a millimeter to an inch longer than the lateral incisors to accomplish this. Ensure not to forcefully push the maxillary incisors forward when their vertical position before treatment is typical for their age. Keep the upper lip from covering the maxillary incisors too much.

Ensure that every orthodontic patient exhibits their vertical incisors at an age-appropriate level while at rest and in regular conversation [27].

47.7.2 Midlines

If you want a practical way to find your face's midline, draw a vertical line from your nose to your philtrum crease. If you want your teeth to look their best, their midlines do not have to be perfectly aligned with your face. Most people can tolerate a little maxillary midline deviation as long as the canting of the central incisor crown is not too severe. Securing the maxillary anterior teeth's connector areas for a more attractive smile is helpful according to the 50-40-30 guideline. A lengthy, vertical, and parallel-to-the-face midline connecting area should join the two maxillary central incisors; this area should be about half the length of their clinical crowns. As far as aesthetics are concerned, the mandibular midline is not crucial [2].

47.7.3 Transverse Dimension

Despite the lack of proof for the most aesthetically pleasing crown inclinations, the following clinical guidelines are helpful: Give each patient a unique, symmetrical, and aesthetically pleasing labio-lingual crown inclination of their canines and premolars. Even in the same patient, there is a common asymmetry in the crown inclination of the premolars and canines on the opposite sides of the mouth. To address these issues, it is necessary to [2] identify them during the initial stages of treatment by observing the teeth from the front and [3] deliberately tighten the archwire (or use individualized bracket torque recommendations) to rectify them. Please do so to avoid an uneven clinical crown inclination in the final product. For a fuller grin, make sure the front teeth are straight. The maxillary first and second premolars will serve as the final teeth in the mouth in around 90% of instances. The aesthetic and functional benefits of the treatment are enhanced by a lateral curve that is smooth and gradual from the front to the back teeth. Adverse effects on aesthetics will result from any interference [2].

Refrain from lingual tipping of the mandibular canines, premolars, and molars during orthodontic treatment. Mastering the art of seeing critical dentition details before, during, and after treatment is the key to successful orthodontics [2, 27].

References

1. Correa BD, Bittencourt MA, Machado AW. Influence of maxillary canine gingival margin asymmetries on the perception of smile esthetics among orthodontists and laypersons. Am J Orthod Dentofacial Orthoped. 2014;145(1):55–63.
2. Patankar K, Khatri J. Smile esthetics in orthodontic: a review article. Int J Appl Dent Sci. 2021;7(4):223–7.
3. Morley J, Eubank J. Macroesthetic elements of smile design. J Am Dent Assoc. 2001;132(1):39–45.
4. Goldstein RE. Study of need for esthetics in dentistry. J Prosthet Dent. 1969;21(6):589–98.
5. Roden-Johnson D, Gallerano R, English J. The effects of buccal corridor spaces and arch form on smile esthetics. Am J Orthod Dentofacial Orthoped. 2005;127(3):343–50.
6. Janson G, Branco NC, Fernandes TM, Sathler R, Garib D, Lauris JR. Influence of orthodontic treatment, midline position, buccal corridor and smile arc on smile attractiveness: a systematic review. Angle Orthod. 2011;81(1):153–61.
7. Machado AW. 10 commandments of smile esthetics. Dental Press J Orthod. 2014;19(4):136–57.
8. Van der Geld P, Oosterveld P, Heck GV, Kuijpers-Jagtman AM. Smile attractiveness: self-perception and influence on personality. Angle Orthod. 2007;77(5):759–75.
9. Hulsey CM. An esthetic evaluation of lip-teeth relationships present in the smile. Am J Orthod. 1970;57(2):132–44.
10. Peck S, Peck L, Kataja M. The gingival smile line. Angle Orthod. 1992;62(2):91–100.
11. Rubin LR. The anatomy of a smile: its importance in the treatment of facial paralysis. Plast Reconstr Surg. 1974;53:384–7.
12. Manjula WS, Sukumar MR, Kishorekumar S, Gnanashanmugam K, Mahalakshmi K. Smile: a review. J Pharm Bioallied Sci. 2015;7(Suppl 1):S271.
13. Wolfart S, Thormann H, Freitag S, Kern M. Assessment of dental appearance following changes in incisor proportions. Eur J Oral Sci. 2005;113(2):159–65.
14. Levin EI. Dental esthetics and the golden proportion. J Prosthet Dent. 1978;40(3):244–52.
15. Kokich VO, Kokich VG, Kiyak HA. Perceptions of dental professionals and laypersons to altered dental esthetics: asymmetric and symmetric situations. Am J Orthod Dentofacial Orthop. 2006;13(2):141–51.
16. Machado AW, McComb R, Moon W, Gandini LG Jr. Influence of the vertical position of maxillary central incisors on the perception of smile esthetics among orthodontists and laypersons. J Esthetic Rest Dent. 2013;25(6):392–401.
17. Tjan AH, Miller GD, The JG. Some esthetic factors in a smile. J Prosthet Dent. 1984;51(1):24–8.
18. Kokich VO, Kiyak HA, Shapiro PA. Comparing the perception of dentists and lay people to altered dental esthetics. J Esthet Dent. 1999;11(6):311–24.
19. Suzuki L, Machado AW, Bittencourt MAV. An evaluation of the influence of gingival display level in the smile esthetics. Dent Press J Orthod. 2011;16(5):37–9.
20. Rufenacht CR. Fundamentals of esthetics. Chicago: Quintessence; 1990.
21. Chiche G, Pinault A. Esthetics of anterior fixed prosthodontics. Chicago: Quintessence; 1994.
22. Nascimento DC, Santos ER, Machado AW, Bittencourt MAV. Influence of buccal corridor dimension on smile esthetics. Dent Press J Orthod. 2012;17(5):145–50.
23. Krishnan V, Daniel ST, Lazar D, Asok A. Characterization of posed smile by using visual analog scale, smile arc, buccal corridor measures, and modified smile index. Am J Orthod Dentofacial Orthoped. 2008;133(4):515–23.
24. Zachrisson BU. Esthetic factors involved in anterior tooth display and the smile: vertical dimension. J Clin Orthod. 1998;32:432–45.
25. Sabri R. The eight components of a balanced smile. J Clin Orthod. 2005;39(3):155–67.

26. Isci KD, Bayar Muluk N, Gungor E, Cingi C. Preventive measures for safer orthognathic surgery: key points. Ear Nose Throat J. 2024:1455613241266747. https://doi.org/10.1177/01455613241266747.
27. Sarver DM. The importance of incisor positioning in the esthetic smile: the smile arc. Am J Orthod. 2001;120:98–111.

Aesthetic Jawline Management

48

Songul Demir

48.1 Introduction

Both internal and external elements have a strong influence on the aging process. Delays in wound healing, increased skin fragility, and slower turnover are all consequences of thinning skin layers that occur with age [1–5]. Decreased expression of collagen and other proteins that promote structure and volume is linked to a dermal-epidermal interface that is becoming weaker [6]. Radiation, overall health, alcoholic and cigarette consumption, and gravity are some external elements that can influence these fundamental processes [7]. Loss of skin elasticity, soft tissue fall, muscular atrophy, and bone loss are all results of the aging process, which is influenced by internal and external influences. Excess skin on the lower face can cause jawling, and bone loss along the mandible can limit the chin projection [8]. The drooping of soft tissues that causes a noticeable submental crease is the root cause of chin ptosis, or witch's chin [1, 9].

Facial rejuvenation includes measures to lessen the visible signs of aging on the chin and mandible. This chapter aims to examine the most popular dermal fillers, emphasizing their safety and effectiveness, mechanism of action, indication, technique, and data supporting their use as a nonsurgical method for mandibular rejuvenation. To help clinicians choose the best option for their patients' aesthetic goals, it is important to understand the pros and cons of injectable fillers for jawline rejuvenation [1].

S. Demir (✉)
Department of Otorhinolaryngology, Selahaddin Eyyubi State Hospital, Diyarbakir, Turkey

C. Cingi et al. (eds.), *Minor Interventions, Major Outcomes on the Face*, Comprehensive ENT, https://doi.org/10.1007/978-3-032-01305-7_48

48.2 Anatomy of Lower Face

The lower face is characterized by a downward angle beginning at the upper lip and ending at the lower boundary of the chin. The mandible's angle forms the lower face's lateral border. The lower part of the face is where the jaw, chin, and lips are located [10].

48.2.1 The Lips

The lips stand out among the other features on the lower face. There is a distinct separation between the upper lip and the lower lip. The lips are sensory structures that help with speech articulation, eating, and kissing. Around the lips is the orbicularis oris muscle. The mandible and maxilla supply the orbicularis oris muscle, which inserts onto the lip skin and forms a sphincter. When you speak, kiss, chew, or otherwise change the shape of your lips, the orbicularis oris muscle contracts. Located in the area of the lower face, the risorius muscle begins in the parotid fascia and inserts into the modiolus near the angle of the mouth. The risorius muscle is responsible for drawing the jawline back. The majority of the lower face muscles primarily work on the lower lip. There are two pairs of muscles on the inside of the lower lip. The mentalis and depressor labii inferioris are the names of these muscles. The mentalis muscle attaches to the chin after traveling from the front of the jaw. Muscles such as the mentalis and depressor labii inferioris enter the lower lip, respectively, and work to elevate and wrinkle the jaw skin and protrude from the lower lip. Pressing down on the lips is what the depressor labii inferioris muscle does. You can find the depressor anguli oris muscle where your jaw meets your cheeks. A muscle called the depressor anguli oris inserts into the modiolus of the mouth after it arises from the tubercle of the mouth. The depressor anguli oris is a muscle that contracts to lower the angle of the mouth. The upper jaw (maxilla) and lower jaw (mandible) form the bone components of the lips [10].

48.2.2 Chin and Jaw

Chin or mental protuberance is the bony projection on the mandible's midline. The mandible's lateral parts give rise to the jaw and jawline, and a pre-mental fat pad is near the chin's tip. The inferior jowl fat pad is located on the jawline, close to the side of the pre-mental fat pad. An additional little fat pad, the superior jowl fat pad, sits above the inferior one. The platysma muscle is located on the underside of the jaw and chin. The platysma muscle inserts onto the jaw, cheek, and mouth from its origins in the infraclavicular and supraclavicular regions. It is a superficial muscle. Depressing the corners of the lips and pulling the skin of the neck superiorly are the actions of the platysma muscle. Additionally, the platysma muscle safeguards the underlying systems, including the trachea, esophagus, carotid arteries, jugular veins, and nerves, by providing a muscular covering [10].

48.3 Injectible Fillers

It is essential to have a well-defined mandibular angle and chin area for a face that looks proportionate and young. Particularly appealing to both sexes is a jawline that is well-contoured. As we age, our jaws naturally recede somewhat to the front and lower, creating a wider mandibular angle, and our chins gradually grow shorter and more pointed [11]. A double chin, or jowl, can develop when the fat around the jawbone atrophies and the septum between the jaws decreases. Therefore, to restore a more youthful appearance, nonsurgical face rejuvenation focusing on the lower third of the face aims to target these particular areas. Mild to moderate loss of face volume, laxity, and contour is the ideal candidate for hyaluronic acid (HA) fillers; severe cases may necessitate surgical intervention [12].

Meritonella folds, mental creases, chin apexes, pre-jowl regions, mandibular bodies, and angles are some of the areas that filler injections are most commonly used to treat. For all lower face rejuvenation procedures, it is crucial to know vascular anatomy to prevent vascular problems. By remaining medial to the crease and delivering most of the volume to the upper third of the fold, a linear subcutaneous retrograde method is used to target the melo-mental folds [8, 13]. Similarly, if you want to decrease the depth of the mental crease, you can do that by using an anterograde injection method. Injecting filler into two or three areas in the front of the chin will bring its projection closer to the lower lip [14]. Overfilling the pre-jowl area could make the chin look more expansive. Thus, the injector must be careful when restoring the jawline. An injection into the subcutaneous tissue, administered using a fanning technique to ensure uniform distribution, can achieve this goal. In conclusion, a more defined jawline is possible with mandibular augmentation, which involves a superficial subcutaneous injection over the body and a supraperiosteal injection over the angle [1] (Fig. 48.1).

48.3.1 Hyaluronic Acid (HA)

The soft tissue filler that is most frequently utilized is HA. The extracellular matrix of connective tissues, synovial fluid, and other tissues contains this injectable, big, nonsulfated glycosaminoglycan. It creates hydrogen bonding in water and consists of polymeric disaccharides. So, HA is structurally stable and includes water [15]. One gram of HA can bind as much as six liters of water [16]. From assisting with tissue healing to absorbing shock in joints, HA has multiple purposes in the native human body [17]. Because of its low immunogenicity, HA is a good choice for many people who want to avoid surgery to reduce the appearance of fine lines and wrinkles on their faces [1].

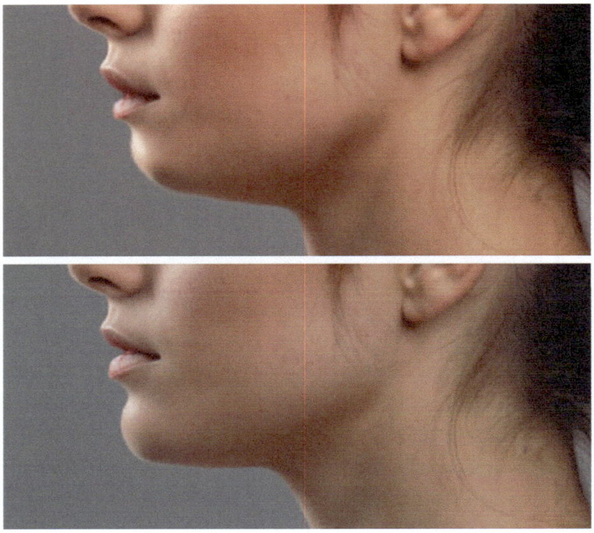

Fig. 48.1 Aesthetic jaw management with fillers Case 1

48.3.2 Calcium Hydroxylapatite (CaHa)

One example of a synthetic, biocompatible, and biodegradable soft tissue filler is CaHa, marketed as Radiesse by Merz Pharmaceuticals GmbH. Its composition is virtually equal to human bone and teeth [18]. CaHa is an innovative product that is a semi-permanent filler with a distinct time-delayed dual function. The filler expands the volume when injected for the first time. Because CaHa microspheres promote collagen ingrowth by inhibiting osseointegration and calcification and increasing fibroblastic growth, they gradually act as a scaffold for freshly produced collagen [19–21]. There is no indication of inflammation, body reaction, or granuloma development with CaHa microspheres since these fillers physiologically imitate the structure and metabolism of bone [22]. Patients do not need to undergo allergy testing before use, which is an advantage [1] (Fig. 48.2).

48.3.3 Poly-L-Lactic Acid (PLLA)

A synthetic polymer known as PLLA has several medicinal applications; it is semi-permanent, biodegradable, and biocompatible. A delayed method of action distinguishes PLLA from other fillers. Once implanted, PLLA particles trigger an inflammatory response, producing lactic acid and its derivatives [23]. Over time, type I collagen is deposited surrounding the foreign body reaction due to the host tissue's response, which involves the induction of collagen, connective tissue, and inflammatory cell development [24]. Biopsies taken after injection show no fibrosis or residual filler material, proving that the foreign body reaction is fully biocompatible despite the immune response [25]. It is recommended that numerous treatments

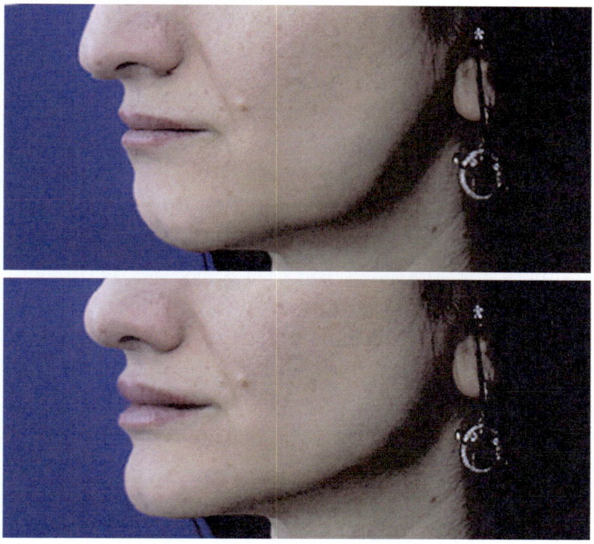

Fig. 48.2 Aesthetic jaw management with fillers Case 2

be undertaken over 1–2 months to fully appreciate the longevity of the effects of tissue growth. However, they have been observed to last up to 2 years [1].

Facial lipoatrophy caused by HIV and nasolabial fold repair are two of the current indications for Sculptra (Galderma). You need to mix the sterile freeze-dried powder with sterile water and lidocaine for anesthesia for at least two hours before applying the filler, which is contained in a glass vial [26]. It is recommended to inject into the superficial subcutaneous fat when approaching the lateral mandible and mandibular angle but to inject into the supra-periosteal space for menton and pre-jowl sulcus augmentation [27]. Nodules can occur if injections are made directly into the fibers of the oral commissure or depressor anguli oris muscles [28]. Full volumetric correction may require numerous sessions; thus, patients should be advised of this. Uneven contouring and nodularity are more likely to occur if the defect area is overfilled. Patients are advised to adhere to the "rule of 5 s" after injections, which involves massaging the injection site for 5 min, five times a day, for five days [29].

48.3.3.1 Polymethyl Methacrylate (PMMA)

PMMA is a long-lasting, biocompatible filler that works in two ways comparable to Radiesse (CaHA). Bovine collagen gel is used to suspend PMMA microspheres, which prompts an immediate increase in volume upon injection and promotes long-term collagen formation following the gel's dissolution within one month [30]. In contrast to macrophage phagocytosis and destruction, PMMA microspheres promote the formation of connective tissue and cells because of their small, smooth, and homogeneous size [25]. In the 1990s, Suneva Medical found that granulomas could develop in as many as 2.5% of patients between 6 and 18 months after receiving the fillers Arteplast and Artecoll, which contained PMMA microspheres [31].

Contemporary PMMA injectables, such as Artefill and Bellafill from Suneva Medical, have been purified to a higher standard and have received FDA approval for treating wrinkles in the face and correcting severe acne scars on the face. The product's bovine collagen base necessitates a four-week lead time for hypersensitivity testing, and any patient showing a positive response is not to be treated [1].

Because there is a limit to how much filler may be implanted into the deep-dermal layer with PMMA, overcorrection is less of an issue than with CaHa. This feature makes it such that adding a second layer above the first injection usually requires a second injection [32]. Easy use, permanent implantation, collagen production, and long-lasting outcomes are other benefits of PMMA. A more uniform dispersion of PMMA can be achieved by injecting it along the pre-jowl sulcus, chin, marionette lines, and mandibular region using the fanning technique. Reports have shown that utilizing a massager while injecting can alleviate some of the pressure patients feel in the pre-jowl area, making the process more comfortable [27].

48.3.4 Advantages of the Injectable Fillers

Among the many benefits of injectable fillers are their low price, quick results, minimal discomfort, and short recovery periods. Patients need not worry about scarring because there will be no surgical incisions. Because the physician can implant material according to patient preference and goals, injectables also allow personalized treatment strategies. An assortment of contours can be achieved for the chin with volume replacement in the anterior, vertical, and transverse dimensions. Filler injections across the masseter muscle might widen the jaw for males who want a more robust jawline [33]. Depending on the material, the effects of fillers can persist for years, and they are usually well-tolerated by the general public. With a therapeutic benefit lasting up to 18 months, HA has been extensively researched as an injectable filler for jawline rejuvenation [34]. Despite this, much of the research on this subject has used single-blind experiments, which could introduce bias when evaluating subjective progress [35, 36].

48.4 Liposuction of the Neck and Jowls

Clinically speaking, liposuction of the jowls and neck is among the most satisfying cosmetic surgery techniques. A patient can get a noticeable makeover with a quick, painless, affordable treatment. The outcomes of liposuction can now compete with those of a facelift in many patients, according to technological advancements in the field [37].

Since liposuction was initially described in the late 1970s, patients have undergone procedures to remove fat from their submental region, neck, and jowl. Before 1979, Illouz used a 5-mm cannula and a lateral route to execute the surgery [38]. Using a single submental incision, Hetter detailed the use of smaller cannulae [39]. In 1984, two further incisions were performed in the sub-ear lobules to enable suctioning at a right angle to the submental suctioning. The likelihood of discernible ridges forming was thereby reduced. Injuries to the marginal mandibular nerve were also less likely to occur. A 2.5-mm cannula had become standard by the mid-1980s. The neck suctioning was supplemented with the cheekbone, jowl, and mandibular border suctioning to attain a balanced outcome. Subplatysmal fat suctioning was also introduced in 1987 [37].

Patients under 40, in whom uniform skin shrinkage was anticipated, were the initial candidates for neck liposuction. Surgeons, however, began to acknowledge the possibility of suction in older patients with an apparent excess of skin in the early 1990s. Typically, the skin will redrape without drooping over the longer distance. The idea here is based on the triangle's length inequality, which states that two sides added together must be longer than the third. Furthermore, surgeons discovered that subdermal liposuction caused skin contraction [37].

By 1990, it was common practice to administer anesthesia and hemostasis via subcutaneous infiltration of the subcutaneous plane, using lidocaine and epinephrine at different dosages. Although this method has fallen out of favor over the past decade, certain surgeons have used internal and external ultrasonography since the late 90s.

Much recent talk has been about how liposuction might tighten the skin. Methods like laser-assisted liposuction and other externally applied energy like fractional lasers, radiofrequency and infrared radiation, and high-energy focused ultrasound (Ulthera) have been tried [40–43]. However, there is still insufficient unbiased evidence to recommend these approaches. Hence, jowl and neck liposuction should only be done when the skin is anticipated to contract naturally. Another option is to provide liposuction with all the necessary cautions and informed permission if the patient is okay with loose, maybe dangling skin [37].

48.4.1 Issue and Resolution

This issue comprises a lack of discernible mandibular contour, extra submental fat, and jowl fat. Obesity is often associated with submental fat. But even people who do not gain much weight can have some fat. Many people experience the development of submental fat deposits as they age, which are unrelated to their weight. As the skin dries out and droops, this could become more noticeable. Similarly, jowl fat could be associated with aging or just plain old extra fat. Impairment of the mandibular boundary visibility has the exact cause [37].

The cervicofacial concavity narrows and finally approaches a convexity as submental fat accumulates. Fat in this region is the "giveaway" sign of obesity, even though overall body fat can be concealed by clothing. The cervicofacial angle is approximately 118 degrees (37 degrees) when the neck is young.

By the time most people reach the age of 50, jowls have become a prominent feature of aging faces. One more thing that happens with age, especially in overweight people, is that the mandibular border gets less defined. Not only does the technique seem to remove fat, but it also gives the impression of skin loss by stimulating the contraction of the skin [37].

Submental fat is already an issue; microgenia and the harder-to-diagnose subplatysmal fat only worsen things. Aesthetic satisfaction depends on a thorough examination of the patient's specific concerns [37].

References

1. Go BC, Frost AS, Friedman O. Using injectable fillers for chin and jawline rejuvenation. World J Otorhinolaryngol Head Neck Surg. 2023;9(2):131–7. https://doi.org/10.1002/wjo2.93.
2. Quan T, Xiang Y, Liu Y, et al. Dermal fibroblast CCN1 expression in mice recapitulates human skin dermal aging. J Invest Dermatol. 2021;141:1007–16.
3. Amano S. Possible involvement of basement membrane damage in skin photoaging. J Investig Dermatol Symp Proc. 2009;14:2–7.
4. Feru J, Delobbe E, Ramont L, et al. Aging decreases collagen IV expression in vivo in the dermo-epidermal junction and in vitro in dermal fibroblasts: possible involvement of TGF-β1. Eur J Dermatol. 2016;26:350–60.
5. Vázquez F, Palacios S, Alemañ N, Guerrero F. Changes of the basement membrane and type IV collagen in human skin during aging. Maturitas. 1996;25:209–15.
6. Roig-Rosello E, Rousselle P. The human epidermal basement membrane: a shaped and cell instructive platform that aging slowly alters. Biomolecules. 2020;10:1607.
7. Mokos ZB, Ćurković D, Kostović K, Čeović R. Facial changes in the mature patient. Clin Dermatol. 2018;36:152–8.
8. Shah AR, Kennedy PM. The aging face. Med Clin North Am. 2018;102:1041–54.
9. Lesavoy MA, Creasman C, Schwartz RJ. A technique for correcting witch's chin deformity. Plast Reconstr Surg. 1996;97:842–6.
10. Nguyen JD, Duong H. Anatomy, Head and Neck: Face. [Updated 2023 Jun 5]. In: StatPearls [Internet]. Treasure Island (FL): StatPearls Publishing; 2024. Available from: https://www.ncbi.nlm.nih.gov/books/NBK551530/
11. Toledo Avelar LE, Cardoso MA, Santos Bordoni L, de Miranda AL, de Miranda Avelar JV. Aging and sexual differences of the human skull. Plast Reconstr Surg Global Open. 2017;5:e1297.
12. Sykes J, Fitzgerald R. Choosing the best procedure to augment the chin: is anything better than an implant. Facial Plast Surg. 2016;32:507–12.
13. de Maio M, Wu WTL, Goodman GJ, Monheit G. Facial assessment and injection guide for botulinum toxin and injectable hyaluronic acid fillers: focus on the lower face. Plast Reconstr Surg. 2017;140:393e–404e.
14. Braz A, Eduardo CCP. Reshaping the lower face using injectable fillers. Indian J Plast Surg. 2020;53:207–18.
15. Vasvani S, Kulkarni P, Rawtani D. Hyaluronic acid: a review on its biology, aspects of drug delivery, route of administrations and a special emphasis on its approved marketed products and recent clinical studies. Int J Biol Macromol. 2020;151:1012–29.
16. Monheit GD, Coleman KM. Hyaluronic acid fillers. Dermatol Ther. 2006;19:141–50.
17. Toole BP. Hyaluronan: from extracellular glue to pericellular cue. Nat Rev Cancer. 2004;4:528–39.
18. Herrmann JL, Hoffmann RK, Ward CE, Schulman JM, Grekin RC. Biochemistry, physiology, and tissue interactions of contemporary biodegradable injectable dermal fillers. Dermatol Surg. 2018;44(suppl 1):S19–31.
19. Marmur ES, Phelps R, Goldberg DJ. Clinical, histologic and electron microscopic findings after injection of a calcium hydroxylapatite filler. J Cosmet Laser Ther. 2004;6:223–6.

20. Yutskovskaya Y, Kogan E, Leshunov E. A randomized, split-face, histomorphologic study comparing a volumetric calcium hydroxylapatite and a hyaluronic acid-based dermal filler. J Drugs Dermatol. 2014;13:1047–52.
21. Berlin AL, Hussain M, Goldberg DJ. Calcium hydroxylapatite filler for facial rejuvenation: a histologic and immunohistochemical analysis. Dermatol Surg. 2008;34(suppl 1):S64–7.
22. Jacovella PF. Use of calcium hydroxylapatite (Radiesse) for facial augmentation. Clin Interv Aging. 2008;3:161–74.
23. Sickles CK, Nassereddin A, Gross GP. Poly-l-lactic acid. StatPearls. StatPearls Publishing; 2022.
24. Cabral L, Teixeira LN, Gimenez RP, et al. Effect of hyaluronic acid and poly-l-lactic acid dermal fillers on collagen synthesis: an in vitro and in vivo study. Clin Cosmet Investig Dermatol. 2020;13:701–10.
25. Lemperle G, Morhenn V, Charrier U. Human histology and persistence of various injectable filler substances for soft tissue augmentation. Aesthetic Plast Surg. 2003;27:354–66.
26. Lee JC, Lorenc ZP. Synthetic fillers for facial rejuvenation. Clin Plast Surg. 2016;43:497–503.
27. Buckingham E, Glasgold R, Kontis T, et al. Volume rejuvenation of the lower third, perioral, and jawline. Facial Plast Surg. 2015;31:070–9.
28. Vleggaar D, Fitzgerald R, Lorenc ZP, et al. Consensus recommendations on the use of injectable poly-L-lactic acid for facial and nonfacial volumization. J Drugs Dermatol. 2014;13:44–51.
29. Kates L, Fitzgerald R. Poly-l-lactic acid injection for HIV-associated facial lipoatrophy: treatment principles, case studies, and literature review. Aesthet Surg J. 2008;28:397–403.
30. Liu MH, Beynet DP, Gharavi NM. Overview of deep dermal fillers. Facial Plast Surg. 2019;35:224–9.
31. Pollack SV. Some new injectable dermal filler materials: hylaform, restylane, and artecoll. J Cutan Med Surg. 1999;3(suppl 4):S4-27–S4-35.
32. Lemperle G, Romano JJ, Busso M. Soft tissue augmentation with artecoll: 10-year history, indications, techniques, and complications. Dermatol Surg. 2003;29:573–87.
33. Vanaman Wilson MJ, Jones IT, Butterwick K, Fabi SG. Role of nonsurgical chin augmentation in full face rejuvenation: a review and our experience. Dermatol Surg. 2018;44:985–93.
34. Ogilvie P, Benouaiche L, Philipp-Dormston WG, et al. VYC-25L hyaluronic acid injectable gel is safe and effective for long-term restoration and creation of volume of the lower face. Aesthet Surg J. 2020;40:NP499–NP510.
35. Beer K, Kaufman-Janette J, Bank D, et al. Safe and effective chin augmentation with the hyaluronic acid injectable filler, VYC-20L. Dermatol Surg. 2021;47:80–5.
36. Ogilvie P, Sattler G, Gaymans F, et al. Safe, effective chin and jaw restoration with VYC-25L hyaluronic acid injectable gel. Dermatol Surg. 2019;45:1294–303.
37. Perry AW. Submental and Jowl Liposuction. In: Narayan D (Ed). Medscape. Updated: Sep 23, 2020. https://emedicine.medscape.com/article/1272432-overview#a9. Accessed online at 8 July 2024.
38. Illouz YG. The origins of lipolysis. In: Hetter GP, editor. Lipoplasty: the theory and practice of blunt suction lipectomy. New York: Lippincott Williams & Wilkins; 1984. p. 25.
39. Hetter GP. Lipoplasty of the face and neck. Lipoplasty: the theory and practice of blunt suction lipectomy. New York: Lippincott Williams & Wilkins; 1984. p. 249.
40. Stebbins WG, Hanke CW. Rejuvenation of the neck with liposuction and ancillary techniques. Dermatol Ther. 2011;24(1):28–40.
41. Collawn SS. Skin tightening with fractional lasers, radiofrequency, Smartlipo. Ann Plast Surg. 2010;64(5):526–9.
42. Sun Y, Wu SF, Yan S, Shi HY, Chen D, Chen Y. Laser lipolysis used to treat localized adiposis: a preliminary report on experience with Asian patients. Aesthetic Plast Surg. 2009;33(5):701–5.
43. Keramidas E, Rodopoulou S. Radiofrequency-assisted liposuction for neck and lower face adipodermal remodeling and contouring. Plast Reconstr Surg Glob Open. 2016;4(8):e850.

Mentoplasty: Overview

49

Aykut Kuru, Nuray Bayar Muluk, and Cemal Cingi

49.1 Introduction

The chin greatly influences aesthetics and facial symmetry. The nose plays a significant role in determining facial equilibrium, mainly when seen in profile. This has been known to surgeons for a long time, so rhinoplasty and genioplasty surgeries performed in conjunction are quite popular [1, 2]. A person's chin says a lot about their face and personality. People with long chins are powerful and assertive, whereas those with short chins are weak and vulnerable [1].

49.2 Anatomy

The chin results from the midline union of the two mandibular processes. The adjacent overlaying mesoderm is the progenitor of the soft tissues' muscular components. Although muscle fusion happens in the middle, it is frequently incomplete and divided into two parts by a fibrous median raphe. Parts of the chin's structure include soft tissue and bone [1].

A. Kuru
Department of Otorhinolaryngology, Merzifon Karamustafa Paşa Devlet Hastanesi, Amasya, Turkey

N. Bayar Muluk
Faculty of Medicine, Department of Otorhinolaryngology, Kırıkkale University, Kırıkkale, Türkiye

C. Cingi (✉)
Eskisehir Osmangazi University, Medical Faculty, Department of Otorhinolaryngology, Eskisehir, Türkiye
e-mail: cemal@ogu.edu.tr

C. Cingi et al. (eds.), *Minor Interventions, Major Outcomes on the Face*, Comprehensive ENT, https://doi.org/10.1007/978-3-032-01305-7_49

Subcutaneous tissues, skin, and muscles are all considered soft tissues because they are located below the labio-mental angle. The thickness of this chin pad might vary, particularly in cases of mentalis muscle hypertrophy. In most people, the mentalis muscle is tiny, inserts into the chin skin, and originates on the mandible beneath the incisors. The seventh cranial nerve is responsible for innervating it [1].

The mandible is responsible for the chin's skeletal structure, including the symphysis menti (the joint between the two parts of the jaw), the mental protuberance (the elevated area above this joint), and the mental tubercles (the bumps on the underside). Chubby cheeks and mental protuberance determine chin projection [1].

The labio-mental angle is the point where the chin and the lip meet. The lip and chin, on the other hand, are very close. Along with the orbicularis oris muscle, the depressor muscles interdigitate and insert on the mental tubercles. Chin procedures can influence the lips [1].

49.3 Fillers

Less invasive procedures have reduced the demand for chin augmentation surgery [3]. The Aesthetic Society recorded a 17% decrease in chin augmentations from 2015 to 2019, with a 7% decrease from 2018 to 2019 [4]. One possible major factor contributing to this trend is the growing acceptance of injectables. According to a 2016 worldwide poll by Allergan, 65% of people think injectable face fillers are more acceptable now than 5 years ago [5]. Injectable therapies were also believed by 57% of respondents to be able to produce outcomes that looked natural. Injectable fillers offer a safe and effective alternative to standard surgeries, which is appealing to more patients [3].

Among the many benefits of injectable fillers are their low price, quick results, minimal discomfort, and short recovery periods. Patients need not worry about scarring because there will be no surgical incisions. Because the physician can implant material according to patient preference and goals, injectables also allow personalized treatment strategies. An assortment of contours can be achieved for the chin with volume replacement in the anterior, vertical, and transverse dimensions. For example, individuals who want to look more manly can choose to have filler placed over the masseter, which will widen the jaw [6]. Depending on the material, the effects of fillers can persist for years, and they are usually well-tolerated by the general public. With a treatment benefit that lasts up to 18 months, HA has been extensively investigated as an injectable filler for rejuvenating the jawline [7]. Nevertheless, most published works on the issue are single-blind studies, which can introduce bias in evaluating subjective improvement [3, 8, 9] (Fig. 49.1).

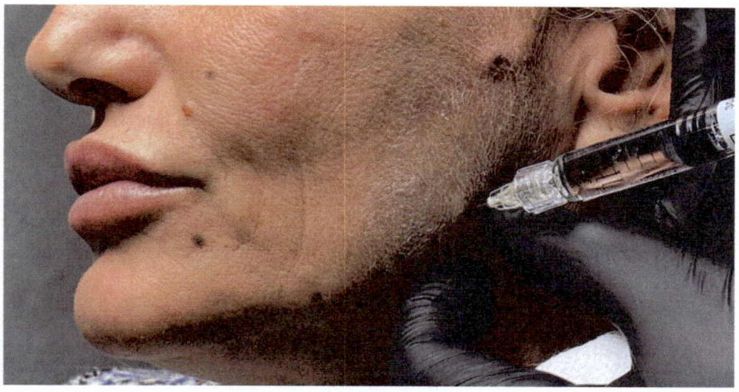

Fig. 49.1 Filler (injection) mentoplasty

49.3.1 Complication of Fillers

Complications, both immediate and distant, are linked to all fillers. Possible injection site responses include redness, swelling, bruises, soreness, and discomfort [10]. To lessen the severity of these usually temporary side effects, injections of lidocaine, avoiding anticoagulants before the surgery, and using a cold compress may be helpful [11]. Applying antiseptic chemicals to the skin and following sterile techniques can reduce the risk of infection [12]. The severity of hypersensitivity reactions to invaded bodily fluids might vary from moderate inflammation to massive blood clots. Medicines that modulate the immune system can ameliorate symptoms, such as ibuprofen, oral corticosteroids, antihistamines, and others [13]. Antibiotics, hyaluronidase, and immunosuppressive medications can treat delayed-onset nodules and foreign-body granulomas, which are long-term problems [14].

Vascular compromise is a worrisome consequence that can cause blindness and skin necrosis. No significant neurovascular structures exist in the subdermal or subcutaneous planes along the jawline, so it is not often used for face rejuvenation [15]. Prior knowledge of the area's anatomy is crucial when injecting fillers, especially the face veins and arteries, marginal mandibular nerve, parotid gland and duct, and masseter muscle [16]. According to consensus guidelines, patients receiving HA should be treated with hyaluronidase and oral aspirin in the event of vascular infiltration [17]. Several strategies have been devised to control this uncommon problem [13, 18, 19], which is a relief.

It is important to note that injectable fillers have several restrictions. Fillers have a great safety record; however, they do not work as well for patients with severe chin retrusion. For patients of average height vertically, chin deficits that are horizontal (i.e., anterior) are commonly corrected with surgically implanted alloplastic implants [20]. On the other hand, genioplasty is a dependable treatment to fix many jawline problems, such as prognathia, vertical deficit, and chin asymmetry. Still, it is more intrusive and comprehensive [21]. Surgical procedures may be better than injectable fillers if you are looking for a long-term solution that will not require any touch-ups or revisions. The long-term results were more stable with genioplasty, according to a clinical comparison study by Bertossi et al. [22] that examined surgical sliding genioplasty, alloplastic implants, and injectable HA filler in 345 patients. If a patient's horizontal chin deficit was more severe (defined as retrusion of the chin more than 4 mm from the real vertical line), genioplasty was performed on them; fillers were used to address less severe deficiencies in patients over the age of 50 with diminished soft tissue volume.

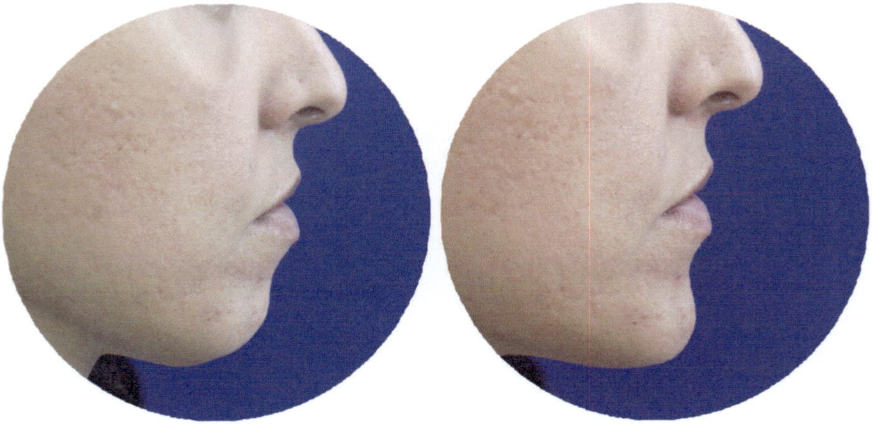

Fig. 49.2 Mentoplasty by intraoral implant

49.4 Genioplasty and Mentoplasty

Patients seeking advice about face cosmetic surgery often concentrate on areas like the eyes, nose, and skin laxity. However, during the assessment, the facial plastic surgeon often points out the lower third of the face as a potential area for surgical modifications to enhance overall harmony and beauty. A chin augmentation or reduction treatment might drastically change a patient's appearance, resulting in a noticeable change in the degree of facial symmetry [23, 24] (Fig. 49.2).

Chin abnormalities can be addressed using a variety of surgical procedures. Two techniques that are now accepted for chin augmentation are sliding genioplasty and alloplastic chin implants. The purpose of this essay is not to permit, however, the discussion of whether osseous genioplasty or alloplastic augmentation is more appropriate. Genioplasty and direct chin reduction are two methods for reducing the size of the lower jaw. Over the years, skeletal surgery has been shown to be a valuable technique for facial surgeons. Several articles in reputable journals have recently validated sliding genioplasty. In 2006 [25], Wolfe released a 28-year history; in 2007, Hoenig released a 10-year experience [26].

49.4.1 History of the Procedure

To treat the retruded mentum, surgeons began employing bony osteotomy procedures in the mid-1940s. Sliding genioplasty is being carried out by surgeons trained in various subspecialties. A sliding genioplasty or an open reduction using a rotary burr are two possibilities for the projecting chin [23].

Various materials have been used for chin augmentation, such as methyl methacrylate, paraffin, ivory, and many more. The figure below depicts the increasing popularity of alloplastic implants, which include silicone, polytetrafluoroethylene, and polyester mesh, due to the pleasure of both patients and surgeons. Mersilene mesh, manufactured by Ethicon in Somerville, NJ, was made famous in the 1980s by Beekhuis and Johnson. Mersilene mesh was found to be safe and well-tolerated for chin augmentation in a recent 14-year study. Placing an alloplastic material is typically less invasive and takes less time than a sliding genioplasty; nevertheless, it is only effective on mild to moderately receded chins [23].

Chin augmentations using autografts, such as iliac crest or rib cartilage, were more common in the past. Additionally, nasal cartilage and bone have been utilized. Using them seems linked to an elevated infection rate, which persists even after 40 years [23].

49.4.2 Problem

Suppose a patient's profile shows facial dysharmony. In that case, the next step is to rule out more serious causes, such as occlusal and skeletal deformity, and focus on correcting the patient's mentum projection. The poor projection must be skeletal in origin for skeletal deformities to be classified as Angle class II. The classification of the Angle skeleton depends on the location of the first molar. If you have retrognathia, the buccal groove of your mandibular first tooth will be directly in front of the mesiobuccal cusp of your maxillary first molar. The term "micrognathia" is more appropriate when merely a hypoplasia of the jaw is present [23].

Retrogenia, microgenia, retruded chin, hypoplastic mentum, and horizontal mandibular hypoplasia are all names for a receding chin without a skeletal abnormality. The case with an over-protruding chin (sometimes called prognathic) is identical. The literature has used all of these phrases without distinction. While mentoplasty typically involves an alloplastic implant, genioplasty typically refers to an osseous movement. Having said that, the two terms are now considered interchangeable [23].

49.4.3 Presentation

The preoperative consultation includes a full medical history, including a dental history and occlusal evaluation, as well as standard facial pictures. Partitioning the face into thirds is a common technique in profile analysis. The typical vertical lines that divide a human face are the hairline, the glabella, the midface, and the subnasal. Examining the chin next will reveal whether it harmonizes with the rest of the face [23].

Utilize preoperative photography, cephalometric imaging, panoramic radiography, and face analysis to learn about skeletal structures and dental occlusion. The patient and doctor should talk about their aesthetic and functional goals. Get more tests done if there are problems with the chin. Take radiographs of the skull from the front, back, side, and occlusal perspectives, as well as cephalometric and anteroposterior (AP) views [23].

Dental models should be made if skeletal or oral abnormalities are detected. Use this data to counsel the patient on their available options for optimizing their outcome. If a skeletal anomaly is detected, recommend orthodontic adjustment or orthognathic surgery. Talk about alloplastic implant augmentation and sliding genioplasty when the patient wants a cosmetic fix only. The severity of the deformity and any other facial treatments being evaluated inform the recommendation of which treatment approach is most suitable, if any, depending on the severity of the abnormality [23].

When making plans for a chin augmentation, be sure to take the mentolabial fold into account. An unbalanced profile and increased depth could result from a big implant. Multiple writers have recommended that people think about ways to avoid creating a deep sulcus when doing a sliding genioplasty. Bertossi et al. used fresh-frozen human bone allografts for grafting, including effacement of the sulcus or fold [27]. In their description of a new shield osteotomy, Triaca et al. aim to stop the labiodental crease from getting deeper [28]. The crease is softened, and a shield effect is created by cutting the buccal cortex high [23].

49.4.4 Indications

Making sure your face has a healthy proportion and having a beautiful contour are two of the main aims of plastic surgery. Reducing a prominent chin or augmenting a poorly projected chin may be part of this procedure [23].

The goal of the augmentation treatment should be to minimize any potential complications during the surgery. There is a minimal complication risk, and alloplastic implants are often not technically demanding. In addition, local anesthetic can make it easy to insert these implants. For chins with mild to moderate microgenia and a shallow labiomental fold, this is a widely recognized method of correction [23].

It has been noted that the success rates of sliding genioplasty are comparable. Another benefit of this method is that it can fix prognathia, vertical macrogenia with retrogenia, and vertical microgenia with or without retrogenia. While alloplastic implant augmentation works wonders for smaller anomalies, more complicated deformities can be treated with surgical expertise via osseous genioplasty. Supporters of the sliding genioplasty operation point out that it may fix problems in three dimensions, which makes it more flexible. When dealing with numerous issues related to alloplastic chin implants, this method has also been employed. Some patients have found relief from problems with alloplastic procedures after undergoing osseous genioplasty [25].

A more direct method of reduction is also possible. The inferior mandible cortex can be burred down using either an intraoral labial technique or an external submental incision [23].

49.5 Chin Implants

Regarding chin surgeries, osteoplastic genioplasty has long been considered the gold standard. Nevertheless, the process is more time-consuming, technically demanding, and hazardous to the inferior alveolar and mental nerves than alloplastic implants. When treating a ptotic chin pad or the pre-jowl sulcus, chin augmentation is frequently done in conjunction with rhinoplasty or rhytidectomy [29]. After a century of sporadic use, implants are all the rage again, largely thanks to the advent of new alloplastic materials [24].

Autogenous materials, such as cartilage from the nose or iliac or rib bones, have a long history of usage in soft tissue and skeletal augmentation procedures. When Aufricht and his colleagues underwent nose-chin plastic surgery, he detailed the use of the osteocartilaginous nasal hump to increase the patient's chin [30]. In 1928, he devised this method and documented a case where the autograft stayed for 27 years. The aesthetic advantage of doing rhinoplasty and genioplasty simultaneously and the ease of employing an autograft led him to recommend this method [1].

Precious metals, acrylic, ivory, and other alloplastics are now mostly of historical significance. Silicone and polytetrafluoroethylene (PTFE) are two more widely used polymers. Nylon mesh and expanded PTFE are examples of softer materials, while high-density polyethylene and hydroxyapatite compounds are examples of tougher materials [1].

The degree to which an implant is biocompatible is dependent on a number of generic characteristics. Crucially, materials that do not cause a persistent inflammatory response or an adverse reaction to foreign bodies can be extremely biocompatible. Another plus for implants is that they are not carcinogenic or immunogenic. To ensure the shape and position of an implant remain unchanged over time, the material used must not degrade yet still be malleable [1].

The human body has been using silicone for almost 40 years. Silicone, a polymer that can exist in both liquid (silicone gel) and solid (suitable for facial augmentation) forms, is formed when the element silicon (period 14 on the periodic table) is bonded with oxygen. Intraoperative carving or custom molding can be used to personalize the solid form. While the formation of a tight fibrous capsule around the implant aids in correctly positioning the implant, no tissue ingrowth happens following implantation. Sterilization, shaping, and removal are all made simple using silicone. It is also easy to work with in case of revision or complications. Silicone implants are well-liked due to their affordability and pleasant sensation [1].

PTFE is an ethylene monomer with four fluorine moieties, giving it a spongy texture. Teflon, Gore-Tex, and Proplast are some brand names under which it is sold as an implant. When facing plastic surgery, only Proplast and Gore-Tex have been utilized. The nonimmunologic and noncarcinogenic polytetrafluoroethylene (PTFE) has been used for over 40 years, much like silicone [1].

Teflon (PTFE) and graphite made up the first Proplast, which was black. Proplast II, a white polymer made of Teflon and alumina, superseded it. Proplast I was black. Fibrovascular ingrowth of the host's tissues is enabled by the material's pores, which range in diameter from 50 to 400 μm. Evidence of delamination under shear stress, particle formation, and inflammatory reaction led to Proplast's discontinuation. A sheet of Gore-Tex is made up of tiny expanded PFTE fibers that are connected by solid expanded PTFE nodes. The porous nature of Proplast II, with pores of 10–30 μm, permits modest fibrovascular ingrowth, and it is simple to cut and trim for contouring purposes [1].

One other alloplastic that is not fluorinated or spongy is high-density polyethylene or Medpor. Because of its pliability, it may be easily warmed in a warm water bath to conform to any shape. Soft tissue and some bone ingrowth are possible due to its porous nature, which has 125–250 μm pores. It remains intact in the body and does not trigger an immune response to foreign bodies. Research comparing the histologic reaction of Gore-Tex and Medpor implants to experimental infection found that the latter provided better protection due to the accelerated fibrovascular development into the former. The bigger holes and enhanced stability caused by the implant integrating with the host tissue might be responsible for this. Implant stability is not assured by fibrous ingrowth into porous materials [1].

The porous block hydroxyapatite is a form of the hard porous compound hydroxyapatite. Its origins are in marine coral, and it has a history of use in cosmetic procedures involving the face. Its pores enable the ingrowth of both fibrous and bone materials. No bone degradation is associated with its application, which is done with a firm attachment to the underlying bone [1].

An acceptable implant can be made from a pliable material called Mersilene mesh, made of non-absorbable polyester fiber sheeting. It was initially introduced for hernia repair and has been used for half a century. The biodegradable polyamide nylon mesh known as Mersilene is an alternative to Supramid. Fraying and shrinkage are not issues when cutting it [1].

Prefabricated implants of varying sizes and shapes are available, made of materials such as expanded PTFE, high-density polyethylene, and silicone. These materials can be shaped and carved to make them unique for each patient [31]. Surgeons' experiences with alloplasts vary, and each device has its own set of pros and cons [1].

49.5.1 Planning

Surgeons have sought inspiration in works of art to create a standard for the ideal chin. Scientific studies have shown that the chin is one of the most important facial features for overall attractiveness and harmony. The way the chin appears about the rest of the face is called chin projection. Several descriptions of analytical methodologies and chin classifications have been made [1].

Microgenia, also known as retrusion of the chin, can be remedied via chin augmentation. Micrognathia, on the other hand, affects the jaw rather than the chin. The surgeon considering chin augmentation does not see the chin as a flat surface but as a three-dimensional prominence with bone and soft tissue components. Also considered is the angle at which the chin meets the nose. Maintaining a balanced face depends on this connection. Rhinoplasty alone might not improve a patient's profile if their chin is too small [1].

49.5.2 Indications

Gonzalez-Ulloa's substantial writings on profile plasty [32, 33] focused on this subject. He established analytical ways to comprehend the relationships between faces based on the fundamental principle that the shape and size of the skull determine attractiveness. The surgeon can increase the likelihood of a successful operation by planning it around the bony skeleton, which supports the soft tissue and is actually the mechanism for achieving optimal aesthetics (81).

When minor microgenia is present, a chin implant may be recommended. Gonzalez-Ulloa used the Frankfort plane and the zero degree meridian as his bases when assessing faces. The horizontal line that extends from the infraorbital rim to the upper external auditory canal is known as the Frankfort plane. The zero degree meridian is delineated in the vertical plane that is orthogonal to the pogonion and the nasion, and perpendicular to the horizontal plane of Frankfort. Retruded means the chin is positioned behind the 0° meridian. The level of retrusion dictates the intervention [1].

Various surgeons have detailed and evaluated numerous methods of analysis. The subnasal and pogonion are perpendicular to Burstone's vertical line. A 3.5 mm anterior upper lip and a 2.2 mm anterior lower lip are present [1].

Gibson finds the sweet spot for the chin concerning the lower face height by utilizing soft tissue landmarks in the lower face triangle [34]. The tragion, subnasale, and chin are its three distinguishing features. Goode marks the perfect chin position at the alar crease by dropping a line perpendicular to the Frankfort horizontal plane. The face convexity angle measured by Legan is 12 degrees, formed by a line perpendicular to the subnasale and pogonion and another line perpendicular to the glabella and subnasale [1].

Merrifield's Z angle is 80° (±5°), defined as the intersection of the Frankfort horizontal plane and a vertical tangent from the upper lip to the pogonion. Ricketts marked the nasal tip and pogonion with a vertical line at a right angle [35]. The upper lip is 4 mm, and the lower lip is 2 mm posterior to this plane. To determine how far forward the lips extend, one uses Steiner's nasal philtrum S. The lower nasal and upper labial profiles come together to form an inverted S, and a vertical line is lowered tangential to the pogonion [1].

Similar to how "the golden rectangle" served as the foundation for the Parthenon in Greece, the phi-based golden proportion governs the relationship between the chin and various facial features. In the golden rectangle, the base is 1.618 times the altitude, and the proportion of the altitude to the base is 1. According to phi, this is the case [1].

Several of the face's height connections exhibit the golden proportion. From forehead to the eye, the proportion is 1, and from eye to menton, it is phi. The proportion is satisfied throughout the face. From the menton to the nasal ala, the measurement is 1, and from the nasal ala to the forehead, it is phi, reversing the golden proportion. The measurement from the eye to the nasal ala is 1, and from the nasal ala to the menton is phi, and the proportion is maintained to the chin. Measuring from the menton to the stomion yields the inverse proportion, whereas measuring from the stomion to the eye yields the value phi. At last, the golden proportion is maintained between the chin and the nose. It is possible to calculate phi by comparing the distances between the menton and the stomion, with the distance between the nasal ala and the eye being 1 [1].

References

1. Doud Galli SK. Chin Implants. In: Meyers AD (Ed). Medscape. Updated: Mar 01, 2023. https://emedicine.medscape.com/article/842915-treatment#d12. Accessed online at 8 July 2024.
2. Sykes JM, Suarez GA. Chin advancement, augmentation, and reduction as adjuncts to rhinoplasty. Clin Plast Surg. 2016;43(1):295–306.
3. Go BC, Frost AS, Friedman O. Using injectable fillers for chin and jawline rejuvenation. World J Otorhinolaryngol Head Neck Surg. 2023;9(2):131–7. https://doi.org/10.1002/wjo2.93.
4. The Aesthetic Society. Aesthetic plastic surgery national databank statistics 2019. https://www.surgery.org/sites/default/files/Aesthetic-Society_Stats2019Book_FINAL.pdf. Accessed 24 Jan 2021.
5. Allergan. The changing faces of beauty: a global report 2016. https://totallyderma.com/wp-content/uploads/2016/10/LIBRARY%201st%20HEADING%20-%20Changing-Faces-of-Beauty-Report-FINAL-INT-0361-2016h.pdf. Accessed 24 Jan 2021.
6. Vanaman Wilson MJ, Jones IT, Butterwick K, Fabi SG. Role of nonsurgical chin augmentation in full face rejuvenation: a review and our experience. Dermatol Surg. 2018;44:985–93.
7. Ogilvie P, Benouaiche L, Philipp-Dormston WG, et al. VYC-25L hyaluronic acid injectable gel is safe and effective for long-term restoration and creation of volume of the lower face. Aesthet Surg J. 2020;40:NP499–NP510.
8. Beer K, Kaufman-Janette J, Bank D, et al. Safe and effective chin augmentation with the hyaluronic acid injectable filler, VYC-20L. Dermatol Surg. 2021;47:80–5.
9. Ogilvie P, Sattler G, Gaymans F, et al. Safe, effective chin and jaw restoration with VYC-25L hyaluronic acid injectable gel. Dermatol Surg. 2019;45:1294–303.
10. Funt D, Pavicic T. Dermal fillers in aesthetics: an overview of adverse events and treatment approaches. Clin Cosmet Investig Dermatol. 2013;6:295–316.
11. Urdiales-Gálvez F, Delgado NE, Figueiredo V, et al. Preventing the complications associated with the use of dermal fillers in facial aesthetic procedures: an expert group consensus report. Aesthetic Plast Surg. 2017;41:667–77.
12. Bailey SH, Cohen JL, Kenkel JM. Etiology, prevention, and treatment of dermal filler complications. Aesthet Surg J. 2011;31:110–21.
13. Heydenrych I, Kapoor KM, De Boulle K, et al. A 10-point plan for avoiding hyaluronic acid dermal filler-related complications during facial aesthetic procedures and algorithms for management. Clin Cosmet Investig Dermatol. 2018;11:603–11.
14. Artzi O, Cohen JL, Dover JS, et al. Delayed inflammatory reactions to hyaluronic acid fillers: a literature review and proposed treatment algorithm. Clin Cosmet Investig Dermatol. 2020;13:371–8.
15. Suwanchinda A, Rudolph C, Hladik C, et al. The layered anatomy of the jawline. J Cosmet Dermatol. 2018;17:625–31.
16. Fang M, Rahman E, Kapoor KM. Managing complications of submental artery involvement after hyaluronic acid filler injection in chin region. Plast Reconstr Surg Global Open. 2018;6:e1789.
17. Cohen JL, Biesman BS, Dayan SH, et al. Treatment of hyaluronic acid filler-induced impending necrosis with hyaluronidase: consensus recommendations. Aesthet Surg J. 2015;35:844–9.
18. Vedamurthy M, Vedamurthy A, Nischal K. Dermal fillers: do's and dont's. J Cutan Aesthet Surg. 2010;3:11–5.

19. Aviv U, Haik J, Weiss N, et al. Treatment algorithm for hyaluronic acid-related complication based on a systematic review of case reports, case series, and clinical experience. Craniomaxillofac Trauma Reconstr. 2020;13:313–28.
20. Sykes J, Fitzgerald R. Choosing the best procedure to augment the chin: is anything better than an implant. Facial Plast Surg. 2016;32:507–12.
21. Sykes JM, Suárez GA. Chin advancement, augmentation, and reduction as adjuncts to rhinoplasty. Clin Plast Surg. 2016;43:295–306.
22. Bertossi D, Galzignato PF, Albanese M, Botti C, Botti G, Nocini PF. Chin microgenia: a clinical comparative study. Aesthetic Plast Surg. 2015;39:651–8.
23. Chang EW. Genioplasty. In: Meyers AD (Ed). Medscape. Updated: Nov 30, 2021. https://emedicine.medscape.com/article/839645-overview#a10. Accessed online at 8 July 2024.
24. Harris WC, Winters R, Raggio BS. Facial Chin Augmentation. 2024 Mar 7. In: StatPearls [Internet]. Treasure Island (FL): StatPearls Publishing; 2024.
25. Wolfe SA, Rivas-Torres MT, Marshall D. The genioplasty and beyond: an end-game strategy for the multiply operated chin. Plastic abd Reconstruct Surg. 2006;117:1435–46.
26. Johannes Franz Hoenig. Sliding osteotomy genioplasty for facial aesthetic balance: 10 years of experience. Aesthetic Plastic Surgery. 2007;31:384–91.
27. Bertossi D, Albanese M, Nocini PF, D'Agostino A, Trevisiol L, Procacci P. Sliding genioplasty using fresh-frozen bone allografts. JAMA Facial Plast Surg. 2013;15(1):51–7.
28. Triaca A, Furrer T, Minoretti R. Chin shield osteotomy – a new genioplasty technique avoiding a deep mento-labial fold in order to increase the labial competence. Int J Oral Maxillofac Surg. 2009;38(11):1201–5.
29. Kridel RWH, Patel S. Cheek and chin implants to enhance facelift results. Facial Plast Surg. 2017;33(3):279–84.
30. Aufricht G. Combined plastic surgery of the nose and chin; resume of twenty-seven years' experience. Am J Surg. 1958;95(2):231–6.
31. Chang PC. Computer-assisted planning and 3D printing-assisted modeling for chin augmentation. Aesthet Surg J. 2017;38(1):1–10.
32. Gonzalez-Ulloa M. Quantitative principles in cosmetic surgery of the face (profiloplasty). Plast Reconstr Surg. 1962;29:186–98.
33. Gonzalez-Ulloa M, Stevens E. The role of chin correction in profileplasty. Plast Reconstr Surg. 1968;41(5):477–86.
34. Gibson FB, Calhoun KH. Chin position in profile analysis. Comparison of techniques and introduction of the lower facial triangle. Arch Otolaryngol Head Neck Surg. 1992;118(3):273–6.
35. Ricketts RM. The biologic significance of the divine proportion and Fibonacci series. Am J Orthod. 1982;81(5):351–70.

Designing the Smile with Botulinum Toxin

50

Ece Ozer

50.1 Introduction

One definition of smile design is developing an aesthetically pleasing smile by adhering to scientific and artistic parameters developed through research, perception, and cultural and racial standards that have been acknowledged over time. Facial aesthetics, lip dynamics, pink and white aesthetics, and personality are all factors considered in smile design, a dynamic discipline constantly growing alongside new trends. Modern smile designers must have a comprehensive grasp of the patient to create the ideal smile for their patients [1].

The moment the doctor meets the patient, the oral examination starts. The first evaluation consists of a broad examination of the head and neck. The examiner should visually inspect asymmetry, bone deformities, and overt anomalies of the head, face, orbits, nose, chin, and neck [2]. The patient's dental, social, and family history should be obtained and recorded [3].

Examiners should palpate each neck area individually while the patient is seated upright, paying particular attention to lymphadenopathy. Palpation should always be organized and sequential [4]. A thorough extraoral examination should include an assessment of the temporomandibular joints and related facial skin, muscles, lips, cervical lymph nodes, and facial features [3].

E. Ozer (✉)
Private Periodontology Clinic, Izmir, Turkey

C. Cingi et al. (eds.), *Minor Interventions, Major Outcomes on the Face*, Comprehensive ENT, https://doi.org/10.1007/978-3-032-01305-7_50

50.2 Evaluation of the Patients

50.2.1 Analysis of the Oral Region

The intraoral examination includes both visual examination and superficial and deep palpation. For a successful intraoral examination, having a reliable light source is necessary [5]. Moisture often changes the appearance of oral lesions; therefore, drying the mucosa will be beneficial [2].

Teeth should be evaluated using inspection, palpation, and percussion to determine the presence of potential dental decay, fractures, mobility issues, faults in restorations, gingival recession, and bone loss. Whether gingivitis or systemic disease is present, changes in the clinical appearance of the gingivae can be a sign of one of these conditions. Moreover, the gingiva is the first place where mucocutaneous disorders manifest themselves, such as lichen planus, mucous membrane pemphigoid, and pemphigus vulgaris [6]. The lack of proper oral hygiene is the most common cause of periodontal disease. When there is periodontal disease, the gums appear red and edematous, bleeding on probing, increased depth of the periodontal pocket due to destruction of the supporting structures of the teeth, and increased tooth mobility [7].

The gingival structure and the tooth length are essential for an aesthetic smile. The mobility and rigidity of the labium superius oris muscles, the vertical height of the lip and the size of the clinical crown, and the skeletal relationship, especially the vertical maxillary tooth length, can cause a difference in the degree of gingival visibility when talking about smiling in individuals. Different disorders, such as malpositioned teeth, tooth eruption, gingival recession, and interdental gingival loss, cause an unaesthetic appearance. Various dental surgical procedures can change the gingival structure in the "smile line" [8–10].

50.2.2 Analysis of the Face

The most often used vertical and horizontal reference planes when considering face symmetry are the interpupillary line and the facial midline. It is widely acknowledged that aesthetic harmony is reached when the dental midline and the face midline coincide and the vertical and horizontal reference planes are perpendicular. An essential reference axis for establishing the ultimate positions of the gingival, occlusal, and incisal planes, respectively, is the interpupillary line [11].

In the frontal plane, the face can be divided into three regions: the "upper third," which includes the area between the hairline and the eyebrow line; the "middle third," which extends from the eyebrow line to the base of the nose; and the "lower third," which includes the area between the base of the nose and the tip of the chin. The lower third appears to be the most essential region in determining the overall face appearance [11].

50.2.3 Analysis of the Lips

The lips' width, fullness, and symmetry should all be noted when examining morphology and degree of mobility. Measuring the amount of anterior tooth exposure in both the resting and active positions of the lips is preferable. It should be known that the level of exposure of the incisal edges decreases with age [12].

This distance represents the length of the upper lip compared to the distance between its subnasal and lower border. The average height of young people is between 20 and 24 millimeters, increasing with age [13]. A less than 20 millimeters measurement deems a patient to have a short lip. Patients with this condition may also exhibit gummy smiles and lip incompetence [14].

The usual interlabial spacing is between 0 and 4 or 3 millimeters at repose [15].

The upper central incisors are displayed while the person is at rest. They must be between 3 and 4 millimeters for young women and 2 millimeters for young men; nevertheless, they decline with age [12].

Doctors should investigate which of the three factors—short lips, dentoalveolar extrusion, or VME—is responsible for the disparity [14].

50.2.4 Smiling

Lip mobility is the amount of lip movement when a patient smiles. The term "smile line" refers to the relationship between the lower edge of the upper lip and the teeth and gingival soft tissues when smiling. Three kinds of lip lines are defined:

"Low smile line" refers to upper lip mobility that does not expose more than 75% of the anterior teeth.
"Medium smile line" refers to lip movement that reveals 75% to 100% of the teeth and interdental papillae.
"High smile line" fully exposes the teeth and gingival tissues beyond the gingival margins, often known as a "gummy smile" [16].

The upper lip should symmetrically expose up to 3 mm of the gum line. Gingiva exposed more than 3 mm during the smile, known as a gummy smile [17]. A high smile line is typically a hallmark of women, while low smile lines are often a male characteristic [18].

Wide lips typically result in a broad smile, with a smile that is seen as visually attractive if it is at least half the breadth of the face. The most frequently seen grin width pattern has been reported to be a smile that displays ten maxillary teeth, including the second premolars [19]. Research indicates that to achieve the best possible aesthetics; the dental hard tissues should fill in the corners of the mouth to form a "full smile," preventing the formation of "negative buccal corridors." The top border of the lower lip should be positioned slightly below the incisal edges, and the lower lip's curvature should ideally be parallel to the incisal margins' curvature [3].

50.3 Smile Aesthetics and Pink Aesthetics

Factors that contribute to the sense of facial beauty are numerous. Aesthetics studies beauty, proportions, and symmetry [20, 21]. It is the study that evaluates and comprehends these concepts. The concept of the perfect grin is challenging to pin down because it combines art and science, and all the factors considered are interdependent and interrelated [22]. To achieve the perfect combination of pink and white aesthetics, smile analysis requires a thorough examination of the teeth, the framework of the lips, and the gingival scaffold. The cosmetic appearance of both the natural and artificial dentition that has been repaired is impacted by the anomalies in the symmetry and contour [17].

The white part of the smile aesthetics consists of the teeth, and the pink part is the gingiva. Restoring the ideal gingiva's proper amount, position, and shape while considering the account of the unpleasant smile is among the purposes of periodontal mucogingival surgery. The position and shape of the free gingival margins, gingival color, gingival excess, gingival recession, and absence/presence of interdental papillae are the determining factors for soft tissue aesthetics [23, 24]. The three-dimensional architecture of hard and soft tissue ridge abnormalities may not be sufficiently recreated despite numerous surgical procedures and modern regenerative techniques, including soft tissue graft, bone graft, and orthodontic displacement. For patients who choose not to have surgery, creating a prosthetic gingiva can provide an aesthetically pleasing and practical alternative for the predictable correction of ridge abnormalities in restorations. In this case, gingival-color-compliant pink ceramics or composites can produce pink aesthetics [25].

The etiology of gummy smiles includes altered passive eruption, upper lip hypermobility, bimaxillary protrusion, gingival enlargement, and vertical maxillary excess. Orthodontic treatments, periodontal surgery (gingivectomy, lip repositioning, etc.), and botulinum toxin injections can all be used to treat such problems [26]. While maintaining the patient's functional stability and optimizing the length of care, the operator should strive for the agreed-upon aesthetic result. Still, it should be essential to follow the minimally invasive treatment method [3].

Botulinum toxin injection is the recommended minimally invasive treatment for gummy smiles resulting from hyperactive lip muscles due to its safety and ease of application [27]. Hwang et al. suggested that the center of the triangle formed by the reference points of the three muscle vectors is a suitable injection point. They named it the "Yonsei point," considering that the levator labii superioris, levator labii superioris alaeque nasi, and zygomaticus minor muscles determine the amount of lip elevation during smiling. The average horizontal distance from the nose wing to this point was measured as 10.4 ± 2.1 mm in men and 10.3 ± 2.1 mm in women, while the average vertical distance from the lip line was calculated as 32.3 ± 4.2 mm in men and 31.5 ± 3.3 mm in women [28]. Injections should be made at a dosage appropriate to the selected botulinum toxin product. If an anterior gingival smile is present (gingiva between canine teeth revealed while smiling extends over

3 mm)—levator labii superioris alaeque nasi is the muscle engaged in this scenario—it can be treated by injecting the toxin lateral to the wing of the nose. In a posterior gingival smile (more than 3 mm of gingiva exposed posterior to canine teeth)—which is associated with the zygomatic muscles—half of the dose should be administered at the level of the tragus line, at the conventional point and 2 cm lateral to it (Figs. 50.1 and 50.2) [27].

With injections made at the right points targeting the right muscle, the activity of hyperactive lip muscles can be limited, and a minimally invasive approach to smile aesthetics can be provided. The literature shows successful results in treatments with botulinum toxin, and these temporary results also make the complications reversible [29].

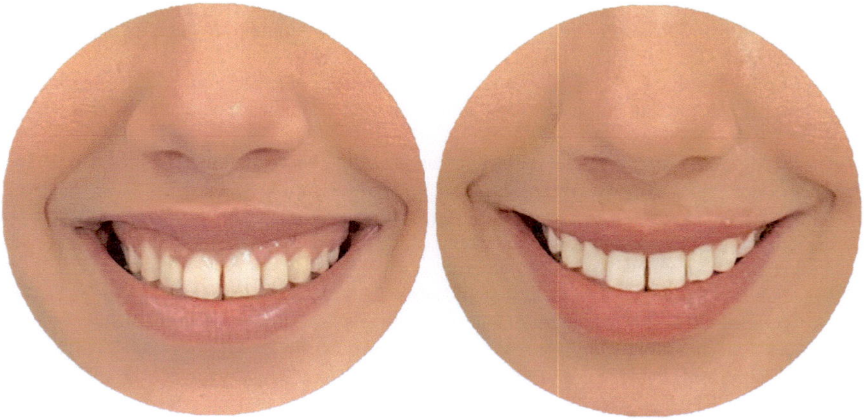

Fig. 50.1 Smiling case 1, before and after botulinum toxin injections

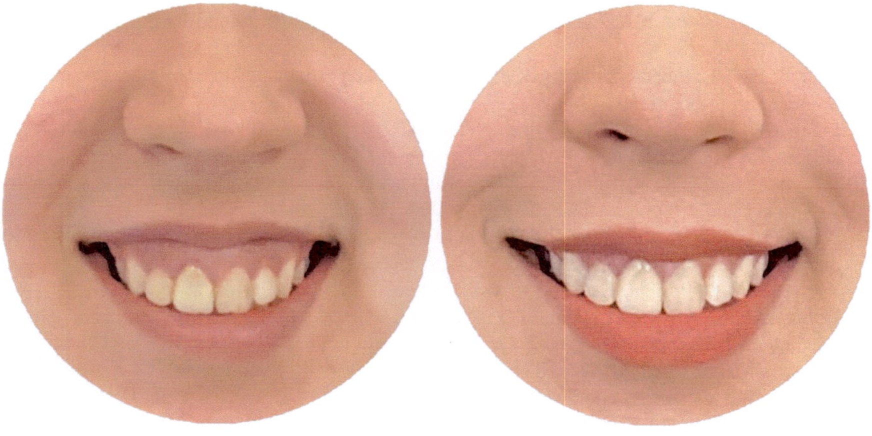

Fig. 50.2 Smiling case 2, before and after botulinum toxin injections

References

1. Sabbah A. Smile analysis: diagnosis and treatment planning. Dent Clin N Am. 2022;66(3):307–41.
2. Agha R, Mirowski GW. The art and science of oral examination. Dermatol Ther. 2010;23(3):209–19.
3. Mehta SB, Banerji S, Aulakh R. Patient assessment: preparing for a predictable aesthetic outcome. Dent Update. 2015;42(1):78–86.
4. Turner JRJS. An overview of the head and neck. In: Clinical methods: the history, physical, and laboratory examinations; 1990.
5. Madani M, Berardi T, Stoopler ET. Anatomic and examination considerations of the oral cavity. Med Clin. 2014;98(6):1225–38.
6. Patel S, Kumar S, Laudenbach JM, Teruel A. Mucocutaneous diseases: oral lichen planus, mucous membrane pemphigoid and pemphigus vulgaris. J Calif Dent Assoc. 2016;44(9):561–70.
7. Kinane DF. Causation and pathogenesis of periodontal disease. Periodontology. 2000;25(1):8–20.
8. Sepolia S, Sepolia G, Kaur R, Gautam DK, Jindal V, Gupta SC. Visibility of gingiva-An important determinant for an esthetic smile. Journal of Indian Society of Periodontology. 2014;18(4):488–92.
9. Dashti M, Zadeh MA. Gingival recession classification and treatment. In: Innovative perspectives in oral and maxillofacial surgery; 2021. p. 155–68.
10. Tajbakhsh N, Delpisheh F, Ghadimi N, Ansari S. Smile management: White esthetic, pink esthetic and facial attractiveness, a review of literature. Open Access Research Journal of Biology and Pharmacy. 2022;5(2):046–50.
11. Fradeani M. Esthetic analysis: a systematic approach to prosthetic treatment. (No Title); 2004.
12. Vig RG, Brundo GC. The kinetics of anterior tooth display. J Prosthet Dent. 1978;39(5):502–4.
13. Jorgensen MG, Nowzari H. Aesthetic crown lengthening. Periodontology. 2000;27(1)
14. Dym H, Pierre R. Diagnosis and treatment approaches to a "gummy smile". Dent Clin N Am. 2020;64(2):341–9.
15. Pavone AF, Ghassemian M, Verardi S. Gummy smile and short tooth syndrome – Part 1: Etiopathogenesis, classification, and diagnostic guidelines. Compend Contin Educ Dent. 2016;37(2):102–7.
16. Tjan AH, Miller GD, The JG. Some esthetic factors in a smile. J Prosthet Dent. 1984;51(1):24–8.
17. Garber DA, Salama MA. The aesthetic smile: diagnosis and treatment. Periodontology 2000. 1996;11(1):18–28.
18. Peck S, Peck L. Selected aspects of the art and science of facial esthetics. Paper presented at: Seminars in orthodontics; 1995.
19. Dong J-K, Jin T-H, Cho H-W, Oh S-C. The esthetics of the smile: a review of some recent studies. Int J Prosthodont. 1999;12(1)
20. Patil AS, Ranganath V, Yerawadekar SA, Kumar CN, Sarode GS. Pink esthetics: a study on significant gingival parameters. J Contemp Dent Pract. 2020;21(2):207–10.
21. Naini FB, Moss JP, Gill DS. The enigma of facial beauty: esthetics, proportions, deformity, and controversy. Am J Orthod Dentofacial Orthoped. 2006;130(3):277–82.
22. Ahmad I. Anterior dental aesthetics: historical perspective. Br Dent J. 2005;198(12):737–42.
23. Batra P, Daing A, Azam I, Miglani R, Bhardwaj A. Impact of altered gingival characteristics on smile esthetics: laypersons' perspectives by Q sort methodology. Am J Orthod Dentofacial Orthoped. 2018;154(1):82–90. e82
24. Rotundo R, Genzano L, Nieri M, Covani U, Peñarrocha-Oltra D, Peñarrocha-Diago M. Smile esthetic evaluation of mucogingival reconstructive surgery. Odontology. 2021;109:295–302.
25. Christian Coachman C. The reconstruction of pink and white esthetics.

26. Mahardawi B, Chaisamut T, Wongsirichat N. Gummy smile: a review of etiology, manifestations, and treatment. Siriraj Med J. 2019;71(2)
27. Mazzuco R, Hexsel D. Gummy smile and botulinum toxin: a new approach based on the gingival exposure area. J Am Acad Dermatol. 2010;63(6):1042–51.
28. Hwang W-S, Hur M-S, Hu K-S, et al. Surface anatomy of the lip elevator muscles for the treatment of gummy smile using botulinum toxin. Angle Orthod. 2009;79(1):70–7.
29. Gürbüz E, Kaçar Z. Botulinum Toksinin Gummy Smile Tedavisinde Kullanımı. Sağlık Akademisi Kastamonu. 9(1):144–56.

Correction to: Fat Injections as Volumizer on the Face: Overview

Çiğdem Fırat Koca, Cemal Cingi, and Codrut Sarafoleanu

Correction to:
Chapter 25 in: C. Cingi et al. (eds.), *Minor Interventions, Major Outcomes on the Face*, Comprehensive ENT,
https://doi.org/10.1007/978-3-032-01305-7_25

The original version of Chap. 25 was inadvertently published with an incorrect author name, Cigdem Firat, instead of Çiğdem Fırat Koca. The chapter has now been updated.

The updated version of this chapter can be found at
https://doi.org/10.1007/978-3-032-01305-7_25

C. Cingi et al. (eds.), *Minor Interventions, Major Outcomes on the Face*, Comprehensive ENT, https://doi.org/10.1007/978-3-032-01305-7_51

MIX
Papier aus verantwortungsvollen Quellen
Paper from responsible sources
FSC® C105338

If you have any concerns about our products,
you can contact us on
ProductSafety@springernature.com

In case Publisher is established outside the EU,
the EU authorized representative is:
Springer Nature Customer Service Center GmbH
Europaplatz 3, 69115 Heidelberg, Germany

Printed by Libri Plureos GmbH
in Hamburg, Germany